Microbiology
for
Surgical
Technologists

Third Edition

Margaret H. Manning Rodriguez,
CST, CSFA, FAST, M.Ed.

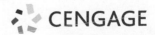
CENGAGE

Australia • Brazil • Canada • Mexico • Singapore • United Kingdom • United States

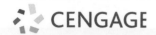

Microbiology for Surgical Technologists,
Third Edition
Margaret H. Manning Rodriguez

SVP, Product: Erin Joyner

VP, Product: Thais Alencar

Product Director: Jason Fremder

Product Manager: Bianca Fiorio

Product Assistant: Dallas Dudley

Learning Designer: Elinor Gregory

Content Manager: Mark Peplowski

Digital Delivery Quality Partner: Andy Baker

VP, Product Marketing: Jason Sakos

Director, Product Marketing: Neena Bali

Product Marketing Manager: Annie Gillingham

Marketing Coordinator: Lindsey Schultz

IP Analyst: Ashley Maynard

IP Project Manager: Haneef Abrar

Production Service: MPS Limited

Designer: Felicia Bennett

Cover Image Source:

© isak55/Shutterstock.com

© sursad/Shutterstock.com

© Jezper/Shutterstock.com

Interior Image Source:

© Ivan Cholakov/Shutterstock.com

© Alexander Raths/Shutterstock.com

© fusebulb/Shutterstock.com

© Jezper/Shutterstock.com

© Tatiana Shepeleva/Shutterstock.com

For product information and technology assistance, contact us at
**Cengage Customer & Sales Support, 1-800-354-9706
or support.cengage.com.**

For permission to use material from this text or product, submit all requests online at **www.cengage.com/permissions.**

Library of Congress Control Number: 2022900582

ISBN: 978-0-357-62615-3

Cengage
200 Pier 4 Boulevard
Boston, MA 02210
USA

Cengage is a leading provider of customized learning solutions with employees residing in nearly 40 different countries and sales in more than 125 countries around the world. Find your local representative at: **www.cengage.com.**

To learn more about Cengage platforms and services, register or access your online learning solution, or purchase materials for your course, visit **www.cengage.com.**

Notice to the Reader

Publisher does not warrant or guarantee any of the products described herein or perform any independent analysis in connection with any of the product information contained herein. Publisher does not assume, and expressly disclaims, any obligation to obtain and include information other than that provided to it by the manufacturer. The reader is expressly warned to consider and adopt all safety precautions that might be indicated by the activities described herein and to avoid all potential hazards. By following the instructions contained herein, the reader willingly assumes all risks in connection with such instructions. The publisher makes no representations or warranties of any kind, including but not limited to, the warranties of fitness for particular purpose or merchantability, nor are any such representations implied with respect to the material set forth herein, and the publisher takes no responsibility with respect to such material. The publisher shall not be liable for any special, consequential, or exemplary damages resulting, in whole or part, from the readers' use of, or reliance upon, this material.

Printed at CLDPC, USA, 04-22

DEDICATION

I dedicate this book to my husband of 39 years, George, who has dedicated his professional life of 42 years to being the quintessential example of what a Certified Surgical Technologist should be. I also dedicate this book in loving memory of our grandson Joseph, taken much too soon. Lastly, I dedicate this to all the victims of the COVID-19 pandemic, their loved ones, and the incredible front-line responders of all types who have heroically cared for those in need.

Contents

Chapter 9
Microbial Disease Transmission 105

Chapter 10
Parasites and Vectors 121

Chapter 11
Mycology 143

Chapter 12
Gram-Positive Cocci 155

Chapter 13
Gram-Positive Bacilli 171

Chapter 14
Actinobacteria 187

Chapter 15
Gram-Negative Cocci and Spirochetes 199

Chapter 16
Gram-Negative Bacilli and
Coccobacilli 215

Chapter 17
Diseases of the Circulatory and Central Nervous Systems 231

Chapter 18
Diseases of the Skin and Internal Tissues 245

Chapter 19
Diseases of the Gastrointestinal and Genitourinary Systems 259

Chapter 20
Diseases of the Eyes, Ears, and Respiratory System   275

Chapter 21
Control of Microbial Growth   289

Chapter 22
Emerging, Recurring, and Reappearing Diseases   309

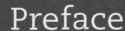

Preface

The Importance of Microbiology for Surgical Technologists

Few healthcare professionals focus as much attention on the war against infectious disease transmission as surgical technologists. Every task, every technique, every procedure, and every movement within the surgical environment of care requires incredible awareness of potential risks and attention to the smallest details to create, protect, and maintain the sterile field—at the center of which is the surgical patient. Equally important is the necessity for surgical technologists and all members of the team to protect themselves from exposure to infectious and pathogenic microorganisms within the operating room suite and the broader outside world in which we live. Without the fundamental knowledge of microbiology and its relationship to healthcare and surgical technology, the concepts and techniques are meaningless ideas and exercises taught in a classroom or lab.

Part of a crucial foundation for perioperative care, *Microbiology for Surgical Technologists*, Third Edition helps surgical technology students understand and prevent disease transmission in clinical settings. In addition to exploring the vast microbial world, learners investigate the infectious disease process and disease pathologies, correlating them with anatomical body systems. Health and safety procedures are important topics, with key procedures for protecting patients, team members, and the students themselves. *Microbiology for Surgical Technologists*, Third Edition is also packed with helpful extras, including colorful photos, realistic case studies, end-of-chapter questions, and special boxed features that call out interesting facts and anecdotes to highlight the importance of aseptic and sterile techniques in various types of surgical intervention.

New Material in the Third Edition of *Microbiology for Surgical Technologists*

In the two decades since the first edition was released, there has been an explosion of scientific and media attention toward topics such as the following: global epidemics of viral diseases jumping from other species to humans; expanding microbial antibiotic resistance; federal insurance regulations regarding healthcare-associated infections; societal debates regarding immunizations and impact on public health; development of bioterrorism agents as weapons of mass destruction; resurgence of previously eradicated diseases; identification of microbial species mutations; and emergence of previously unknown diseases with dramatic impact and mortality rates.

The third edition of *Microbiology for Surgical Technologists* expands on on these topics with:

- Updated content including historical timelines, current world events (including information on COVID-19 in multiple chapters), challenges for healthcare providers, and impact of disease transmission on individuals and society at both the local and global levels.

- Alignment of material with the AST Core Curriculum for Surgical Technology, Seventh Edition.

- Revised chapter Learning Objectives with real-world relevance and broader professional contexts.

- New "Under the Microscope" scenarios and review questions for learning assessment.

- New and diverse images and graphics for enhancement of subject matter materials.

Chapter Overview

Chapters have been developed with emphasis on examination of general and consolidated microbial classifications as well as the correlation between indigenous microflora and body systems with a wide selection of color photos, graphics, and tables to illustrate subject materials. A progression of information includes the following: introduction to the science of microbiology and the laboratory; classifications of microbes into eukaryotes, prokaryotes, viruses, parasites, Gram-positive cocci and bacilli, Actinobacteria, Gram-negative cocci, spirochetes, and bacilli; microbial growth and viability; genetics and mutations; disease transmission; control of microbial growth; microbiologically-linked pathology of specific body systems; and emerging, reappearing, and recurring diseases.

Key Features for Students and Instructors

Careful attention has been given to the correlation of all content with the Core Curriculum for Surgical Technology, Seventh Edition so instructors are assured of compliance with current education and accreditation requirements and students are prepared for certification examination content questions.

Textbook Features:

- Big Picture questions guide students' focus and attention toward general subject areas of discussion.
- Clinical Significance Topics (CSTs) link the chapter material to specific surgical technology skills, techniques, and responsibilities.
- Under the Microscope case studies at the end of chapters use relevant scenario questions to assess comprehension and critical thinking about the material and its connection to the perioperative environment.
- Micro Notes provide quirky and novel tidbits of information about the microbial world and our relationship with it.

MindTap Features:

- Microbes in the Media get students engaged with a short news video showing how microbiology is relevant in the world today.
- Concept Checks in the ebook assess students' understanding of key concepts as they read.
- Flashcards help students learn key terms.
- PowerPoint Reviews summarize key concepts from the chapter.
- Video Quizzes show how chapter concepts apply in the real-world and assess students' understanding.
- New Branching Activities present real-world scenarios in which students choose an action and react to the consequences.
- End of Chapter Quizzes assess students' understanding of key concepts.
- Certification Exam Review provides a practice assessment to help prepare students for the certification exam.

Student Outcomes

Surgical technology students will gain an understanding of the methods of identifying, classifying, and testing for various groups of microbes that determine the appropriate course of treatment for the pathological conditions created by the various infectious agents. Topics such as personal protective equipment (PPE) use, hand hygiene, surgical conscience, care and handling of culture specimens, prevention of surgical site infection (SSI), and healthcare-associated infection (HAI) are discussed. Important correlations between the types of pathogenic microbes commonly encountered in surgery and the potentially life-threatening results are covered. This knowledge will enhance performance as allied healthcare professionals and provide real-world concepts for infection prevention strategies in day-to-day life in the operating room and the local or global community. Additionally, for those interested in future medical/surgical humanitarian relief work in foreign countries, the covered topics of diseases and prevention methods available are important considerations for health maintenance.

Teaching and Learning Package

Additional instructor resources for this product are available online. Instructor assets include an Instructor's Manual, Educator's Guide, PowerPoint® slides, a test bank powered by Cognero®, and more. Sign up or sign in at www.cengage.com to search for and access this product and its online resources.

- Instructor Manual—provides chapter outlines with instruction and activity ideas.
- PowerPoint slides—support lectures with definitions, key concepts, and examples.
- Guide to Teaching Online—offers tips for teaching online and incorporating MindTap activities into your course.
- Educator's Guide—offers suggested content from MindTap by chapter to help you personalize your course.
- Cengage Testing, powered by Cognero®—a flexible, online system that allows you to access, customize, and deliver a test bank from your chosen text to your students through your LMS or another channel outside of MindTap.
- Transition Guide—outlines changes between the Second and Third editions of the textbook.

About the Author

Margaret Rodriguez has been a Certified Surgical Technologist (CST) since 1980 and a Certified Surgical First Assistant (CSFA) since 1992. She graduated from the El Paso Community College Surgical Technology program in 1980 and immediately began private-scrubbing for a neurosurgeon who took her under his wing from a busy private practice to the world of medical school academia. Following his retirement, she returned to general surgical practice. After obtaining her Associate of Applied Science (AAS) degree in Surgical Technology, she began teaching in the EPCC surgical technology program with her mentor, Cynthia A. Rivera RN, BS. Changing course from nursing studies, she earned her Bachelor of Science (BS) in Occupational Career Training and Development from Texas A&M University, Corpus Christi in 2002 and subsequently received her Master's of Education in Higher Education Leadership from the University of Texas—El Paso in 2018. She is a tenured Professor and Program Coordinator at El Paso Community College.

Professionally, Mrs. Rodriguez served on the CSFA Exam Review Committee of the National Board of Surgical Technology and Surgical Assisting (NBSTSA) and is now serving as a member of the Board of Directors. She has been a site-visitor for the Accreditation Review Council on Education in Surgical Technology and Surgical Assisting (ARC-STSA). She served on the Texas State Assembly of AST Board before being elected to national office in the Association of Surgical Technologists (AST) in 2005. During her eight years on the national AST Board of Directors, she served as Director, Vice-president, and as AST President from 2011 to 2013 and earned the title of Fellow of the Association of Surgical Technologists (FAST). During that time, she also served as Chair of the Council on Surgical and Perioperative Safety (CSPS) from 2012 to 2013 and as the AST Commissioner to the Commission on Accreditation of Allied Health Education Programs (CAAHEP) in 2012 to 2013. She is the first and currently the only CST or CSFA faculty consultant for Ethicon, a division of Johnson & Johnson Medical Devices.

She has been a contributor to the AST Exam Review Study Guide, three editions of Surgical Technology for the Surgical Technologist, Surgical Instrumentation, Alexander's Surgical Procedures, an upcoming Surgical Assisting textbook, as well as writing numerous AST journal articles and contributing to publications by AORN, NBSTSA, and Outpatient Surgery magazine.

Mrs. Rodriguez has been married for 39 years to George Rodriguez, also a CST, and together they have four children and twelve grandchildren.

Acknowledgments

I thank my husband, family, and friends for their unwavering encouragement and understanding of the considerable time needed to complete this project.

I thank my mentor Cynthia A. Rivera, RN, BS, for giving me the foundation for my professional surgical technology career and owe my first employer and dear friend, the late William J. Nelson, MD, enormous gratitude for giving me the freedom to expand my skills and develop my passion for the world of surgery and healthcare education.

I appreciate every student I've had the honor to instruct over the past 26 years for reminding me to step back and look at things from the perspective of someone new to the mysteries and complexities of the perioperative environment.

I sincerely thank the members and staff of AST for their dedication to quality surgical patient care and giving me the opportunity to serve our professional organization and Ethicon for recognizing surgical technologists and first assistants as valuable and irreplaceable surgical team members and partners with industry for deliverance of quality patient care.

Finally, I am forever grateful to all of the wonderful members of the Cengage Learning team who guided me through the complex world of publishing with patience and understanding.

Reviewers

The author thanks the following individuals for their careful reviews and recommendations for improvements in the manuscript. Their comments were most helpful in making this text market-ready.

Kathy Patnaude, CST, BA, FAST
Midlands Technical College
West Columbia, SC

Lisa Day, CST, CSFA, FAST
Lord Fairfax Community College
Warrentown, VA

Mark Wilms, CST, CRCST, CHL, M. Ed.
Pima Medical Institute
Denver, CO

Michael Sells
Kirkwood Community College
Cedar Rapids, IA

Robert Blackston, M. ED., CST, CSFA
North Idaho College
Coeur d'Alene, ID

Sugey F. Briones, CST, BHA
American Career College
Los Angeles, CA

CHAPTER 1

Introduction to Microbiology

Learning Objectives

After completing the study of this chapter, you will be able to:

1. Define key terms.
2. Discuss the responsibilities of surgical technologists and other sterile surgical team members in prevention of disease transmission.
3. Discuss significant historical contributions from pioneers in microbiology.
4. Relate notable discoveries and events of the twentieth century from the historic timeline to current, twenty-first century public health concerns.
5. Explain how the theories of spontaneous generation and abiogenesis were disproved and the impact on the work of future researchers.
6. Discuss the scientific impact of Koch's postulates, including the exceptions to them.
7. Apply critical thinking skills in relating chapter material to the surgical environment of care or broader global community.

Key Terms

Abiogenesis

Aerobic

Anaerobic

Antibiotic

Aseptic technique

Bioterrorism

Blood-borne pathogens (BBPs)

Cell theory

Chemotherapy

Conjugation

Endemic

Epidemic

Etiology

Germ Theory of Disease

Germ warfare

Gram stain

Immunity

Immunocompromised

Inoculation

Koch's postulates

Other potentially infectious materials (OPIMs)

Pandemic

Pasteurization

Penicillin

Personal protective equipment (PPE)

Petri dish

Puerperal fever

Pure culture technique

Quarantine

Sterilant

Surgical conscience

Vaccination

The Big Picture

History and microbiology may not be your favorite subjects, especially learning about a bunch of long-dead scientists who made discoveries that we now take for granted. The COVID-19 pandemic upended global life starting in 2020 and showed us how events of the past can repeat in the present with both remarkably similar and quite different impact and responses. Keeping an open mind may actually help you find the information interesting and broaden your understanding of the wonders and interconnectedness of the world around us from microscopic to macroscopic points of view.

During your examination of the topics in this chapter, consider the following questions:

1. Which pioneers of microbiology had the biggest impact on surgical patient care?

2. What types of discoveries in this century, in your opinion, equal those made by the pioneers?

3. Do patterns exist for disease outbreaks, treatment, eradication, and recurrence and in what ways are those patterns beneficial or detrimental to global health responses?

4. How does awareness and understanding of the mechanisms of disease transmission help to break the chain of infection?

5. Based on your study of the topics covered, do you feel that public health and prevention of disease transmission will become a larger focus in daily life and what would that focus look like?

Microbiology and Surgical Technology

The most fundamental component of surgical technology is providing the best possible care for the patients who come into our operating room suites. Many surgical procedures are increasingly complex and technical, but no matter what type of procedure or variety of instruments and equipment used, the delineation between what is sterile and what is unsterile is of

> **Clinical Significance Topic**
>
> Surgical technology is a profession heavily dependent on scientific research. It is the cumulative knowledge of all the scientists who have studied microorganisms and diseases that gives validity to our professional practice and dedication to the principles of asepsis. Without knowledge of the incredible efforts of these pioneers, we might not understand the reasons we are taught to pay such close attention to the importance of sterile technique. It is not possible to simply see whether an item is sterile or unsterile, but we can have reasonable assurance that if our technique is stringent and we use our surgical conscience, then the patients in our care will have the best outcomes possible. *Aeger Primo*—the patient first!

paramount importance and may determine the ultimate outcomes for these patients. The concept of a **surgical conscience**, to which surgical technologists hold so tightly, is largely based on a broad educational foundation and understanding of microbiology and its relation to disease transmission from recognized or undetected sources of contamination. This guiding principle ensures that patients entering the surgical environment will receive optimal care with the goal of positive postoperative outcomes. Microbial contamination of a surgical wound, cross-contamination between patients or the environment, and the emergence or re-emergence of diseases among the general population may be minimized through a thorough understanding of:

- Classes of microorganisms and their ability to cause disease

- Various mechanisms for the spread of pathogenic microorganisms

- Aseptic and sterile techniques designed to prevent contamination

- Appropriate diagnosis and pharmacological treatment of disease

- Personal and community responsibility for utilization of resources to prevent **endemic, epidemic**, or **pandemic** outbreaks of disease

A minor bacterial or viral infection may be merely an annoyance to a healthy individual; however, to **immunocompromised** patients such as those who routinely enter the surgical environment of care, it may become literally a matter of life and death. Surgical technologists must also be responsible for their own health and safety.

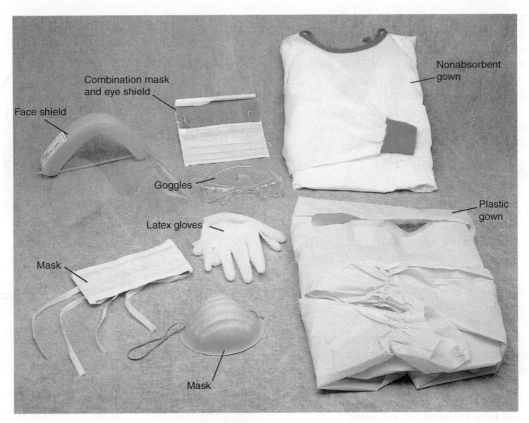

Figure 1-1 Examples of personal protective equipment (PPE).

Personal protective equipment (PPE) and knowledge of practices that reduce or prevent exposure to **blood-borne pathogens (BBPs)** or **other potentially infectious materials (OPIMs)** are important tools in the surgical technologist's professional armamentarium (see Figure 1-1).

The news media covers the outside world with a much broader focus and stories of topics such as:

- The global COVID-19 pandemic and its morbidity and mortality statistics
- Debates over the development and efficacy of vaccinations
- The impact of politicization of public health initiatives
- Mechanisms for disease transmission and preventative measures
- Food recalls after consumers are sickened
- Fears of use of biological weapons of mass destruction
- Exposure of patients to contaminated drugs or surgical instruments
- Cases of diseases turning up in travelers to foreign countries and then returning to the United States, potentially exposing fellow passengers over long distances in close spaces
- Re-emergence of childhood diseases previously thought eradicated due to lack of parental compliance in immunization schedules
- Cases of diseases spreading from animal populations to humans

Whether in the smaller, controlled operating room environment or on a more global scale, surgical technologists are uniquely qualified and skilled to fight the battle against microscopic armies of invaders. Breaking the chains of infection requires surgical technologists to practice standard techniques and utilize the comprehensive education gained through the core curriculum (including the study of microbiology) each day and on every procedure.

Early Pioneers of Microbiology

Taking time to look back in history to examine the origins of a science, especially from a twenty-first century perspective, demonstrates that the enormity of the accomplishments of the trailblazers in microbiology. This section examines the most prominent examples of these early scientists and their determination to give proof to theory by replacing mysticism and folklore with experimentation and scientific methodology.

Girolamo Fracastoro

There have been a number of individuals over the centuries who have studied and tried to demonstrate the existence of living organisms responsible for the spread of disease. One of the earliest pioneers was a physician from Verona, Italy, named Girolamo Fracastoro.

Fracastoro published his research regarding syphilis in 1530. In 1546, he published his findings regarding epidemic diseases in a paper entitled, *De Contagione et Contagiosis Morbis* (*On Contagion and Contagious Diseases*). He theorized that tiny, unseen organisms were spread by several means including contact between an infected host and others, indirect contact, carried on clothing, or carried through the air. Fracastoro was the first to apply scientific principles to his theory. Although his findings were generally accepted at that time, following his death in 1553, they soon fell out of favor and scientific focus until the late 1800s.

Robert Hooke

A pivotal event occurred in the mid-seventeenth century when a prolific English scientist, Robert Hooke, designed and built a compound microscope. He built telescopes to study the heavens and later used his talents to focus on much smaller bodies. In 1665, he published a work entitled "Micrographia" (small drawings) in which he was the first to use the term "cell" to describe the small, honeycomb-like spaces found in cork. Hooke's discovery was the beginning of **cell theory**—that all living things are composed of cells. Hooke was better known for his subsequent research in which he postulated that the ability of something to be deformed by application of stress forces and return to its original size, shape, or form when those forces are removed is the property of elasticity. Hooke's Law in its mathematical equation was published in 1676 and is still in use today.

Antonie van Leeuwenhoek

Dutch amateur scientist Antonie van Leeuwenhoek was the first to observe and record bacteria and protozoa in 1673. He used a single-lens microscope and a variety of sources such as rainwater, saliva, and even his own semen, to examine what he termed "animalcules" (see Figure 1-2). He reported his results to the Royal Society of London between 1673 and 1723, including the first accurate drawings of various types of bacteria, using only a simple microscope (see Figure 1-3). These drawings served as the basis for modern depictions of the previously "invisible" world.

Francesco Redi

Francesco Redi, an Italian physician and biologist set out to disprove the theory of **abiogenesis** in 1668, even before Leeuwenhoek's findings were reported. Redi, openly critical of the theory, devised an ingenious experiment in which he filled three jars with decaying meat and sealed them with a lid. He also placed meat in three other jars but left those open. Maggots soon appeared on the meat in the open jar, but no maggots were present in the sealed jars. Redi concluded that given ready access to the meat, the flies had laid their eggs there and could not do so on the meat in the other jars because they were sealed. His opponents were undaunted and scoffed at the results of the experiment, arguing that fresh oxygen was a requirement of spontaneous generation.

Redi then conducted a second experiment. Again, meat was placed in three open jars, but this time the other three jars were sealed with fine mesh gauze to satisfy his critics. The

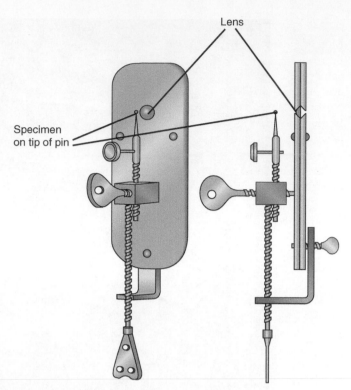

Figure 1-2 Antonie van Leeuwenhoek's microscope. The specimen was placed on top of the point in front of the small lens.

results were the same as the first experiment. This provided a strong basis for refuting abiogenesis, but the scientific community was still not ready to give up its long-held belief.

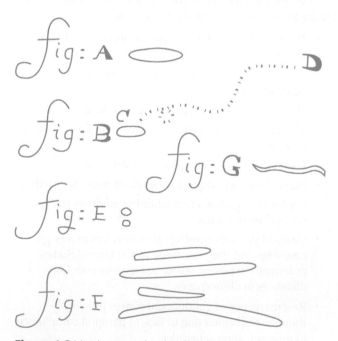

Figure 1-3 Van Leeuwenhoek's drawings of cells that were later identified as bacteria.

John Needham and Lazzaro Spallanzani

Most scientists believed in the theory of spontaneous generation, or abiogenesis, until the second half of the nineteenth century. This theory claimed that life could spontaneously arise from non-living material. An English priest, John Needham, had performed experiments in 1749 with meat broths that became infested with microbes, spurring his belief in a "vital force" that was responsible for the spontaneous generation of life. Other scientists were interested in finding the origins of these seemingly spontaneously generated cells after the discoveries of Hooke and Leeuwenhoek. Italian scientist and priest, Lazzaro Spallanzani, one of these skeptical researchers, sought to disprove abiogenesis through his own experiments years later showing that boiling was able to kill or prevent microbial growth but failed to sway Needham or the rest of the scientific community.

Edward Jenner

Smallpox had become a major cause of death in many parts of the developing world by 1798. Early attempts at vaccinating healthy individuals with small amounts of fluid from the pustules of infected hosts proved ineffective. The practice that originated in India and China known as variolation did not induce mild cases and immunity as hoped but instead, often caused serious infections that spread to others by contact exposure.

An Englishman, Edward Jenner became a pupil of John Hunter, a renowned physician and surgeon at St. George's Hospital in London. Hunter instilled in Jenner a scientific curiosity telling him, "Why think (speculate)—why not try the experiment?"

Jenner witnessed first-hand the devastation of smallpox throughout all areas of the country and segments of the population. He noted that individuals who became infected with a much less serious disease, known as cowpox, a disease transmitted from exposure to cattle, would easily recover and those individuals never contracted smallpox, even after intentional exposure. Jenner put his critical thinking and experimentation talents to use when he **inoculated** an 8-year-old boy with fluid from the blisters of a milkmaid with cowpox. The boy became mildly ill and recovered. Jenner then inoculated the same boy with smallpox; however, he never displayed any signs of infection. Jenner was eventually recognized prior to his death in 1823 as having been the first to effectively provide **immunity** through **vaccination**, despite problems including others trying to take credit for Jenner's work as well as difficulty in creating and then transporting properly prepared cowpox vaccine doses to the rest of Europe and America.

Ignaz Semmelweis

Another mid-nineteenth century pioneer was Ignaz Semmelweis, a Hungarian physician, who worked in an obstetrics clinic in Austria and witnessed a 25–30 percent maternal fatality rate from **puerperal fever**. After he experienced the death of a friend from a wound infection, he focused his observations on the practices of staff members and students in the clinic. He discovered that the patients attended to by midwives had much lower infection rates than those who were seen by medical students who would often participate in autopsies and anatomical dissections prior to examining the patients on the obstetrics ward. His investigation showed that the midwives took great care to wash their hands often and between patient examinations, whereas the medical students took no such steps.

Once determining the root cause, Semmelweis implemented practices of routine hand washing with chlorinated lime solutions. The result was a dramatic reduction of maternal mortality from more than 18 percent down to just over 1 percent. Unfortunately, the dedication to routine hand washing was not embraced by other physicians. Following years of working at other obstetrical hospitals in other countries, the physician population remained resistant to Semmelweis' findings and recommendations. He eventually was institutionalized after a mental breakdown and ironically, died in 1865 from a surgical wound infection following a minor procedure in 1865.

The Golden Age of Microbiology

The 60 years between 1855 and 1915, saw major strides in the study of microbiology in an increasingly enlightened era that embraced experimentation and the scientific method of proving new, or disproving old and commonly accepted, beliefs about the origins and spread of diseases.

Louis Pasteur

One of the most recognized figures of the Golden Age of Microbiology is Louis Pasteur, a French scientist, who earned his doctorate in physical sciences with a focus on chemistry and physics. As an educated scientist, Pasteur felt compelled to dispute the theory of abiogenesis, which had been widely accepted up until the latter part of the 1800s (see Figure 1-4).

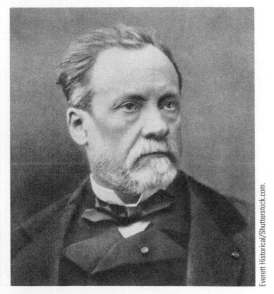

Figure 1-4 Louis Pasteur, 1822–1895.

Pasteur conducted a controlled experiment by using short-necked flasks. He filled several of the flasks with beef broth and boiled the broth. Some of the flasks were left open and, consequently, microbes were found thriving in the broth. As expected, the sealed flasks remained free of microbes.

Next, using flasks with necks bent into the shape of an "S," Pasteur again boiled beef broth and allowed it to cool in the flasks without sealing them (see Figure 1-5). Microbes never appeared in the S-shaped flasks, allowing Pasteur to conclude that the curve in the neck of the flasks had trapped

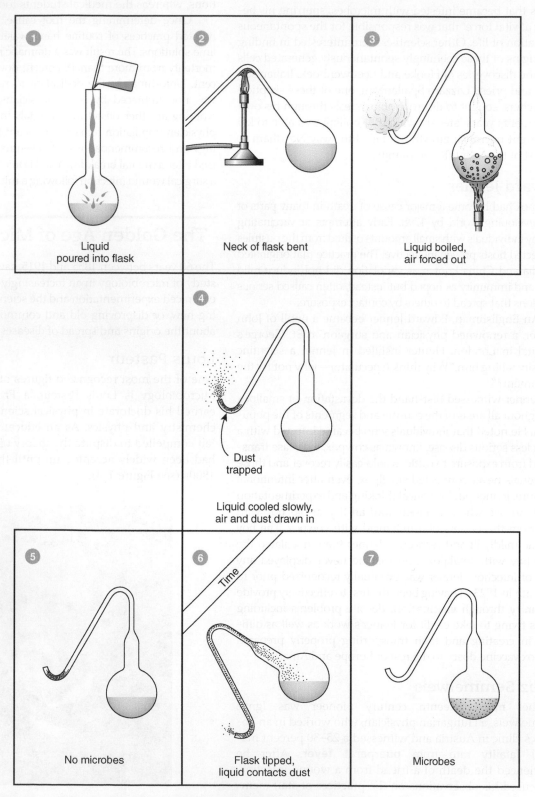

1. Liquid poured into flask

2. Neck of flask bent

3. Liquid boiled, air forced out

4. Dust trapped

Liquid cooled slowly, air and dust drawn in

5. No microbes

6. Time — Flask tipped, liquid contacts dust

7. Microbes

Figure 1-5 Pasteur's experiment disproving the theory of spontaneous generation.

the airborne microbes, preventing the contamination of the broth. Pasteur had successfully refuted Needham's "vital force" theory, permanently dismantling the theory of spontaneous generation.

Louis Pasteur is probably most notably credited with developing experiments leading to the Germ Theory of Fermentation. French Emperor Napoleon III commissioned a study of distilling processes. Pasteur's experiments showed that bacteria were the agents responsible for the spoilage of beer and wine. He was able to demonstrate that the bacteria changed the alcohol into acetic acid, otherwise known as vinegar. He identified for the

first time that microorganisms can be categorized into either **aerobic** or **anaerobic** classifications after unexpectedly arresting the fermentation process by passing air through the liquids, demonstrating that certain types of microbes cannot survive in the presence of air.

His solution to the problem was to use just enough heat to kill the bacteria without affecting the taste of the product. The same heating process is used today to kill bacteria in milk and is referred to as **pasteurization** (see Figure 1-6). Pasteur's proof of the relationship between food spoilage and microorganisms was a major contribution to the establishment of the connection between disease and microbes.

MINNESOTA DEPARTMENT OF HEALTH

Division of Sanitation

ESSENTIALS FOR A SAFE MILK SUPPLY

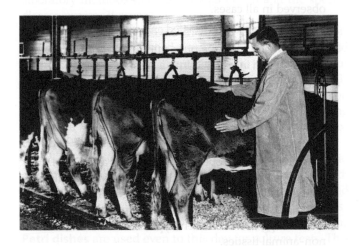

Healthy Dairy Cows

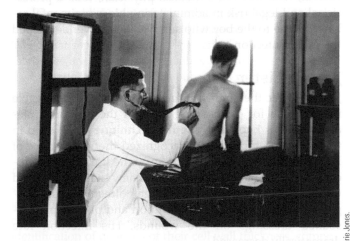

Healthy Dairy Workers

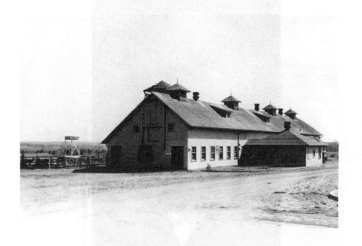

Sanitary Production

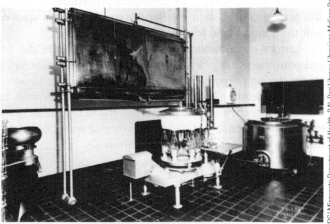

Pasteurization

Figure 1-6 1934 instructional flyer for maintenance of a safe milk supply, from the Minnesota Health Department.

Koch felt the pressure to remain relevant among his peers following his success with his refined laboratory techniques. In 1890, Koch culminated his extensive research on tuberculosis with news of a treatment that was seized by the media as a"cure." A small percentage of patients with mild skin symptoms caused by the tubercle bacilli gained some therapeutic benefit from Koch's remedy that he called tuberculin. Most patients saw little to no benefit and some actually suffered fatal allergic reactions. Koch's reputation suffered further when it was discovered that he had a significant financial interest in the production of tuberculin.

Despite the trouble with his research on tuberculosis, Koch continued his studies and subsequently began to focus his attention on the deadly cholera infection. Controversy plagued Koch again in the form of public challenge by Emanuel Klein, a British microbiologist, on Koch's findings and recommendations regarding quarantine of cholera victims. The scientific community ultimately agreed to acknowledge value in the work of both men and, in turn, they were able to accept components of each other's recommendations. Koch was eventually awarded the Nobel Prize for Physiology or Medicine in 1905.

Just as Koch was influenced by his teachers, several of his students went on to achieve recognition for their work as well. Emil von Behring won the Nobel Prize for Physiology or Medicine in 1901 for his work with serum therapy and application against tetanus and diphtheria, 4 years before his mentor was awarded the prize. August von Wassermann became famous in 1906 for his work with Albert Neisser to create a universal blood-serum test to detect syphilis.

Paul Ehrlich, another student of Robert Koch, would go on to become a Nobel Prize winner in 1908. He was given the name of "father of **chemotherapy**" for his work with chemical agents for the treatment of pathological microbes which were previously isolated and categorized by his scientific peers and predecessors. Ehrlich worked with derivative forms of the poison arsenic to develop what he called the first "magic bullet," a chemical therapy capable of destroying a pathogen without harming the host. Salvarsan was version 606 of the numerous arsenical compounds developed and was initially tested on rabbits infected with syphilis. Ehrlich later developed Neosalvarsan, version 914 of the drug, as a more soluble and easily administered alternative, although its curative effects on syphilis were less than the more potent original.

The Modern Era of Microbiology

The foundations for modern science had been firmly established by the time Koch and his students and colleagues had achieved public recognition for their extensive research and findings.

Ruth Ella Moore

In 1933, African-American bacteriologist, Dr. Ruth Ellen Moore was the first African-American to receive a Ph.D. in bacteriology. She also was the first African-American to join the American Society for Microbiology in 1936. Her doctoral research focused on treatments for tuberculosis, which at the time was the second highest cause of death in the United States. She later expanded her work to immunology and blood type-associated pathology in African-Americans. She became the head of the Howard University's Department of Bacteriology.

Moore's dissertation research contributed to eventually treating tuberculosis, which was the second leading cause of death in the U.S. at that time. She has also published work on immunology, dental caries, and blood types in African-Americans. She lectured in bacteriology at variety of universities, including teaching at and being the head of the Department of Bacteriology at Howard University. Eventually in 1986, she was recognized by the ASM Minority Committee for her exemplary service as a mentor, leader, and activist in the microbiology science community.

Elizabeth Bugie

Elizabeth Bugie, an American microbiologist and biochemist was part of a team of Rutgers University research scientists who developed the antibiotic streptomycin in 1944. The discovery of the ability of streptomycin to fight *Mycobacterium tuberculosis*, the microorganism that causes tuberculosis was a medical breakthrough in the fight of an often-fatal disease. The other all-male team scientists were awarded the Nobel Prize for Medicine for the discovery, however, the lead scientist, Professor Selman Waksan chose to exclude Dr. Bugie's name from the streptomycin patent based on their reasoning that she would "get married and have a family" so it was not necessary for her to be recognized for her work. Bugie continued her work with antimicrobial substances that advanced the development of effective antibiotic treatments.

June Almeida

June Hart Almeida was a Scottish-born immigrant to Canada who, although she never completed her formal undergraduate education, became a lab technician who gained professional recognition for her skills and techniques of identification of microscopic particles. Following her return to the United Kingdom to take a position at a London medical school, Almeida used antibodies to pinpoint viral particles. The antibodies from previously infected individuals were introduced into samples and were drawn to their antigen-counterparts, congregating around the viruses, making them visible under the microscope and opening up a new way to diagnose viral infections in patients. In 1964, using the electron microscope, June Almeida was the first to identify the coronavirus, the pathogen we are well-familiar with after the COVID-19 pandemic.

A Century of Scientific Breakthroughs in Microbiology

As the twentieth century progressed, discoveries in microbiology, bacteriology, virology, and genetics seemed to develop exponentially and have continued into the twenty-first century. Some of the notable discoveries, advances, and events in microbiology during the past 120 years include the following timeline.

1902: Cambridge, Massachusetts enacted a mandatory smallpox vaccination program following an outbreak of the disease. Following a failed challenge to the city health department's mandate by an individual who refused to be vaccinated, the case was heard by the U.S. Supreme Court which ruled in 1905 that the state of Massachusetts had the right to make vaccination compulsory as a public health protection against communicable disease.

1904: William Gorgas brought mosquito control methods to construction sites of the Panama Canal including netting, screens, fumigation, and draining of stagnant water. The following year, the last case of mosquito-borne yellow fever was reported in Panama City, Panama.

1905: The last case of the yellow fever epidemic in North America was reported in New Orleans, Louisiana.

1905: Polio, also known as infantile paralysis, was reported to be a contagious disease transmitted from person-to-person contact following epidemic in Sweden.

1906: The first diphtheria antitoxin was produced by Ernst Lederle who founded Lederle Laboratories which later became part of Wyeth Laboratories.

1906: Belgian scientists Jules Bordet and Octave Gengou were the first to isolate *Bordetella pertussis* responsible for pertussis, also known as whooping cough.

1907: Mary Mallon, later given the name "Typhoid Mary" was placed in forced confinement when investigators found that her employment history as a cook had exposed numerous individuals who contracted typhoid fever and at least two died. The "healthy carrier" concept of disease transmission was recognized and accepted. Though she was released in 1910 with the promise to not work as a cook, Mary used a pseudonym and began to work at a hospital as a cook and was again identified as the probable infective carrier when numerous patients contracted typhoid fever. She was again forced into **quarantine** on North Brother Island in New York until her death in 1938.

1908: Karl Landsteiner, MD and Erwin Popper, MD determined that a virus is the cause of polio. The physicians from Vienna used cerebrospinal fluid of a patient who died from polio, passed it through special filters, and injected into a laboratory monkey which subsequently developed the infection.

1910: Paul Ehrlich published his findings of a successful treatment for syphilis in the November issue of *The Journal of Cutaneous Diseases*.

1913: Bela Schick produced a widely used "Schick test"—a skin test that shows whether an individual is susceptible or immune to diphtheria. A massive immunization program for those who tested positive resulted in a dramatic decrease in diphtheria cases.

1918: In March, 46 soldiers at Fort Riley, Kansas, died from an outbreak of influenza. With the onset of World War I, soldiers from Ft. Riley were deployed to fight in Spain. Soon, troops from all of the countries involved in the conflict came down with the same disease. Soldiers returned to the United States as well as to the other countries. What was later named the Spanish Flu Pandemic of 1918 spread worldwide and killed an estimated 20–50 million. The combined official death toll of WWI was 16 million. One in four people in the United States was afflicted with the virulent mutated flu virus.

1928: Scottish bacteriologist Alexander Fleming accidentally discovered a mold later identified as *Penicillium notatum* while throwing out contaminated Petri dishes. He noticed that there was a clear line of demarcation between the mold and where the bacteria had stopped growing. Fleming was responsible for naming the secretion of the mold **penicillin**, the first **antibiotic**.

1933: Rebecca Lancefield proposed a system for classifying streptococci based on how antigens in the walls of cells reacted with the human immune system. She was able to classify streptococci into various serotypes.

1937: The disease West Nile virus was first documented in Uganda. It resulted in fatal encephalitis in humans.

1942: A covert Japanese program called Unit 731 performed horrific experiments on human subjects, exposing them to anthrax, cholera, typhus, and bubonic plague to perfect **germ warfare** tactics. It is believed that the unit was responsible for releasing insects coated with these diseases from war planes flying over provinces in China over several years. An estimated 270,000 were victims of the attacks.

1943: During WWII in Europe, one million diphtheria cases, with 50,000 deaths, accompanied other disruptions of life during the war and disruption in Europe.

1944: Oswald Avery, Colin MacLeod, and Maclyn McCarty confirmed that deoxyribonucleic acid (DNA) is the carrier of hereditary information.

1945: The first influenza vaccines using inactivated influenza A and B strains were developed by Dr. Thomas Francis, Jr. and Dr. Jonas Salk and approved for military use. A year later, it was released for use by the public.

1946: Joshua Lederberg and Edward Tatum discovered the process of **conjugation**, in which the genetic material from one bacterium could be transferred to another.

1947: The first case of penicillin-resistant *Staphylococcus aureus* was reported.

1949: A Texas woman who had the last reported case of smallpox in the United States died.

1953: James Watson and Francis Crick established the model for the double helix structure and replication of DNA.

1954: Dr. Jonas Salk began a mass vaccination campaign against poliomyelitis, a viral attack of the central nervous system that could cause paralysis and asphyxiation, for children in Philadelphia. By 1955, the vaccinations were being given nationwide.

1955: Dr. Thomas Peebles was first to isolate the measles virus at Boston Children's Hospital from an infected 13-year-old student.

1958: The Food and Drug Administration (FDA) fast-tracked approval of a compound later called vancomycin to treat growing numbers of penicillin-resistant *S. aureus.*

1960: Interferon was discovered. Interferon is manufactured by specific cells of the immune system of the human body. Interferon "interferes" with the ability of viruses to replicate.

1960: Methicillin, a new antibiotic to fight resistant *S. aureus*, was released for use.

1961: Jacques Monod and Francois Jacob discovered messenger ribonucleic acid (mRNA); the chemical involved in the process of protein synthesis.

1961: First cases of methicillin-resistant *S. aureus* (MRSA) were documented.

1963: Measles vaccine developed in 1958 was widely distributed to the public.

1967: First cases of the Marburg hemorrhagic virus were reported. Laboratory workers in Marburg, Germany, were exposed while performing polio experiments with Ugandan monkeys.

1969: US President Richard Nixon announced an unconditional renunciation of biological weapons.

1971: First vaccine against meningitis was developed.

1971: The United States discontinued routine smallpox vaccination programs due to eradication of the disease.

1976: An epidemic of swine flu broke out in an Army base in New Jersey. A nationwide vaccination program prevented further spread; however, the vaccines were linked to cases of paralysis so they were discontinued by year's end.

1976: Legionnaire's disease broke out in a hotel in Philadelphia. The cause was identified as *Legionella pneumophila*, which contaminated the hotel's ventilation system.

1976: Zaire (Congo), Africa—280 people died of the Ebola virus, a hemorrhagic fever that prevents clotting.

1979: Anthrax spores leaked from a germ warfare plant in Sverdlovsk, Russia, causing more than 100 deaths in the surrounding town over a 2-month period.

1979: Australian Dr. J. Robert Warren first identified *Helicobacter pylori* in biopsy specimens of the lower stomachs of patients. In 1982, Dr. Barry Marshall grew the slow-growing bacterium in cultures.

1979: Acquired immunodeficiency syndrome (AIDS) was diagnosed for the first time. The chief sign and associated disease was Kaposi's sarcoma lesions visible on the skin of infected and dying patients.

1984: French researchers identified the human immunodeficiency virus (HIV) as the causative agent of AIDS. Robert Gallo, a US scientist, was also credited with research findings of workers in his laboratory around the same time, so credit is generally shared between the two countries. In the late 1970s, Gallo had discovered the first retrovirus, human T-cell leukemia virus (HTLV).

1987: The FDA approved the sale of AZT for treatment of HIV and AIDS. They also approved the antibiotic Cipro.

1988: Vancomycin-resistant enterococcus (VRE) was first reported in Europe. The potent antibiotic Vancomycin had been in use since 1958 as treatment for Gram-positive bacteria such as *Clostridium difficile.*

1989: The hepatitis C virus was first documented.

1995: The FDA approved the first chicken pox vaccine.

1996: The World Health Organization (WHO) warned of a growing number of highly resistant tuberculosis infections in South Africa.

1997: The CDC began work on a vaccine for avian "bird flu" virus (H5N1) after deaths in Hong Kong and fear of possible spread.

2001: Letters laced with anthrax were mailed to the New York Post and NBC, and later to several US Senators and Congressmen. Office workers who had come into contact with the letters contracted cases of cutaneous anthrax, and several US postal workers died from inhalation anthrax. **Bioterrorism** had become a reality in the United States. A governmental scientist was eventually charged with the crimes.

2002: Findings published, which were later found to be erroneous, proposed a link between childhood vaccinations and risk of autism. Parents began refusing vaccinations for their children, despite evidence of the tainted research, and cases of childhood diseases mostly eradicated began to rebound over the following years.

2002: Concerns grew over cases of Cipro-resistant gonorrhea and erythromycin-resistant group A streptococci.

2002: Two cruise ship lines dealt with outbreaks of gastrointestinal illness among large numbers of passengers.

2002: Vancomycin-resistant strains of *Staphylococcus* were identified.

2003: Cases of severe acute respiratory syndrome (SARS) began to appear in Hong Kong, Vietnam, and parts of China.

2003: MRSA was now being spread to healthy individuals through skin contact.

2003: A new strain of "mad cow disease" was identified in a young bull in Japan.

2005: French and South African researchers reported that circumcision reduced the risk of AIDS by 70 percent.

2005: Two cows in the United States died from mad cow disease, as did one in Austria.

2006: The number of cases of blindness caused by a rare fungal infection in persons who wore contacts and used commercial saline solutions increased to 122.

2006: Consumers were warned about eating spinach after 173 people became sickened by *Escherichia coli* traced back to a farm in California.

2006: The CDC warned travelers to Africa and Asia of a mosquito-borne disease, Chikungunya fever, which has symptoms similar to Dengue fever, including severe headaches, muscle pain, and joint swelling that may take months to resolve. The disease has been found in the intervening years in the islands of the Caribbean and even in the United States in 2014.

2006: *Coccidiomycosis*, better known as valley fever in California, infected 5,500 people and resulted in 33 deaths. Spores spread by disturbed soil in the Southwest were found to be the origin of the epidemic.

2006: The FDA approved a vaccine for Human Papillomavirus (HPV).

2007: An attorney from Atlanta ignored warnings about exposure of the public when he traveled to Italy by airline, despite being aware that he had a dangerous multi-drug-resistant form of tuberculosis. Government officials in the United States and Italy tried to advise all passengers of their exposure risk. Upon his return, he was forcibly quarantined in the first such action since the 1960s.

2009: A former Army nurse anesthetist pleaded guilty to assault after having infected 15 patients with hepatitis C (HCV). During surgical procedures, he would inject narcotic drugs himself and reuse the contaminated needles on patients, thus passing on his infected blood to patients in his care.

2009: A surgical technologist in Colorado exposed nearly 6,000 patients and infected 26 with HCV by stealing anesthesia narcotics and replacing them with contaminated syringes of saline.

2009: From the initial outbreak in Mexico in April through December, the CDC and WHO reported that more than 10,000 people died from and approximately 200,000 were infected with the H1N1 "swine flu" virus pandemic. In mid-June 2010, the death toll had increased to more than 18,000.

2010: Scientists in Britain showed concern about cases of patients returning from hospitals in South Asia or India with an antibiotic-resistant "superbug" called New Delhi metallo-lactamase-1 (NDM-1). One patient had died of the infection, spurring concerns about possible spread. Later, a Japanese patient treated in India also became infected with the same disease.

2010: A cholera epidemic in Haiti spread following the devastating earthquake in January that left much of the population homeless and living in squalor. In December, the death toll had reached more than 2,000, with more than 80,000 having suffered with the disease. The strain of cholera was traced back to infected United Nations troops from Nepal who had come to help with disaster relief and was spread through poorly designed sanitation facilities that contaminated the Artibonite River with human waste.

2011: US scientists cited an increase of 225 percent in oral cancers, mainly in white men between 1974 and 2007. The evidence pointed strongly to human papillomavirus (HPV) as the likely cause of the cancer increases.

2011: An Australian anesthesiologist infected 50 female patients with hepatitis C at an abortion clinic.

2011: The WHO determined that the strain of *E. coli* responsible for nearly 50 fatalities was a new variant not seen before.

2011: Health officials reported three deaths from a "brain-eating" disease, *Naegleria fowleri*, an amoeba found in water. The CDC stated that there had been 120 cases, mostly fatal since the amoeba was identified in the 1960s.

2011: An outbreak of *Listeria* found in cantaloupe from Colorado killed 33 in the United States.

2011: There were 8.7 million new cases of tuberculosis (TB) reported during the year, with 400,000 being multi-drug-resistant strains.

2012: Middle East Respiratory Syndrome (MERS), a disease similar to SARS, was identified in a Saudi Arabian man who died from severe pneumonia-like symptoms and renal failure.

2012: Seventeen people in Texas died from West Nile virus, a mosquito-borne illness.

2012: Park rangers in Yosemite closed cabins after six people became sickened and three died from hantavirus, a disease carried by deer mice and disseminated through their urine and feces.

2012: The death toll increased to 19 for patients at the National Institutes of Health (NIH) infected with an antibiotic-resistant strain of *Klebsiella pneumonia*. The outbreak was apparently attributed to a single individual.

2012: Hundreds of patients who had been given steroid injections for back pain were warned of the fungal contamination of the medication, which resulted in 30 deaths and 419 cases of meningitis. The fungus was identified as *Exserohilum rostratum*. A compounding pharmacy in Massachusetts was found to be the sole distributor of the tainted steroids but had distributed them to at least 18 states.

2012: A traveling medical technician was charged with having infected at least 39 patients with hepatitis C through stolen drugs and syringes.

2013: British officials revealed a 25 percent increase in antibiotic-resistant gonorrhea.

2013: Britain's Health Minister warned that the emergence and worldwide spread of antibiotic-resistant diseases may pose a catastrophic threat to patients in health-care settings as well as the general population.

2014: Two cases of MERS were diagnosed in patients returning from the Middle East. Since its discovery in 2012 there have been 538 cases, with 145 deaths in 17 countries.

2014: A study of healthy placentas showed a potential link between microbes typically found in the mouth to those found in placentas, in opposition to the previously held belief that the fetus grows in a sterile environment. Preliminary results may point to a benefit to the placenta from these microbes, possibly even in preventing pre-term labor.

2014: The Centers for Disease Control and Prevention in Atlanta revealed that at least 84 laboratory workers might have been inadvertently exposed to live anthrax bacteria, sparking a US Congressional investigation regarding standardization of laboratory procedures and oversight.

2014: Thousands of people were infected with Ebola hemorrhagic fever (EHF) in Guinea, Sierra Leone, and Liberia, Africa. Since its discovery in 1976, there have been 18 outbreaks of Ebola infections and a total of 11,193 fatalities through June 2015. Two nurses contracted the disease in Dallas, Texas, while treating a patient infected with Ebola while visiting Africa who died of the disease in October.

2015: Measles spread quickly in 24 states following a December 2014 outbreak originating in Disneyland in California with 117 cases linked to that source and a total of 178 cases by June 2015. California passed a mandatory vaccination law in response to the outbreak.

2015: MERS in South Korea caused shutdowns of schools and large quarantines following 166 cases through June.

2016: The World Health Organization (WHO) Emergency Committee announced a strong association between Zika virus infection in pregnant women and microcephaly and other birth defects in their infants. The virus is spread by mosquitos and was found to be transmissible by human sperm. Approximately 600,000 cases were recorded in North, Central, and South America.

2018: CDC's PulseNet that includes public health departments in all 50 states was able to use whole-genome sequencing for subtyping pathogens that cause foodborne illness including: *Salmonella, Yersinia, Vibrio, Shigella, and Cronobacter*.

2019: The Centers for Disease Control and Prevention (CDC) reported 704 cases of measles in the U.S., the largest number of cases in a single year since 1994.

2019: On December 31, health officials from Wuhan in China's central Hubei province confirmed an outbreak of dozens of pneumonia cases from an unknown pathogen.

2020: Public health agencies responded in January to the outbreak caused by a novel coronavirus first identified in Wuhan. The WHO subsequently gives the new SARS-CoV-2 disease the name COVID-19.

2020: On March 11, 2020, the WHO declared COVID-19 a world-wide pandemic. China began administering the first vaccine trials to volunteers.

2020: In March and April, the U.S. began administering vaccine trials in two doses.

2020: In August, the African continent was declared free of wild poliovirus although a small number of vaccine-derived polio infections persist.

2020: On December 8, 2020, the U.S. reached the 15 million case total. On December 8, a British 90-year-old woman became the first person in the world to receive a clinically approved vaccine. On December 11, the U.S. FDA approved use of the Pfizer vaccine for emergency use and the rollout began a few days later. The Moderna vaccine was approved for emergency use on December 18.

2021: According to the Johns Hopkins Coronavirus Research Center, by mid-May, the global number of COVID-19 infections reached nearly 163 million with 3.4 million deaths. The U.S. recorded 33 million cases with nearly 590,000 deaths. The vaccination rate skyrocketed on a global scale to nearly 1.5 billion doses given and, in the U.S., nearly 270 million doses given.

2021: Concerning COVID-19 variants from the United Kingdom, South Africa, and Brazil spread globally, worrying researchers about the effectiveness of current vaccines against mutations.

Learning from the Past

The value in examining the preceding historic timeline is not in the useless memorization of dates and facts, but rather to recognize the enormous strides that have been made in science in a relatively short period and to see how interconnected we are as individuals to the rest of humanity and the planet on which we live. One brief century after the 1918 Spanish Flu global pandemic, the world was again caught off guard by the COVID-19 pandemic. Each of us will remember the impact of the pandemic going forward but it raises the question of how much did we learn on an individual, societal, or global health scale about personal and collective responsibility, critical disaster planning for future outbreaks, and the fragility of the human species?

The microbial world is incredibly resourceful in its survival methods and, for good or for bad, the human race must find a way to coexist with it. As the relative size of the planet shrinks through global travel and access, the expanding problems and diseases that plague other countries now find their way onto our own doorsteps and from our shores to theirs. These shared experiences should unify us and magnify our need to work collectively as a species to be just as resourceful as the innumerable members of the natural microbial world to ensure our survival.

Breaking the Chain of Disease Transmission

There are many ways by which pathogenic microorganisms can be transmitted. In the timeline of the previous section, some examples of how diseases can spread include:

- Human to human
- Animal to human
- Environment to animal or human
- Insect to animal or human
- Laboratory specimens to human
- Bioterrorist attacks with various dissemination methods

Transmission of disease cannot always be prevented; however, those who work in healthcare have tools at their disposal that allow them to simultaneously protect themselves from exposure to patients and protect patients from exposure to personnel (see Figure 1-9). These tools include use of personal protective equipment (PPE) including gowns, gloves, masks, shoe covers, goggles/ face shields, N-95 respirators, aprons, etc. as well as sets of guidelines that guide their professional work practices. The COVID-19 pandemic

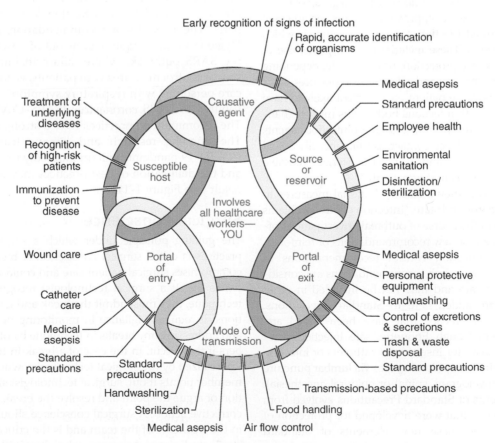

Figure 1-9 Components of the chain of infection with ways it can be broken.

brought a never-before-seen focus on the need for massive amounts of PPE during a global pandemic response and how critical but fragile that supply chain can be when not maintained or managed effectively.

Standard Precautions

An awareness of diseases and their transmissibility is a good start; however, without definitive guidelines that outline professional best practices for everyone working within the various healthcare settings, consistency cannot be achieved (see Figure 1-10).

A special section within the Centers for Disease Control and Prevention (CDC) is the Healthcare Infection Control Practices Advisory Committee (HICPAC). The members of this committee are charged with making and reviewing guidelines, and advising the CDC, the US Secretary of Health and Human Services (HHS), and other agencies regarding a broad scope of public health issues. In Section III.A of the *2007 Guideline for Isolation Precautions: Preventing Transmission of Infectious Agents in Healthcare Settings which was updated in 2019*, the HICPAC members state "Standard Precautions combine the major features of Universal Precautions (UP) and Body Substance Isolation (BSI) and are based on the principle that all blood, body fluids, secretions, excretions except sweat, non-intact skin, and mucous membranes may contain transmissible infectious agents. Standard Precautions include a group of infection prevention practices that apply to all patients, regardless of suspected or confirmed infection status, in any setting in which healthcare is delivered. These include: hand hygiene; use of gloves, gown, mask, eye protection, or face shield, depending on the anticipated exposure; and safe injection practices. Also, equipment or items in the patient environment likely to have been contaminated with infectious body fluids must be handled in a manner to prevent transmission of infectious agents (e.g., wear gloves for direct contact, contain heavily soiled equipment, properly clean and disinfect or sterilize reusable equipment before use on another patient)."

In Section III.A.1, they include additional measures to augment the standards and state, "Infection control problems that are identified in the course of outbreak investigations often indicate the need for new recommendations or reinforcement of existing infection control recommendations to protect patients. Because such recommendations are considered a standard of care and may not be included in other guidelines, they are added here to Standard Precautions. Three such areas of practice that have been added are: Respiratory Hygiene/Cough Etiquette, safe injection practices, and use of masks for insertion of catheters or injection of material into spinal or epidural spaces via lumbar puncture procedures (e.g., myelogram, spinal or epidural anesthesia). While most elements of Standard Precautions evolved from Universal Precautions that were developed for protection of healthcare personnel, these new elements of Standard Precautions focus on protection of patients."

Transmission-Based Precautions

Standard Precautions are used in all circumstances and presume that all patients are potential carriers of undiagnosed disease. When a specific disease process or pathogenic condition has been identified, additional work practices are used to address the method by which it is spread. The (July 2019 updated) 2007 HICPAC report states in Section III.B, "There are three categories of Transmission-Based Precautions: Contact Precautions, Droplet Precautions, and Airborne Precautions. Transmission-Based Precautions are used when the route(s) of transmission is (are) not completely interrupted using Standard Precautions alone. For some diseases that have multiple routes of transmission (e.g., SARS), more than one Transmission-Based Precautions category may be used. When used either singly or in combination, they are always used in addition to Standard Precautions."

In the six listed developments included in the Executive Summary of the updated HICPAC report, only months before the beginning of the COVID-19 outbreak, Section 2 stated "The emergence of new pathogens (e.g., SARS-CoV associated with the severe acute respiratory syndrome [SARS], Avian influenza in humans), renewed concern for evolving known pathogens (e.g., *C. difficile*, noroviruses, community-associated MRSA [CA-MRSA]), development of new therapies (e.g., gene therapy), and increasing concern for the threat of bioweapons attacks, established a need to address a broader scope of issues than in previous isolation guidelines." As if almost foreseen for the year ahead (2020), in Section 3 the report states, in part, "The need for a recommendation for Respiratory Hygiene/Cough Etiquette grew out of observations during the SARS outbreaks where failure to implement simple source control measures with patients, visitors, and healthcare personnel with respiratory symptoms may have contributed to SARS coronavirus (SARS-CoV) transmission. The recommended practices have a strong evidence base." The ongoing research and lessons learned from the COVID-19 pandemic will undoubtedly reach far and wide and the delineation of best practices may be modified as a result (see Figure 1-11).

Surgical Conscience

The guiding principle under which a surgical technologist practices is called surgical conscience. A break in technique compromises surgical patient care and could threaten the patient's life. If a surgical technologist recognizes a break in technique, they must admit the break and take corrective actions. It requires vigilance in monitoring of the sterile field and addressing any breaks in technique by other team members if they occur. In the case of a break in technique that is not realized by the surgical technologist, when another team member points it out, surgical technologist should not question or argue the point and resolve the break with immediate corrective action. A surgical conscience should be imbedded in the members of the team and is the critical foundation of sterile technique. A person who does not have a strong

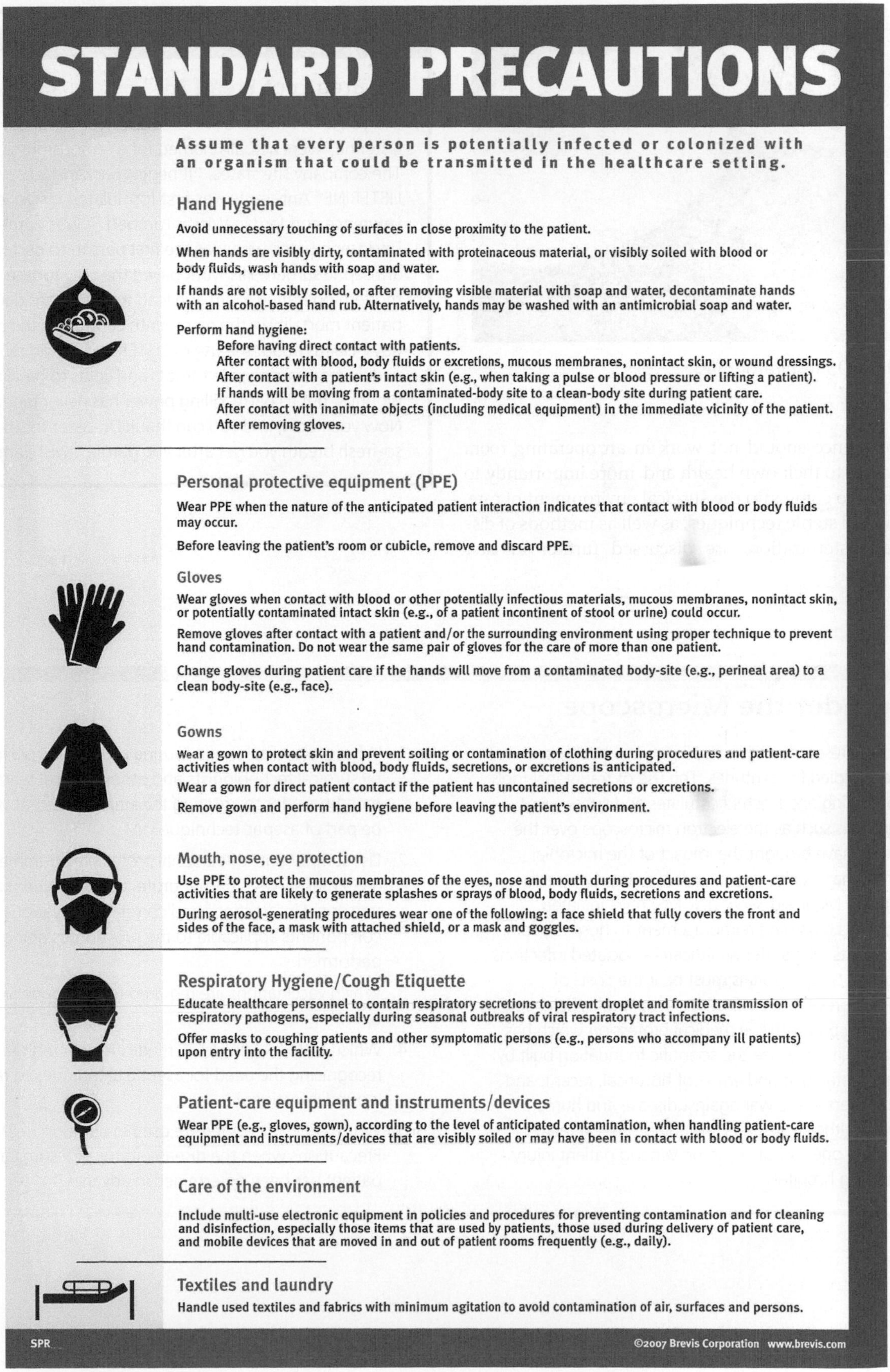

STANDARD PRECAUTIONS

Assume that every person is potentially infected or colonized with an organism that could be transmitted in the healthcare setting.

Hand Hygiene

Avoid unnecessary touching of surfaces in close proximity to the patient.

When hands are visibly dirty, contaminated with proteinaceous material, or visibly soiled with blood or body fluids, wash hands with soap and water.

If hands are not visibly soiled, or after removing visible material with soap and water, decontaminate hands with an alcohol-based hand rub. Alternatively, hands may be washed with an antimicrobial soap and water.

Perform hand hygiene:
Before having direct contact with patients.
After contact with blood, body fluids or excretions, mucous membranes, nonintact skin, or wound dressings.
After contact with a patient's intact skin (e.g., when taking a pulse or blood pressure or lifting a patient).
If hands will be moving from a contaminated-body site to a clean-body site during patient care.
After contact with inanimate objects (including medical equipment) in the immediate vicinity of the patient.
After removing gloves.

Personal protective equipment (PPE)

Wear PPE when the nature of the anticipated patient interaction indicates that contact with blood or body fluids may occur.

Before leaving the patient's room or cubicle, remove and discard PPE.

Gloves

Wear gloves when contact with blood or other potentially infectious materials, mucous membranes, nonintact skin, or potentially contaminated intact skin (e.g., of a patient incontinent of stool or urine) could occur.

Remove gloves after contact with a patient and/or the surrounding environment using proper technique to prevent hand contamination. Do not wear the same pair of gloves for the care of more than one patient.

Change gloves during patient care if the hands will move from a contaminated body-site (e.g., perineal area) to a clean body-site (e.g., face).

Gowns

Wear a gown to protect skin and prevent soiling or contamination of clothing during procedures and patient-care activities when contact with blood, body fluids, secretions, or excretions is anticipated.

Wear a gown for direct patient contact if the patient has uncontained secretions or excretions.

Remove gown and perform hand hygiene before leaving the patient's environment.

Mouth, nose, eye protection

Use PPE to protect the mucous membranes of the eyes, nose and mouth during procedures and patient-care activities that are likely to generate splashes or sprays of blood, body fluids, secretions and excretions.

During aerosol-generating procedures wear one of the following: a face shield that fully covers the front and sides of the face, a mask with attached shield, or a mask and goggles.

Respiratory Hygiene/Cough Etiquette

Educate healthcare personnel to contain respiratory secretions to prevent droplet and fomite transmission of respiratory pathogens, especially during seasonal outbreaks of viral respiratory tract infections.

Offer masks to coughing patients and other symptomatic persons (e.g., persons who accompany ill patients) upon entry into the facility.

Patient-care equipment and instruments/devices

Wear PPE (e.g., gloves, gown), according to the level of anticipated contamination, when handling patient-care equipment and instruments/devices that are visibly soiled or may have been in contact with blood or body fluids.

Care of the environment

Include multi-use electronic equipment in policies and procedures for preventing contamination and for cleaning and disinfection, especially those items that are used by patients, those used during delivery of patient care, and mobile devices that are moved in and out of patient rooms frequently (e.g., daily).

Textiles and laundry

Handle used textiles and fabrics with minimum agitation to avoid contamination of air, surfaces and persons.

SPR

©2007 Brevis Corporation www.brevis.com

Figure 1-10 Standard Precautions.

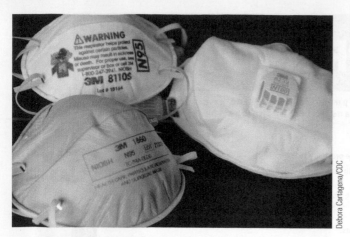

Debora Cartagena/CDC

Figure 1-11 N-95 respirator masks.

surgical conscience should not work in an operating room and poses a risk to their own health and, more importantly, to the patients who come into the surgical environment of care.

Aseptic and sterile techniques, as well as methods of disinfection and sterilization, are discussed further in later sections.

 ## Under the Microscope

Microbiology research and its application to healthcare have been studied for centuries. The use of traditional tools of Gram staining and Koch's Postulates and subsequent advanced tools such as the electron microscope over the past century have brought the impact of the microbial world on human health into clear focus. The Centers for Medicare and Medicaid Services (CMS) have initiated revised policies regarding reimbursement to hospitals for care of patients who suffer healthcare-associated infections (HAIs) such as SSIs. Hospitals must bear the costs of treatment of preventable infections acquired in the course of their interaction with the medical profession which has the responsibility to utilize the scientific foundation built by the experimental trials and errors of historical, recent, and current pioneers in the war against disease and human suffering. Healthcare workers, including surgical team members, are one critical key in preventing patient injury and protecting hospitals.

1. What are examples of a routine procedures performed by surgical technologists and other surgical team members prior to entering the sterile field that would be part of aseptic technique?

2. List components of personal protective equipment (PPE) that serve as barrier protection for patient and personnel interactions and correlate the various components applicable to the procedures being performed.

3. Which vaccinations are required for personnel in the operating room and why?

4. Which historical figures in medicine are credited with recognizing the need for aseptic techniques to reduce wound infections?

5. Which set of measures are used in addition to Standard Precautions when the disease status of a surgical patient has been determined in advance?

CHAPTER 2

The Science of Microbiology

Learning Objectives

After completing the study of this chapter, you will be able to:

1. Define key terms.
2. Distinguish between normal flora and pathogenic microbes.
3. Compare the various classification systems of living organisms.
4. Discuss characteristics of the prokaryotes.
5. Describe how viruses and prions become pathogenic.
6. Discuss the systems of nomenclature and taxonomy to classify microbes.
7. Apply critical thinking skills in relating chapter material to the surgical environment of care or broader global community.

Key Terms

Acellular

Archaea

Capsid

Capsomere

Cladistics

Creutzfeldt-Jakob disease (CJD)

Eukaryotes

Genome

Microbiology

Microbiome

Morphology

Normal flora

Osmotrophic

Pathological condition

Phenetics

Phylogeny

Prions

Prokaryotes

Protoplasm

Retrovirus

Surgical site infection (SSI)

Taxonomic hierarchy

Taxonomy

Transmissible spongiform encephalopathy (TSE)

Viruses

The Big Picture

Surgical technologists are keenly aware of the existence of microbial life in the surgical environment and even on our own skin. Transient microbes also known as microflora are the temporary passengers that we each acquire as we touch surfaces or that deposit on our skin or hair from the environment around us. Our resident or indigenous microbes are normal microflora that live deep in our skin layers. The same holds true for the patient's skin. Invasive procedures require that the skin is cleansed with antimicrobial soap prior to the incision.

During your examination of the topics in this chapter, consider the following:

1. How do we, as surgical technologists, deal with our own resident microbes before going into the operating room to prepare for surgery?

2. Why do we go to such lengths if microbes are everywhere?

3. Why is it important to determine the characteristics and classifications of microbes?

4. What are aseptic and sterile techniques?

Clinical Significance Topic

There is a saying, "In the eyes of the law, if it isn't documented, it didn't happen." The idea may be stated in other words, but the lesson is the same: scientific research and healthcare require documentation of every procedure, outcome results, steps taken, and identity of all persons involved in clinical studies or in surgical procedures. Science, like surgery, relies on critical procedural steps, accurate documentation, clear communication, professional collaboration, technical skill, and personal integrity. Standards of care are foundational principles based on those criteria. Patients rely on best practices in scientific research and in the surgical arena.

What Is Microbiology?

Encyclopaedia Britannica defines **microbiology** as, "The study of microorganisms, or microbes, a diverse group of minute, simple life forms that include bacteria, archaea, algae, fungi, protozoa, and viruses. The field is concerned with the structure, function, and classification of such organisms and with ways of both exploiting and controlling their activities." In the surgical environment of care, controlling the microbial populations encountered is of paramount importance in prevention of **surgical site infections (SSIs)**.

Overview of Microbes

Microbes, often referred to as microorganisms, are extremely small living beings or bits of material that actually may not be alive at all in the traditional sense. As their names imply, they are invisible to the naked eye and were only accepted by scientists after Van Leeuwenhoek created the microscope, began observing these tiny populations, and then recorded and published his findings. His single-lens microscope was sufficient to view some of the larger microbes he found in rainwater, saliva, and sperm. Long after that initial critical invention, much stronger magnification systems such as the electron microscope have been developed that allow scientists to explore the even more elusive world of viruses and other microbial life that would otherwise remain unseen. This chapter outlines the various forms and classifications of microbes as well as the scientific classification systems used to categorize and name them.

Ancestors of Life on Earth

Microbes are typically associated with disease, and they are the purveyors of many terrible **pathological conditions**. The reality however is that no living organism on the planet would exist or continue to survive without the smallest and most populous life forms—microbes. They can be found everywhere on Earth, including inhospitable environments such as deep inside ancient glaciers and geothermal hot springs.

Most of the millions of types of microbes on the planet pose no threat to our species. Humans and animals depend on the **normal flora** or bacterial populations of the gastrointestinal tract and skin to fend off invading or competitive pathogenic microbes. Normal flora allows our bodies to synthesize nutrients from our food while it travels through the various regions of the gastrointestinal tract. Unfortunately, even these beneficial inhabitants can cause problems if they escape their normal environment, or **microbiome**, and become invaders themselves.

Scientists have been able to identify evidence of microbial life dating back to more than 3 billion years by some estimates, making them most likely the first living things on the planet. Microbes are able to adapt to their environment to ensure survival and certain species can even live without oxygen. Viruses and prions are examples of microbes that are not considered living organisms, but they are able to invade healthy cells and tissues and spread through the host's normal cellular division and growth.

Scientific Classifications of Microbes

Since ancient times, humans have devised ways in which to classify the things around them. In the fourth century BC (BCE), the Greek philosopher Aristotle wrote about a classification system of living beings based on observations of the similarities and differences between species. His system had two components referred to as kingdoms: plantae (plants) and animalia (animals). It was many centuries later before anyone modified this long-accepted system.

Ernst Haeckel, a German biologist, added a third class in 1894 as the scientific community explored microorganisms. His addition to the kingdoms of plantae and animalia was the kingdom Protista. This group included single-cell **eukaryotes** and bacteria (**prokaryotes**).

In 1956, American biologist Herbert Copeland split the kingdom Protista that Haeckel had described into two distinct parts, thereby adding a fourth kingdom: bacteria. He observed that there were enough substantial differences between single-cell eukaryotes and bacteria that it merited creating a new separate kingdom.

Robert Whittaker, an American plant ecologist, was the next to revise the kingdom classification system. He first proposed his Five Kingdom classification in 1959, which he later refined in 1969. The Five Kingdom classification system was used widely in scientific circles and may still be found in current literature. Whittaker's classifications were:

- Plantae (plants)
- Animalia (animals)
- Protista (single-cell eukaryotes)
- Monera (single-cell prokaryotes)
- Fungi (single-cell or multi-cell **osmotrophic** eukaryotes)

In 1977, Carl Woese, an American biophysicist and evolutionary microbiologist at the University of Illinois, along with his colleagues announced the discovery of a category of microbes, distinctly different genetically from eukaryotes and prokaryotes. They called this new category **archaea**. Dr. Woese spent years studying the genetic sequences of microbial ribosomes and ribosomal DNA (protein building structures in cells). He was able to determine through this research that these archaea found in some of the harshest environments including glaciers and hot springs, shared a single genetic ancestor with the prokaryotes and eukaryotes, but that they had each evolved to be very different from one another. He initially proposed a Six Kingdom classification system in 1977, which modified Whittaker's system. He changed Monera to Eubacteria and added Archaebacteria, which was defined as including prokaryotes that were genetically different from other prokaryotes and actually more closely resembled eukaryotes.

Three Domains System of Classification

Recognizing the potential for confusion from so many versions of classification systems, Dr. Woese proposed an entirely new system in 1990—the Three Domains system. He simplified the groups and defined them as:

- Bacteria (single-cell prokaryotes)
- Archaea (prokaryotes that differ from bacteria in their genetic transcription and translation and are more similar to eukaryotes)
- Eukarya (multi-cell plants and animals; single-cell eukaryotes; single-cell and multi-cell osmotrophic eukaryotes)

The first four classification systems were devised from **phenetics**, the scientific observations of the similarities between organisms. Dr. Woese's research dealt with **cladistics** and **phylogeny**, studies that map out the evolution of a genetically related group of organisms, creating a type of genetic microbial family tree (see Figure 2-1).

In a 1996 New York Times interview, Dr. Woese said, "It's clear to me that if you wiped all multi-cellular life-forms off the face of the earth, microbial life might shift a tiny bit. If microbial life were to disappear, that would be it—instant death for the planet." He also stated that microbes accounted for more of the living **protoplasm** on Earth than every plant, animal, and human being combined.

Two Empires and Three Domains

Researchers have continued to strive for explanations to complex questions regarding the connections between all life forms on Earth. Comparative genomics called into question the accepted theory of an ancestral "tree of life" encompassing all living cells. Scientists studying nucleotide sequences for the genomes of the three domains of life, bacteria, archaea, and eukarya, theorized in 2010 that a better representation would be that of two major groups or empires, one for cellular organisms (including the three domains) and one for viruses (including plasmids, transposons, and other particles of genetic material). These researchers proposed replacing graphic models of family trees with network connections for the prokaryotes and viruses that contained complex genetic crosslinks or horizontal gene transfer. The genome researchers discovered evolutionary changes that combined traits of both bacteria and archaea and may explain the emergence of antibiotic-resistant strains of bacteria. Ultimately, genomic researchers have come to the conclusion that the empire of

Bacteria	Archaea	Eukarya
• Cyanobacteria • Flavobacteria • Gram-Positive Bacteria • Green Non-sulfur Bacteria • Green Sulfur Bacteria • Purple Bacteria • Spirochetes • Thermatogales	• Crenarchaeota • Euryarchaeota • Halophiles • Methanobacteriales • Methanococcales • Thermophiles	• Alveolates • Animals • Ciliates • Diplomonads • Entamoebae • Flagellates • Fungi • Microsporidia • Plants • Protists • Rhodophytes • Slime molds • Trichomonads

Figure 2-1 Three Domains classification of organisms.

viruses, tiny though they may be individually, far surpasses the empire of cellular life in size and diversity.

Eukaryotes

Humans, mammals, plants, birds, and insects are living organisms composed of eukaryotic cells. Each eukaryote's cells have membrane-bound organelles and a nucleus that contains deoxyribonucleic acid (DNA). Single-cell eukaryotes include protozoa, algae, and fungi. Cell structures of eukaryotic microbes are discussed further in Chapter 5.

Prokaryotes

All bacterial cells are prokaryotes. These microbes contain genetic material but they do not have a nucleus as part of their cell structure. A specific type of prokaryote is cyanobacteria. Once called blue-green algae, cyanobacteria are aquatic and photosynthetic, meaning they live in water and produce their own food. Fossils of them have been found that date back more than 3.5 billion years. The oxygen produced by photosynthesis of cyanobacteria changed the Earth's atmosphere early in the planet's history and created the more hospitable environment that allowed for life to form. Prokaryotic cell structure is discussed further in Chapter 4.

Archaea

Archaea are the newest forms of prokaryotes to be studied, but they may actually pre-date any other forms in the historical timeline of our planetary evolution. These single-cell organisms share similar cellular structure with bacteria; however, they have distinct genetic differences. Archaea show an affinity for unusually extreme environments, including glaciers, geothermal springs, and salt marshes.

Non-Living Pathogens

In addition to the eukaryotes, prokaryotes, and archaea, there are types of pathogens that do not fit the description of living microorganisms but are covered under the general heading of microbes. These special exceptions include viruses and prions.

Viruses

Viruses are extremely small bundles of genetic material, either DNA or ribonucleic acid (RNA), only visible with the use of an electron microscope. They can be 10,000 times smaller than some bacteria. They are **acellular** and consist of nucleic acid wrapped in a coating called a **capsid** made of proteins called **capsomeres**. Some viruses will also have an additional wrapping called an envelope. **Retroviruses** utilize and spread only RNA genetic material and are responsible for the disease human immunodeficiency virus (HIV). Viruses are incapable of performing reproductive functions on their own and are sometimes referred to as obligate intracellular parasites. Without a host cell that can reproduce, viruses are metabolically inert and incapable of multiplying. The empire of viruses is discussed in depth in Chapter 8.

Prion Diseases

Transmissible spongiform encephalopathies (TSEs) are found in both animals and humans and comprise a group of diseases caused by infectious agents found mainly in structures of the central nervous system, most often the brain. These agents are called **prions** (from proteinaceous infectious particles) and have no nucleic acids and no cellular structure. The mechanism of infection is thought to be an abnormal folding of these normal prion proteins that destroy brain tissue and create holes, resulting in the appearance of a sponge (spongiform). Animal TSE infections are called bovine spongiform encephalopathy (mad cow disease), ovine spongiform encephalopathy (scrapie), and chronic wasting disease (CWD) in North American hooved animals such as deer, elk, and moose.

The prion infections in humans are **Creutzfeldt-Jakob disease (CJD)** and variant Creutzfeldt-Jakob disease (vCJD), Gerstmann-Straussler-Scheinker syndrome, fatal familial insomnia, and Kuru.

These diseases are discussed further in Chapter 8.

Taxonomy

The system of classifying every living organism is called **taxonomy**. The objectives of taxonomy are to:

1. Establish relationships between like organisms
2. Differentiate between two groups of organisms
3. Classify a previously unknown organism

Taxonomy is especially important in the identification of a microbe that is capable of, or actively causing a disease. The bacterium is isolated from a patient and its characteristics compared to the characteristics of microbes already classified. After the pathogen has been identified, the course of treatment can be prescribed.

The last important purpose of the science of taxonomy is that it establishes a universal language of communication used by scientists and microbiologists around the world. Taxonomy establishes a system of categories called taxa (singular, taxon) that reveal the degree of relationship among microbes; in other words, the taxa show the phylogenetic (common ancestor) relationships. It is from this foundation that scientists can communicate on a mutual, standardized basis concerning the complex world of microbes.

Nomenclature

In the eighteenth century, Carolus Linnaeus developed a scientific nomenclature that standardized the naming and classification of organisms. He used Latin names because the scholars of his time wrote in Latin.

Binomial Nomenclature

The system is referred to as binomial nomenclature. Every living organism has two names: genus name and species name. Both names are underlined or italicized when written. The genus name is always capitalized and the species name is in lowercase. Additionally, the genus name is always a noun and, typically, the species name is an adjective. In written text, the first time the name is used, it must be fully spelled out. Subsequent uses of the genus name can be abbreviated by using the first capitalized letter of the name. The species name, however, is never abbreviated. Consider the following examples:

1. *Homo sapiens* (human species); *Homo* is the genus and means "man"; *sapiens* is the species and means "wise." It is abbreviated as *H. sapiens*.
2. *Klebsiella pneumoniae* (one type of bacteria that causes pneumonia); *Klebsiella* is the genus and is derived from the name of scientist Edwin Klebs, who discovered the microbe; *pneumoniae* is the species and specifically describes the disease it causes. It is abbreviated as *K. pneumoniae*.

3. Bacteria are sometimes referred to using a shortened portion of the genus name with the species name or even just the shortened genus. Examples include *Staph aureus* and staph or strep.

The International Committee on Systematics of Prokaryotes establishes the rules for assigning a name to a new classified bacterium and to which taxa the bacterium is assigned. The rules are published in the *International Code of Nomenclature of Prokaryotes* (commonly referred to as the Bacteriological Code). The descriptions of bacteria and the evidence for their chosen classification are published in the *International Journal of Systematic and Evolutionary Microbiology*. After this has taken place, the bacterium can be placed in the most well-known and standardized reference, *Bergey's Manual of Systematic Bacteriology*, discussed later in this section.

Taxonomic Hierarchy

All living organisms are placed in a system of subdivisions that comprise what is called the **taxonomic hierarchy**. Beginning at the top of the classification is the species, closely related organisms that interbreed and are the basic grouping unit of living organisms. Next is the genus, which comprises species that are related by descent but differ from each other in particular ways. Related genera (plural of genus) comprise a family. A group of families comprise an order and a group of similar orders constitute the next group, called a class. Related classes comprise a division or phylum, and all divisions that are similar to each other constitute the last grouping, called a kingdom. Revised models of the taxonomic hierarchy include the three-domain system (archaea, bacteria, and eukarya) as well (see Figure 2-2).

In summary, the order of the divisions from largest group to smallest is as follows: kingdom, division (phylum), class, order, family, genus, and species.

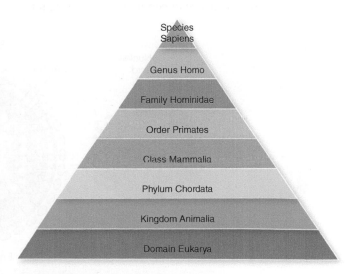

Figure 2-2 Taxonomic hierarchy of humans (including domain).

Standardized Classification of Prokaryotes

As previously mentioned, the taxonomic classification for bacteria is published in *Bergey's Manual of Systematic Bacteriology*. The first edition of the reference had four separate volumes with publication dates from 1984 to 1989. The current reference, the second edition, has five volumes focusing on the following areas:

- Volume 1 (2001)   The *Archaea* and the deeply branching and phototrophic *Bacteria*
- Volume 2 (2005)   The *Proteobacteria*
- Volume 3 (2009)   The *Firmicutes*
- Volume 4 (2011)   The *Bacteroidetes, Spirochaetes, Tenericutes (Mollicutes), Acidobacteria, Fibrobacteres, Fusobacteria, Dictyoglomi, Gemmatimonadetes, Lentisphaerae, Verrucomicrobia, Chlamydiae,* and *Planctomycetes*
- Volume 5 (2012)   The *Actinobacteria*

Bergey's Manual of Systematic Bacteriology was preceded by the 1936 publication of *Bergey's Manual of Determinative Bacteriology*. Realizing the value of having a resource for the scientists working in the field of microbiology, the Bergey's Manual Trust was established in 1936 as a nonprofit group charged with continually reviewing and updating research materials that provide an established classification system for the identification of bacteria (prokaryotes). Information is obtained from the analyses of DNA and RNA, chemical analyses, and other laboratory tests to create the phylogenetic models. Microbiologists from around the world contribute to the research and preparation of new reference volumes.

The challenge to the publishers of the manual is keeping pace with the explosion of information submitted by researchers. By the time a volume is distributed in print, it may be seriously deficient in the most current findings of the community. In the digital age of communications, electronic versions may provide a way in which to update outdated material more expeditiously. *Bergey's Manual of Systematics of Archaea and Bacteria* (BMSAB) was made available online for the first time in 2015. The digital edition is described as an extensive reference for microbiology with over 1750 articles that provide descriptions of the taxonomy, physiology and biological properties of over 600 new species and 100 new genera of prokaryotic taxa per year and an authoritative collection of archaeal and bacterial diversity.

Viral Taxonomy

One of the most challenging areas of microbiology is that of identifying and classifying viruses. These nonliving cellular invaders are so tiny an electron microscope is necessary to visualize them. The methods of classifying viruses include **morphology**, nucleic acid type, mode of replication, the types of host organisms invaded, and type of disease they cause. Viruses invade living organisms, large and small. Three general classifications are based on the types of host cells they penetrate. Those that infect members of the animal kingdom are termed zoophaginae. If they infect plants, then they are considered phytophaginae. Viruses will even invade prokaryotes and are classified simply as phaginae (see Figure 2-3).

ICTV Viral Taxonomy

The International Committee on Taxonomy of Viruses (ICTV) is responsible for identifying and classifying viruses in the same way that the International Committee on Systematics of Prokaryotes classifies bacterial species. The committee comprises six subcommittees that are responsible for covering fungal viruses (including algae), plant viruses, invertebrate viruses, prokaryotic (including archaea) viruses, and vertebrate viruses. The sixth subcommittee manages ICTV data and websites.

The 2021 *ICTV 10th Report* lists nine groups of viruses or viral agents:

- Double strand DNA viruses (dsDNA)
- Single strand DNA viruses (ssDNA)

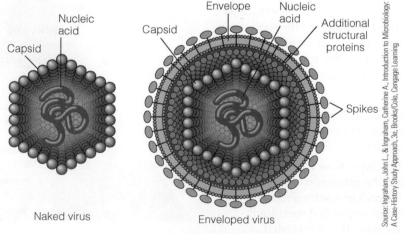

Naked virus

Enveloped virus

Source: Ingraham, John L., & Ingraham, Catherine A., Introduction to Microbiology: A Case-History Study Approach, 3e, Brooks/Cole, Cengage Learning

Figure 2-3 Examples of viruses.

- Single strand DNA/Double strand DNA viruses (ssDNA/dsDNA)
- Positive sense RNA viruses
- Negative sense RNA viruses
- Double strand RNA viruses (dsRNA)
- Reverse transcribing DNA and RNA viruses
- Subviral agents
- Unclassified viruses

The taxonomic hierarchy for viruses does not include domain or kingdom classifications because they are not considered living organisms, but they do have genetic codes and characteristics that allow for grouping into the taxa: order, family (or sub-family), genus, and species. The species name may be more than one word but must clearly describe the virus. For example, the HIV is a common name with sub-species given a number, such as HIV-1. The common names are not underlined or italicized. If the virus has been given a genus, then it is italicized (as in *Papillomavirus*, human wart virus, which is in the family *Papovaviridae*).

The genus name will end in the suffix *-virus*. The sub-family taxon is used when naming a complex group of genera and written with the suffix *-virinae*. The suffix used for the family taxon is *-viridae*. Order names will end in *-virales* (see Figure 2-4).

The ICTV is governed by the Virology Division of the International Union of Microbiological Societies (IUMS). In an explanation of its process of determining how to assign viral species into specific taxa on the ICTV website, they state, "As defined therein, 'a virus species is a polythetic class of viruses that constitute a replicating lineage and occupy a particular ecological niche.' A 'polythetic class' is one whose members have several properties in common, although they do not necessarily all share a single common defining property."

Baltimore Classification System

American virologist and Nobel Laureate, David Baltimore, devised a system of classifying viruses in seven groups on the basis of the virus' **genome** and messenger RNA (mRNA). The viruses will carry either single or double strands of genetic strands of DNA or RNA. In addition, the Baltimore classification takes into consideration whether there is a positive (+) or negative (−) sense component. This designation has to do with the ability of the viral mRNA to interact with the host cell's cytoplasm and through a process of translation, creating the proteins and enzymes necessary for replication of its genome. The chapters listed in the previously discussed *ICTV 10th Report* follow this classification system.

The seven groups of the Baltimore classification of viruses are:

- Group I: Double-stranded DNA (dsDNA)
- Group II: Single-stranded DNA (ssDNA)
- Group III: Double-stranded RNA (dsRNA)
- Group IV: Positive-sense single-stranded RNA [(+)ssRNA]
- Group V: Negative-sense single-stranded RNA [(−)ssRNA]
- Group VI: Reverse-transcribing diploid single-stranded RNA (ssRNA-RT)
- Group VII: Reverse-transcribing circular double-stranded DNA (dsDNA-RT)

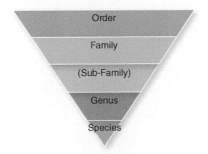

Figure 2-4 Viral taxonomic hierarchy.

Under the Microscope

Dev, a student taking the microbiology course pre-requisite to enter the surgical technology program, was intrigued by a surgery-related article. As neurosurgery was Dev's favorite surgical specialty, he chose this topic for his research paper to discuss the connection between microbiology and his future profession. The case in the article involved a craniotomy for biopsy in which the neurosurgeon advised the staff that the patient was being assessed for symptoms of ataxia (loss of muscle coordination) and relatively sudden onset of dementia. Tumors and any other intracranial lesions had been ruled out by radiographic studies. The patient had lived in England approximately 10 years ago when there had been an outbreak of "mad cow" disease.

1. What condition or disease process might the neurosurgeon suspect based on the patient's history as given?

2. Using binomial nomenclature and taxonomy taught in the microbiology course, how would Dev describe the other groups of organisms affected by this particular type of pathogen and general category of disease?

3. What type of infective agent is the cause for this form of transmissible spongiform encephalopathy?

4. Which scientific microbial classification system (if any) would contain this type of pathogen?

5. How would Dev describe the characteristics of the infective agents in this case as compared to the other classes of microbes studied in his course?

The Microbiology Laboratory

Learning Objectives

After completing the study of this chapter, you will be able to:

1. Define key terms.
2. Describe the parts of a compound light microscope as discussed in the chapter.
3. Describe other types of microscopes used in a hospital or research microbiology laboratory.
4. Describe various forms of culture media as outlined in the chapter.
5. Describe the procedure for performing a Gram stain analysis.
6. Discuss the possible findings of a Gram stain test and what they indicate.
7. Discuss the variety of laboratory studies available for classification of microorganisms.
8. Apply critical thinking skills in relating chapter material to the surgical environment of care or broader global community.

Key Terms

Acid-fast stain
Agar
Anaerobic chamber
Antibodies
Antisera
Blood agar
Chocolate agar
Condenser
Culture

Culture media
Differential media
Enriched media
Enzyme
Enzyme-linked immunosorbent assays (ELISAs)
Fastidious
Flagella staining

Hybridization
Immunofluorescence
MacConkey agar
Metric system
Mordant
Ocular lenses
Oil immersion objective
Phage typing
Plaques

Reducing media
Refractive index
Resolution
Selective media
Simple stain
Slants
Spores
Virulence

The Big Picture

Surgical technologists rarely have the opportunity to visit and explore the microbiology laboratory in the hospital. Maybe it would be interesting to arrange a "shadowing" experience for lab and surgical personnel to follow one another for a day to see what each position does. Intraoperatively, the surgeon may request cultures to be taken of tissue or fluid for testing.

During your examination of the topics in this chapter, consider the following:

1. Why are two culture tubes typically used and sent for analysis?

2. Which types of microbes might be found in different tissues/areas of the body and why?

3. How might an individual's performance of laboratory studies impact the accuracy of results?

4. Why does final determination of antibiotic sensitivity of bacteria take so long?

Clinical Significance Topic

Surgical technologists must know how to deal with specimens collected during surgery. However, to assure accurate analysis, everyone involved with the care and handling of surgical specimens must be aware of the importance and proper preparation procedures of the various types of samples sent for study. During your surgical technology education and later in your career, you will deal with frozen sections, bacterial cultures, tissue specimen staining and marking, appropriate containment of tissue, amputated limbs, foreign bodies, cancerous tumors, and bizarre anomalies. You will be making sure these specimens are properly identified, gently and appropriately handled, and prepared with (or without) fixatives. All surgical specimens must be transported to the lab in a safe and timely manner. It is a team effort that makes the difference between whether a patient is receiving or not receiving a correct diagnosis.

Microbiology Lab Personnel

The US Department of Labor Bureau of Statistics states that "microbiologists study microorganisms such as bacteria, viruses, algae, fungi, and some types of parasites. They try to understand how these organisms live, grow, and interact with their environments." The physicians and scientists are only one component of the microbiology laboratory. Just as in the operating room, there are technologists and technicians who do a large part of the day-to-day work. They function under the broad direction of research scientists, pathologists, or laboratory directors, although much of the testing and processing for which they are responsible is done largely unsupervised. This requires that these personnel be well-educated and possess the same type of moral and ethical principles that should guide all allied health professionals. Accurate diagnostic test results and reliable experimental research studies require both microbiologists and technicians to be exacting, thorough, accurate, organized, and dedicated to the scientific method (see Figure 3-1).

This chapter explores various microscopes, staining techniques, culture media, and other specialized testing methods to determine the identity and classification of microorganisms.

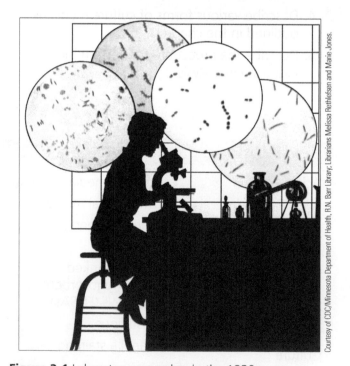

Courtesy of CDC/Minnesota Department of Health, R.N. Barr Library; Librarians Melissa Rethlefsen and Marie Jones.

Figure 3-1 Laboratory researcher in the 1930s.

Introduction to the Microscope

Microbes cannot be seen without the use of a microscope. The development of microbiology could not have gone beyond the advances of the nineteenth century if it were not for the invention of sophisticated microscopes that allow the smallest of organisms to be seen. This section first discusses the metric system and its use in measuring microbes.

Units of Measure

The standard unit of length in the **metric system** is the meter (m). One of the advantages of the metric system is that it is based on units of 10. The breakdown is as follows: 1 m = 10 decimeters (dm) = 100 centimeters (cm) = 1,000 millimeters (mm) (see Table 3-1).

Microbes are measured in even smaller metric units of length such as micrometers, nanometers, angstroms, and picometers. The old term micron has been replaced with micrometer and the old term millimicron has been replaced with nanometer. A micrometer (μm) is equal to 0.000001 m or 1 mm = 1,000 μm. The prefix "micro" indicates that the unit following it should be divided by one million. A nanometer (nm) is equal to 0.000000001 m (1 m = 1 billion nm) or 1 mm = 1,000,000 nm. The prefix "nano" indicates that the unit after it should be divided by one billion. An angstrom (Å) is equal to 0.0000000001 m (1 m = 10 billion Å), and 0.1 nm = 1 Å or 1 nm = 10 Å. A picometer (pm) is equal to 0.01 Å (1 Å = 100 pm) and 1 nm =1000 pm. The angstrom (Å) is no longer considered an official unit of measure, but due to its prevalent use in scientific literature it should be familiar to the student of microbiology.

Table 3-1 Measuring Microorganisms

Unit of Measurement	Equal To
1 meter (m)	10 decimeters (dm)
10 decimeters (dm)	100 centimeters (cm)
100 centimeters (cm)	1,000 millimeters (mm)
1 micrometer (μm)	0.000001 meter (m)
1 nanometer (nm)	0.000000001 meter (m)
1 angstrom (Å)	0.0000000001 meter (m)

Examples of sizes of microbes include the following:

1. Bacteria can range in size from 3 μm to as small as 0.2 μm.
2. Erythrocytes (red blood cells) are approximately 7 μm in diameter.
3. Many viruses range in size from 10 to 300 nm.
4. Most protozoa measure 2–200 μm in length.

Types of Microscopes

Scientists utilize various types of microscopes to visualize the microbial world. Microscopes described in this section include compound, dark-field, phase-contrast, transmission electron, and scanning electron microscopes (see Table 3-2).

Table 3-2 Types of Microscopes

Microscope	Special Features
Compound light	• Two-lens system with light source • High-dry lens for viewing large microbes • Oil immersion objective for viewing bacterial characteristics
Dark-field	• Used when microbes are not visible with light microscope or cannot be stained (*Treponema pallidum*) • Motility is not easily visualized
Phase-contrast	• Allows detailed visualization of internal structures of microbes • Eliminates need to fix or stain microbes
Fluorescence	• Allows visualization of naturally fluorescent microbes or those stained with fluorochromes
Electron	• Used for visualization of viruses, internal structures of cells in detail, and other objects smaller than 0.2 μm
Transmission electron	• Can resolve objects as close in proximity as 2.5 nm • Can magnify objects 10,000× − 100,000×

Scanning electron	• Offers two advantages over TEM:
	  1. Specimen does not have to be thinly sliced.
	  2. Three-dimensional views are obtained.

Compound Light Microscope

The compound light or bright-field microscope is a multi-lens system combined with a light source (see Figure 3-2). The light passes through the specimen and lenses and then returns back up to the eyepiece. The condenser lens controls the light aimed at the specimen from its bottom. The objective lens is adjusted to be near the specimen from the top. The most proximal lenses to the viewer are called the **ocular lenses** and are located in the binocular eyepieces. The multi-lens compound system can magnify 40× to 2,500×. The magnification is indicated by the numeral preceded by ×, such as "1,000×," in which the × means "times."

The 40× lens is called the high-dry lens and is used to view algae, protozoa, and other large microbes. The 100× lens is the **oil immersion objective** used for viewing the unique characteristics of various bacteria. The oil immersion objective must be used with a drop of oil between the specimen and the objective lens. The immersion oil aids in reducing the scattering of light.

The light must be focused to obtain a clear view of the specimen. The **condenser**, located below the fixed stage, is used to focus light onto the specimen, adjust the amount of light emission, and shapes the light beam that is entering the objective. Usually, the higher the magnification used, more light is needed.

Magnification alone is ineffective unless the image seen produces structure and fine detail. The clarity of the image is dependent on the microscope's **resolution**, which is the ability of the lens to distinguish two objects at a particular distance apart. For example, if a microscope has a resolving power of 0.2 μm, the viewer will be able to distinguish two bacteria that are separated by a distance of 0.2 μm or more.

A principle that applies to the use of the compound light microscope is that the shorter the wavelength of light, the greater the resolution. A compound microscope is able to image a bacterium but not a virus. A bacterium is typically 0.5–5.0 μm (500–5,000 nm) and viruses are usually around 0.02 μm (20 nm) in size. The shortest or smallest wavelength of visible light is approximately 0.4 μm (400 nm); therefore the compound microscope is unable to create a clear resolution of the much smaller virus.

Another important principle of microscopy is the **refractive index**. A clear, detailed image of an object under the microscope requires that there be a relatively dramatic or substantial contrast between the specimen being examined and type of medium in which it is suspended. The refractive index of the specimen must be changed to achieve a clear contrast from that of the medium. The refractive index is a measure of the relative velocity at which light passes through a material. The refractive index of microbes is changed through the use of staining procedures, discussed in the next section. Light rays travel in a straight line through a single medium, but staining causes the light rays to pass through a specimen and its medium with different refractive indexes. This causes the light rays to change direction from a straight path to an angle or refractive path at the boundary of the specimen and medium. This refraction of the light increases the contrast between the two. As the light rays travel away from the specimen, they spread out to achieve resolution. The light rays continue to pass through the objective lens, and the image is magnified.

Dark-Field Microscope

The dark-field microscope is actually a bright-field or compound microscope fitted with a dark-field condenser. The dark-field microscope is used when (1) microbes are not visible with the use of the light microscope, (2) the microbes cannot be stained by standard methods, or (3) the staining process distorts the microbes.

The dark-field microscope uses a dark-field condenser that contains an opaque disc in place of the normal condenser. The opaque disc is either inserted below the condenser or is a permanent component of the condenser. The disc blocks light that would enter the objective directly and only permits peripheral rays of light to enter (see Figure 3-3).

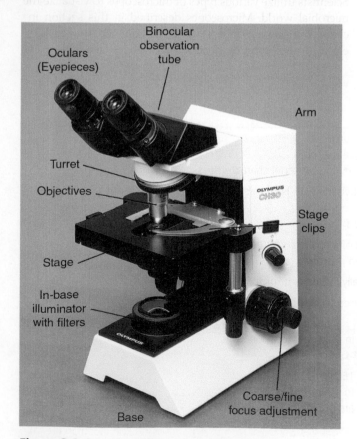

Figure 3-2 Compound light microscope.

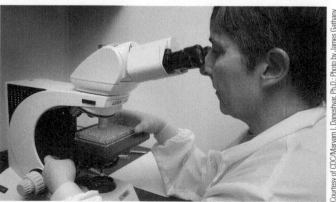

Figure 3-3 CDC researcher reading a microscope agglutination test (MAT) by using dark-field microscopy.

Courtesy of CDC/Maryam I. Daneshvar, Ph.D.; Photo by James Gathany

Phase-Contrast Microscope

The phase-contrast microscope is particularly useful because it allows detailed visualization of the internal structures in living microbes. Flagella, granular microbes, and other types of bacteria are examples of organisms that are more effectively examined with the phase-contrast microscope. The degree of detail also eliminates the need to fix or stain the microbes because these are procedures that may alter or kill the microbe.

The microscope is equipped with a special condenser that contains a ring-shaped diaphragm. The light passes through the diaphragm and focuses on the specimen, forming a halo of light around it. The light is also simultaneously focused on the second ring-shaped diffraction plate in the objective lens. The undiffracted and diffracted light rays are then brought into phase or synchronization with each other to produce the image of the specimen.

The principle of phase-contrast microscopes is based on the refractive index. The velocity of light rays is altered by the various internal structures of the microbe as they pass through the specimen. The light rays are bent, or diffracted, and travel in various pathways. This is referred to as being "out of phase," and the differences in phases are seen through the microscope as varying degrees of brightness. The internal structures therefore appear as degrees of brightness against a dark background, allowing an observer to identify the details of the structures.

Fluorescence Microscope

Some microbes are fluorescent, meaning that they absorb ultraviolet light. After absorbing the energy, they emit a longer wavelength of light that is seen with the use of special filters. Some microbes have a natural property of fluorescence and others can be stained with one of a group of dyes called fluorochromes. Microbes stained with a fluorochrome appear as a bright object against a dark field when an ultraviolet light source is used (see Figure 3-4).

One of the primary uses of fluorescence microscopy is a diagnostic technique called **immunofluorescence**. This technique is useful in detecting bacteria and other pathogens within cells and tissues. It is frequently used in diagnosing the pathogens that cause rabies and syphilis. The following steps are examples of how the immunofluorescence technique is performed:

1. An animal is injected with an antigen, such as a specific type of bacteria.
2. The animal's immune system begins producing specific antibodies against that antigen.
3. The antibodies are removed in a laboratory setting from the serum of the animal.
4. A fluorochrome dye is added and chemically combines with the antibodies.
5. The fluorescent antibodies are then placed on a microscope slide that contains unknown bacteria.
6. If the unknown bacteria are of the same type as those originally injected into the animal, the fluorescent antibodies will bind to the antigens on the surface of the bacteria, causing it to fluoresce.

Fluorochromes have an attraction to specific microbes. Two common dyes are fluorescein and rhodamine. Fluorescein produces a yellow-green fluorescence and rhodamine produces a reddish orange color. The fluorochrome Auramine O is highly absorbed by *Mycobacterium tuberculosis*, causing it to glow yellow when exposed to ultraviolet light. Consequently, the bacteria are visualized as a bright yellow organism against a dark background. *Bacillus anthracis* appears apple green against a dark background when the fluorochrome fluorescein isothiocyanate is absorbed by the bacterium's cell wall.

Electron Microscope

The invention of the electron microscope created the ability to visualize viruses, the internal structures of cells, and other objects smaller than 0.2 μm. The electron microscope uses a beam of electrons instead of light; therefore, the resolving power of the electron microscope is much higher than it is for other types of microscopes (see Figure 3-5). The improved resolution is due to the much shorter wavelength of the electrons.

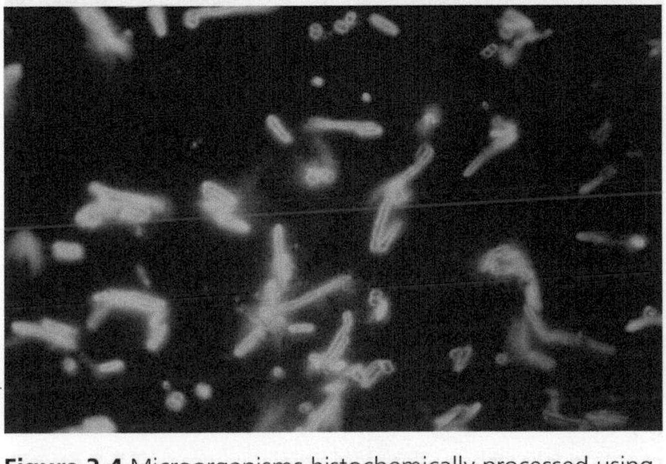

Figure 3-4 Microorganisms histochemically processed using the fluorescent antibody (FA) staining method. Visible are both rod-shaped bacilli and small round cocci bacteria.

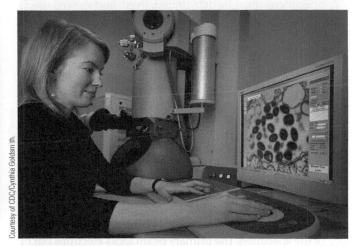

Figure 3-5 CDC intern using a transmission electron (TEM) microscope.

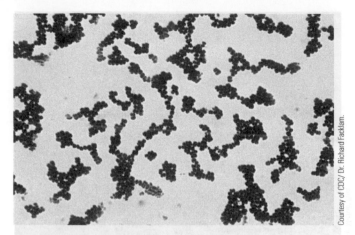

Courtesy of CDC/ Dr. Richard Facklam.

Figure 3-10 Magnified 320×, this photomicrograph revealed the presence of many Gram-positive *Micrococcus mucilaginosis* bacteria. Note that micrographically, these bacteria closely resemble staphylococcal organisms.

3. After 30 seconds the iodine is gently rinsed off with water. Gram-positive and Gram-negative bacteria both appear dark purple.

4. The slide is then coated with the decolorizing agent called ethanol, an organic compound also known as ethyl alcohol. The ethanol removes the purple stain from some bacteria and not from others.

5. The ethanol is rinsed off.

6. The slide is next stained with a basic red dye called safranin. The safranin is termed as a counterstain because it has color contrasting to the primary stain. The stain is left on the slide for 1 minute.

7. The slide is finally rinsed with water, blotted dry, and examined under immersion oil.

Gram-positive bacteria remain purple (or dark blue) from uptake of the crystal violet. The purple color is removed by the ethyl alcohol in Gram-negative bacteria, and they appear red or pink from the safranin counterstain (see Figure 3-11). As previously mentioned, some types of

bacteria do not consistently stain purple or red and are referred to as Gram-variable bacteria. Examples of Gram-variable bacteria include *Mycobacterium tuberculosis*, *Clostridium tetani*, and *Yersinia pestis*.

Acid-Fast Stain

The **acid-fast stain** binds only to bacteria that have a waxy chemical material in their cell wall. The stain is used to identify all the bacteria that are classified in the genus *Mycobacterium* (see Figure 3-12).

The following steps state the procedure for applying the stain:

1. The bright red dye carbolfuchsin is applied to a fixed smear. The microscope slide is heated for several minutes. The heat aids the stain in penetrating the cell wall.

2. The slide is allowed to cool and is rinsed with water.

3. A mixture of acid and alcohol, which acts as a decolorizer, is used to treat the slide. Bacteria (such as the mycobacteria) that retain the red color are said to be acid-fast. The other bacteria that do not retain the stain and appear colorless are non-acid-fast.

4. Methylene blue can be used as a counterstain to stain the non-acid-fast bacteria.

The acid-fast mycobacteria are visualized as red organisms against a blue background in a sputum specimen obtained from a patient positive for tuberculosis.

Special Stains

Special stains are used to stain specific structures of microbes, such as spores or flagella, and aid in identifying the presence of a capsule. The three most common special stains are negative staining for capsules, spore staining, and flagella staining.

Negative Staining for Capsules

A capsule is a gelatinous-like covering that many microorganisms contain. The capsule often protects pathogenic

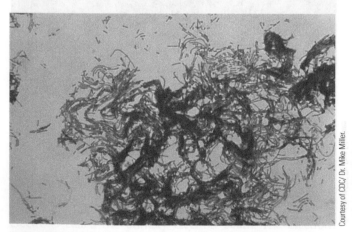

Courtesy of CDC/ Dr. Mike Miller.

Figure 3-11 Under magnification of 1,200×, this Gram-stained photomicrograph revealed the presence of numerous Gram-negative *Haemophilus ducreyi* bacteria.

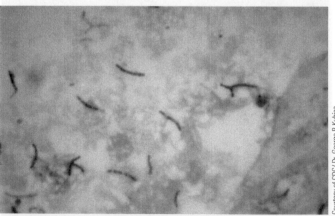

Courtesy of CDC/ Dr. George P. Kubica.

Figure 3-12 The photomicrograph reveals *Mycobacterium tuberculosis* bacteria using acid-fast Ziehl-Neelsen stain. Magnified 1,000×. The acid-fast stain is retained by *M. tuberculosis*.

microbes from the process known as phagocytosis performed by the protective phagocytes in the host's body. **Virulence**, the degree to which a pathogen can cause disease, can be determined by confirming if a microbe has a capsule.

Capsule staining is difficult because the material that forms the capsule is soluble in water, and rinsing can cause the capsule to be removed. The procedure involves mixing the bacteria in a solution of India ink, a colloidal suspension that provides a dark background for viewing the bacteria. The bacteria can then be stained with a simple stain such as safranin. Because of its chemical composition, the capsule does not absorb the simple stain and a halo appears around the stained bacterial cell.

The India ink is used to demonstrate a negative-staining technique. The stain does not penetrate the capsule, causing the colorless bacteria to appear against a colored background. This provides a sharp contrast between the capsule and the surrounding dark medium.

Spore Staining

A select group of bacteria can form a structure called a **spore**. The spore is a dormant structure found within the cell. The cell forms the spore as a way of self-preservation when environmental conditions that allow the cell to live do not exist. The spore is highly resistant to difficult environmental conditions, such as heat, and is very difficult to destroy. When the environmental conditions improve and can support the cell, the spore is released. More discussion on spores is found in later sections.

Spores cannot be stained by methods previously presented because the stains cannot penetrate the wall of the spore (see Figure 3-13).

The following is the procedure used to stain a spore:

1. The primary stain is malachite green. It is applied to a heat-fixed smear and heated approximately 5 minutes until the stain is steaming. The heat aids the stain in penetrating the spore wall.

2. The slide is washed for 30 seconds to remove the malachite green from all the portions of the cell except for the spore.

3. The counterstain safranin is applied to stain the portions of the cell other than the spore.

4. The spore appears green within a red cell.

Flagella Staining

The flagella of bacteria, which aid in motility of the cell, cannot be seen through a compound light microscope without staining. **Flagella staining** is a tedious staining procedure that uses a mordant and the stain carbolfuchsin to thicken the flagella. The flagellum can be seen through the light microscope as soon as its diameter is large enough (see Figure 3-14).

Culture Media

Pure cultures of bacterial species are grown in the laboratory with the use of **culture media**. The culture media (medium is singular) provide a method in which the appropriate nutrients can be delivered to the bacteria in a controlled environment. The microbiologist can easily control the amount of oxygen, heat, and pH available to the bacteria. Optimal conditions for growth are created for the bacteria when combined with the culture medium.

Some types of bacteria can proliferate on almost any type of culture medium, whereas others require special media. The microbial colonies that grow and multiply in or on a culture medium are referred to as the **culture**.

The culture medium must meet the following criteria to be useful:

1. It must contain nutrients, and often species-specific nutrients, to encourage the growth of the microbe that is being cultured.

2. It must contain enough moisture and the proper level of pH.

3. It must be able to be either exposed to or not exposed to oxygen, depending on the requirements of the microbe.

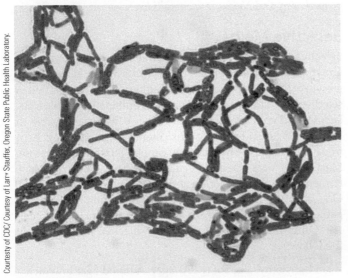

Courtesy of CDC/ Courtesy of Larry Stauffer, Oregon State Public Health Laboratory.

Figure 3-13 *Bacillus* sp., Malachite Green spore stain, at a 1,000× magnification.

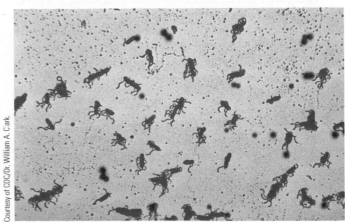

Courtesy of CDC/Dr. William A. Clark.

Figure 3-14 *Bacillus alvei*, Leifson flagella stain.

4. It must be sterile, meaning no other microbes are growing on the medium prior to the addition of the microbes that are being grown.

5. It must be able to withstand the temperature conditions created during incubation.

Growth media can be used in broth (liquid) form, which is available in tubes, or in a solidified form, created by the addition of **agar** that is poured into Petri dishes. The bacteria can then be grown on the solid surface of the agar medium. Agar is a complex polysaccharide and has a long history of use as a thickener in foods such as jellies, soups, and ice cream.

Robert Koch and his associate Walter Hesse are credited with the discovery of agar. The actual credit, however, belongs to Hesse's wife, who knew that her husband and Koch were struggling to find an improved method of growing pathogens without the use of gelatin. She told Walter about a substance her grandmother used in the tropics to make jams and jellies remain solid in the hot, humid tropical temperature. The substance is agar, obtained from red marine algae growing along the coasts of southern California, China, Japan, and Malaysia.

Agar is a solidifying agent that is added to the medium. It has valuable properties that make it irreplaceable in the laboratory and no other satisfactory substitute has ever been found. Agar remains solid because few microbes have the ability to break it down. Agar melts at the boiling point of water and then solidifies at approximately 40°C. In the laboratory, agar is maintained at approximately 50°C and it does not injure the bacteria. The solidified agar can be incubated up to 100°C before it liquefies. This is especially useful when thermophilic, or heat-preferring bacteria are to be grown.

Agar media are contained not only in Petri dishes but also in test tubes. The test tubes are called **slants** because the agar is allowed to solidify with the tube positioned at an angle. This slanted agar surface provides the bacteria with a larger surface area for growth. Agar solidified in a tube in a straight, vertical fashion is referred to as a "deep" (see Figure 3-15).

There are three categories of media: enriched, selective, and differential. There are different types of agar within each category that serve particular uses in the laboratory. The various categories of media are not mutually exclusive. Some of the media fall into two or more categories according to their action.

Enriched Media

Enriched media can be either a solid or a broth that contains a supply of nutrients that promote the growth of fastidious organisms. Bacteria that are recognized as having complex nutritional requirements are referred to as **fastidious**. They will not grow outside of living cells and must be cultured in living animals, cell cultures, or chicken egg embryos.

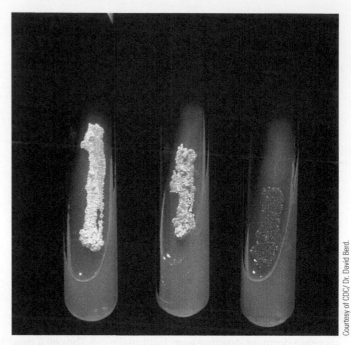

Courtesy of CDC/ Dr. David Berd.

Figure 3-15 Slant cultures demonstrating variations in colonial appearance among aerobic *Actinomycetes* spp. White indicates *A. madurae*; yellow indicates *Nocardia asteroides*; and red indicates *Micromonospora* sp.

Blood agar and **chocolate agar** are two popular types of solid enriched media. Blood agar is a combination of nutrient agar and sheep erythrocytes, otherwise known as red blood cells. It is used to cultivate certain microorganisms, including *Staphylococcus epidermidis*, *Diplococcus pneumoniae*, and *Clostridium perfringens*.

Chocolate agar, which is both an enriched and a selective medium, is a combination of nutrient agar and powdered hemoglobin. The name is given only due to the brown color of the agar. Microorganisms commonly cultivated with the use of chocolate agar include *Haemophilus influenzae*, *Neisseria gonorrhoeae*, and *Neisseria meningitidis*.

Selective Media

Selective media have chemical inhibitors that prevent the growth of particular species of microbes while allowing the growth of the desired species. **MacConkey agar**, which is both a selective and differential medium, is a combination of bile salts, lactose, and crystal violet. Gram-negative bacteria are able to ferment lactose and produce pink colonies, distinguishing them from the colorless bacteria that cannot ferment the lactose. MacConkey agar specifically differentiates between lactose-fermenting (LF) and non-lactose-fermenting (NLF) bacteria. One important use of the agar is distinguishing between the pathogenic *Salmonella* bacteria and other types that are related.

Other frequently used types of selective media include the following:

1. Phenylethyl alcohol (PEA) agar: A blood agar to which inhibitory substances have been added. Selective for Gram-positive bacteria.

2. Thayer-Martin agar: A type of chocolate agar that contains extra nutrients and an antimicrobial agent. It is selective for *N. gonorrhoeae.*

3. Mannitol salt agar (MSA): Only allows salt-tolerant bacteria to grow.

4. Colistin-nalidixic acid (CNA): Also a blood agar to which inhibitory substances have been added. Selective for Gram-positive bacteria.

5. Eosin methylene blue (EMB): A differential and selective medium. It contains substances that indicate fermentation of sugars and the resulting change in pH. It also contains crystal violet to inhibit the growth of Gram-positive microorganisms.

Differential Media

Differential media can make it easier to distinguish specific colonies of bacteria from other colonies that are growing on the same Petri dish. Blood agar, which is also an enriched medium, is frequently used to identify bacteria that destroy erythrocytes. For example, *Streptococcus pyogenes*, the bacteria responsible for causing strep throat, display a clear ring around the colony where the bacteria have lysed the surrounding erythrocytes.

MSA is used to identify *Staphylococcus aureus*, which grows readily on MSA and also ferments mannitol. Fermentation turns the MSA medium to a yellow color.

Reducing Media

The cultivation of anaerobic bacteria is difficult for the microbiologist. Special media called **reducing media** must be used to prevent the destruction of the bacteria by oxygen. The reducing medium contains chemicals, such as sodium thioglycolate, that combine with oxygen to eliminate it from the environment. To grow pure cultures of anaerobes, the reducing medium must be stored in tightly capped test tubes. The medium is then heated immediately before use so that the absorbed oxygen is eliminated.

When the culture must be grown in a Petri dish so that individual colonies can be observed, special jars are used that can contain several Petri dishes in an oxygen-free environment.

The oxygen is removed through the following process:

1. A chemical combination of sodium bicarbonate and sodium borohydride is placed in the jar, and moistened with just a few milliliters of water. The jar is tightly sealed.

2. The chemical reaction with the water produces hydrogen and carbon dioxide.

3. Next, the hydrogen and oxygen combine together in a chemical reaction and forms water.

4. The result is the disappearance of oxygen in a short period of time.

The carbon dioxide that is produced aids the growth of many types of anaerobic bacteria.

Microbiologists who work with anaerobes on a daily basis use an **anaerobic chamber**. The chamber is equipped with air locks and filled with inert gases. Researchers are able to handle and manipulate the equipment by inserting their hands into airtight gloves that are fixed to the wall of the chamber.

Rapid Identification Testing

A number of manufacturers have developed kits for use by healthcare providers to allow for expedited test results for certain types of pathogens. In response to the HIV/AIDS epidemic, screening efforts have been greatly expanded over time. One of the ways in which to encourage testing by individuals was to make access and results easy and discreet. Physicians in pediatric offices utilize rapid result tests for Streptococcal infections to begin immediate pharmacological treatment rather than having to wait for 24- to 48-hour culture results.

In the laboratory setting, manufactured kits have also been developed that incorporate multiple types of culture media in one device for inoculation. The Enterotube™ II Prepared Media Tube was developed by Becton Dickinson (BD) (see Figure 3-16). Another test kit designed for detection of anaerobic Gram-negative bacilli is the Rapid ID 32A tray by bioMérieux (see Figure 3-17).

Serology

When a microorganism enters an animal's body, it stimulates the host's immune system to produce **antibodies**. Antibodies are proteins located in the circulatory system that bind with the specific bacterium or antigen that was the cause of their production. **Antisera** (singular, antiserum) are solutions of

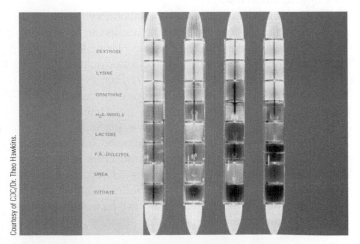

Figure 3-16 The Enterotube® identification kit is a multi-test system designed to confirm the identification of different isolates. Each tube contains eight different agar preparations, allowing a diagnostician to perform a number of simultaneous biochemical tests.

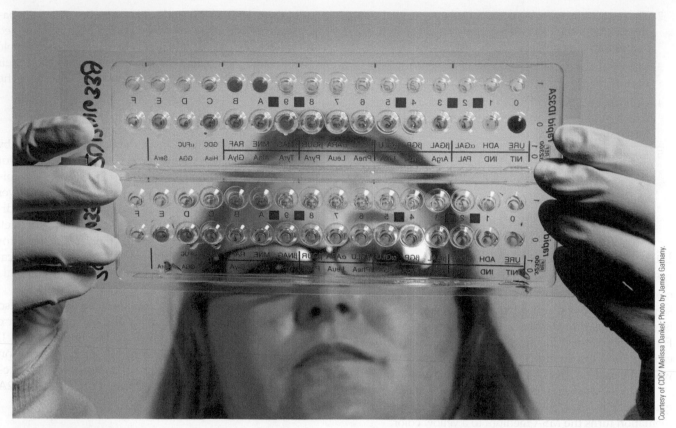

Figure 3-17 Centers for Disease Control (CDC) laboratorian holding a multi-well Rapid ID 32A tray (biomérieux, Inc.) used for the identification of anaerobic Gram-negative bacilli.

antibodies that are commercially produced and used to identify microorganisms. An unknown bacterium that is isolated from a patient can be tested against the antisera and identification can be achieved. Two popular tests using antisera are the **enzyme-linked immunosorbent assays (ELISAs)** and slide agglutination test.

ELISA is used extensively in the laboratory because test results can be quickly obtained and the results can be analyzed by a computer scanner. The test involves placing known antibodies in the depressions or wells of a microplate. The unknown bacteria are placed in each well. A reaction between the bacteria and antibodies identifies the type of bacteria. ELISA is commonly used in the diagnosis of HIV (see Figure 3-18).

The slide agglutination test involves placing samples of an unknown bacterium in a drop of saline on several microscope slides. Next, a different known antiserum is placed in each sample. If the bacteria agglutinate (clump together), a positive test result is achieved. The agglutination is caused by the combination of the bacteria that have an affinity for the antiserum that was added.

Specialized Laboratory Analyses

Numerous other forms of laboratory analyses are performed to identify microorganisms. Routinely, computers are tasked

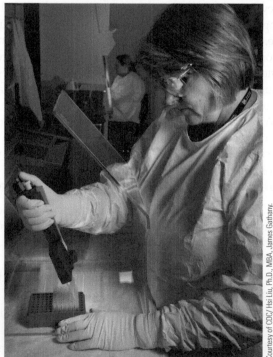

Figure 3-18 CDC microbiologist using an enzyme-linked immunosorbent assay (ELISA) test to develop a method for the rapid detection of HIV p24 antigen in blood samples.

with compiling the complex results and creating comprehensive reports for scientists and physicians to develop their research protocols or treatment plans. Some of the specialized testing methods are included in this section.

Catalase Test

Catalase is an **enzyme** produced by many living cells, including a number of species of bacteria. Hydrogen peroxide is a by-product of some normal cellular metabolic processes. The enzyme allows for the rapid breaking down of hydrogen peroxide (H_2O_2), a toxic chemical to cells, into harmless molecules of water (H_2O) and oxygen (O_2). Many organisms survive, in part by having defense mechanisms that allow them to escape or repair the oxidative damage caused by hydrogen peroxide. Some species of bacteria are able to perform cellular detoxification by producing catalase and are classified as being either catalase-positive or catalase-negative. The presence or absence of catalase in bacterial cultures provides an easy identification marker for clinicians.

The laboratory test involves placement of a carefully obtained sample from a culture onto a microscope slide placed into a Petri dish (optional but recommended). The technician takes care not to inadvertently pick up culture media, especially if using a blood agar, which might create a false-positive result. A single drop of 3 percent hydrogen peroxide is placed onto the bacterial sample and the cover of the Petri dish is positioned to prevent catalase aerosols. If effervescence (bubbling) is seen, then the test result is positive. In some weak responses, it may be necessary to examine the slide under the microscope. The test can also be performed using test tubes. *N. gonorrhoeae* produces vigorous bubbling reactions. *S. aureus* produces positive catalase reactions, and *Staphylococcus pyogenes* exhibits a negative reaction. *Streptococcus* and *Enterococcus* species usually are catalase-negative.

Coagulase Test

Coagulase is another enzyme produced by some bacterial species that coagulates (clots) blood plasma. The coagulase test is a laboratory study performed on Gram-positive, catalase-positive species of bacteria to definitively identify the coagulase-positive *S. aureus* species. Coagulase is considered a virulence factor of *S. aureus* because formation of a clot around the site of infection caused by these bacteria likely protects it from the body's natural inflammatory process of phagocytosis.

Two versions of the coagulase test are also used for definitive identification of *Staphylococcus* species. A laboratory slide preparation is inoculated with the bacterial specimen and a specific type of prepared plasma. In a matter of seconds, the positive reaction is observed as a clumping together of the bacterial cells. This provides a presumptive reading of *S. aureus*, due to the property of positive coagulase reaction. If, however, the slide test is negative, then further testing by the tube method is performed. The bacteria is introduced into prepared plasma in a test tube and allowed 24 hours to develop. At that time if there remains no reaction, the organism is deemed coagulase-negative and, if other studies agree, the species is determined to most likely be *S. epidimidis* or another coagulase-negative *Staphylococcus* (CoNS) and *S. aureus* is ruled out.

Amino Acid Sequencing

DNA is responsible for the encoding of the proteins that contain the base sequence of amino acids. Amino acid sequencing is based on the evolutionary course of two organisms. The changes in the DNA sequence that encodes the proteins in the two organisms will be either similar or dissimilar depending on the length of time that has taken place between the evolution of two microbes. The similarity of the DNA sequence can aid in determining the evolutionary closeness of the microbes by comparing the amino acid sequences from proteins of two different microbes. The more similar the proteins, the more related the microbes are.

Phage Typing

Phage typing, like serologic testing, is useful in determining the origin and course of a disease, such as healthcare-associated infections (HAIs). Phage typing indicates to which phages a bacterium is susceptible. Bacteriophages are bacterial viruses that are responsible for the lysis of bacteria they invade. The phages infect only specific types of bacteria in a particular species. Phage typing is used most often to identify strains of *S. aureus*, *Vibrio cholerae*, *Salmonella typhi*, and *Pseudomonas aeruginosa*.

To perform phage typing, a Petri dish is covered with bacteria on the agar growth medium. Drops of different phages are placed on the bacteria. Clear spaces called **plaques** subsequently appear on the dish. These areas indicate where the phages have lysed the bacteria. Phage typing is important in establishing the source of a surgical wound infection that may have been caused by an individual on the surgical team. The bacteria that are isolated from the surgical wound can be shown to have the same sensitivity to phages as those bacteria isolated from a member of the surgical team. This establishes the source carrier, whether the surgeon, nurse, surgical assistant, or surgical technologist as the source of infection or clears them.

As an example, if a staphylococcal infection appears to be associated with the surgery department, then all surgery personnel could be cultured for *S. aureus*. Positive cultures would be phage-typed and compared with the phage type of the cultures from the infected surgical patients. This would identify the colonized individual responsible for the spread of the infection and allow them to seek treatment for what may have been an unrecognized, asymptomatic infection.

Flow Cytometry

Flow cytometry is unique in that a culture of bacteria is not needed to identify the type. The process involves the flow of fluid through a small opening at the bottom of the tube. Bacteria are detected by the difference in electrical conductivity between the bacterial cells and the fluid. If a laser is used to illuminate the fluid as it travels through the opening, then the reflection or scattering of the light provides information pertaining to the size of the cell, its density, and morphology. The information is analyzed by a computer.

Nucleic Acid Hybridization

The double strands of DNA are held together by hydrogen bonds. If the strands are exposed to heat, then the bonds break and the two strands separate. When the single strands are cooled, they rejoin to form a double strand similar to the original. This technique is used on separate DNA strands from two different microorganisms to determine the similarity between the DNA base sequences of the two microbes.

The assumption of the test is that if two species are similar, their nucleic acid sequence will also be similar. The test reveals the extent of the DNA strands' ability from one microorganism to hybridize (bind) with the DNA strands of the other microorganism. The stronger the degree of **hybridization** is, the greater the similarity.

Another method of hybridization involves RNA. RNA is a single strand and is transcribed from one of the double strands of the DNA. Therefore, the strand of RNA should hybridize with the separated strand of DNA from which it was transcribed. The DNA–RNA hybridization can then be used to determine the degree of relationship between the two microorganisms in the same manner as the DNA–DNA hybridization.

Nucleic Acid–Base Composition

Another effective method for classifying microbes with evolutionary relationships is the determination of the nitrogenous-base composition of DNA. The base composition is expressed as a percentage of guanine plus cytosine, or G+C. The base composition in a single species is fixed and does not change. Therefore, by comparing the G+C content of different species, the degree of interrelationship can be investigated.

Two microbes that are similar will have many identical genes and similar amounts of the various bases in their DNA. However, if the difference is more than 10 percent in their percentage of G–C pairs, then the two microorganisms are most likely not related. For example, if one bacterium's DNA contains 30 percent G–C and the other has 65 percent G–C, then these two microbes are probably not related.

The base sequences of different microorganisms are compared by using the restriction enzyme test. The DNA from two microorganisms is treated with the same restriction enzyme. The restriction fragments are separated by the process of electrophoresis on a layer of agar. The number and sizes of restriction fragments produced by the different microbes are compared to reveal information about their genetic likeness or difference. The patterns are called DNA fingerprints, and the more similar the DNA fingerprints, the more closely related the microorganisms.

DNA fingerprinting is very important in determining the source of healthcare-associated infections. As an example, a high percentage of patients undergoing coronary artery bypass grafting at a hospital in the Midwest were developing postoperative infections caused by *Rhodococcus bronchialis*.

The DNA fingerprints of the patients' bacteria and the bacteria of a nurse were discovered to be identical. The infections were stopped by identifying the infected nurse and making sure that proper aseptic technique was practiced.

The real-time polymerase chain reaction (PCR) test, also known as a quantitative polymerase chain reaction (qPCR), works to amplify, as well as quantify, a specific or targeted DNA molecule. The detection of the DNA molecule in question occurs in real-time, rather than having to wait until the end of the conventional test. In critical cases of drug-resistant strains of pathogens, this allows therapeutic measures to be prescribed more quickly and efficiently.

The SARS-CoV-2 novel coronavirus that causes the COVID-19 infection is widely believed to have been first recognized in the latter months of 2019 in Wuhan, a city in the Hubei Province in China and subsequently became a worldwide pandemic. The incredible speed of global transmission required researchers to develop laboratory test methods that should be rapid and accurate and could be performed in a multitude of conditions throughout the world. The nucleic acid amplification tests (NAATs) and antigen tests were used as diagnostic tests to detect SARS-CoV-2 infections. The requirement of 1–3 days for laboratory NAATs was a barrier to quick diagnosis and recommendations for immediate isolation or quarantine of infected individuals to reduce transmission. Quicker, less expensive, and relatively equally accurate, point-of-care antigen tests were developed with results available in about 15–45 minutes. Current diagnostic tests for coronavirus, based on its genomic characteristics include reverse transcriptase polymerase chain reaction (RT-PCR), real-time reverse transcription PCR (rRT-PCR), reverse transcription loop-mediated isothermal amplification (RT-LAMP), and real-time RT-LAMP. The RT-LAMP tests rely on slightly heating cells in the specimen sample, causing cell lysis and nucleic acid release, which can be used as template for the visible color change indicating amplification of nucleic acids. The diagnostic test gives results in approximately 30 minutes (see Figure 3-19).

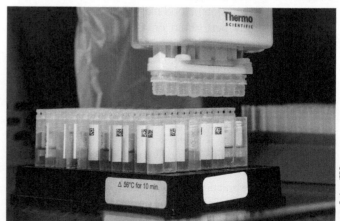

Figure 3-19 Samples for SARS-CoV-2 antibody testing. Serological testing is used to detect antibodies, which indicate past infection with the virus that causes COVID-19 and is important to the understanding of disease prevalence within a population.

Alternative Biosensor Technology

A diagnostic challenge for healthcare providers treating patients in a pandemic, such as COVID-19, has been that the clinical manifestations of COVID-19 are often non-specific. Biosensor technology, including Clustered Regularly Interspaced Short Palindromic Repeats (CRISPR), CRISPR-Cas9 or the newer CRISPR-Cas-13 DNA and RNA genome editing, and diagnostic tools are being explored as potential alternatives in traditional diagnosis and therapeutic approaches.

Another technology designed to quickly detect specific viral pathogens such as SARS, COVID, and MERS utilizes a binding protein that attaches to coronavirus fragments. The resulting protein bound viral nanobody is treated with a series of biochemical linkers that adhere it to a thin layer of gold which acts as a semiconductor. An electrical charge is applied to the plate and a device known as an organic electrochemical transistor measures the levels of and changes in current flow in response to the presence of the viral nanobody-bound particles. Researchers are seeking to develop user-friendly devices that are capable of rapid, inexpensive, and accurate diagnostic results in anticipation of potential future viral global pandemics.

Hanging Drop Technique

Bacterial motility (ability to move) can be assessed using the hanging drop technique of observing live bacteria. Robert Koch first utilized this method of studying bacteria in the late 1800s. A special laboratory slide with a concave depression in the center is used along with a coverslip prepared with petrolatum around the edges to keep it securely attached to the slide. A sterilized loop is used to transfer a drop of fluid to be studied onto the coverslip. The slide with the depression is placed over the cover slip and then turned over carefully so that the drop remains suspended from the coverslip over the center well of the slide. An advantage of this type of laboratory test is that the specimen does not dry out due to the intensity of the microscope light as quickly as a standard wet mount slide preparation (see Figure 3-20).

Numerical Taxonomy

Numerical taxonomy involves the comparison of morphologic and biochemical characteristics, amino acid sequence, percentage of G–C pairs, and many other characteristics of microbes to aid in determining relationships. A similarity index is calculated with the use of a computer to determine the similarities. Essentially, the computer matches the characteristics of each microorganism against other microorganisms. The greater the number of characteristics shared by two or more organisms, the greater the chance they are related. A match of 90 percent or more of these characteristics usually indicates a single species.

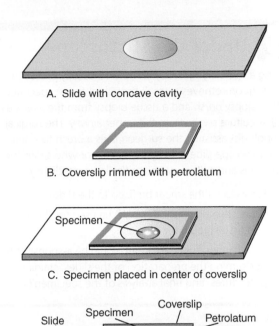

A. Slide with concave cavity

B. Coverslip rimmed with petrolatum

C. Specimen placed in center of coverslip

D. Invert slide so coverslip is on top

Figure 3-20 Preparation of a hanging drop slide. This technique is used to study living bacteria.

MICRO NOTES

"This Is Just a Test"

The CDC's section on Laboratory Quality Assurance and Standardization Programs states, "More than a billion laboratory tests that identify and measure chemicals, such as lead or cholesterol, are performed each year in the United States. The test results have a significant influence on medical decisions. Given the importance of laboratory test results, the Centers for Disease Control and Prevention's (CDC) National Center for Environmental Health has programs to help assure the quality of these data so patients and healthcare providers (as well as researchers and public health officials) can be confident that laboratory test results they receive are accurate." As members of the surgical team, we understand the importance of accurate microbial testing of surgical specimens as well as in monitoring of the instrument sterilization processes we rely on to prevent SSIs. Evaluation of the testing is an important quality control measure for all involved, from the CDC down to a local hospital laboratory or sterile processing department.

Under the Microscope

During a microlaryngoscopy and bronchoscopy procedure, the surgeon retrieves a small bronchial tissue specimen with a biopsy brush and a tissue biopsy from the larynx as well as culture swabs from the upper airway. The surgical technologist assisting the surgeon uses a brush to smear the microscope slide held by the circulator who sends the specimens and culture swabs to the lab immediately.

1. How would the smear be fixed to the slide?

2. What staining methods might be used for this smear and tissue biopsy?

3. Which laboratory personnel would be responsible for performing the preparation of the slides, staining procedures, and final analysis of the specimen?

4. What types of organisms might be identified by the various staining procedures?

5. What type of microscope would be necessary to visualize the organisms found in the smear and tissue biopsies?

6. How would the culture swabs be prepared for incubation?

7. Which other types of serological or specialized analysis tests might also be performed to provide a full diagnosis for this patient?

CHAPTER 4

The Prokaryotes

Learning Objectives

After completing the study of this chapter, you will be able to:

1. Define key terms.
2. Distinguish between archaea and bacteria.
3. Compare and contrast different bacterial morphologies.
4. Discuss characteristics of prokaryotic cell structure.
5. Describe how bacteria are classified.
6. Discuss the significance of bacterial spore formation.
7. Apply critical thinking skills in relating chapter material to the surgical environment of care or broader global community.

Key Terms

Aerotolerant	Extremophiles	Microaerophile	Pili
Anoxygenic	Facultative	Obligate	Sterilization
Capnophiles	Glycocalyx	Organelles	Susceptibility
Desiccation	Greenhouse gases	Pathogenicity	Synthesizing
Ecosystem	Macromolecule	Permeable	Viability
Exotoxins	Meningitis	Pneumonia	

The Big Picture

We are a product of our genes, so they say; however, we are also populated by microbes. Some we cannot live without, but others wait around until our defenses are down and then they strike.

During your examination of the topics in this chapter, consider the following:

1. Which characteristics of bacterial cells allow them to cause disease in humans?

2. What types of relationships do we have with the microbial world?

3. How do bacteria get around?

4. What do these microscopic invaders look like up close?

Clinical Significance Topic

Bacteria are on the "most wanted" list of the healthcare environment. Our sterilization methods and techniques are designed to kill ALL microbes. Aseptic techniques and principles including proper hand washing, surgical scrubbing or chemical surgical hand antisepsis, environmental sanitation, patient skin preps, and antibiotic administration are all designed to kill MOST bacteria, or at least as many as possible. Microbes are found everywhere; however, those found deep inside the human body's tissues are more likely pathogenic invaders. Our efforts are focused on trying to prevent these unwanted opportunists from gaining access to where they can do serious damage. Scientists must understand bacterial characteristics and how they behave to find ways to neutralize them, reduce the potential for surgical site infections, and manufacture the antimicrobial agents and sterilization methods we rely on for the war on infection.

Two Domains: Archaea and Bacteria

As discussed in Chapter 2, the basic ancestors of life on Earth are the prokaryotes: archaea and bacteria. These tiny microorganisms are more similar to complex eukaryotes, but their genetic material, usually DNA is not contained in a cell nucleus, a characteristic of prokaryotes.

Bacteria have literally been the focus of scientists' attention for centuries, as demonstrated in the timeline in Chapter 1. Despite our fascination with these microbes, it is estimated that researchers have been able to identify only a few thousand species of prokaryotes out of the probable millions existing almost everywhere in, on, and around us. Surgical technologists and other surgical team members direct their attention to the care of the patient during surgery; however, they must also understand the microbial world and how it impacts those efforts.

Archaea

The research into the classification of archaea is ongoing; however, after a few decades of focus on these unique ancient microbes, the data still lag far behind what has been discovered about the larger domain of bacteria or eubacteria otherwise referred to as "true bacteria."

What researchers know about archaea is that these organisms are fundamentally separate from both bacteria and eukaryotes. When initially identified in the 1970s, scientists created a new classification of "archaebacteria" due to the similarities in metabolism and cell structure with bacteria. The ways these organisms produce proteins from genetic encoding more closely resemble eukaryotes. The classification was changed to simply archaea to reflect their unique design characteristics and reproductive functions. Archaea are believed to have derived from ancient anaerobic organisms that emerged approximately 4 billion years ago and thrived in the hot, toxic, oxygen-poor atmosphere.

The descendants of archaea have been isolated in modern times, primarily in extreme environmental conditions such as boiling hot springs, volcanic steam vents, salt marshes, and under glacial ice in Antarctica. They are sometimes termed **extremophiles** because of the exceptional circumstances of their survival in such hostile conditions. Despite that reputation, archaea have also been found in more common and ordinary areas, living in similar conditions with present-day common bacteria and eukaryotes. Archaea have been found in soil, ocean plankton, and even in animal and human intestinal tracts. Their microscopic forms vary and resemble the morphological shapes of most bacteria. Their genomes have been found to be smaller than those of bacteria; however, the individual genes appear unlike any other known organism's DNA or RNA.

The genetic coding of archaea changed over billions of years from anaerobic to aerobic or **facultative** to match the evolution of the planetary surfaces and atmospheric conditions. They have been classified into groups including:

- Methogenes: methane gas-producing anaerobes
- Halophiles: salt-loving aerobes
- Thermoacidophiles: hot, acidic environment-loving aerobes

The Basics of Bacteria

Bacteria are grouped into different categories based on certain characteristics that can be established by the microbiologist in the laboratory. The surgical technologist must have a working knowledge of various types of bacteria as the predominant causes of healthcare-associated infections (HAI) in broad terms, and, more specifically in our environment of care, to prevent the potential for cross-contamination and surgical site infection (SSI).

The identification of specific characteristics aids in identifying the type of bacteria and establishing relationships among the microbes based on their genetic and structural makeup. Examples of these characteristics include the presence or absence of a cell wall, ability to thrive in the presence of air, and specific variations of size and shape. Microscopic examination of these tiny lifeforms is performed to provide detailed information for the process of identification and classification based on the following:

- Morphology
- Staining
- Growth
- Motility
- Nutritional requirements
- Oxygen requirements
- Pathogenicity
- Metabolism
- Proteins
- Genetics

Morphology

A standard compound light microscope can be used to view bacteria to determine the morphology: size, shape, and arrangements of bacterial microbes. Bacteria can vary widely in size, ranging on average from 0.2 μm (micrometer) to 10.0 μm.

The three basic shapes of bacteria first identified by van Leeuwenhoek are:

1. Coccus: round-shaped. The plural of coccus is cocci.
2. Bacillus: rod-shaped. The plural of bacillus is bacilli.

- Coccobacillus: very short rod that resembles a coccus.

3. Spiral or corkscrew-shaped

- Spirillum (plural is spirilla) is a rigid, thickened spiral.
- Spirochetes are flexible, thin spirals.
- Vibrios are comma-shaped or C-shaped rods.

Additional forms that have been identified in more recent years include:

- Pleomorphic or L-form: ability to change shape based on adverse environmental conditions.
- Mycoplasma: lobulated "spherules," ring-shaped, star-shaped, or fried egg-shaped. These bacteria have cell membranes, but no cell walls, and vary in shape.

Bacterial Arrangements In addition to the basic shape of individual microbes, arrangements of bacteria further determine the species and are indicated by adding a descriptive prefix to the morphological name. Cocci can be further described as:

- Monococcus (single sphere; also called micrococcus)— rarely found in singular form
- Diplococci (pairs)—example: *Neisseria gonorrhoeae*— bacterial meningitis
- Tetracocci (groups of four)—example: *Micrococcus luteus*—normal (indigenous) microflora of the upper respiratory tract
- Sarcinae (cubic groups of eight)—example: *Sarcina ventriculi*—gastric ulcers, septicemia
- Streptococci (chains or filament forms)—example: *Streptococcus mutans*—endocarditis
- Staphylococci (clusters or sheets)—example: *Staphylococcus aureus*—normal (indigenous) microflora on skin, causative agent for SSIs, pneumonia

Bacilli also vary in their basic shapes; they can be short or long, have pointed or curved ends, and can be thin or wide in diameter (see Figure 4-1). Typically, bacilli are described as straight, cylindrical, and rod-shaped. As with cocci, they can further be categorized by their arrangements:

- Monobacillus (single)—example: *Escherichia coli*— normal indigenous microflora of the intestines; causes urinary tract infections, septicemia, and diarrheal diseases
- Diplobacillus (paired)—Morax-Axenfeld diplobacillus (*Moraxella lacunata*)—causes blepharoconjunctivitis
- Streptobacillus (in chains or filament form)— example: *Streptobacillus moniliformis*—causes rat-bite fever and septic arthritis
- Palisade (in the shape of a stack of rods)— example: *Corynebacterium diphtheriae*—causes the upper respiratory disease diphtheria

Coccus	Rod	Spiral
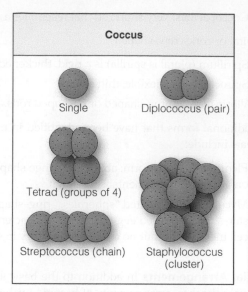	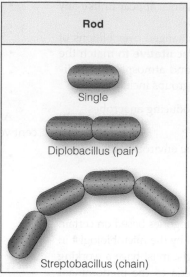	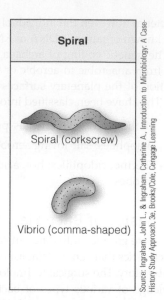

Figure 4-1 Bacterial classification and morphology.

Spirochetes and spirilla are, as their names imply, spiral-shaped or coiled bacteria. They can be found in single form or in chains and vary in length, rigidity of their cell walls, and number of spirals or coils along the length of the individual bacterium. They are small and very fine, making them difficult to see, even with magnification. One of the most common sexually transmitted diseases, syphilis, is caused by the spirochete *Treponema pallidum*.

Campylobacter bacteria are spirilla-shaped and, according to the Centers for Disease Control and Prevention (CDC), *Campylobacter* is the most common cause of bacterial diarrheal infections and affects approximately 1.5 million individuals each year in the United States. Antibiotic resistance is increasing with these bacterial populations.

Vibrio bacteria are comma-shaped, slightly curved bacteria responsible for deadly diseases from *Vibrio cholerae* and *Vibrio vulnificus*. These organisms are found in water supplies and, in the case of cholera, an individual may contract it by drinking water or eating food contaminated with the cholera bacterium usually due to inadequate sewage treatment. *V. vulnificus* is in the same family as *V. cholera* but is found in warm saltwater supplies and is contracted by eating contaminated seafood or through open wounds exposed to contaminated water. Individuals who are immunocompromised are at risk for development of septic shock, which has a 50 percent fatality rate.

Various bacteria have been identified as having the ability to lose their normal shape when faced with adverse environmental conditions, but they continue to reproduce in a new "L-form." The first documentation was recorded in 1948 at the Lister Institute in London, where it received the name L-form. These bacteria are categorized as being cell wall–deficient (CWD) and termed "stealth pathogens."

Mycoplasmas are very small bacteria that have no cell walls, only flexible cell membranes. They present in a variety of shapes under the microscope and are often difficult to detect.

The lack of a cell wall often makes antibiotic therapy ineffective. For otherwise healthy patients who contract *Mycoplasma pneumoniae*, responsible for atypical or "walking" **pneumonia**, antibiotics may be prescribed for an extended course, or it is possible that no pharmaceutical treatment may be given to allow the infection to run its course.

Staining

Staining methods discussed in Chapter 3 are used to identify microbes and their special characteristics. Selection of the proper methods for culturing specific types of microbes can only occur when the identity of the bacteria has been determined. Simple, differential, and Gram staining techniques are just a few methods utilized to determine bacterial identities.

Gram stain results (Gram-positive or Gram-negative) provide one of the standard methods of determining the preliminary identity and **pathogenicity** of bacteria. Microbes that turn purple or dark blue when exposed to Gram staining are called Gram-positive, and those that do not take on the stain and appear red or pink are Gram-negative. Physicians can prescribe preliminary antibiotic therapy based on Gram stain results and a generalization of bacterial **susceptibility** to various classes of pharmacologic agents. After full culture and sensitivity (C&S) techniques have been completed in 24 to 48 hours, the prescribed treatment may be changed if results determine that the type of infection detected would be unresponsive to the routine prescribed antibiotics.

Growth

Bacterial colonies isolated, incubated, and studied in the laboratory setting grow at different rates depending on factors such as the type of agar medium, nutrients used, and staining agents applied to them. Bacteria require specific nutrients and environmental conditions to proliferate or multiply. Note that growth of colonies refers to the numbers of cells within a

Source: Ingraham, John L., & Ingraham, Catherine A., Introduction to Microbiology: A Case-History Study Approach, 3e, Brooks/Cole, Cengage Learning

microbial population, not the size of the individual microbial cells. The cycle of bacterial colony life is described in four phases and is discussed in detail in later sections along with the specific physical and chemical requirements for **viability** of microorganisms.

Motility

The ability of a microbe to move itself is called motility. Bacterial motility is accomplished by use of two types of cell structures: flagella and axial filaments (see Figure 4-2). Not all microorganisms are motile. Most spiral-shaped bacteria are motile, whereas only a few species of bacilli are motile. Cocci are typically non-motile. A fast and relatively easy laboratory test used to determine the motility of a specimen is the hanging-drop technique described in Chapter 3. Standard wet-mount methods can also be used; however, motility may be more difficult to observe with the sample compressed between the slide and coverslip, and the wet-mount samples may also dry out under the microscope light more quickly than hanging-drop samples.

Nutritional Requirements

Another tool for classifying microbes is to determine their nutritional requirements or sources of energy and carbon.

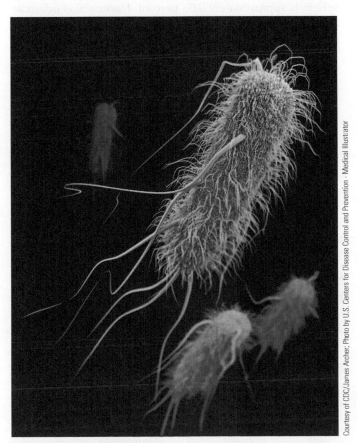

Figure 4-2 3D computer-generated image of a group of *Enterobacteriaceae* with long, whip-like peritrichous flagellae as well as numerous shorter and finer fimbriae, giving the bacteria a furry appearance.

Courtesy of CDC/James Archer; Photo by U.S. Centers for Disease Control and Prevention - Medical Illustrator

Bacteria, fungi, and algae are some of the original recyclers on the planet. They recycle essential life elements such as carbon, oxygen, nitrogen, hydrogen, and sulfur as well as **greenhouse gases** in the atmosphere.

There are a number of terms that are used to describe the mechanism by which prokaryotes acquire the energy to survive and reproduce. The suffix -troph means "feeder" which indicates the nutritional source. The prefix used describes the source of energy with which the bacteria need to live.

Prokaryotes are classified as either autotrophs (self-feeders) or heterotrophs (different or other-feeders). Autotrophs do not eat in the traditional sense and utilize light or chemicals to produce their own nutrients; further they are sub-classified as phototrophs (light feeders) or chemotrophs (chemical feeders). Those capable of converting light energy into chemical energy are classified as photosynthetic organisms. Autotrophs use carbon dioxide (CO_2) as their source of carbon. Heterotrophs are also known as organotrophs due to their ability to consume organic materials such as dead and decomposing plants and animals. Lithotrophs use inorganic compounds, usually of mineral origin, to meet their carbon needs.

As shown in Table 4-1, terms can be combined to indicate an organism's energy and carbon source. Photoautotrophs, such as eukaryotic plants, algae, and prokaryotic cyanobacteria, use light as their energy source and CO_2 as a carbon source. Photoheterotrophs (photoorganotrophs), such as purple non-sulfur and green non-sulfur bacteria, use light as an energy source and organic compounds such as alcohols and carbohydrates as sources of carbon. They are **anoxygenic**. Chemoautotrophs, such as hydrogen, iron, and sulfur bacteria, use chemicals as energy sources and CO_2 as their carbon source. Chemolithotrophs are organisms that derive their energy from the oxidation of inorganic compounds and their carbon from CO_2.

Chemoheterotrophs (chemo-organotrophs) include most bacteria and all fungi, protozoa, and animals that use chemicals as their energy source and organic compounds for a carbon source. Heterotrophs are further classified according to their source of organic compounds. Saprophytes obtain organic nutrients from dead organic matter, and parasites obtain nutrients from a living host. The majority of medically significant microbes discussed in this text are chemoheterotrophs.

Table 4-1 Nutritional Classification of Microorganisms

Source of Carbon	Source of ATP	
	Chemical Reaction	Source of Light Energy
Organic Compounds	Chemoheterotrophs	Photoheterotrophs
CO_2	Chemoautotrophs	Photoautotrophs

The interactions between prokaryotes and eukaryotes maintain the delicate balance of our **ecosystem**, which is defined as a community of all of the living (biotic) organisms in conjunction with the non-living (abiotic) components of their shared environment. Dead animals and plants and other debris would collect on the surface of the earth without this balance and if the chemoheterotrophic saprophytic decomposers, such as fungi and bacteria, did not break down the dead organic material into inorganic compounds for use by the photolithotrophs. The inorganic compounds include CO_2, phosphates, and nitrates. The photolithotrophs complete the cycle through the process of photosynthesis. The light energy from the sun is used by the photolithotrophs to synthesize organic compounds such as proteins, carbohydrates, and nucleic acids from the inorganic compounds. The benefit of photosynthesis for the animal kingdom, including *Homo sapiens*, is that the hydrogen atoms of water are used to reduce CO_2 and life-sustaining oxygen is released for the critical purpose of respiration.

Oxygen Requirements

Bacteria are classified according to their oxygen and carbon dioxide requirements (see Table 4-2). A bacterium can be classified into one of six main groups:

1. **Obligate** aerobe
2. **Microaerophile**
3. Facultative anaerobe
4. **Aerotolerant** anaerobe
5. Obligate anaerobe
6. **Capnophiles**

Obligate aerobes require a level of oxygen that is similar to that found in ambient room air: 20 to 21 percent oxygen. Examples of obligate aerobes are *Pseudomonas aeruginosa* and *Mycobacterium tuberculosis*.

Microaerophiles require oxygen, but at a much lower level than that found in room air, requiring only approximately 5 percent O_2 and increased amounts of CO_2 (8–10 percent). *Campylobacter jejuni* and *Helicobacter pylori* are examples of microaerophiles.

Facultative anaerobes are able to survive with or without oxygen. They can grow even in zero percent O_2 or in an atmosphere containing oxygen in concentrations comparable to that found in ambient room air. The family of bacteria called *Enterobacteriaceae* (including *E. coli*) is an example of facultative anaerobes.

Aerotolerant anaerobes do not necessarily require oxygen and actually grow better in the total absence of oxygen. They can survive, however, in atmospheres that contain the amount of oxygen found in a CO_2 incubator. Some strains of *Clostridium* are classified as aerotolerant anaerobes.

Obligate anaerobes will not grow in an environment in which any amount of oxygen is present. The anaerobes will not grow, even in a CO_2 incubator because it contains approximately 15 percent O_2. *Clostridium perfringens*, which causes gas gangrene, and *C. tetani*, which causes tetanus, are examples of obligate anaerobes.

Capnophiles are types of bacteria that grow better in higher concentrations of CO_2, usually in concentrations of 5 to 10 percent. The average percentage of CO_2 in the atmosphere is approximately 0.03 percent. *Haemophilus infuenzae* and *Neisseria gonorrhoeae* are examples of anaerobes that are classified as a capnophiles.

Pathogenicity

There are millions and millions of microbes that inhabit every corner of the earth and comprise the majority of the cells in the human body. Only a few thousand species of those microbes are pathogenic, or able to cause disease. Classification of microbes includes the pathogenicity of microbial life. Digestion and protein synthesis required for us

Table 4-2   Bacteria and Oxygen Relationships

Microbial Class	Response to Oxygen	Catalase	Superoxide Dismutase	Example
Obligate aerobes	Require oxygen	Present	Present	*Pseudomonas aeruginosa*
Facultative anaerobes	Can grow with or without oxygen	Present	Present	*Escherichia coli*
Microaerophile	Grow best with low oxygen	Present	Present	*Campylobacter jejuni*
Aerotolerant anaerobes	Grow without oxygen but not killed by it	Absent	Present	*Streptococcus pneumoniae*
Obligate anaerobes	Killed by oxygen	Absent	Absent	*Methanococcus vannielli*

Adapted from Ingraham J. L., & Ingraham, C. A. (2000). *Introduction to Microbiology* (2nd ed., p. 217). Pacific Grove, CA: Brooks/Cole.

to survive and grow would not be possible without our indigenous (native) microbial populations. When the normal resident microflora or invading transient microflora gain access through various portals of entry into tissues and organs where they are not normally present, and the conditions for their survival and growth are favorable, they become pathogenic and cause infections. Some microbes cause infections and diseases by secreting **exotoxins**. It is often less the actual presence of microbes that causes harm and more the body's normal immune system reaction to the pathogens that causes damage to the host's tissues.

Specific types of bacteria known as spore-forming microbes form protective capsules or coats that protect them from unfavorable environmental conditions and chemical agents such as antibiotics (see Figure 4-3). These species of bacteria are of particular interest in healthcare and the perioperative environment of care. The goal of surgical instrument sterilization processes hinges on the ability to kill all living microorganisms, including spores. The process of infection and disease transmission is discussed in greater detail in subsequent sections.

Metabolism

Metabolism is defined by *Encyclopaedia Britannica* as "the sum of the chemical reactions that take place within each cell of a living organism and that provide energy for vital processes and for **synthesizing** new organic material. Living organisms are unique in that they can extract energy from their environments and use it to carry out activities such as movement, growth and development, and reproduction." Nutritional requirements and food sources as the first part of the metabolic cycle were discussed previously.

Bacteria, as with other living organisms, expel waste products and other secretions, such as enzymes, as they grow. The enzymes enable the bacteria to invade their host's cells and tissues and subsequently cause disease. *Staphylococcus* and *Streptococcus* species are identified according to the enzymes they secrete. Certain types of bacteria are classified according to their production of substances such as oxygen, methane, or carbon dioxide.

The metabolic activities on a cellular level of prokaryotes and eukaryotes are nearly identical in most cases and are discussed more in the sections on eukaryotes.

Proteins

Proteins are organic compounds that consist of large molecules composed of single or multiple chains of amino acids. Some proteins within a bacterium or microbe are specific for that species. The microbiologist can examine the amino acid sequence of the proteins to determine how closely that species is related to other types of bacteria as another method of classifying them. The sequencing of amino acids determines the final structure and function of a protein. The specific types of proteins found in prokaryotic cells and eukaryotic cells are outlined in other sections.

Genetics

Instructions for the synthesis of proteins are encoded in the genetic material of both prokaryotic and eukaryotic cells. The chemical reactions inside individual cells are programmed by genes and, when combined with the unique intracellular and extracellular environmental conditions present, determine the cell's structural and physical characteristics. The topics of genetics and genomics are complex, and the basics are discussed in other sections.

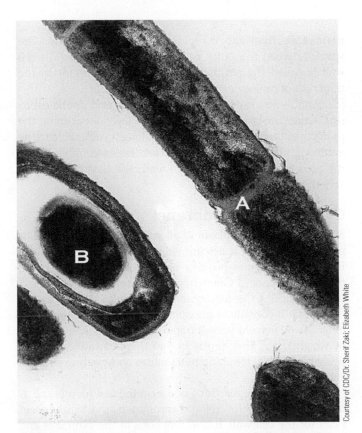

Figure 4-3 Transmission electron micrographic image of *Bacillus anthracis* from an anthrax culture showing cell division (A) and spores (B).

Courtesy of CDC/Dr. Sherif Zaki; Elizabeth White

Anatomy of a Prokaryote

All bacteria and archaea are prokaryotes. Prokaryotes are single-cell organisms and the oldest forms of life on Earth. Prokaryotes range in size from 0.2 μm to 2.0 μm and have no true nucleus; that is, the nucleus is not enclosed within a membrane (see Figure 4-4). Their **organelles** are not membrane-bound and their cell walls are chemically complex. The flagellum of the eukaryotic cell is composed of microtubules (long tubes made up of the protein tubulin) and propels the cell with wave-like motions. The plasma membrane of the prokaryotic cell does not contain the sterols and carbohydrates that comprise the eukaryotic cell's plasma membrane.

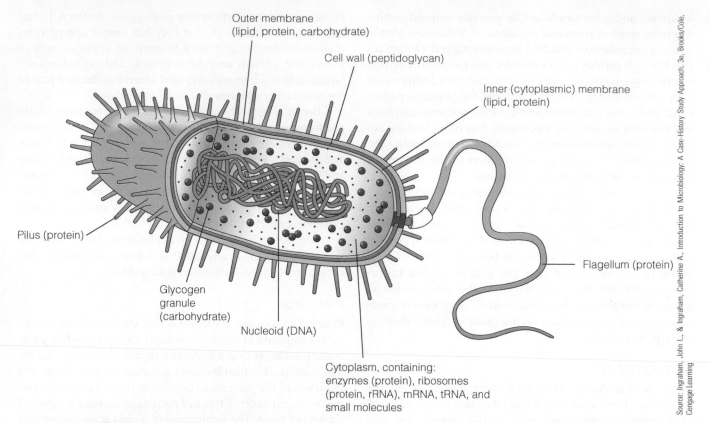

Figure 4-4 Structures of a bacterial cell.

Although prokaryotes are less complex than eukaryotes, they are still complex enough to complete the necessary functions for life. The prokaryotes divide by the process of binary fission, which is a simple division that results in two cells. The following bacterial structures are discussed: cell wall, cell membrane, capsules, cytoplasm, cytoplasmic particles, chromosomes, flagella, pili, and endospores.

Bacterial Cell Wall

The cell wall of the typical bacterium is rigid. It gives shape to the cell and forms a physical barrier to the outside of the cell. The chemical composition of the wall is complex. The main component of the cell wall is the large polymer **macromolecule** called peptidoglycan (abbreviated as PGN), also called murein. It consists of polysaccharide chains connected by protein chains that form a mesh-like structure. PGN is found in all bacterial species except the mycoplasmas and ureaplasmas, which have no cell walls. The thickness of the cell wall varies between Gram-positive and Gram-negative bacteria.

Gram-positive bacteria have a thick layer of peptidoglycan (up to 90 percent of the structure). The Gram-negative bacteria have a much thinner wall that is also composed of peptidoglycan (5–20 percent of the structure). Gram-negative bacterial cells have a thin layer of lipid macromolecules in addition to the cell wall, referred to as the outer membrane. The outer membrane of Gram-negative bacterial cells is composed of lipopolysaccharides (LPS) generally considered to be toxins. This membrane is less

permeable than the cytoplasmic inner membrane. The space between the outer cell membrane and the thin cell wall is called the periplasm, a structure important in the transport of molecules into and out of the cell.

Antibiotics, especially the penicillins and cephalosporins, target the cross-links of the PGN layer, weakening the protective structure of the cell and making it vulnerable to the antibiotic. Gram-negative bacteria are less susceptible due to the presence of the outer LPS membrane that protects the very thin layer of PGN.

Cytoplasmic Membrane

Surrounding the cytoplasm of all bacterial cells is the cell or plasma membrane. It lies immediately within the cell wall's PGN layer in Gram-positive bacteria and adjacent to the periplasmic space in Gram-negative bacteria.

Chemically, the membrane is similar to the eukaryotic cell in that it consists of phospholipids embedded with proteins (30–60 percent phospholipid and 50–70 percent protein by weight). It is also similar in that the membrane is selectively permeable, retaining metabolites and ejecting external substances.

The metabolic reactions occur on the cell membrane. It contains enzymes for cellular respiration and synthesis of PGN for the cell wall. It also functions in the synthesis and secretion of bacterial toxins. It provides a barrier in which membrane potential can be accumulated and used for propulsion by flagella. Cellular respiration for bacteria takes place within the cell membrane. Proteins embedded within the cytoplasmic membrane are involved in the active transport of molecules into the cytoplasm. These carrier proteins are called permeases.

Mesosomes are invaginations (folding inward to form a pouch-like cavity) within the cytoplasmic membrane, extending into the cytoplasm thereby increasing the surface area for enzyme synthesis of energy molecules. The process within the mesosomes is similar to the process within the mitochondria of the eukaryotic cells in which nutrients are broken down to produce energy in the form of adenosine triphosphate (ATP) to be used for cellular functions. However, the bacteria do not contain a Golgi complex or endoplasmic reticulum found in the eukaryotic cells.

Capsules

Some types of bacteria have a capsule composed of **glycocalyx** located outside the cell wall. The layer is referred to as a capsule if it is strongly attached to the cell wall; it is called a slime layer if it is loosely attached. Different species of bacteria have different chemical compositions that are used by microbiologists to identify particular species of bacteria. Several species of *Haemophilus influenzae*, the bacteria responsible for bacterial **meningitis** in children, are identified by their capsular types.

Capsules and slime layers serve different functions. They provide protection against **desiccation** and penetration of environmental toxins. They provide the bacterial cell motility or the ability to move on solid surfaces. Some capsules allow the bacteria to anchor to mucous membranes or the enamel surface of teeth so they are not flushed away by mechanical means or normal bodily secretions.

The material that comprises the capsule is usually antigenic, and its detection serologically is made with the Quellung (German for swelling) test developed in the early 1900s by German physician Friedrich Neufeld, an assistant to Robert Koch. It is used to identify the human pathogens *Streptococcus pneumoniae*, *H. influenzae* type b, *Klebsiella pneumoniae*, and *Neisseria meningitidis* serogroups (see Figure 4-5).

Cytoplasm

The gelatinous cytoplasm is contained within the plasma membrane. It is composed of a mixture of the materials needed by the cell to complete metabolic functions. Cytosol is the semi-liquid portion of the cytoplasm and is composed of mainly water. It also contains organic and inorganic material such as waste products, food nutrients, carbohydrates, proteins, and enzymes. Also found in the cytosol is the nucleoid—the genetic material or DNA of the cell. The majority of important chemical reactions responsible for survival of the cell occur within the cytosol.

Cytoplasmic Particles

Inclusions are tiny packets of reserve nutrients or chemicals found within the cytoplasm. In certain marine bacteria,

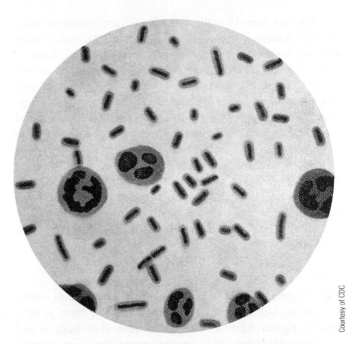

Courtesy of CDC

Figure 4-5 This illustration depicts a photomicrographic view of a Hiss capsule-stained culture specimen revealing the presence of numerous *Klebsiella pneumoniae* bacteria.

inclusions may contain gases that provide cell buoyancy and the ability to remain floating.

Ribosomes are tiny, non-membranous organelles that are found in both prokaryotic and eukaryotic cells. Prokaryotic ribosomes are found in fewer numbers, although they still may be in the thousands, and are responsible for protein synthesis or translation.

In recent years, scientists have found the presence of cytoskeletons in rod-shaped bacteria and some archaea. The cytoskeleton is a network of protein fibers playing a role in cell division and supporting the cell structure; however, it was previously thought to be present only in eukaryotes. Cocci (round-shaped) bacteria are not believed to contain cytoskeletons.

Chromosomes

The chromosomes in the prokaryotic cell are not surrounded by a nuclear membrane, contain no protein material, and do not maintain a stable shape. The chromosome contains a single strand of DNA that controls the functions of the cell. It contains the genetic information needed to synthesize proteins and enzymes. The chromosome also guides the process of binary fission.

Flagella

Many bacteria have flagella attached to the cell that are responsible for movement through the cell's environment. They are typically found in rod-shaped, Gram-negative bacteria, although certain motile Gram-positive rods have them as well. They are long, snake-like appendages that are produced from the basal body of the cytoplasmic membrane, extending through the cell wall into the area outside of the cell.

The number of flagella that a bacterium contains is used for classification. There are four types of flagella: peritrichous, lophotrichous, amphitrichous, and monotrichous. Bacteria that have flagella that surround their entire surface are referred to as peritrichous. Those with multiple flagella at one or both ends are called lophotrichous. Bacteria with a single flagella at each pole of the cell are called amphitrichous, and those with a single flagellum at one pole are referred to as monotrichous (see Figure 4-6).

Some species of spirochetes have two flagella called axial filaments; one is attached to each pole of the cell. The filaments point toward each other and wrap around the microbe between the cell wall layers, overlapping in the middle. The result is that the spirochete can move in a spiral manner.

Pili

Pili (singular, pilus) are hair-like structures that occur mainly on Gram-negative bacteria. Another term is fimbriae (singular, fimbria). They are thinner than flagella and are more rigid; they do not provide motility. They are produced from the cytoplasm and travel through the plasma membrane, layers of cell wall, and capsule. The functions of pili are as follows:

1. Serve as a site for the attachment of particular types of bacteria.
2. Provide bacteria that have a sex pilus the ability to transfer genetic material to another bacterial cell through a process called conjugation.
3. Provide bacteria the ability to attach to other bacteria or surfaces, such as the lining of the intestine.

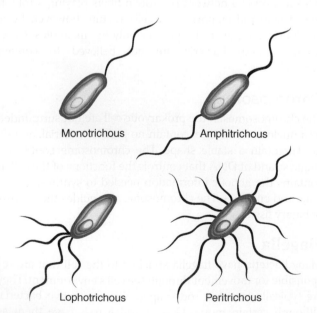

Monotrichous   Amphitrichous

Lophotrichous   Peritrichous

Figure 4-6 Four basic types of flagella for bacteria: monotrichous, amphitrichous, lophotrichous, and peritrichous.

Spore Formation

Seven known species of bacteria are capable of forming spores, a process referred to as sporulation. *Clostridium* and *Bacillus* groups are examples of spore-forming bacteria. When environmental conditions are not favorable or conducive to the support of the microbe's life functions, the bacterial cell forms an endospore as a means of survival. During the process of sporulation, the genetic material of the cell is enclosed in a capsule of several protein coats that are highly resistant to heat, dry conditions, and many chemicals. Endospores can survive for long periods of time until conditions are favorable for germination, reverting back into vegetative cells—active bacterial cells that undergo metabolic activity (see Figure 4-7). Sporulated *Bacillus anthracis* and *Clostridium tetani* bacteria can remain dormant for decades to centuries until the surrounding area provides temperatures in the normal body temperature range and changes occur in the cell wall surface tensions to allow diffusion of water and nutrients through the protective cell walls.

Bacteria in the genus *Methylosinus* form exospores, which are spore coats similar to endospores; however, they develop by budding from one end of the bacterium and have different proteins. Exospores are similar to endospores in their durability.

Another type of protective coating developed by the genera *Azotobacter*, *Bdellovibrio*, *Myxococcus*, and *Cyanobacteria* is a cyst coat. Cysts are less durable than endospores or exospores.

Microsporidia, a group of parasitic protozoa, are spore-forming single-cell eukaryotes. These protozoa remain dormant and protected until swallowed by a host. Once in the digestive tract, they create a tube-like structure through its spore coat, which pierces the mucosal lining of the host and transfers its genetic material into the surrounding cells and begins to replicate.

Spore formation should not be confused with reproduction. It is just a method of bacterial survival. Only one spore is produced in a bacterial cell; therefore, only one bacterium germinates.

Small samples of spore-forming bacteria are used to test the various methods of **sterilization** used in hospitals, clinics, and industries. Due to their resistance to heat and chemicals, the method of sterilization must be able to kill all of the bacterial spores, which can be an approved, effective method of sterilization. If a sterilization method can kill bacteria but not their spores, then it is not considered a reliable method for sterilization. The biological test for the steam sterilization process utilizes a small vial of the bacteria *Geobacillus stearothermophilus*, a spore-forming type of bacteria capable of surviving and actually thriving in high temperature environments, but not pathogenic in humans. The proof that the steam sterilization process is effective lies in the ability to inactivate and kill the type of bacteria that could otherwise withstand the high heat used

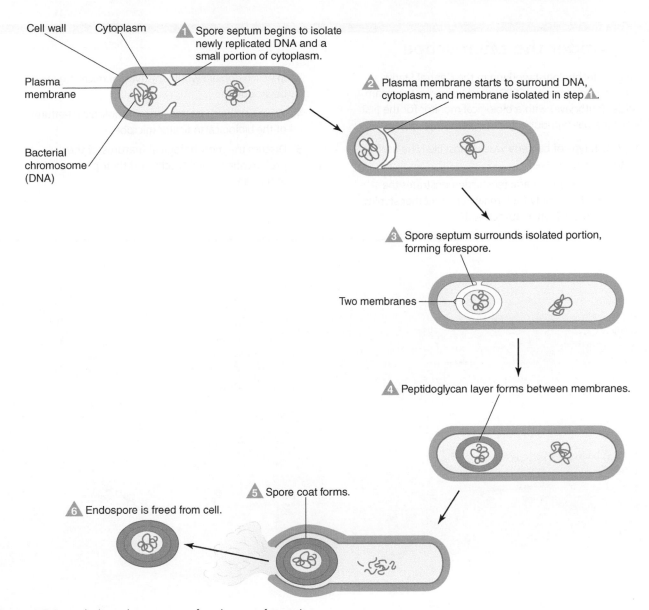

Cell wall   Cytoplasm

1 Spore septum begins to isolate newly replicated DNA and a small portion of cytoplasm.

Plasma membrane

2 Plasma membrane starts to surround DNA, cytoplasm, and membrane isolated in step **1**.

Bacterial chromosome (DNA)

3 Spore septum surrounds isolated portion, forming forespore.

Two membranes

4 Peptidoglycan layer forms between membranes.

5 Spore coat forms.

6 Endospore is freed from cell.

Figure 4-7 Sporulation, the process of endospore formation.

in steam sterilizers. Other bacterial species are used for validation of chemical sterilization processes and are discussed further in Chapter 21.

Chemical agents that kill most bacteria but not their spores are referred to as a high-level disinfectants and render items "surgically clean" or disinfected. This method of decontamination and disinfection may be used for orifices, areas of the body that have natural openings to the outside, such as the mouth or nose. The surgical technologist should remember that all instruments and equipment used in invasive surgical procedures must be sterile, or free from all microbes, including those that are capable of forming spores.

MICRO NOTES

"Give Up, We've Got You Outnumbered!"

Scientists in different specialties studying the human genome and various microbiomes have concluded that bacterial cells outnumber our "human" cells 10 to 1. In other words, of the trillions of cells that comprise a human, 90 percent are prokaryotes that live in our mouths, noses, stomachs, intestinal tracts, vaginas, and within every inch of our skin.

Under the Microscope

A surgical technologist working in the Central Sterile Processing Department (CSPD) is asked to run the steam sterilizer (autoclave) with a biological monitor for the first load of the day without any instrument trays or items.

1. Which type of bacteria would most likely be used to test the autoclave?

2. Which bacterial characteristic demonstrates the required capability for lethality and whether sterility was achieved when autoclaved?

3. In which domain would this type of microorganism be included?

4. What are the characteristic morphological features of the biological indicator microbes?

5. Discuss the morphological features of the prokaryotic bacterial cells and their pathogenicity in humans.

CHAPTER 5

The Eukaryotes

Learning Objectives

After completing the study of this chapter, you will be able to:

1. Define key terms.
2. Distinguish between prokaryotes and eukaryotes.
3. Discuss characteristics of eukaryotic cell structures.
4. Describe the various microbial relationships.
5. Compare and contrast the three types of eukaryotic microbes.
6. Apply critical thinking skills in relating chapter material to the surgical environment of care or broader global community.

Key Terms

Adenosine
    triphosphate (ATP)

Amoebas

Centrioles

Chloroplasts

Chromosomes

Ciliates

Diatoms

Dinoflagellates

Endosymbiotic

Fermentation

Flagellates

Lichens

Microtubules

Motility

Osmosis

Oxidative
    phosphorylation

Photosynthesizers

Ribosomes

Sporozoans

The Big Picture

The human body is very good at housekeeping chores. When foreign material or bacteria enter tissues following an injury, specialized cells attack the invader and try to isolate or remove it.

During your examination of the topics in this chapter, consider the following:

1. What type of cell is responsible for the task of engulfing foreign matter?
2. Which cell structures in eukaryotes differ from those found in prokaryotes?
3. Which types of eukaryotes can become opportunistic pathogens in humans?
4. What types of cellular transport mechanisms do eukaryotic cells use?

Clinical Significance Topic

A surgeon performing a breast biopsy procedure may request that the specimen be sent to pathology "fresh." This means that a fixative such as formalin would not be placed in the container with the specimen. One reason for sending breast tissue suspected of being cancerous this way (fresh) is to allow the pathologist to initiate hormonal receptor studies. There are various implications for the prognosis of how effective adjuvant cancer treatment modalities might be based on the hormonal receptor presence or absence in those eukaryotic breast cancer cells. The surgical technologist should verify with the surgeon how a biopsy specimen should be handled prior to handing it off the field and given to the circulating nurse.

Empire: Cellular, Domain: Eukarya

Throughout human history, man has sought to find order in his world. Natural curiosity led to exploration and a need to categorize and classify everything observable. Over time and with the aid of innovations such as the microscope, even the previously unseen entities of microbial life could be studied and classified. Living organisms have evolved over the millennia and the process of researching and understanding the microscopic world has evolved over time as well.

The complicated science of classifying microorganisms was discussed in Chapter 2, including the separation of microbial life into kingdoms and domains. The concept of an alternative classification model has developed that divides the domains into two larger groups called empires (cellular and viral) has emerged. The cellular empire contains domains of prokaryotes and eukaryotes, while a separate empire was established to cover viruses and other "non-living" substances such as prion proteins. This chapter discusses the eukaryotes and how they differ in form and function from prokaryotes. Viruses and other non-living microbes are discussed in Chapter 8.

Eukaryotic Cell Structure

Eukaryotes range from one-celled microbes to the largest and smallest living organisms on the planet: plants and animals, including humans. Eukaryotic cells are more complex when compared to prokaryotic cells and also include protozoa, fungi, and algae (green, brown, and red).

Eukaryotic cells range in size from 10 μm to 100 μm and unlike prokaryotes, have a true nucleus that is enclosed within a membrane. The specialized structures called organelles found within the cytoplasm of the cell are also membrane-bound and their cell walls are relatively simple in chemical composition (see Figure 5-1).

Plasma Membrane

The internal structures of the cell are held in place by the plasma membrane (also called the cell membrane) that encloses the cytoplasm and forms the outer boundary of the cell. It is only approximately 7 nm thick, yet it is a complex, orderly structure that keeps the cells intact.

The plasma membrane is composed of a combination of large molecules of proteins and phosphate-containing fat lipids called phospholipids. Cholesterol, another lipid, is also contained within the cell membrane and helps to stabilize and fortify the other phospholipids. Protein molecules are scattered throughout the framework of the cell. These molecules provide structural support and act as receptors that lock onto specific molecules within the salt-water solution that surrounds the cell (interstitial fluid)

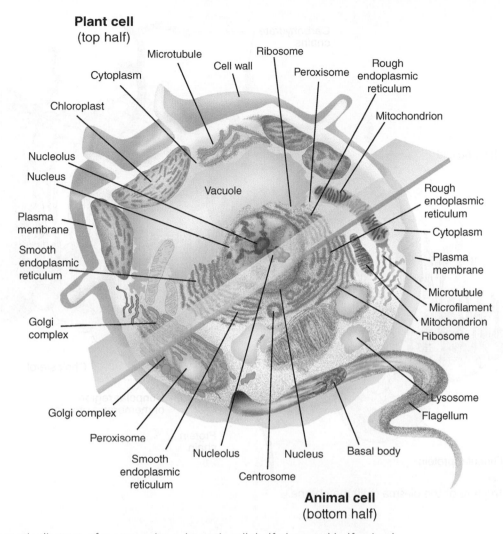

Plant cell
(top half)

Microtubule
Cytoplasm
Chloroplast
Cell wall
Ribosome
Peroxisome
Rough
endoplasmic
reticulum
Mitochondrion

Nucleolus
Nucleus
Plasma
membrane
Smooth
endoplasmic
reticulum

Vacuole

Rough
endoplasmic
reticulum
Cytoplasm
Plasma
membrane
Microtubule
Microfilament
Mitochondrion
Ribosome

Golgi
complex

Golgi complex
Peroxisome
Smooth
endoplasmic
reticulum
Nucleolus
Centrosome
Nucleus
Basal body

Lysosome
Flagellum

Animal cell
(bottom half)

Figure 5-1 Schematic diagram of a composite eukaryotic cell: half plant and half animal.

that comes into contact with them and creates a change in cell function (see Figure 5-2).

The plasma (cell) membrane functions to create selective permeability, meaning that only certain substances are allowed to enter and leave the cell. The molecules of the membrane are responsible for managing the inflow and outflow of waste products, nutrients, and other types of cell secretions.

Materials move across plasma membranes of both eukaryotes and prokaryotes by using two processes: active and passive. In active processes, the cell uses ATP (**adenosine triphosphate**) to move substances from an area of low concentration to an area of high concentration. In passive processes, substances move through the plasma membrane from an area of high concentration to an area of low concentration without the cell using any ATP energy. The passive processes include simple diffusion, facilitated diffusion, and **osmosis**. The process of osmosis is the focus of this discussion.

Osmosis is defined as the movement of solvent molecules across a selectively permeable cell membrane from an area that

has a high concentration of solvent molecules to an area of low concentration. The primary solvent in living things is water. Living cells are exposed to three kinds of osmotic solutions: isotonic, hypotonic, and hypertonic. An isotonic solution is one in which the concentration of solutes equals the number found inside a cell (the prefix iso- means "equal"). Water exits and enters the cell at the same rate, therefore the cell's water content is equivalent to the environment outside the cell wall.

A hypotonic solution means the concentration of solutes outside the cell is lower than inside the cell. The majority of bacteria live in hypotonic solutions but survive because the swelling created by the imbalance is contained by the cell wall. However, cells with a weak cell wall, such as Gram-negative bacteria, will rupture (burst) or in other words, osmotic lysis will occur due to the excessive intake of water by the cell. Certain types of antibiotics work in this manner. The antibiotic damages the cell wall. The bacterial cell that already contains a high concentration of solutes cannot control the additional water that enters the cell or contain the swelling, and the cell lyses (ruptures).

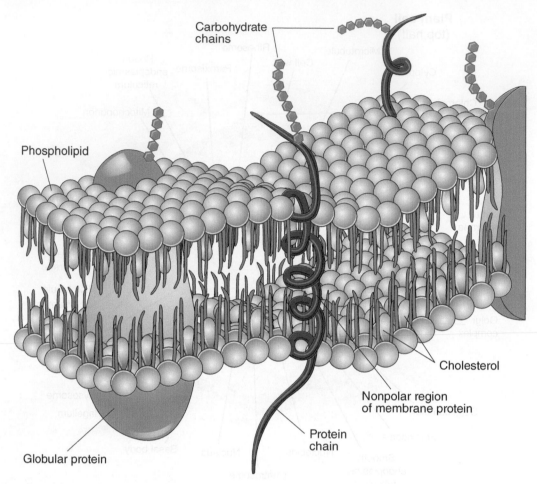

Carbohydrate chains

Phospholipid

Globular protein

Cholesterol

Nonpolar region of membrane protein

Protein chain

Figure 5-2 The structure of the plasma (cell) membrane.

A hypertonic solution is the opposite of hypotonic; the medium in which the cell lives has a higher concentration of solutes in the extracellular fluid than inside of the cell. The majority of bacterial cells that are placed in a hypertonic solution shrink as the cell wall collapses and the intracellular water exits the cell by osmosis, causing cell death.

The plasma membrane of eukaryotic cells, including animal cells, is covered by a glycocalyx, a protective layer of adhesive carbohydrates that strengthens the cell's surface and helps to attach cells together.

Cell Wall

The eukaryotic cell wall is found only in algae, fungi, and plant cells. It is primarily composed of cellulose but can contain other substances such as lignin and mineral salts (found in the cell wall of algae). Eukaryotic cell walls do not contain peptidoglycan (PGN), the framework of the prokaryotic cell wall. Peptidoglycan is a type of polysaccharide that is attached to short, cross-linked peptides. The polysaccharides that make up cell walls of eukaryotes are complex, insoluble simple sugar chains such as glucose.

The cell walls of molds contain some cellulose but the chief substance is chitin, which is the same organic substance that encases insects with an exoskeleton (outer shell).

Cell walls provide rigidity and shape that protect the internal structures of the eukaryotic cell. Only certain types of bacteria can break down cellulose. Termites have a symbiotic relationship with bacteria that live in their digestive system and allow them to break down wood (cellulose) for nutrition.

Protozoa may have alternative structures of calcium shells instead of cell walls. Another way that some protozoa maintain an osmotic balance in water environments is with a specialized compartment called a contractile vacuole that fills with water and then contracts to expel it. Additionally, some species of protozoa are surrounded with alveoli, small air sacs, instead of cell walls.

Amoebas are tiny, single-cell protozoa. Their structure consists of cytoplasm separated into two parts. The outer layer, or ectoplasm, is a clear, gel-like layer that acts like a cell membrane. The inner material is a watery, grainy substance called the endoplasm, which contains the organelles and one or more nuclei.

Nucleus

The nucleus is a small, spherical structure within the central portion of the eukaryotic cell. It acts as a control center for all activities of the organelles. The nucleus is surrounded by a nuclear envelope (nuclear membrane) that is composed of two separate membranes and encloses the cell material, called the nucleoplasm. The nucleoplasm contains two important structures: the nucleolus and the chromatin granules.

In the center of the nucleus is a dark area called the nucleolus. The nucleolus designs and oversees the construction of **ribosomes** within the nucleus. Once constructed, the ribosomes migrate through the nuclear envelope into the cytoplasm of the cell and begin the production of proteins.

Chromosomes are hereditary structures within the nucleus. A gene is the specific structure at a particular location on the chromosome that determines each individual trait of a species. When the DNA of a eukaryotic cell is not reproducing, it appears as a thread-like mass called chromatin, which is suspended in the nucleoplasm. The strands of chromatin condense into tight coils of chromosomes prior to the division of the cell. Chromatin granules are stick-like structures within the nucleus of the cell and are made of proteins and DNA (deoxyribonucleic acid). DNA determines the variations of the body, such as brown eyes instead of blue, tall instead of short, or large instead of small. DNA contains the "blueprint," or genetic information for the cell to produce the proteins needed for proper function and viability (see Figure 5-3). Ribonucleic acid (RNA), a nucleic acid that controls cellular protein synthesis and replaces DNA as a carrier of genetic codes in some viruses, is manufactured in the nucleolus before traveling to the cytoplasm of the cell.

Cytoplasm

The portion of the cell where the majority of the cell's work is performed is the cytoplasm, sometimes referred to as endoplasm or the "living material" of the cell. The organelles (little organs) contained in the cytoplasm actually perform the functions of the cell, which are controlled by the DNA.

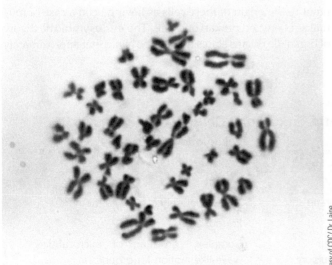

Courtesy of CDC/ Dr. Laine.

Figure 5-3 This image depicts a karyotype, or chromosomal profile, created by performing a chromosomal analysis on a sample of human peripheral blood, revealing the full complement of 46-chromosomes, or 23-pairs.

The cytoplasm matrix is merely a semifluid nutrient material located within the cell membrane and outside the nuclear membrane. The organelles directing the vital cellular functions within the cytoplasm include the endoplasmic reticulum (ER), ribosomes, Golgi complex, mitochondria, centrioles, microtubules, and lysosomes.

Endoplasmic Reticulum The ER is a system of membranes that form a series of tubules that twist through the cytoplasm, connecting it to the outside of the nucleus. The majority of ER has a rough appearance due to the presence of ribosomes attached to the surface of the structure (sometimes called rough ER). Smooth ER does not have ribosomes, appearing smooth to the observer when examining the cellular structures using a microscope. The endoplasmic reticulum is responsible for the manufacture of fats, carbohydrates, and proteins that comprise the cell membrane. The ribosomes are responsible for the synthesis of proteins that are needed for the cell to function and chemical synthesis and are carried from one part of the cytoplasm to another by the membranous canals. The ER is also responsible for the transport of nutrients to the nucleus.

Golgi Complex The Golgi complex or apparatus, also known as the Golgi body, consists of small, flattened sacs stacked atop one another, resembling a stack of pancakes. The apparatus connects and communicates with the ER. Small sacs called vesicles that contain protein molecules break away from the smooth ER and carry them to the Golgi complex. Proteins are synthesized and packaged into these vesicles so that they can be stored or transported to the cell membrane where they fuse with the cell membrane, open, and release their contents into the interstitial fluid.

Lysosomes Lysosomes are another type of small vesicles produced by the Golgi complex. They contain the enzyme lysozyme that lyses (destroys or dissolves) foreign substances ingested by the cell. The process of ingestion is called phagocytosis and is performed by a particular type of leukocyte (white blood cell) called a phagocyte. The enzymes also break down deteriorated native structures of the cell as well as destroy invading microbes. If the powerful enzymes were able to escape from the lysosomes into the cytoplasm, they could destroy the cell itself.

Mitochondria The mitochondria are the "power plants" of the cell and are composed of two membranous sacs, one contained inside the other. Mitochondria produce energy through use of ATP, the cell's main energy source. This process combines oxygen and simple sugars to create ATP from ADP (adenosine diphosphate) and inorganic phosphate through a process called **oxidative phosphorylation**. The mitochondria are responsible for the formation of ATP by the process known as aerobic or cellular respiration. During cellular respiration, energy is released from glucose molecules (simple sugars) by enzymes that use oxygen to provide energy for the other cellular functions. The number of mitochondria present in the cytoplasm varies according to the functions and specific activities performed by the eukaryotic cell.

Centrioles Centrioles lie perpendicularly (at a right or 90° angle) to the nucleus. Their main purpose is to form spindle fibers that aid in cell division. The process of eukaryotic cell division is called mitosis, which results in two "daughter cells" with the same number of chromosomes as the parent cell. Two centrioles exist within every cell and are arranged so that they lie at right angles to each other. The centrioles may also be involved in the manufacture of eukaryotic flagella and cilia because their protein composition is similar to the centriole.

Flagella and Cilia Some types of eukaryotic cells have long, thin structures attached to the outside of the cell called flagella or cilia. Their whipping motion provides the cell a means of **motility** to travel through liquid environments. Therefore, the flagella are said to be an organelle of locomotion or cell movement. Cells may have one or two flagella located at the poles of the cell.

Cilia are very fine, hair-like extensions on the surfaces of some cells. They are much shorter than flagella and more numerous around the outside of the cell. Cilia move with a coordinated, rhythmic movement. Examples of cilia are those found on some types of protozoa and particular types of human cells such as the epithelial cells that line the bronchus.

Eukaryotic flagella are more complex than those of the prokaryotic cells. They consist of multiple **microtubules**, unlike the prokaryote's flagella that consist of only two protein building blocks. The individual, single prokaryotic flagellum rotates, whereas the eukaryotic flagellum moves back and forth in a wave-like motion (see Table 5-1).

Inclusion Bodies

Inclusion bodies are cellular structures that are commonly found in prokaryotic cells and are used for storage of inorganic substances, carbon compounds, or energy. Inclusion bodies in eukaryotic cells are an abnormal finding and may indicate the presence of a viral invader or even a genetic disorder. Numerous animal species have been found to have inclusion bodies in various tissue cells. Scientists have discovered several types of inclusion bodies in humans including:

- Russell Bodies: found in plasma cells; thought to be a possible cause of cancer or alternately, an indicator of the presence of cancer
- Negri Bodies: found in nerve cells of individuals exposed to the rabies virus
- Guarnieri Bodies: found in cells of individuals exposed to vaccinia (smallpox)
- Cowdry Bodies: type A is associated with herpes viruses and type B is associated with polio

Microbial Relationships

The focus in microbiology is chiefly on the smallest members of the eukaryotic domain; however, of great interest is how both eukaryotic and prokaryotic microbes interact with possibly the most complex eukaryotic organisms—humans. Symbiosis is the relationship between two species living in close approximation, including those living in or on the other.

Mutualism or a mutualistic relationship is between two organisms where both parties benefit, as described in the previous section. When one species benefits from an association and the other species is unaffected (neither harmed nor benefitted), it is termed commensalism or a commensal relationship. These interspecies living arrangements may be beneficial to one (invader) and detrimental to the other (host), and this is called parasitism or a parasitic relationship.

Endosymbiotic Theory

Unicellular eukaryotes have existed for millennia and have found their way to nearly every corner of the planet. Theories point to the origin of these cells as having been a case of mutualism between prokaryotic cells. The **endosymbiotic** theory of organelle origins states that it is possible that approximately

Table 5-1 **Comparison Between Prokaryotic and Eukaryotic Cells**

Characteristic	Prokaryotic	Eukaryotic
Cell division	Binary fission	Mitosis
Membrane-bound organelles	Absent	Present
Nucleus	No true nucleus; nuclear membrane absent	True nucleus enclosed by a membrane
Nucleolus	Absent	Present
Flagella	Simple, consisting of two protein building blocks; rotates for propulsion	Complex, consisting of microtubules; wave-like motion for propulsion
Cell wall	Complex with peptidoglycan	Simple
DNA	Circular chromosome, singular; no chromatin	Linear chromosome, multiple; chromatin

1.5 billion years ago, prokaryotes combined with one another and began to work in unison, changed their structures and eventually evolved into what we now recognize as the eukaryotic cell structures such as mitochondria. Researchers propose that this happened when one prokaryotic bacterium (or possibly an archaea) ingested another and instead of destroying it, the consumed microbe took up residence in its host and began a mutually beneficial relationship—endosymbiosis. They believe that this theory explains why mitochondria developed and compartmentalized within the cytoplasm, giving rise to the new type of microbe—the eukaryote. This event is theorized to have been a singular incident from which all mitochondria in every subsequent organism is descended.

Scientists studying archaea also speculate about the ways in which these "new" microbes may have combined with cyanobacteria to create the first eukaryotic **photosynthesizers**. From that process, plastids developed. The organelles called chloroplasts present in eukaryotic plant cells are derived from plastids. Researchers point to the closer similarities in the DNA of mitochondria and **chloroplasts** to prokaryotic DNA than to the eukaryote genome. They also note that the organelles are enclosed in inner membranes and they divide and reproduce by binary fission, the same way prokaryotes do.

Scientific discoveries and theories come and go quickly as the branches of scientific sub-specialization direct their attention and advanced technological tools to our shared microbial ancestors. In recent years, researchers have also been reviewing, and in some cases revising, classification models after discovery of ultra-small eukaryotes less than 20 μm in size. These formerly unknown microbes break the previously accepted morphological criteria of single-cell eukaryotes always being much larger than tiny bacteria and archaea.

Eukaryotic Microbes

Research of microbial populations has been driven in large part by the need to understand, treat, and prevent disease based on these relationships with our microbial partners in life. Three of the eukaryotic microbial populations that we have somewhat complicated relationships with are protozoa, algae, and fungi.

Protozoa

The name protozoa comes from Greek meaning "first animal." A single microbe is a protozoan. An individual protozoan is typically extremely small, typically ranging from 10 μm to 200 μm, although there have been some protozoa that are found to be visible to the naked eye, measuring nearly 3 mm. Fossilized remains measuring 20 mm were also discovered. Scientists have identified more than 50,000 species.

Protozoa are classified as heterotrophs, relying on food sources of organic and inorganic materials. They use specialized cellular organelles called vacuoles for digestion. Protozoa have a nucleus, a basic criterion for being classified as eukaryotic, and some species have multiple nuclei.

They have developed mitochondria for energy production but relatively primitive cell walls. They can live solo lives or in large populations. Water is a key requirement for protozoa. When conditions are unfavorable, such as when there is a lack of moisture as in environmental drought conditions or tissue dehydration, they are able to enter into a dormant phase with a protective coating called a cyst (see Figure 5-4).

Movement or motility for protozoa is accomplished by the use of flagella, cilia, or pseudopods (false feet). Types of motile protozoa include: **flagellates**, **amoebas**, **ciliates**, and **sporozoans**. There is some debate in scientific communities regarding these classifications and species relationships. Diseases caused by protozoa are discussed in later sections.

Algae

Algae or the singular alga, like protozoa, require wet environments for survival. Many species of algae exist and include both single-celled algae and multicellular forms such as seaweed. Most species are classified as autotrophs (self-feeders) through photosynthesis performed by organelles in their cytoplasm called chloroplasts or plastids. Chloroplasts contain pigments that determine the color of the algae: green, red, or brown.

Cyanobacteria are prokaryotic microbes that have been incorrectly referred to as blue-green algae. Newer research models point to the possibility that billions of years ago cyanobacteria, which utilizes photosynthesis for energy, partnered with primitive forms of eukaryotic algae and evolved into their modern cell structures.

Red and brown algae are mostly marine species, whereas green algae may be the ancestors of plants on land. Symbiotic combinations of algae and fungi have created species of **lichens** that can withstand hostile environmental conditions such as deserts and extreme cold.

Sea plankton, also called phytoplankton, are microbes of mainly cyanobacteria, but they include algae and are essential parts of the ocean's food chain. Two forms of algal phytoplankton are **diatoms** and **dinoflagellates** (see Figure 5-5).

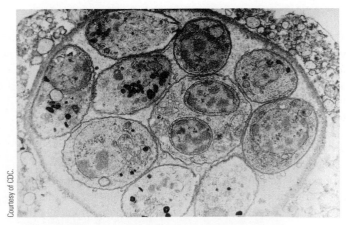

Courtesy of CDC.

Figure 5-4 Transmission electron micrograph (TEM) reveals *Toxoplasma gondii*, a protozoan parasite that forms cysts in skeletal muscle, myocardium, brain, and eyes. These cysts may remain throughout the life of the host.

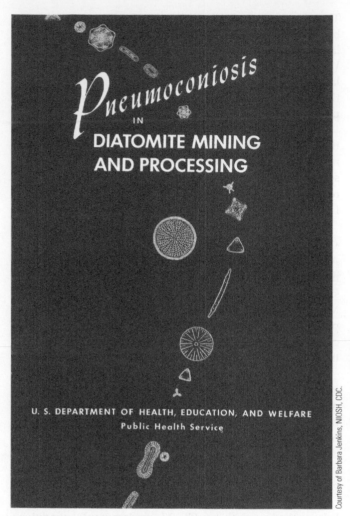

Figure 5-5 1958 US Public Health Service (USPHS) report cover, *"Pneumoconiosis in Diatomite Mining and Processing"* depicting just a few of many forms of diatoms. The report contained results of a study of miners who were exposed to airborne particulates in diatomaceous earth mining and processing plants and suffered respiratory, ocular, and dermal disorders.

These species have a delicately impressive appearance when viewed microscopically. These lacy organisms are responsible for destructive algal "blooms" in bodies of water such as lakes and streams that kill large populations of sea plants and creatures. Overgrowth of algae in ponds on a smaller scale is termed pond scum. In larger areas, the cause is usually large amounts of nitrogen from fertilizer used on land that gain access to waterways and pour into lakes, river deltas, and ocean waters. This overabundance of nitrogen causes a population explosion of the algae, and they harm marine life by depriving them of oxygen and sometimes by producing toxins released into the water supply. Algae are typically not directly responsible for disease in humans; however, fish and shellfish take in the toxins released from the algae and humans consume the fish and shellfish, thereby indirectly causing illness through contamination of the food chain.

Fungi

When fungi are mentioned, what comes to our minds is almost always the various types we see growing in dark, moist areas that we harvest for food called mushrooms. The word fungus (singular for fungi) is the Latin word for mushroom. The medical prefix myco- is from the Greek word for mushroom. While mushrooms are indeed fungi, the more predominant forms of fungi are microbial and known as molds, mildews, and yeasts. Scientists theorize that there are at least a million species of fungi and have identified approximately 100,000, of which only approximately 400 species are known to cause disease in humans. Conversely, 5000 species of fungi cause diseases in plants (see Figure 5-6).

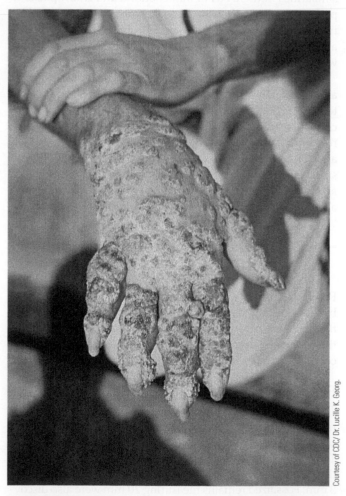

Figure 5-6 Brazilian patient's right hand infected with *Phialophora verrucosa* fungal organisms.

Even though fungi have been considered plants, they are classified as heterotrophs, not autotrophs. They cannot photosynthesize their energy from the sun and, in fact, often grow very well in dark places. Enzymes are released from fungi that break down organic matter into absorbable nutrients. For humans, we utilize yeasts to produce bread and alcohol by a process called **fermentation**.

The first antibiotic, penicillin, was created from a type of mold. Yeasts produce spores but molds create filaments called hyphae, which tangle together into a mycelium. Fungi can take on either a round or a mycelium form, depending on the environmental conditions faced. The spores released by fungi and mycelium fragments released from mold are responsible for allergic reactions for many people (see Figure 11-1). Diseases attributed to fungi are further discussed in Chapter 11.

MICRO NOTES

"The Needs of the Many Outweigh the Needs of the One."

Apoptosis is the term for biological suicide. Eukaryotic human cells release proteins from mitochondria, causing organelles to break down. The cells break into pieces and are consumed by phagocytes. Why do they kill themselves? If cells have DNA damage or are infected by certain substances, they sacrifice themselves for the good of all. If you are a fan of the 1960s science fiction series *Star Trek* or its numerous spin-off movies and series, you may remember the quote from Mr. Spock when he chooses to sacrifice himself by performing a selfless act to save the lives of the entire ship's crew.

 ## Under the Microscope

During certain surgical procedures, such as those for malignancy, the surgeon may request that sterile water be used for irrigation instead of normal saline following excision of the cancerous mass.

1. How is water different from saline in terms of its tonicity?

2. In this scenario, what effect on the residual malignant cells is the surgeon trying to achieve by use of the sterile water?

3. Compare and contrast the osmotic reactions that occur between eukaryotic and prokaryotic cells when placed in hypertonic or hypotonic solutions.

4. Discuss the other differences between eukaryotic cells and prokaryotic cells.

CHAPTER 6

Microbial Viability and Growth

Learning Objectives

After completing the study of this chapter, you will be able to:

1. Define key terms.
2. Describe the conditions or physical requirements necessary for microbial growth.
3. Discuss methods used in the laboratory to determine bacterial population size.
4. Discuss the chemical requirements for microbial survival.
5. Describe biofilms.
6. Apply critical thinking skills in relating chapter material to the surgical environment of care or broader global community.

Key Terms

Alkaline
Autoinducers
Biofilms
Bioleaching
Denatured

Desiccator
Equilibrium
Gas gangrene
Granulation tissue
Inoculum

Optimum
Pheromones
Plasmolysis
Purines
Pyrimidines

Smelting
Solute

The Big Picture

Just as with most living beings, bacteria require the proper conditions to grow, thrive, and reproduce. Rarely are bacterial cells found alone; so, you could say they are social beings.

During your examination of the topics in this chapter, consider the following:

1. Which types of bacteria prefer optimal or extreme environmental temperatures?

2. What are the specific categories of oxygen preference or requirements for bacteria?

3. What is meant by generation time in the microbiology lab setting?

4. How do bacteria communicate with one another?

Clinical Significance Topic

When surgeons encounter an infected area during a surgical procedure, they may ask for culture tubes to swab the fluid or tissue. Two samples are taken so that separate processing can be performed in the microbiology lab under aerobic and anaerobic conditions. These collected samples should be sent to the lab immediately and not left sitting on the back table until the end of the case. If the organisms are anaerobic, which many that are found deep in body tissues tend to be, prolonged exposure may kill the organisms before they can be incubated and processed for culture and sensitivity results. Pass off the culture tubes and advise your circulating nurse from where they were collected and that they need to go to the lab immediately.

Requirements for Microbial Viability

When scientists discuss microbial growth, they are referring to the number of cells in a culture sample, not the growth in the size of individual cells. Microbial growth means the cells are increasing in number and forming colonies. A colony may consist of cell populations that number in the billions.

This chapter discusses the requirements for cell growth, maintenance, and division. The growth requirements can be divided into two categories namely physical and chemical. The physical requirements include temperature, pH, and osmotic pressure. The chemical requirements include carbon sources, nitrogen, sulfur, phosphorus, trace elements, oxygen, and growth factors.

Physical Requirements

Temperature, pH, and osmotic pressure are essential elements for the growth of a microorganism, and in order to study them, microbiologists manipulate these factors to sustain growth.

Temperature

Microbes are placed into one of three categories based on the range of temperature in which growth can occur: psychrophiles that thrive in cold temperatures; mesophiles that grow best at moderate temperatures or temperatures that are close to the normal temperature of the human body (37°C); and thermophiles, which are heat-loving microbes.

Each type of microbe has a range of temperatures referred to as minimum (lowest temperature at which the species will grow), **optimum** (temperature at which the best growth occurs), and maximum growth temperatures (highest temperature at which growth is possible). A graph of a particular microbial colony's temperature range typically reveals that the optimal growth temperature is near the top of the maximum limit. Temperatures above the optimum result in a rapid decrease in microbial growth. This most likely happens because the heat has inactivated or **denatured** the enzymes of the cells.

Two groups of organisms are capable of growth at 0°C: psychrotrophs and psychrophiles, also known as cryophiles. Psychrotrophs have an optimum growth at temperatures from 20°C to 30°C and cannot grow in temperatures above 40°C. Psychrotrophs are more common than psychrophiles and are the most likely to be responsible for the spoilage of food in the low-temperature refrigerator because they grow well at refrigerator temperatures. Food scientists recognize that 65 to 70 percent of spoilage of raw milk products is from the species *Pseudomonas*.

The second group of cold-loving microbes, psychrophiles, can grow at 0°C, but the optimum growth temperature is approximately 15°C. The microbes placed in this group are highly sensitive to higher temperatures and will not grow in temperatures above 25°C. The researchers discovered that these cold-loving microbes contain higher concentrations of polyunsaturated fats in their cell membranes than do warmer climate microbes. The polyunsaturated fats allow the cell membranes to remain more flexible with temperature changes, thereby preventing rupture.

Mesophiles, the most common type of microbe, have an optimum growth at temperatures in the range of 25°C to 40°C. Many species of bacteria that are pathogenic to humans have an optimum temperature of 37°C (98.6°F, or normal body temperature) that allows them to survive in our host cells.

Thermophiles are microbes that can grow at high temperatures. Many of these microbes have an optimum growth temperature of 50°C to 60°C, approximately the temperature of hot water from an average household faucet. This optimum temperature range can also be achieved in sun-heated soil and thermal springs. The proteins found in microbial thermophiles are thermophilic and able to withstand the high temperatures without denaturing. Some species can actually partially denature at or above 80°C and then re-nature when more favorable conditions return.

Certain archaea have an optimum growth temperature of 80°C or higher. These bacteria are referred to as hyperthermophiles or extreme thermophiles. Most of these types of microbes live in hot springs that are fueled by volcanic activity such as deep-sea hydrothermal vents. Sulfur, discussed later in the section about chemical requirements, is highly important in the metabolic activities of hyperthermophiles.

pH Levels

Most bacteria grow best between a pH level of 6.5 and 7.5. This accounts for why foods are not destroyed by acids produced by bacterial fermentation. A small percentage of bacteria are acidophiles, which are able to grow in an acid environment of pH 4. An example is *Acidithiobacillus thiooxidans*, which grows best at a pH of 2 to 4.

Massachusetts Institute of Technology (MIT) created "Mission 2015: Biodiversity," which involves the problems and solutions of the many ecological communities, also called biomes present on planet Earth. One of their proposed solutions for reducing pollution from the mining industry and from nuclear waste sites is a process called **bioleaching**. The process utilizes acidophile organisms, chiefly *Acidithiobacillus thiooxidans* and *Leptospirillum* bacteria, to break down metal or mineral ores in safer, non-polluting ways than the traditional method of smelting which liberates toxic chemicals into the air. These "rock-munching" acidophilic microbes show promise in also breaking down dangerous stores of uranium ore that threaten pollution of waterways through soil erosion.

The process of bioleaching yields 80 to 90 percent of copper from ore at an estimated half the cost of traditional methods. The technology industry has exploded in the past few decades and, with it, so has the need for copper used in most electronic devices (e.g., computers, circuit boards, cell phones) due to its excellent properties of electrical conduction. Copper that exists in low-grade ore that would previously be inaccessible through traditional mining and **smelting** methods is made accessible through bioleaching (see Figure 6-1.)

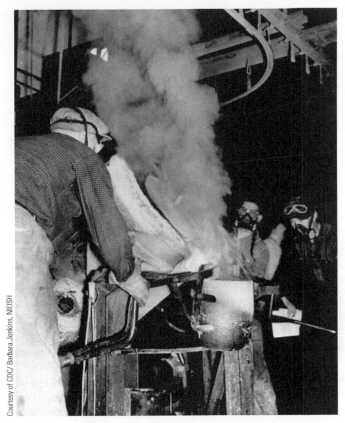

Courtesy of CDC/ Barbara Jenkins, NIOSH

Figure 6-1 This historical photograph was provided by the Center for Disease Control's (CDC) National Institute for Occupational Safety and Health (NIOSH). The image depicts three men working in a foundry, processing molten metal. All three men were properly wearing respirators, although only two had their goggles in place. In the enclosed building, the indoor air pollutants given off as a result of the smelting process were quite visible.

Alkalinity also inhibits microbial growth but is not used as a means of preserving food. Alkaliphiles grow best under **alkaline** conditions, usually at a pH of 8. *Thermomicrobium roseum*, found in hot springs, thrives in a pH of 8.2 to 8.5. Scientists have successfully described the full genome of *Bacillus halodurans* C-125, an alkaliphilic species used extensively in industrial production of detergents. These detergents work by utilizing the extracellular enzymes: protease, amylase, cellulase, and lipase commonly produced by the bacilli.

Bacteria that are grown in the laboratory usually produce acids that will interfere with growth. To counteract the acid, chemical buffers such as peptones, amino acids, and phosphate salts are added to the growth medium. The chemical nutrient phosphorus is derived from phosphate salts.

Osmotic Pressure

Microbes obtain most of their required nutrients from water in the environment. Water, required for growth, comprises approximately 70 percent of the cell. A basic generalized correlation made about osmotic movement is that water follows salt. High osmotic pressure has a detrimental effect on a cell by causing the passage of intracellular water to the exterior, extracellular space. For a cell that is in a hypertonic solution, cellular water passes through the plasma membrane to the area of high **solute** concentration. The resulting osmotic loss of water is called plasmolysis, in which the plasma membrane shrinks and pulls away from the cell wall (see Figure 6-2).

Plasmolysis inhibits the growth of the cell, and this is important in the preservation of foods. By adding solutes such as salt or sugar to a solution to increase the osmotic pressure, water is drawn out of the microbial cells and prevents their growth. Salted fish, salted beef jerky, and honey are preserved through plasmolysis.

Some microbes, called extreme or obligate halophiles, require a high salt concentration for growth. For example, microbes from the high-saline waters of the Dead Sea require approximately 30 percent salt for survival. The inoculating loop used in a laboratory to transfer these microbes must be dipped in a high-salt solution before use. Many microbes are facultative halophiles and do not require a high salt concentration but can grow at a concentration of up to 2 percent.

A low osmotic pressure, hypotonic solution such as distilled water allows water to enter higher salt internal space of the cell, rather than exit it. Microbes that exhibit a weak cell wall are subject to lysis, or breaking apart, when placed in a hypotonic solution.

Chemical Requirements

The chemical requirements of microbes include an energy source as well as carbon, nitrogen, sulfur, phosphorus, trace elements, oxygen, and growth factors.

The classification of microbes based on their sources of energy and carbon was discussed in Chapter 4. To review, microbes are given the following classifications based on those general or combined sources of energy and carbon:

- Autotroph
  - Phototroph
    - Photoautotroph
  - Chemotroph
    - Chemoautotroph
- Heterotroph (also known as organotroph)
  - Photoheterotroph
  - Chemoheterotroph
- Lithotroph
  - Photolithotroph
  - Chemolithotroph

Carbon

Carbon is the basic building block for life on Earth. Its production and use by every living being is described as the carbon cycle. Within the carbon cycle are sources and reservoirs or "sinks" that produce and use or accumulate and store carbon dioxide. Examples of carbon dioxide sources include forests, fossil fuels, oceans, and the atmosphere. Sources are things that provide more carbon than they use. Conversely, carbon dioxide sinks include forests as well. Additional sinks are plants and animals. A sink is anything that uses or accumulates and stores more carbon (or carbon dioxide) than it produces. This demonstrates the way in which carbon, as the fundamental building block, is constantly recycled and how ubiquitous (present or found everywhere) it is.

Carbon is necessary for the production of proteins, carbohydrates, lipids, and nucleic acids—from which DNA is formed. Along with water, it is one of the most important requirements for microbial growth. It is a requirement for the synthesis of all the organic compounds of a cell. Approximately 50 percent of the dry weight of a bacterium is carbon.

Hypertonic solution	Hypotonic solution	Isotonic solution
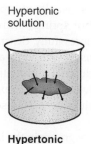		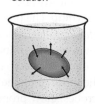
Hypertonic solution (seawater) A red blood cell will shrink and wrinkle because water molecules are moving out of the cell.	**Hypotonic solution (freshwater)** A red blood cell will swell and burst because water molecules are moving into the cell.	**Isotonic solution (human blood serum)** A red blood cell remains unchanged because the movement of water molecules into and out of the cell is the same.

Figure 6-2 Movement of water molecules in isotonic, hypertonic, and hypotonic solutions. Osmotic pressure is the pressure on a cell membrane exerted by solutions inside and outside the cell. A solution that is isotonic has the same osmotic pressure as the solution in the cell. The cell is unchanged. A hypertonic solution has greater osmotic pressure than the solution within the cell, causing the cell to shrink (crenate) because water is drawn out of the cell. A hypotonic solution has osmotic pressure lower than that of the solution in the cell, causing water to be drawn into the cell and causing the cell to swell.

Nitrogen, Sulfur, and Phosphorus

Approximately 14 percent of the dry weight of a bacterial cell is nitrogen and 4 percent is sulfur and phosphorus. A large amount of nitrogen and some sulfur are required for the synthesis of protein. Nitrogen and phosphorus are required for the synthesis of DNA, RNA, and ATP, the molecule required for the transfer and storage of intracellular chemical energy.

Microorganisms use nitrogen to form the amino acids of proteins. To accomplish amino acid synthesis, some bacteria will decompose protein-containing substances and use the amino acids to synthesize proteins. Other bacteria obtain nitrogen from ammonium ions that are found in organic cellular material. A few types of bacteria derive nitrogen from nitrates, chemically stable forms of inorganic nitrogen.

Photosynthetic microorganisms known as cyanobacteria use gaseous nitrogen (N_2) obtained from the atmosphere in a process called nitrogen fixation. Some microorganisms that use this method live in symbiosis with the roots of legumes, such as soybeans, peas, beans, and alfalfa. The atmospheric nitrogen is used by both the bacterium and the plant for their nutritional requirements.

Bacteria use sulfur to synthesize sulfur-containing amino acids and vitamins such as thiamine. Bacteria can use natural sources of sulfur such as sulfate ions and hydrogen sulfide.

Phosphorus is required for the synthesis of nucleic acids and phospholipids, which are constituents of the cell membrane. It is also part of the energy bonds of ATP. A primary source of phosphorus is phosphate ions.

Trace Elements

The trace elements—referring to the fact that only small amounts are required by microbes for normal enzyme functioning—are iron, copper, zinc, and molybdenum. Because the amount of trace elements present in the tap water used to create various culture media is sufficient, additional amounts are not required to be added to a culture medium.

Oxygen

It is often assumed that oxygen is a necessary ingredient for life to sustain itself. As previously discussed in Chapter 4, this is not true for all organisms. Many exist in low levels of oxygen or require no oxygen and are actually harmed by it. Most heterotrophic organisms obtain oxygen from the same molecule that serves the dual purpose of being a carbon source. Some oxygen is also obtained from water.

Aerobes or aerobic microorganisms are the terms used to describe microbes that use oxygen to produce their required nutrients. Anaerobes or anaerobic microorganisms do not need oxygen. Obligate aerobes require sufficient oxygen concentrations to synthesize the nutrients needed to live and reproduce. Microaerophiles require oxygen and are classified as aerobic, but they grow best in the presence of a much lower level of oxygen. For example, in a test tube or on a Petri dish, the microbes will grow below the surface of the medium where small amounts of oxygen have penetrated; they will not grow in the oxygen-rich environment at the surface level of the medium. Microaerophiles produce the toxic substances superoxide free radicals and peroxides when placed under oxygen-rich conditions.

Facultative anaerobes have developed the ability to continue growth in the absence of oxygen. The facultative microbe will use oxygen when present but uses the process of fermentation or anaerobic respiration for growth when oxygen is absent. This is accomplished by the ability of the microbe to substitute other electron acceptors, such as nitrate, for oxygen. The disadvantage is that energy is not produced as efficiently in the absence of oxygen.

Obligate anaerobes are bacteria that cannot use molecular (atmospheric) oxygen and are harmed by its presence. The bacteria obtain oxygen atoms from water. Aerotolerant anaerobes grow without oxygen but are not killed by its presence. Many of these types of microbes ferment carbohydrates into lactic acid. The lactic acid prevents the growth of aerobic microbes and establishes a favorable environment for lactic acid producers such as *Lactobacillus*, which is used in the production of acidic fermented foods such as pickles and cheese. A laboratory culture is handled and grown the same as any other culture; however, the microbes make no use of the atmospheric oxygen. These bacteria possess superoxide dismutase (SOD), which neutralizes the toxic forms of oxygen.

As mentioned, aerobic metabolism produces highly toxic by-products and microbes have developed enzymes to protect themselves from destruction. All aerobes produce SOD, which destroys superoxide free radicals formed during normal microbial respiration. SOD converts the free radicals into oxygen and hydrogen peroxide.

Hydrogen peroxide is also toxic; therefore, microbes have developed enzymes to neutralize it. The first type of enzyme is catalase, which converts hydrogen peroxide to oxygen and water. The action of catalase is easily recognizable. When hydrogen peroxide is added to a colony of catalase-producing bacterial cells, oxygen bubbles are formed and released. This is also evident when hydrogen peroxide is placed in a wound in human tissue whose cells contain catalase. Another enzyme produced by microbes is peroxidase. Peroxidase also breaks down hydrogen peroxide but differs from catalase in that it does not produce oxygen.

A third toxic substance is hydroxyl radical, another intermediate form of oxygen formed in the cellular cytoplasm when hydrogen peroxide reacts with metal ions. No enzymes are produced to destroy hydroxyl radical, but when it comes into contact with any organic compound, it immediately reacts and is neutralized.

It is important for surgical personnel to understand the difference between the aerobic and anaerobic microbial species. For example, when free oxygen is not available, particular diseases caused by anaerobic bacteria, such as tetanus, lockjaw, and **gas gangrene** (all caused by a species of *Clostridium*), can develop deep in surgical wounds. Therefore, such wounds may be kept open and exposed to air, killing the anaerobic bacteria and allowing the wounds to heal by second or third intention (see Figure 6-3). Second intention healing is when **granulation tissue** fills in a wound from the bottom upward (see Figure 6-4). Third intention healing is often referred to as delayed primary closure and involves sub-

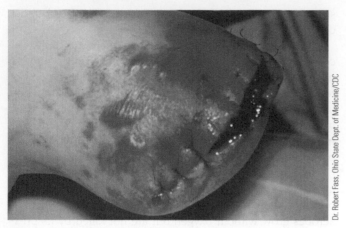

Dr. Robert Fass, Ohio State Dept. of Medicine/CDC

Figure 6-3 Post-operative view of a patient's leg that had undergone an amputation after having a cellulitis infection, also known as clostridial myonecrosis or gas gangrene.

sequent closure of a wound following granulation formation and resolution of bacterial contamination.

Growth Factors

Many microbes can synthesize compounds, amino acids and nucleotides, needed to build macromolecules. The molecules are synthesized from the elements previously discussed. Some essential organic compounds however cannot be synthesized by certain types of microbes and must be obtained directly from the environment. These organic compounds are called growth factors. Growth factors can include amino acids, **pyrimidines**, vitamins, and **purines** depending on what the organism cannot synthesize internally.

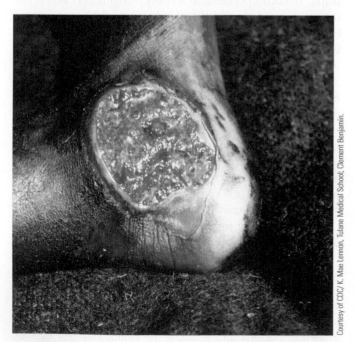

Courtesy of CDC/ K. Mae Lennon, Tulane Medical School; Clement Benjamin.

Figure 6-4 Left foot of patient in New Guinea with an acute tropical ulcer following debridement. Note healthy, pink granulation tissue lining the ulcerative base.

Microorganisms vary widely in their requirements for growth factors. For example, *Escherichia coli* requires no growth factors but *Leuconostoc citrovorum*, a lactic acid bacterium responsible for the fermentation of cabbage, requires all 20 amino acids, several purines, pyrimidines, and 10 vitamins.

Microbial Growth

Bacterial growth, as discussed previously, refers to an increase in the number of bacteria in a microbial colony, not the size of the individual cells. Most bacterial species reproduce by individual cellular binary fission. A few reproduce through the process of budding. The discussion of generation time and bacterial growth presumes that the growth occurs through a most common method of binary fission rather than less common method of budding.

Generation Time

The time required for a bacterial cell to divide and double its population numbers is called generation or doubling time. Therefore, one cell's division produces two cells, and then two cells produce four cells, four doubles to eight, and so forth. The generation time varies with each type of organism and with the environmental conditions that can change, such as temperature and water. The generation time for most bacteria is approximately 1 to 3 hours. A very large number of cells would be produced if binary fission continues uncontrolled. After 20 generations, an initial solitary cell could increase to more than 1 million cells in a matter of hours. An example of a bacterium with a relatively slow generation time is *Mycobacterium leprae*, the causal agent of leprosy. This microorganism has a doubling time of approximately 2 weeks within the infected tissue.

Due to the ability of most bacteria to grow rapidly, a disease can quickly spread from being a local or regional infection, such as a surgical site infection (SSI), to a systemic infection involving multiple body systems and ultimately threatening the life of the patient.

Logarithmic Graphing of Microbial Growth

Logarithms are used to plot large numbers of growth on a graph as opposed to arithmetically plotting the information. A plotted graph of cell growth versus time using an arithmetic scale (plotting cell numbers directly) would reveal a sharply rising curve which would not be practical for reporting large numbers of cells. A better method is to express the cell numbers as powers of 2. For example, the growth of 16 cells in 1 hour would be reported as 2^4 (or $2 \times 2 \times 2 \times 2 = 16$). Graphing the logarithmic number would result in a straight-line graph, which is much more practical. The scale represents a doubling in cell numbers, and the time needed for the doubling is easier to read. In a more practical sense, it is better to use $\log_{10}$ when graphing the growth curve. Again, a straight line will be plotted on the graph, allowing a large number of cells to be plotted using relatively little graph space.

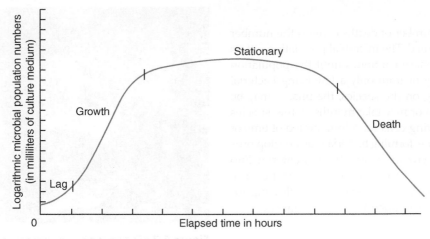

Figure 6-5 Population growth curve of living organisms. The logarithm of the number of bacteria per milliliter of medium is plotted against time. (A) Lag phase. (B) Logarithmic growth phase. (C) Stationary phase. (D) Death phase.

Phases of Bacterial Growth

There are four phases of bacterial growth: lag, log (logarithmic growth), stationary, and death. A bacterial growth curve can be plotted that shows the growth of cells over a period of time related to the four phases (see Figure 6-5).

Lag Phase

For a short period of time, as cells become accustomed to their environment (culture medium in a Petri dish or culture tube) and make intercellular adjustments, the number of cells changes very little, if at all. The cells do not immediately reproduce in the medium. This period of little or no cell division is called the lag phase and can last for 1 hour to several days. However, the cells are not dormant. The microbes are experiencing intense microbial activity involving DNA and enzyme synthesis and preparing for colony or population growth.

Log Phase

The next step of the process is when cells begin to divide and enter the logarithmic growth phase or log phase, also called the exponential growth phase. Cellular reproduction and the metabolic activity of individual microbes are at their peak during this phase. The straight, upward line on a generation time graph, as discussed in the previous section, represents the log phase.

During the log phase, microbes are most vulnerable to unfavorable conditions. This is when antibiotics are most effective because they interfere with the microbial steps of growth and are harmful to the cells.

As a comparative, the world population of humans is in the log phase of its growth curve. The generation time is approximately 35 years. Populations of various organisms, including *Homo sapiens* do not indefinitely continue in this phase of growth unless the food supply, waste products, and birth rate are constant and controlled. More likely, events such as food shortages, war, build-up of toxic waste products, and the spread of diseases (from endemic to pandemic) will force the world population to enter the stationary growth phase and hopefully not proceed to the resultant population death phase.

Stationary Phase

Eventually, the growth rate slows and the number of microbial deaths equals the number of new cells that are produced. This phase is called the stationary phase and the population stabilizes.

The reasons for this period of **equilibrium** include depletion of nutrients, changes in the pH, and accumulation of cellular waste products. Laboratory studies may use a device called a chemostat to keep the microbial population in the log phase by draining the medium of waste products and dead cells and adding fresh medium. This prevents the microbial culture from entering the stationary phase. Chemostats are used in industrial fermentation (see Figure 6-6).

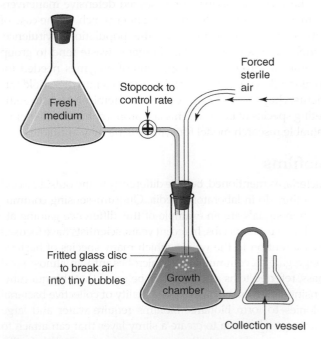

Figure 6-6 Chemostat used for continuous cultures. Rate of growth can be controlled either by controlling the rate at which new medium enters the growth chamber or by limiting a required growth factor in the medium.

Death Phase

As time proceeds, the number of deaths exceeds the number of new cells that are formed. The microbial population enters the death phase. This phase continues until the population has died out completely or until only a few living bacterial cells are left. Depending on the species, the phases may be completed in a few days or may take months. A few species may retain some surviving cells for a long period of time or possibly indefinitely. Spore-forming bacteria may develop protective spore coats to survive the death phase by entering into a type of dormant or hibernation period and wait for ideal environmental conditions to be re-established, allowing for return to normal metabolic functions and reproduction.

Quorum Sensing

Scientists have discovered that there is a community dynamic even among species of bacteria. Bacteria are frequently encountered in groups, whether clusters, chains, or geometric figures. This congregating of bacteria helps researchers identify species because larger groups provide greater variety of collective clues and characteristics to identify the microbial species.

When bacteria are studied "in the wild," in their normal environment and not in the controlled laboratory setting, they exhibit signs of coordinated gathering called quorum sensing. Each individual bacterium releases signaling molecules called **autoinducers**, sometimes alternately called **pheromones**. The bacteria are able to interpret the number of signals present in any given area from nearby bacteria; similar to the ability of animals to sense or interpret chemical signals excreted by other individuals of the species and which may influence social behaviors.

Bacteria can perform orchestrated defensive maneuvers in an almost social networking manner which, in the case of pathogenic bacteria, increases the population's virulence. *Myxobacteria* found in soil and organic waste tend to group together to produce large amounts of enzymes needed for breaking down environmental substances into digestible nutrients. They also collectively produce chemicals toxic to competing species of bacteria. This last property has made them a valuable research model for synthesizing new antibiotics.

Biofilms

Bacteria, as mentioned, behave differently in the outside world than they do in laboratory media. Quorum-sensing communication signals are an example of this difference gaining attention in research labs. In recent years, scientists have focused their attention to the way in which many species of bacteria congregate as communities of microbes into an almost solid mass, referred to as a **biofilm**. It is believed that this quorum-sensing ability is the basis for the ability of collective bacterial colonies to form biofilms. Biofilms require water and large numbers of bacteria to create a slimy layer that can attach to almost any surface, whether organic or inorganic. This fortification of the microbial population protects the group from the dangers of the outside world: sun, wind, rain, temperature extremes, toxins, and outside invaders (see Figure 6-7).

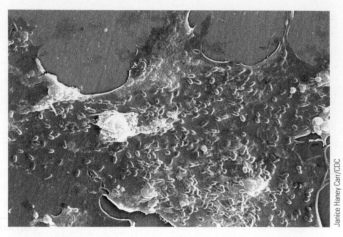

Figure 6-7 SEM image of an untreated wild stream water specimen showing the presence of unidentified organisms including bacteria, protozoa, and algae enmeshed in a mass of gelatinous biofilm.

The biofilm starts with a few individual free-floating bacteria that adhere to a surface by secreting a sticky mixture of sugars and proteins. Through use of quorum-sensing autoinducers, additional bacteria (sometimes even different species) gather into dense groupings along the same surfaces. Researchers have discovered incidents where some bacterial community members break away from the group because of depletion of resources or to establish new biofilms on other surfaces.

Biofilms have gained attention in the surgical environment of care as well. Patients with indwelling urinary drainage catheters used for prolonged periods frequently experience associated urinary tract infections (UTI). Biofilms may be responsible for failure of antibiotic treatment of the infections. Foley urinary catheters and other indwelling medical devices may be available with antimicrobial coatings to prevent biofilm formation on device surfaces.

Ineffective methods of decontamination of surgical instruments or patient care items allow biofilms to remain intact and create barriers to sterilization methods. Biofilms can also adhere to tissues, often making treatment with antibiotics or antimicrobial agents unsuccessful.

Laboratory Bacterial Counts

The number of cells in a colony can be measured using many different methods. The methods utilize either direct or indirect measurements. The count is based on small samples because colonies involve very large numbers, and mathematical calculations are used to determine the estimated total count of the population.

Direct Measurement Methods

Direct methods of measurement include: plate counts, filtration, most probable number, and direct counts.

Plate Counts The plate count is the most frequently used method of measuring a bacterial population. The main advantage of the plate count is that it measures the number of viable cells. The primary disadvantage is that a waiting period, sometimes up to 24 hours, is necessary before visible colonies are formed.

A plate count is reported as a colony-forming unit (CFU). Bacteria most often grow in clumps or chains. A colony is created as a result of segments of bacterial chains or clumps in groups. The CFU is able to reflect this aggregation or clustering by providing a more accurate count.

When the plate count method is used, only plates with approximately 25–250 colonies are counted. If overcrowding occurs, then some cells will not fully develop and this will skew the count. Only a limited number of colonies are allowed to develop to prevent the miscalculation.

Plate counts are accomplished by one of two methods: pour plate or spread plate method. The pour plate method involves pouring a diluted bacterial suspension into a Petri dish. The agar in the medium is maintained at liquid state by placing the dish in water heated at approximately 50°C, and then the bacterial suspension and medium are gently mixed together. The agar is allowed to then solidify and the plate is incubated. Colonies subsequently grow both within the nutrient agar and on the surface.

Major drawbacks can occur with the use of the pour plate method. Heat-sensitive microbes are damaged by the heated melted agar. Additionally, distinctive colonies must form only on the surface. Colonies that form beneath the surface of the pour plate will not provide an accurate diagnosis.

The spread plate method was developed to address the two challenges presented by the pour plate method. A 0.1-mL sample is poured onto the surface of a solidified agar medium. The **inoculum** is then spread in a uniform manner over the surface of the medium with a sterile glass rod. This method spreads the bacteria on the surface of the medium, preventing penetration into the medium, and the heat-sensitive bacteria are saved from destruction by avoiding contact with melted agar.

Filtration When only a small quantity of bacteria requires counting, such as a sample of water from a river, the filtration method is used. A minimum of 100 mL of water is poured through a thin filter that has pores (openings) too small for bacteria to pass through. The filter is placed in a Petri dish that contains a pad that was pre-soaked in a liquid nutrient medium. The colonies of bacteria can then grow on the surface of the filter. This relatively easy and effective method is frequently used in developing countries to determine whether fecal contamination of water supplies has occurred.

Most Probable Number A statistical estimation method for determining the number of bacteria in a sample is the most probable number (MPN) method. The MPN method is based on the principle that the greater the number of bacteria present in a sample, a higher dilution rate, or numbers of times the sample is diluted, would be required to eventually reduce the number of cells to a point at which no bacteria are left

remaining to grow in the series of tubes used in the dilution series. The MPN method determines, with 95 percent probability, that the population is within a certain numerical range and is statistically the most probable number. This technique is used when the microbes to be counted cannot grow on solid media.

Direct Count The direct count involves using a known volume of bacterial suspension that is placed within a defined area on a microscopic slide. The laboratory technician can then count the bacteria. The following is a description of a direct count method using the Petroff-Hausser cell counter.

1. In the center of the microscopic slide, the surface is etched with a grid of squares of a known area. Above this is a slight indentation or space of known volume that is covered with a glass cover slip.

2. The space is filled with the bacterial suspension.

3. The cells are counted within several squares and the results are averaged. A calculation then determines the number of cells present in 1 mL or other specified known volume.

The primary advantage of this technique is that no incubation is required. This advantage also holds true for the Coulter counter, a type of electronic cell counter that automatically counts the number of cells in the known volume of fluid. Limitations of the direct count method include the following:

1. Motile bacteria are difficult to count

2. Dead and live cells are counted (total cell count)

3. A high concentration of cells is required to be counted, approximately 10 million bacteria per milliliter.

Indirect Measurement Methods

Direct measurement methods are not always required to count microbial cells to estimate the number present in a culture. The following indirect methods are often just as useful and often more practical in many situations.

Turbidity Turbidity refers to how turbid (cloudy or hazy) a liquid medium appears as the bacterial cells multiply. The instrument used to measure turbidity is called a spectrophotometer. A beam of light shines through a tube of bacterial suspension and strikes a light-sensitive detector on the spectrophotometer. The more turbid a solution, referring to the fact that the bacterial cell count is high, the less light reaches the light detector. The amount of light is registered on the spectrophotometer's instrument scale as the percentage of transmission and on another scale as a logarithmic expression called the absorbance. The absorbance is used to plot the bacterial growth. When the absorbance is compared to plate counts of the same bacteria, a correlation can be made to assist in future estimations of the bacterial count when measuring turbidity.

Approximately 10 million to 100 million cells per milliliter are required in a suspension for turbidity to be measured using the spectrophotometer. This makes the use of turbidity for measuring contaminated liquids, such as river water, impractical due to the small number of bacteria present in a large volume of water. Turbidity does not distinguish between dead and living cells. It cannot be used with bacterial cells that aggregate (clump together) because they settle and the turbidity is eliminated (see Figure 6-8).

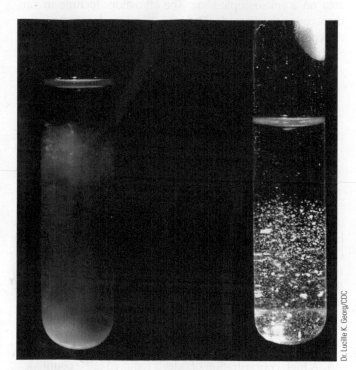

Dr. Lucille K. Georg/CDC

Figure 6-8 Two test tubes, each containing a thioglycolate broth growth medium, inoculated with the gram-positive bacterium, *Actinomyces odontolyticus* on the left, and *Actinomyces israelii* on the right. Note the turbid appearance in the tube on the left, while the tube on the right displayed a colonial morphology appearing clumpy, or granular.

Metabolic Activity A second indirect method measures a population's metabolic activity. The presumption is that the quantity of particular metabolites such as CO_2, is in direct proportion to the number of bacteria present in the medium. For example, the amount of acid produced by a population can be used to determine the amounts of vitamins that are present.

Dry Weight Routine methods of measurement are not conducive (productive) to filamentous organisms; therefore, dry weight is used to measure their growth. This method involves removing the fungus or mold from the culture medium, placing it through a filter to remove debris, and into a special weighing bottle. The sample is dried in an oven at 105°C for approximately 24 hours, cooled in a **desiccator**, and finally weighed. The same method can be used with bacteria, except that the bacteria are removed from the culture medium by use of a centrifuge.

MICRO NOTES

"Freeze Frame"

Ricardo Cavicchioli, a scientist from New South Wales in Australia, studies microbes in Antarctica called psychrophiles or cryophiles. According to Cavicchioli, it makes sense to study this "cold biosphere" because more than 80 percent of the planet never gets over 5°C (41°F). These cold-loving microbes reproduce only six times per year as compared to *E. coli* bacteria, which reproduce approximately every 20 minutes. Other scientists from McGill University discovered *Planococcus halocryophilus* in the Canadian permafrost, which can grow at −15°C (5°F) and stay metabolically active at −25°C (−13°F). Brrrrrrr.

Under the Microscope

Dr. Mehta ordered an exchange of Foley catheter for her patient who was on high doses of corticosteroids after kidney transplantation. She ordered a urine culture, then the replacement of the catheter with a coated Foley to resist microbial invasion and prevent urinary tract infection (UTI).

1. What type of coating should make the urinary catheter be a safer choice for this patient?

2. Which type of bacterial counts would most likely demonstrate the extent of the UTI?

3. Which types of physical or chemical requirements provided by the patient's body would be optimal and increase their population growth?

4. What type of resistant bacterial contamination or colonization is common on implantable devices?

5. Why would the prolonged time the catheter is left in place contribute to the risk of serious UTI in this immunosuppressed patient?

CHAPTER 7

Microbial Genetics and Mutations

Learning Objectives

After completing the study of this chapter, you will be able to:

1. Define key terms.
2. Discuss the mechanisms by which eukaryotic and prokaryotic cells pass on traits.
3. Describe the structure and appearance of DNA in microorganisms and humans.
4. Compare and contrast natural and artificial transformation in bacteria.
5. Describe the role of various mutagens in genetic mutations.
6. Discuss the sources of exposure to mutagens for surgical personnel or other healthcare workers.
7. Apply critical thinking skills in relating chapter material to the surgical environment of care or broader global community.

Key Terms

Auxotrophic	Covalent bonds	Induction	Photoreactivating
Bacteriophages	Dimer	Ionizing radiation	Recombinant
Codon	Double helix	Lysogeny	Replicon
Conjugation	Fluoroscopy	Macerated	Teratogen
Counterbalancing	Frameshift	Mutagen	Ultraviolet light

The Big Picture

Genes determine what traits will be expressed, whether it may be humans or microbes, and when there is a mutation that occurs, the altered trait may be repeated in all subsequent generations.

During your examination of the topics in this chapter, consider the following:

1. How do the basic genetic structures of RNA or DNA differ between organisms?

2. What might the potential impact be on patient care if a pathogenic bacterium with a mutation for antibiotic resistance multiplies?

3. In what ways could some mutations be beneficial?

4. What factors or things are able to cause genetic mutations?

5. Which microbial species are known to develop the genetic mutation for antibiotic resistance?

Clinical Significance Topic

Genetic mutations can occur naturally or due to exposure to mutagens. Surgical personnel are exposed to a number of mutagenic conditions or substances during their careers and must have an awareness and understanding of the potential hazards to protect themselves. Ethylene oxide (EO) used for sterilization of heat and moisture-sensitive items is a known carcinogen and mutagen, so much so that many hospitals have stopped using the method. Large manufacturing plants, however, still use EO as a reliable method of killing microorganisms. Ionizing radiation from x-ray and fluoroscopy machines can cause cellular mutations, especially in developing fetuses. Every exposure to ionizing radiation is cumulative over a lifetime, so surgical technologists and all team members in the exposure zone must take precautions and wear leaded aprons, thyroid collars, glasses, and other protective gear to reduce that exposure. These are just a few examples; numerous other mutagens exist. Awareness of exposure potential and personal protection will minimize risk and ensure a safer work environment for each of us.

Basics of Genetics

Gregor Mendel, an Austrian monk who lived in the mid-1800s, is considered the father of the study of genetics. His observations of the variations in appearance of pea plants became the basis for the modern science that studies genotypes (the genetic make-up of an organism) and phenotypes (the observable characteristics of an organism as a result of the interactions between its genotype and surrounding environment).

Since that early research, scientists have successfully mapped the complete genomes of several bacterial species as well as *Homo sapiens*—humans. The National Institutes of Health (NIH) *Genetics Home Reference* states that:

"A genome is an organism's complete set of DNA, including all of its genes. Each genome contains all of the information needed to build and maintain that organism. In humans, a copy of the entire genome—more than 3 billion DNA base pairs—is contained in all cells that have a nucleus."

The genomes of over 100,000 species of microbes have been sequenced since the first genomes completed in 1995. Bacteria are, in general, much less complicated than most eukaryotes. Their life cycles are also much shorter, allowing for extensive study in much shorter timelines.

The fundamental unit of information in the genome is the individual gene. Each gene is a segment of DNA, or deoxyribonucleic acid, a type of nucleic acid. Every organism contains genetic material that allows for its ability to replicate in new generations. An individual DNA segment is responsible for encoding proteins that eventually determine the unique phenotypes of that organism.

Chromosomes are strands of DNA that may present in cells as singular strands that are straight or circular or as cross-linked pairs in a spiral configuration. In human DNA, this configuration is expressed as the **double helix**. Humans typically have 46 chromosomes arranged in 23 pairs. There are four chemicals (nitrogenous bases) that attach to a phosphate and carbon sugar backbone called a deoxynucleotide. The nitrogenous bases are adenine (A), guanine (G), cytosine (C), and thymine (T), which are referred to by their respective letters when studying DNA sequencing. These chemicals pair or link with each other by hydrogen bonding. These pairings follow a rule: A (adenine) always pairs with T (thymine) and C (cytosine) always pairs with G (guanine).

It is difficult to imagine, but there are 3 billion base pairs responsible for creating the 30,000 genes that, in turn, create the 23 paired chromosomes found in the nucleus of every single human cell (see Figure 7-1). The units of measure used to describe the numbers of base pairs in DNA are the kilobase (Kb), which is 1,000 bases, and the megabase (Mb), which is 1,000,000 bases. Human DNA has 23 linear pairs of chromosomes with 3,000 Mb pairs or 3 billion base pairs. For purposes of comparison, the DNA found in *Escherichia coli* comprises a single circular 4.6 Mb chromosome. The small size, coupled with the fast population growth cycle (20 minutes), makes the study of bacterial genetics much more manageable in the research laboratory setting.

Considering the staggering numbers of genomes found in nature, there is always the potential for variations or mistakes that subsequently may result in mutations that change the entire outcome, for good or for bad. These changes can be artificially engineered in laboratories to manipulate genetic expressions. Genetic mutations and mutagens are discussed later in this chapter.

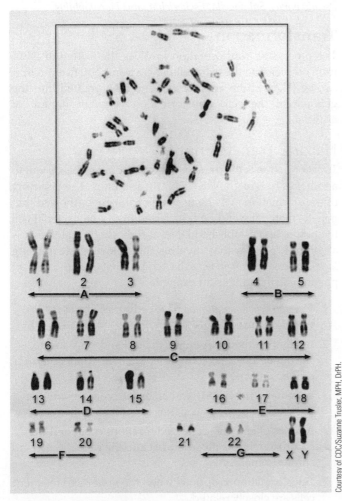

Courtesy of CDC/Suzanne Trusler, MPH, DrPH.

Figure 7-1 This karyogram depicts a complete complement of condensed human chromosomes.

Bacterial Genetic Exchange

Genetic exchange does occur among bacteria, but not through sexual reproduction, as with the eukaryotes. Only a portion of the DNA of the donor cell is transferred to the recipient cell when genetic exchange takes place. In addition, the genetic transfer is a one-way process; the recipient does not transfer any DNA back to the donor.

The portion of donated bacterial DNA cannot replicate by itself. The only way in which the DNA can be replicated is if it is incorporated into one of the existing **replicons** in the cell—the chromosome or plasmid, a small circular DNA molecule. The method of incorporating donated genes into a replicon involves the process of recombination, also called crossing over.

Recombination, a key feature of genetic transfer among prokaryotes, is the formation of a new combination of genes through either natural or artificial means. Recombination also occurs in sexual reproduction: offspring acquire a different combination of genes as compared to either parent because the offspring receives half its chromosomes from each parent, resulting in a combination of parental genes.

During the recombination of prokaryotes, the genes on the same chromosome recombine by crossing over. The chromosomes or DNA molecules break apart and a fragment joins another fragment, resulting in a **recombinant** molecule or a new entity created from a combination of source materials. The recombination will only occur between chromosomes and DNA that are homologous (have the same structure) to facilitate the hydrogen bonding of the two single strands of DNA into a double strand.

Genetic transfer occurs in one of four methods in bacteria: conjugation, transduction, transformation, and lysogenic conversion. Each process allows DNA to leave one bacterium and enter another, but the mechanism of transfer is different.

Conjugation

The process of **conjugation** is completed by specialized plasmids called conjugative plasmids. The plasmids are able to transfer themselves to another bacterial cell. The best-known example of conjugative plasmid is the F plasmid that occurs in *E. coli*, a natural inhabitant of the intestinal tract or large colon. The F plasmid encodes for at least 13 known genes. Bacterial cells that carry an F plasmid are called F+, and those that lack an F plasmid are called F−. One of the genes of the F plasmid encodes for a pilus or hair-like appendage called a sex or F pilus. The sex pilus allows the F+ cell to attach to the F− cell. After attachment, the pilus retracts and the two cells come in direct contact. Next, the plasmid DNA is nicked, meaning one strand of the double helix is broken. Replication occurs at the site of the nick, and one linear strand of plasmid DNA is produced that subsequently enters the F− cell. Inside the F− cell, the plasmid DNA forms a circle and duplicates. The result of the transfer is that the F− cell becomes an F+ cell, capable of conjugation. The original donor cell remains an F+ cell because it retains a copy of the conjugative plasmid.

A majority of other plasmids, such as R plasmids, are transferred in a similar fashion. Some plasmids are referred to as being promiscuous (non-selective) because the bacterial cells that contain them will connect with most other bacterial cells. For example, promiscuous plasmids are transferred among most of the Gram-negative bacterial species, whereas the F plasmid is specific to strains of *E. coli* and related species.

Transduction

Transduction occurs when bacteriophages, viruses that infect bacteria, reproduce themselves. Based on the type of reproduction, there are two kinds of phages and, therefore, two kinds of transduction. Virulent phages always lyse (break apart) the host cell during the production of new bacteriophages and are responsible for generalized transduction.

Temperate phages are transported within the host without harming it and bring about specialized transduction, generalized transduction, or both. In this case, the viral genome does not take over the host cell, thereby preserving the cell. As compared to transformation and conjugation, only small segments of DNA are transferred from cell to cell. The relationship between the bacteriophage and the host cell is called **lysogeny**. Infected bacteria are called lysogenic bacteria. The inactive viral genome is referred to as a prophage. When the right environmental conditions occur, such as heat, chemicals, or ultraviolet light, the prophage is stimulated to produce complete phages and the bacterial cell is lysed. This process is called **induction** of the lytic cycle.

Virulent Phages

Virulent phages attach to the bacterial cell wall and inject their DNA to infect the cell. The infectious DNA controls the cell to make more DNA and protein. The two components combine into mature phage particles that are released from the host cell and proceed to actively infect other bacterial cells.

Occasionally, an error occurs approximately 1 in 100,000 times, when the phage particles are forming. Instead of phage DNA being combined with protein, the bacterial cell DNA is combined. The abnormal phage particles, called transducing particles, can attach to another cell and inject bacterial DNA. The result is a genetic exchange of the errant or deviant DNA. The injected DNA fragment will survive in the host cell as long as it is recombined into the host's genome. This type of transfer is called generalized transduction because any portion of the bacterial chromosome is transferred from one cell to another. Generalized transduction has been observed in species of *Streptococcus*, *Staphylococcus*, *Salmonella*, and in *Vibrio cholerae*.

Temperate Phages

Two life cycles exist for temperate phages: lysogenic cycle and lytic cycle. During the lysogenic cycle, the phage DNA is latent (inactive) and is called a prophage. Some prophages are plasmids, which are extra molecules of DNA floating freely in the cytoplasm of the cell and are separate from the bacterial chromosome. Other prophages become a part of the host cell's chromosomes and are responsible for mediating specialized transduction.

When an environmental condition such as heat or **ultraviolet light** stimulates the prophage, it enters the lytic cycle and begins producing complete phages by producing DNA and proteins. Specialized transducing particles are formed when an error occurs during reactivation of the prophage. Small pieces of bacterial DNA remain attached to the new phage DNA. When the phage particles are produced, bacterial genes can be incorporated into some of the mature bacteriophages. When the phages are released due to cell lysis, they can infect other cells, injecting both the bacterial genetic material and viral genes. Consequently, the prophage exits and a few bacterial genes also leave.

When the specialized transducing particles attach to another host bacterial cell and inject its DNA, the bacterial genes and phage genes are injected. The genetic exchange occurs between the host bacterial cell in which the specialized transducing particles were formed and the cell that is subsequently infected. The term specialized transduction is used to refer to the process because the prophages are inserted at a specific site on the bacterial chromosome. This is the way that genetic phenotypic characteristics such as antibiotic resistance are transduced to other bacteria. Specialized transduction has been confirmed in the laboratory in species of *Bacillus*, *Pseudomonas*, *Salmonella*, *Escherichia*, and *Haemophilus*.

Transformation

The process of transformation involves the exiting of DNA from one cell into the extracellular environment. Eventually it can be taken up by another cell and incorporated into the genome of the cell. Transformation is either natural or artificial.

Natural Transformation

Transformation is the transfer of genes from one bacterium to another as free, or "naked," DNA in a solution. The discovery of transformation in 1928, nearly a century ago, showed that genetic material could be transferred from one bacterial cell to another and established DNA as the genetic material. It is a complex process that involves the following steps using *Streptococcus pneumoniae*, a bacterium that is the cause of pneumonia in humans for example:

1. *Streptococcus pneumoniae* have cell surface receptors to which the free DNA binds.

2. A strand of the DNA enters the cell and, once inside, is surrounded by a protein protective coat to shield it from cellular enzymes.

3. Eventually, the new DNA comes into contact with the cell's genome, which contains homologous genes.

4. A series of enzyme-catalyzed reactions occur and the absorbed DNA is incorporated into the cell's chromosome.

5. Transformation is optimal when the donor and recipient cells are closely related.

Even though only one strand of the DNA enters the host cell, it is a large fragment that is attempting to pass through the cell wall and membrane. A cell that can take up the donor DNA is said to be competent. Competence is the result of changes in the cell wall that make it permeable to the large DNA fragment.

Natural transformation may take place when bacterial cells are lysed after death. The cell's DNA is released into the environment, exposing another bacterium to the DNA. This bacterium takes up the fragments to be integrated into the host cell's chromosomal structure by recombination. This cell with the new genes is a hybrid or recombinant cell. As the cell divides, the subsequent cells are identical (see Figure 7-2).

Natural transformation only occurs in a small number of bacterial species, including *Bacillus, Haemophilus,*

Neisseria, and certain strains of *Staphylococcus* and *Streptococcus.* Natural transformation developed to make genetic exchange a possibility among bacterial cells, but it does not explain the limit on the number of species capable of the process.

Artificial Transformation

The development of artificial transformation was essential to the advancement of **recombinant** technology (also called genetic engineering). *E. coli* is not a competent cell, so it is not genetically programmed in nature for transformation. However, the process of artificial transformation is used to enable *E. coli* to take up the DNA strand.

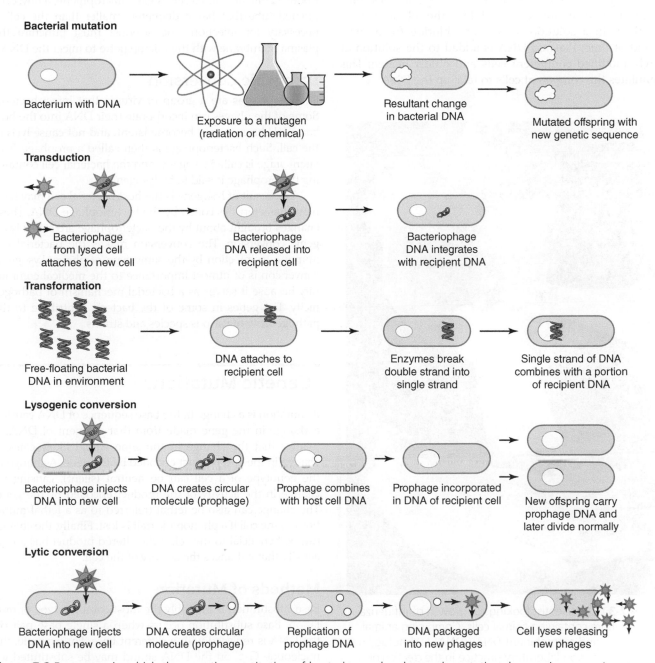

Figure 7-2 Four ways in which the genetic constitution of bacteria may be changed: mutation, lysogenic conversion, transduction, and transformation.

Genetic engineering requires DNA to be handled outside of the cell and returned to the inside of a living cell. Several methods are used to place the DNA into the cell. The method used is determined by the type of vector (carrier) and host cell to be combined. The vector is either a plasmid or a virus specifically used in genetic engineering to insert the DNA genes into the cell. The most important property of the vector is that it must be capable of replicating once in the cell. Any DNA that is cloned in the vector will be replicated during the process making vectors important to the scientist who wants to replicate a desired DNA sequence (see Figure 7-3).

Although *E. coli* does not naturally transform, a simple laboratory chemical treatment makes these cell types competent. The procedure involves chilling the cells and soaking them in a solution of calcium chloride for a short period of time. Plasmid DNA is added to the solution of newly-modified competent cells and mildly heated. This stimulates the competent cells to take up the DNA.

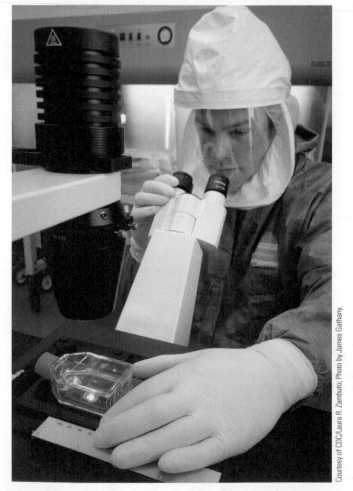

Figure 7-3 CDC scientist looking for growth of influenza virus in culture containing animal cells. Combining animal cell cultures and recombinant DNA (rDNA) technology has become a common laboratory practice in the creation of viral vaccines as well as other biomanufactured products, including hormones, enzymes, and anticancer agents.

Another way of transferring the DNA to cells is called electroporation. An electrical current is used to create pores in the cell membrane, allowing the DNA to enter through the pores. Electroporation can be used on any cell. Cells with a cell wall must be converted to protoplasts. Protoplasts are created by removing the cell wall with special enzymes, allowing a more direct path to the plasma cell membrane.

A third method involves the use of a gene gun that literally "shoots" foreign DNA into plant cells that contain a thick cellulose wall. Microscopic pieces of gold or tungsten are coated with DNA and shot forward by helium through the plant cell wall.

Another popular method of genetic engineering is called microinjection. Using this treatment, DNA can be directly introduced into an animal cell. A glass micropipette, a tiny, cannulated tube that has a diameter smaller than the cell is necessary for injection. The scientist must puncture the plasma membrane with the micropipette to inject the DNA.

Lysogenic Conversion

Bacteriophages are a group of viruses that infect bacteria. Some of the phages can incorporate their DNA into the host bacterial chromosome, become latent, and not cause lysis of the cell. Such bacteriophage is then called a prophage. This latent stage is called lysogeny, and the bacterial cell containing the prophage is said to be lysogenic.

The result of lysogeny is the host bacterial cell may have new characteristics coded by the bacteriophage DNA. These changes brought about by the bacteriophage are called lysogenic conversion. The conversion makes the bacterial cell immune to infection by the same type of phage. Lysogenic conversion is of utmost importance to the medical community because it serves as a bacterial mechanism of pathogenicity. The genes in some of the bacteria contribute to the pathogenicity of various species and strains.

Genetic Mutations

A mutation is a change in the base sequence of DNA causing a change in the gene made from that segment of DNA. It follows that the change in the gene would likely cause a change in the end product encoded by the gene. A change in the genotype of a cell can be neutral (silent), causing no change in the activity of the product encoded by the gene. The change can also be lethal (referred to as a lethal mutation) to the cell if a phenotypic trait is lost. Finally, the change can be beneficial to the cell if the altered product has a new activity that enhances the activity of the cell.

Methods of Mutation

Base substitution is probably the most common type of mutation. Base substitution occurs when a single base pair on the DNA is replaced with a different base. For example, the nucleotide G-C on the DNA strand may be substituted for C-G. Two types of base substitution are recognized: missense mutation and nonsense mutation.

Missense mutation occurs inside a gene that codes for a particular type of protein. The messenger RNA (mRNA) transcribed from the gene will carry the incorrect base at that position on the DNA strand. After the mRNA is translated into a protein, the incorrect base could cause the insertion of an incorrect amino acid into the protein. This type of base substitution is the result of an amino acid substitution in the synthesized protein.

Nonsense mutation involves the creation of a nonsense, or "stop," **codon** in the middle of the mRNA molecule. This type of base substitution results in preventing the complete synthesis of a protein so only a portion of the protein is synthesized.

Changes in the DNA are referred to as **frameshift** mutations. The result of this mutation is the deletion or insertion of one or more nucleotide pairs in the DNA strand. The mutation results in a shift of the triple nucleotide groupings that are recognized by transfer RNA (tRNA) during translation. For example, if a nucleotide pair in a gene was deleted, the amino acids further down from the site of the original mutation will be changed. The result is the production of an inactive protein due to the mutated gene and the change produced in the amino acid. Most often, a nonsense codon will eventually be met and the translation will cease.

The various types of base substitutions and frameshift mutations can occur randomly due to mistakes during the replication of DNA. Referred to as spontaneous mutations, these occur without any interference from a mutation-causing agent, and the cause of the mutation is unknown.

Agents that can cause mutations are called mutagens. The types of mutagens that individuals are exposed to in surgery are chemical agents, biological agents, and ionizing radiation.

Mutagens

A **mutagen** is an agent that induces genetic mutation. On a larger scale, mutagens are often found in the operating room and central sterile supply department, and surgical technologists must be aware of what they are, what they can do, and what precautions must be taken to prevent or minimize exposure. On a microscopic scale, mutagens affect changes in both individual prokaryotic and eukaryotic cells.

Chemical Mutagens

Mutagens alter DNA at various locations on the strand. The alterations can occur by base-pair substitutions, insertions, or deletions resulting in a **frameshift** mutation. Frameshift mutagens produce changes by **counterbalancing** the two strands of DNA, which leaves a space in one or both strands. When the DNA strands are synthesized, one or several pairs of nucleotides are deleted or inserted in the new double strand of DNA.

A good example of a chemical frameshift mutagen is benzopyrene, a chemical that is present in industrial smoke. An example of an agricultural chemical frameshift mutagen is the fungus (sometimes called a mold) *Aspergillus flavus*, responsible for the food and cattle feed pathogen, aflatoxin. Both mutagens are potent carcinogens, as are most frameshift mutagens.

The chemical mutagen ethylene oxide (EO) is also a frameshift mutagen. Ethylene oxide is used as a chemical sterilant that is converted from a liquid form to a gas by the ethylene oxide gas sterilizer. It is highly effective in the sterilization of heat-sensitive and moisture-sensitive surgical instruments, equipment, and supplies. However, ethylene oxide has been proven to be a potent carcinogen and mutagen. EO gas and toxic by-products can cause liver toxicity and cancers of the liver, prostate, and bone. Items that have been sterilized with EO must be aerated in isolated rooms for a specific amount of time before they are considered safe for use.

Polymethyl methacrylate (PMMA), also called methyl methacrylate, is another chemical that may be mutagenic and carcinogenic. PMMA is commonly referred to as "bone cement" and is sometimes used to cement the prosthesis in place during a total joint arthroplasty or replace lost or fractured cranial bone in a cranioplasty. It is a combination of a liquid and powder that the surgical technologist mixes together during the surgical procedure. PMMA beads are tiny, round, smooth particles that are not absorbed by the body and used as permanent soft tissue fillers. More recently approved for use by the FDA, PMMA beads are suspended in a bovine-derived collagen gel and injected into the face. It has not been proven that PMMA is dangerous, despite a long-standing belief that it is a **teratogen** or causes hepatic carcinoma, however, the noxious fumes produced by the chemical substance are capable of producing airway irritation, especially in individuals with upper respiratory conditions such as asthma. Surgical personnel should use mixing containers that evacuate the fumes with the use of suction.

Ionizing Radiation

Ionizing radiation sources in the operating room include portable x-ray machines and **fluoroscopy** (C-arm) units. In the radiology department, x-rays of various forms as well as CT scanners and PET scanners all emit potentially dangerous doses of human-made **ionizing radiation**. Outside of the hospital setting, sources of radiation include the sun, cosmic rays, radioactive elements found in soil, and radon gases that leach out of the earth. Basically, no living organisms are able to completely escape exposure to natural ionizing radiation.

Ionizing radiation is considered a mutagen because of its ability to ionize atoms and molecules in the cells of the body. The external ionizing rays cause the release of electrons from the atomic shell in which they are contained. The electrons assault other molecules, resulting in the formation of ions and free radicals. Free radicals are molecules with unpaired electrons that can combine with the bases in DNA, causing mistakes in DNA replication and producing mutations. A more serious consequence results when the **covalent bonds** of the sugar-phosphate molecules in DNA are broken, causing breaks in the chromosomes.

Ultraviolet Light

Ultraviolet light is another type of mutagenic radiation. Ultraviolet (UV) light is a component of normal sunlight (see Figure 7-4). The atmospheric ozone layer of the earth is important because it is responsible for screening out the most mutagenic component of UV light. UV light has an effect on DNA by stimulating the formation of detrimental bonds

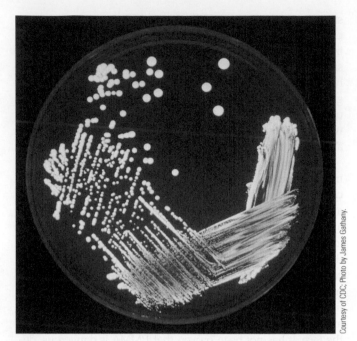

Courtesy of CDC; Photo by James Gathany.

Figure 7-4 *Legionella* sp. colonies cultivated on an agar-cultured plate and illuminated with ultraviolet light.

between thymine in DNA chains called thymine dimers. A **dimer** is a compound formed by the union of two free radicals. The thymine dimers can cause permanent damage or cell death because they inhibit the replication of the DNA.

Bacteria and other cells have enzymes called **photoreactivating** enzymes that can repair the damage done by the UV light. The enzymes bind to the thymine **dimers** and, with the use of light energy, break the bonds to form the dimers. When the bond is broken, the enzymes fill in the space with newly synthesized DNA that fits in the undamaged strand of DNA. This restores the original base-pair sequence. The name of the enzyme responsible for this last bonding step is DNA ligase.

On occasion, an error occurs during the repair process, and the base-pair sequence is not restored. The result of the error is a mutation. Individuals who spend large amounts of time in the sun are exposed to UV light, which can result in a large number of thymine dimers in the cells of the skin. Errors in the repair process result in the increase of additional mutations that contribute to the development of various forms of skin cancer.

Biological Mutagens

Laser plume (smoke) is a mutagenic source in the surgical environment of care. The debate regarding laser plume revolves around the possibility that it might contain viable particles of cellular DNA that could be inhaled during a surgical procedure utilizing a laser, causing later manifestation of disease in the exposed individuals. Surgical smoke contains approximately 95 percent water or steam and the remaining 5 percent is comprised of cellular debris in the form of particulate materials including chemicals, blood and tissue particles, viruses, and bacteria.

In a study cited in the *Journal of Cancer* in 2019, researchers used bovine papillomavirus to test the theory that viral particles present in plume could transmit disease to healtcare workers exposed to it. In this study, the tissue was vaporized with a CO_2 laser and the particles liberated into the plume were captured, cultured, and injected into test animals. The animals developed tumors found to have the same DNA as the original viral tissue, demonstrating that laser plume is a potential biological hazard to surgical team members if smoke evacuator systems and components of personal protective equipment (PPEs) are not used appropriately. The authors found research study citations of only four cases of gynecologic surgeons with extensive occupational exposure to laser plume from cervical ablation procedures have developed HPV-16-positive oropharyngeal squamous cell cancers. Other risk factors for the disease were eliminated as possible causes. Although they were unable to state with absolute certainty that the cancers were a direct result of the inhalation of laser-generated smoke plume, they made a strong recommendation for appropriate prevention strategies based on the evidence gathered from the study.

Studies related to the smoke produced by electrosurgical units as a biological hazard have been less conclusive. Very few studies have been performed on electrosurgical smoke that proves biological risk; however, there is little debate about potentially toxic particles present in ESU smoke plume. In the absence of policies directing use of high-filtration suction evacuators for all cases in which smoke plume is generated, surgical personnel may be somewhat benefitted by the engineering control mechanism in operating rooms with 15–20 room air exchanges per hour. These exchanges remove many of the potential contaminants in the air as well as smoke and anesthesia gases that may escape breathing circuits.

Mutation Rate

The mutation rate is not how often a mutation occurs, but rather the probability that a gene will mutate when a cell divides. The rate of mutation is stated as a power of 10. The number is always negative because mutations are rare. For example, spontaneous mutations occur in DNA replication once in approximately 10^9 replicated base pairs (a mutation rate of 10^{-9}).

Mutations occur randomly along a chromosome. For a species to adapt to its environment, mutations must only occur randomly and infrequently. For example, if a type of bacteria has a large population size, then a small number of mutant cells will always be produced in each new generation. Most mutations are harmful to cells and are removed when the cells die; however, some mutations are beneficial to cells. For example, mutations give some bacterial cells the ability to resist certain antibiotic agents. The cells are able to survive and reproduce and an evolutionary change has then occurred because the new bacterial cells have the mutated gene. This presents a problem to surgical patients who develop a surgical site infection because the bacteria responsible for the infection could be resistant to the routinely prescribed antibiotics.

Laboratory Identification of Mutants

A wide range of microbiology laboratory testing techniques was discussed in Chapter 3. In this section, four general tests specifically designed to identify mutant strains of microorganisms are examined. These laboratory tests are direct selection, counterselection, replica plating, and site-directed mutagenesis. The tests utilize a culture that has been treated with a mutagen to increase the number of mutations to include the one type of mutant organism being sought.

Direct Selection

Direct selection is effective in the isolation of antibiotic-resistant mutant strains. In the laboratory, conditions are created that are conducive to the growth of the mutant strain. For example, if a strain of bacteria is smeared on a Petri dish containing penicillin, only the penicillin-resistant mutant cells will reproduce and grow, forming colonies.

Counterselection

Counterselection, or indirect selection, is the opposite of direct selection. Two environmental conditions are established in the laboratory: (1) one that prevents the growth of the desired mutant strain and (2) one that is used to kill the growing cells. The mutant cells cannot proliferate; however, they are able to survive the conditions that were used to kill the non-mutated cells. This results in a large percentage of mutant cells among the surviving population of microbes, allowing for easier isolation.

Counterselection is used to isolate and study **auxotrophic** mutant strains. Recall that a lethal mutation occurs when a gene product that is required for the survival of the cell is not present, regardless of the environmental conditions. For example, if polymerase is eliminated by mutation, the cell cannot survive due to an inability to synthesize DNA.

However, a mutant microbe that possesses a nutritional requirement that was not possessed by the parent is known as an auxotroph. This is not lethal to the cell as long as the required growth factor is present in the nutrient medium.

Humans have multiple auxotrophs. Many of our nutritional pathways are defective, including those pathways that make several vitamins and amino acids. We compensate for the deficiencies by providing the needed amino acids and vitamins through dietary means.

A mutation can also be responsible for destroying an enzyme that aids in the metabolism of a carbon or nitrogen source. As long as the carbon or nitrogen source is provided through other nutrient means, the mutant strain will survive and grow.

Replica Plating

Replica plating is another method used to detect mutated strains of bacteria. It provides the researcher with the ability to transfer large colonies and track them in a relatively easy way. For example, replica plating can be used to detect antibiotic resistance of bacteria such as E. coli.

The process of replica plating uses multiple agar plates, half inoculated with streptomycin antibiotic and half with only nutrient agar. A piece of sterilized velveteen cloth is stretched across a wooden block or other stabilizer to use as a stamp press. A bacterial specimen to be analyzed is incubated in a Petri dish and considered the "master dish." The block with velveteen is pressed into the sample and then onto the other prepared solid agar Petri dishes with and without streptomycin.

The small fabric threads act like numerous inoculating needles. The subsequent plates are incubated and analyzed. If visible growth is negative on the antibiotic plate, then it is an expected one. Subsequently, the same plate is pressed with a new sterile cloth and, in turn, onto an untreated agar plate. If growth is seen on the last plate, then it demonstrates that mutated E. coli bacteria, with the ability to resist destruction by streptomycin, have survived.

Site-Directed Mutagenesis

Site-directed mutagenesis is related to recombinant DNA technology. The technique involves selection and allows the researcher to mutate one specified gene. Recombinant DNA technology is used to create the desired mutant.

Use of Mutants in Lab Screening Tests

Strains of mutant microbes are used in laboratory tests to discover biochemical pathways and to screen substances to determine if they are carcinogenic. One such test is the Ames test developed by Bruce Ames at the University of California, Berkeley (see Figure 7-5). In the past, animals were used as test subjects to determine if a substance was carcinogenic. This was time-consuming, expensive, and controversial. The Ames test is one example of a faster and less expensive procedure that does not involve animal testing.

The Ames test uses histidine auxotrophic mutants. Through direct selection, the test determines the ability of the mutagen to cause reversions. Reversions are mutations that can reverse the original mutation. The histidine auxotroph can grow in the absence of histidine. The chemical to be evaluated is mixed with **macerated** rat liver, which contains enzymes that convert non-carcinogenic chemicals into carcinogens. If the test is negative, then the chemical is most likely harmless. However, 90 percent of the chemicals tested that demonstrate mutagenic characteristics using the Ames test are subsequently shown to be carcinogenic.

MICRO NOTES

"Raise the Shields!"

Ionizing radiation, the kind that x-ray and fluoroscopy units produce, can cause damage to cells. When the cells try to repair themselves, changes made by the injury may result in mutations of the genes that may be passed down to the next generation of cells. Just to be safe, surgical technologists working where ionizing radiation is used should take special precautions to limit exposure. Lead-lined gloves, glasses, aprons, and thyroid collars are forms of PPE available for protection against radiation exposure. X-ray dosimeter badges that measure radiation exposure should also be worn, however, care must be taken to not leave the badge in an area where x-rays are being performed but not on the individual and to not leave them in a car where the heat and sunlight could mistakenly register as occupational radiation exposure.

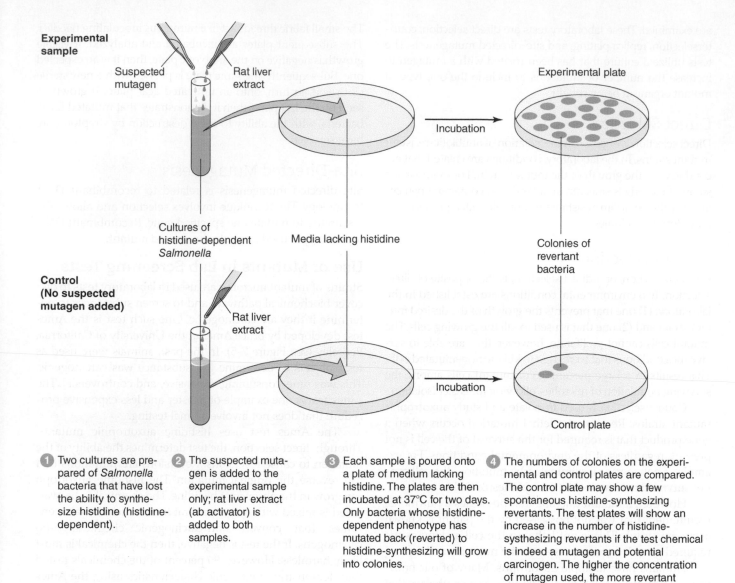

Experimental sample

Suspected mutagen

Rat liver extract

Cultures of histidine-dependent *Salmonella*

Control (No suspected mutagen added)

Rat liver extract

Media lacking histidine

Experimental plate

Incubation

Colonies of revertant bacteria

Incubation

Control plate

1. Two cultures are prepared of *Salmonella* bacteria that have lost the ability to synthesize histidine (histidine-dependent).

2. The suspected mutagen is added to the experimental sample only; rat liver extract (ab activator) is added to both samples.

3. Each sample is poured onto a plate of medium lacking histidine. The plates are then incubated at 37°C for two days. Only bacteria whose histidine-dependent phenotype has mutated back (reverted) to histidine-synthesizing will grow into colonies.

4. The numbers of colonies on the experimental and control plates are compared. The control plate may show a few spontaneous histidine-synthesizing revertants. The test plates will show an increase in the number of histidine-systhesizing revertants if the test chemical is indeed a mutagen and potential carcinogen. The higher the concentration of mutagen used, the more revertant colonies will result.

Figure 7-5 The Ames test is used to screen mutagens suspected of causing cancer in humans.

 ## Under the Microscope

Gabriela is a surgical technologist who often scrubs in orthopedic procedures. She recently found out she is 10 weeks pregnant and is thrilled because she has been trying for some time. She has informed her supervisor but finds herself scheduled to do a total hip replacement procedure with a surgeon who uses UV light for control of microbial contamination in the operating room, PMMA (bone cement) for stabilization of the joint prosthesis, and fluoroscopy to check the prosthetic implant placement.

1. Is Gabriela or the fetus at risk by scrubbing in on this type of procedure?

2. Which factors represent potential at risk for her and why?

3. Based on the normal mechanisms of bacterial genetic exchange, how would the use of ultraviolet light affect bacteria present in the OR?

4. What are examples of precautions that could be taken to minimize risk and still scrub in and do the case?

5. Which risk factors from mutagens would exist even if she was not pregnant? Please explain.

CHAPTER 8

The Empire of Viruses

Learning Objectives

After completing the study of this chapter, you will be able to:

1. Define key terms.
2. Discuss the mechanisms by which non-living viruses, viroids, or prions reproduce.
3. Describe the structure and appearance of viruses, viroids, and prions.
4. Compare and contrast viruses, viroids, and prions.
5. Describe various routes of transmission of viruses, viroids, and prions.
6. Discuss the types of disease or infection caused by viral, viroid, or prion pathogens.
7. Describe the role and impact of viruses, viroids, and prions in disease transmission.
8. Apply critical thinking skills in relating chapter material to the surgical environment of care or broader global community.

Key Terms

Angiogenesis	Dementia	Jaundice	Prodromal stage
Arthropod vectors	Dermatomes	Leukocytes	Rhinovirus
Ataxia	Dormant	Lymphadenopathy	Shingles
Capsomere	Endocytosis	Lymphocytes	Steroids
Cirrhosis	Enteroviruses	Mosaic	Syncytial
Comatose	Icosahedral	Neuralgia	Viroid
Conjunctivitis	Interferons	Pharyngitis	

The Big Picture

Viruses are considered non-living microbes, and yet they are responsible for many major disease outbreaks in humans, animals, and even plants.

During your examination of the topics in this chapter, consider the following:

1. How are these non-living microbes able to reproduce without metabolic functions?

2. How can viruses be exploited to help humans fight bacterial pathogens?

3. Which viruses are commonly able to stay dormant in the human body and reactivate later in life or when immune defenses are compromised?

4. What impact might traveling outside of the United States have in blood, tissue, or organ donation?

5. Armed with an understanding of transmission routes of viral pathogens, what preventative measures can be used to mitigate viral spread?

6. Which viruses or viral infections are of particular concern to surgical personnel?

Clinical Significance Topic

There is a conundrum (riddle, puzzle, or difficult question) with viruses, viroids, and prions: how do you kill something that isn't living in the first place? Unfortunately, the routine practice of giving antibiotics for infections that turn out to be viral has spawned the surge of antibiotic-resistant bacterial infections. Despite the fact that viruses cannot reproduce on their own, they are experts at highjacking other cells to do their bidding. The result is that viral infections can spread like wildfire. Nowhere has this been more evident than with the COVID-19 pandemic. In hospitals, where the majority of patients are immunocompromised or at least vulnerable, it is crucial for healthcare workers who are ill with viral infections to avoid exposing other personnel or patients to infection. A preventative antiviral vaccination is beneficial for many infectious viral diseases; however, prudence, strict adherence to aseptic principles, and good judgment are critical tools in breaking the chain of viral infections.

Basic Virology

The study of viruses, virology, began in a similar fashion to the study of bacteria. An observable disease process was causing destruction of crops. It was in 1890 when a Russian microbiologist, Dimitri Ivanovsky, was asked to investigate the reason why valuable tobacco crops were dying. Ivanovsky performed laboratory studies common in that era and theorized that the disease was caused by an extremely small type of bacteria. He published his findings and later described them in a 1902 dissertation entitled *Mosaic Disease in Tobacco*.

At almost exactly the same time, a Dutch microbiologist, Martinus Beijerinck, researched the same tobacco plant disease, ultimately proposing that a new type of microbial pathogen was responsible. He was first to name these microbes as viruses, based on the Latin words for slimy liquid or poison. The plant disease that both scientists were studying was given the name tobacco **mosaic** virus (TMV).

In 1898, while studying foot-and-mouth disease, Loeffler and Frosch also discovered an infectious agent that was smaller than a bacterium. This was the first recorded evidence of a virus infecting an animal. It is understandable that scientists had difficulty identifying the existence of viruses because they were not able to be viewed until after the invention of the electron microscope in the 1930s (see Figure 8-1).

The scientific community has struggled with and debated the classification of viruses. Initially, under the Kingdom taxonomy, they were included with Monera (prokaryotes). Under the Three Domains system, they were included with bacteria. Finally, when the Two Empire system was proposed, they found equal, although opposite, standing with living cellular organisms. Viral taxonomy and the Baltimore Classification System are discussed in detail in Chapter 2.

Viruses are the causative agents for many diseases in eukaryotes. Examples of human viral diseases include the common cold, influenza (flu), acquired immunodeficiency

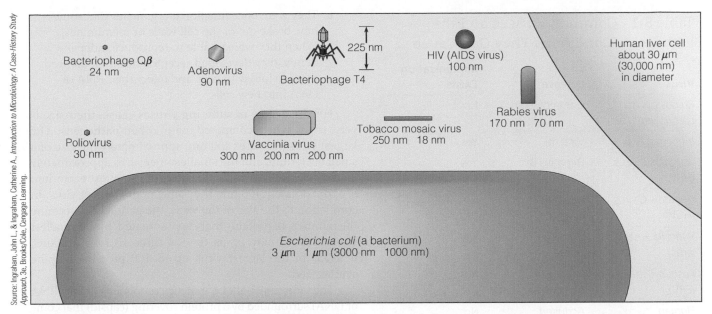

Source: Ingraham, John L., & Ingraham, Catherine A., *Introduction to Microbiology: A Case-History Study Approach*, 3e, Brooks/Cole, Cengage Learning.

Figure 8-1 Relative sizes of viruses, bacteria, and human cells.

syndrome (AIDS), rotavirus, rabies, herpes, and polio (see Figure 8-2). More frightening viral diseases such as Ebola and Marburg viral hemorrhagic fevers took center stage in the media and public awareness in the last decade.

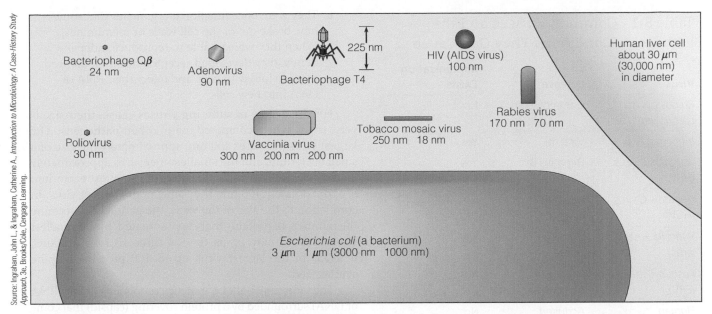

Figure 8-2 Three-dimension graphical representation of rotavirus virions. Note the characteristic wheel-like appearance that gives the rotavirus its name, which is derived from the Latin rota, meaning "wheel".

These emerging and re-emerging pathogenic diseases are discussed in later sections. Without question, the novel SARS-CoV-2 coronavirus responsible for the COVID-19 pandemic and its subsequent variant forms disrupted nearly every aspect of normal life beginning early in 2020.

Reports published in the journal *Microbiome* in July 2021 revealed the discovery of 33 viruses found in Himalayan glaciers, 28 of which were previously unknown. Ice core samples ranging in depths correspond to between 350 to nearly 15,000-years ago. The researchers believe the viruses represent environmental microbes found in dust and rain deposited onto and layered into glacial strata over past centuries. New methods of extraction that prevent or effectively deal with contamination during sampling have allowed scientists to expand their knowledge regarding the previously elusive ancient planetary viral populations.

Characteristics of Viruses

Viruses are not alive by the standard definitions we use to describe life functions. They are tiny particles of nucleic acids (RNA or DNA), surrounded by a protective capsule. They contain none of the cellular components of eukaryotes and prokaryotes, other than the genetic codes necessary for making new copies of themselves. They are obligate parasites, meaning they cannot replicate on their own. Viruses are only able to pass on their genetic material by invading other eukaryotic or prokaryotic cells and depositing their DNA or RNA into them. When those invaded cells reproduce, they also reproduce the viral genes.

Factors taken into consideration when trying to classify viruses include the diseases they cause, method of replication, structural design, genetic material, and types of hosts they invade (see Table 8-1).

Table 8-1   Common Viruses and the Pathogenic Conditions They Can Cause

Virus	Disease	Immunization Exists
Rhinovirus or coronavirus	Common cold	No
Influenza A, B, C	Viral flu	Yes
Hepatitis B virus (HBV)	Hepatitis B	Yes
Hepatitis C virus (HCV)	Hepatitis C	No
Varicella zoster virus	Chicken pox and shingles	Yes
Epstein-Barr virus (EBV)	Infectious mononucleosis	No
Human immunodeficiency virus (HIV)	Acquired immunodeficiency disease syndrome (AIDS)	No
Human papilloma virus (HPV)	Genital warts	Yes
Herpes simplex type 1	Fever blisters	No
Herpes simplex type 2	Genital herpes	In progress
Respiratory syncytial virus (RSV)	Croup bronchitis	No

Viruses are distinguished from other living cells by the following characteristics:

1. Replication of the virus is directed by viral nucleic acid within the host cell. They do not replicate by binary fission or mitosis.

2. Their nucleic acid genome may be single-stranded, double-stranded, linear, or circular ribonucleic acid (RNA) or deoxyribonucleic acid (DNA). They never have both RNA and DNA. RNA viruses are called retroviruses. An example of a retrovirus in humans is human immunodeficiency virus (HIV).

3. Viruses do not possess the enzymes needed to produce energy. They depend on the protein production machinery of the host cell.

4. Prior to 2021, no evidence of fossilized viruses had been found, making the determination of their origin difficult to answer. Two theories of viral origin have been:

   a. They were once independent life forms, possibly prokaryotes, which combined with other cells and gave up all of their properties of independence except their genomes.

   b. They were once functional organelles that somehow broke out of the cell walls or membranes. When they were unable to reproduce independently, they developed receptor sites that allowed them to join with cells and inject their RNA or DNA into new cells.

For the degree of suffering viruses cause, their size is very small when compared with other pathogens. The largest virus measures 400 nm, approximately the size of a small bacterium, and the smallest measures approximately 25 nm (the poliovirus). In contrast, the smallest bacterium is approximately 400 nm, the same as the largest virus. In correlation to the size of the virus, the genomes determine the numbers of proteins that can be created. In the smallest viruses, there may be as few as three to four proteins, whereas in the largest virus up to 100 proteins may be synthesized.

The virus consists of a genetic component (either RNA or DNA) surrounded by a protein covering (capsid) that comprises many individual protein molecules (**capsomeres**). This protein coat protects the genetic component from nucleases and has components for attachment to the host cell (see Figure 8-3).

This specialized unit of nucleic acid and capsid is called the nucleocapsid. There are a variety of structural designs possible. These include variations of **icosahedral** (20 sided) geometric shapes, helical, or complex. Some viral particles (virions) have a nucleocapsid surrounded by an outer membrane (lipid bilayer) borrowed from the cell membrane of the host into which viral proteins were attached or inserted (see Figure 8-4). This lipid bilayer is called an envelope.

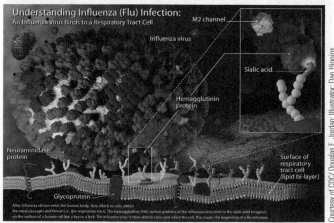

Figure 8-3 Three-dimension image illustrates the very beginning stages of an influenza (flu) infection. The viruses attach to cells within the nasal passages and throat of the respiratory tract. The influenza surface proteins designed to fit the sialic acid receptors of the human cell, like a key to a lock, bind to the sialic acid receptors on the surface of a human respiratory tract cell. The influenza virus is then able to enter and infect the cell, marking the beginning of a flu infection.

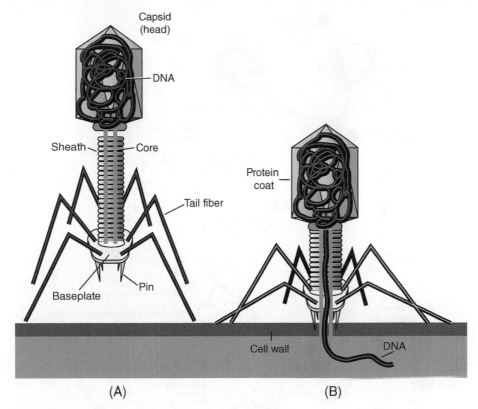

Figure 8-4 T-even bacterial virus (bacteriophage). (A) The head (capsid) is filled with DNA. (B) To replicate, the bacteriophage must penetrate a host cell to allow viral DNA to enter the cell and use the cell's metabolic processes.

Infection by Viruses

Viruses enter the body by inhalation of respiratory droplets, through an exchange of body fluids such as blood (HIV, HBV), by ingesting food or water, or through bites by **arthropod vectors**. Viruses first attach themselves to the host cell with the aid of receptors on the capsomere. The virus then enters the cell either by directly penetrating the cytoplasmic membrane or through receptor-mediated **endocytosis**. The viral nucleic acid is then uncovered and viral replication begins.

The following illustrates the steps of infection by a rhinovirus, the causative agent for the common cold:

1. An infected person sneezes in an area near others, aerosolizing (ejecting) thousands of viral particles into the ambient air.

2. Another person, unmasked and unprotected by PPE, inhales some of the viral particles.

3. The viral particles bind to cells lining the individual's nasal passages and sinuses, an excellent environment for them to begin invasion and replication.

4. The host cells lyse due to the overcrowding of the newly replicated viral particles.

5. Mucous secretions created in response to the invasion by the immune system carry virions down the airway to the lungs of the host, implanting into cells along the nasopharynx and bronchial tree.

6. Irritation of tissues occurs as a result of the body's natural inflammatory response. Additionally, pyrogens cause the body temperature to rise in response.

7. The increased host temperature eventually slows the replication rate of the virus.

Lysogenic and Lytic Cycles

Once inside the host cell, some viruses, such as herpes simplex or HIV, do not reproduce right away. Once they have infected the host cell, they begin mixing their genetic material and instructions for replication into the host cell's genetic material. When the host cell reproduces, the viral genetic instructions get copied into the host's daughter cells. This continues until some environmental or predetermined genetic signal causes the viruses to begin rapid replication and to begin infecting other cells. This cycle is referred to as the lysogenic cycle, one that occurs when the viral genetic material remains latent in the host cell and is transferred to each individual daughter cell as the host cell divides.

When the genetic material of the virus takes over the metabolic machinery of the host cell and begins producing virions, it has officially entered the lytic cycle of viral infection. During the lytic cycle, the virion releases its genetic instructions into the host cell's genetic instructions, which begins recruiting the cell's enzymes for constructing new virus particles. Protein capsids are synthesized and new viral particles are assembled. The host cell lyses and viral particles are released to infect nearby cells (see Figure 8-5).

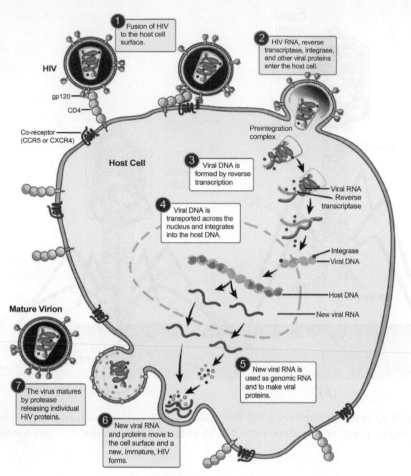

Figure 8-5 Infection stages of a host's cell and replication of a virus. Several thousand viruses particles may be formed from each cell.

Some virions are released from the host cell in a budding process. Envelopes are acquired as they pass through the cytoplasmic membrane of the host cell (see Figure 8-6).

In some types of viral infections, such as hepatitis B infection, the host cell remains alive and slowly releases viral particles over time, leading to chronic infection that becomes active when the host is immunocompromised or under stress.

Viruses can disrupt the metabolic machinery of a host cell enough to transform it into a malignant cell. The behavior and biochemistry of the host cell change significantly, and controlled growth is no longer maintained. These cells become invasive, initiate **angiogenesis**, and develop into tumors. For example, hepatitis C virus is known to cause hepatic carcinoma (cancer of the liver).

Bacteriophages

Viruses that invade bacteria as mentioned in Chapter 7 are called **bacteriophages**. Whereas animal viruses bond with the host cell through the cell's cytoplasmic membrane, bacteriophages bind to receptor sites on the bacterial host's cell wall or its fimbriae or flagella. Bacteriophages are thought to be as numerous in nature as bacteria.

Bacterial viruses are frequently complex structures and therefore are called complex viruses. Many have capsids that

have additional structures attached. The viral replication cycles of the bacteriophage, consisting of lytic and lysogenic cycles, are the best understood of all the viruses because of the extensive research performed with bacterial genome sequencing.

Bacteriophages can be classified as either virulent or temperate. Virulent bacteriophages work immediately upon entry of a bacterial cell to reproduce as rapidly as possible, eventually causing the bacterium to rupture (lyse), releasing new phages (abbreviated form of bacteriophage) into the environment. This is basically the same process as the lytic stage described previously.

Temperate phages take their time. These slower phages may combine with the host's chromosomes or become plasmids within the host cytoplasm, making new copies along with the host cell's plasmids. When the phage senses that the host bacterium is close to death, the phage causes lysis of the cell, releasing new phages to seek out new homes in other bacteria. This mirrors the lysogenic cycle previously discussed.

Harnessing Bacteriophages

An old axiom states, "The enemy of my enemy is my friend." In the case of bacteriophages, this may have come to fruition in the fight against mutant strains of bacteria. Almost a

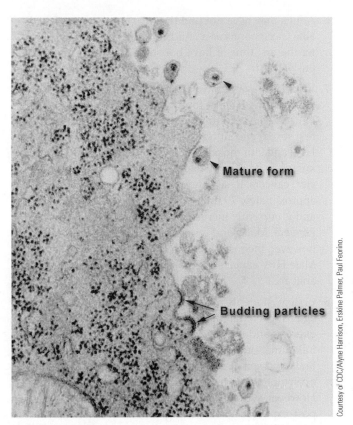

Figure 8-6 This transmission electron micrograph (TEM) depicts HIV-1 budding and free virions.

century ago, scientists took great interest in studying phages as potential therapeutic treatments against bacterial infections. Once antibiotics came to the forefront in medicine, these phages and their abilities to act against bacteria were abandoned for the most part.

In the intervening years and with that explosion of antibiotic therapy, often used inappropriately, bacteria have learned new coping skills such as mutating in their fight for survival. Antibiotic resistance has begun to increase at alarming rates, with fewer and fewer viable alternative pharmaceutical formulations available to fight these mutant strains.

In a return to the potential promise of effective use of genetic engineering and phage programming, scientists are developing and experimenting with the enzymes that phages produce and lyse their host bacterial cells. Nasal sprays containing these specialized enzymes are capable of causing destruction of the pathogenic bacteria without causing any harm to host cells.

Researchers have also focused attention on the problems of biofilms and directed studies to utilize phages for treatment of these difficult infections. They have had to deal with the unique binding factors in biofilms and the problem of getting phages through these resistant microbial barriers. In one report to the National Academy of Sciences of the United States of America, scientists proposed the use of synthetic biology along with genetic engineering to design phages specific to a bacterial biofilm but bolstered with chemical properties that allow it to penetrate the adhesive structure of the colonizing bacterial population. Achievement of this dual capability would expand future possibilities for a broad range of clinical applications. The combination of synthetic components with natural ones also greatly reduces cost and intensiveness of processing large quantities of natural phages.

Latent Viral Infections

Some viruses remain in the host for a lifetime and only emerge to cause symptoms of the disease when conditions are opportune. These types of infections are called latent infections. The human herpes virus can be reactivated in the immunocompromised individual and can cause death in certain situations. The herpes simplex virus that produces cold sores lives in the nerve cells of the host. Heat, ultraviolet rays, or stress can reactivate the virus and cause recurrence of the disease.

The chickenpox virus (varicella) may also migrate from blood to enter nerve cells after the initial infection. Changes in the immune response may also reactivate the virus, causing a painful condition called herpes zoster (shingles) (see Figure 8-7).

Cytomegalovirus (CMV) is an extremely common virus present in 60 percent to 70 percent of humans by the age of 40. Normally, CMV remains dormant and undetected; however, when its human host's immune system becomes compromised from factors such as advanced age, HIV/AIDS, or induced suppression following organ transplantation to prevent rejection, it reactivates and proliferates.

Anti-Viral Vaccinations

Contrary to popular belief, antibiotics have no effect on a virus. Antibiotics are designed to interfere with bacterial reproduction, by either inhibiting new genetic instructions or interfering with the construction of new cell walls. Viruses use the host cell's reproduction machinery; they do not carry out their own biochemical reactions, therefore, antibiotics do not affect them.

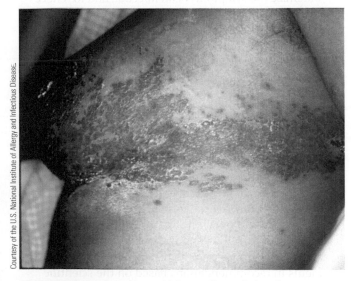

Figure 8-7 Zoster rash and blisters (lateral chest).

Until recently, viral infections could not be cured, so research focused on prevention. Immunizations work because they cause the body to produce the antibodies specific to the infecting virus just as it begins reproducing.

Because of rapid viral replication, mistakes are sometimes injected into their genetic instructions. These mutations might alter the protein coat slightly, so one year's vaccine formulation might not be as effective against the same type of virus the following year.

Many people think that only children need to be vaccinated against diseases. This is definitely a fallacy. It was thought for many years that adults maintained lifetime immunity from certain diseases either if they had been immunized as a child or if they actually had an infection from which they recovered. It is now known that this is not correct. Adults can have serum titers drawn to determine whether their immune status is active or they can have booster vaccinations to restore their protection. There are numerous reasons for children and adults to maintain their vaccination status, including:

1. Protection of babies and young children with whom unvaccinated children and adults may come in contact.

2. The shingles vaccine for herpes zoster is recommended for adults older than 50. Shingles is caused from a previous outbreak of chicken pox caused by the varicella virus. The virus remains **dormant** in the body's neural network until conditions such as stress or immune status change, causing an outbreak of extremely painful blisters on the skin. These often follow peripheral or spinal nerve tracks in their distribution pattern.

3. When traveling to foreign countries, especially developing nations, one should check the World Health Organization (WHO) or Centers for Disease Control and Prevention (CDC) website to determine if pre-travel immunizations are recommended.

4. It is recommended for everyone older than age 6 months to have an annual seasonal flu shot to help minimize the symptoms of an infection and to reduce the spread among the population. It is imperative that the formulation be from the current year or the viral strains may be different and protection may be less effective.

5. As of 2021, the efforts to get all individuals age 6 and over vaccinated for prevention of COVID-19 has met with resistance because of an unfortunate campaign of misinformation and politicization of the pandemic and its impact on global and national public health. Booster doses are recommended for the different vaccine formulations that do not demonstrate lasting effectiveness or are less able to protect against the mutant coronavirus variants such as the highly contagious delta and omicron variants. The research is ongoing with COVID-19 and all major viral diseases that affect large groups and the results may require adjustments in recommendations based on the scientific findings at that particular point in time.

6. Adults may have not had the full complement of available vaccinations as a child, so they should have them for the first time or have booster doses for those previously given.

7. Vaccines may not have been previously available. The HPV vaccine against four strains of the human papilloma virus is recommended for pre-teens prior to their first sexual encounters. There are 150 known strains of HPV and 2 of those strains, HPV 16 and HPV 18, are known to be responsible for up to 75 percent of all cervical cancers. Researchers conclude that HPV affects approximately 79 million people in the United States and is currently increasing by 14 million new cases per year. Males and females are equal carriers of HPV; however, their risk is much lower than that for females. Male HPV cancers develop in the oropharynx, penis, or anal area.

8. College students may be required to be vaccinated against bacterial meningitis because of close living quarters and classroom contact. Bacterial meningitis, an inflammation of the dural membranes that cover the brain and spinal cord, can progress extremely fast from no symptoms to a **comatose** state and possible death. However, symptoms typically develop over 3 to 7 days post-exposure. Viral meningitis is most commonly caused by non-polio **enteroviruses** and are much less aggressive than bacterial infections. There are no specific vaccinations against viral meningitis and most individuals recover on their own.

9. Healthcare workers are required to maintain current vaccinations to protect patients and their families. The CDC vaccination recommendations for healthcare workers include:
   - Hepatitis B (verified by positive serum titer)
   - Influenza (annually)
   - Measles, Mumps, Rubella (MMR) (verified by positive serum titers)
   - Varicella (Chickenpox) (verified by positive serum titers)
   - Tetanus, Diphtheria, Pertussis (Tdap) (booster every 10 years and/or during every pregnancy)
   - Meningococcal (if routinely exposed to isolates of *Neisseria meningitidis*)

10. Sexually active individuals should also be vaccinated against strains of hepatitis as blood-borne pathogens spread through unprotected sex.

Vaccinations available for bacterial diseases and the mechanisms of acquired immunity are discussed in later sections on immunology.

Interferons

Interferons (INFs) are glycoproteins that interrupt replication of both RNA and DNA viruses. They are produced by the host cell as a defense mechanism against virus infection, and each is effective against a wide variety of viruses.

Humans produce two types of INFs and three main groups: alpha (α), beta (β), and gamma (γ). Type I is produced by **leukocytes** (INF-α) and fibroblasts (INF-β). Type II (INF-γ) is produced by **lymphocytes** during an immune response.

Interferon that is released from the infected cell binds to the surface of a neighboring cell, and a signal is sent to the cell's nucleus, activating a gene coding from antiviral protein that acts to inhibit the translation of messenger RNA into proteins. This may kill the host cell, but viral spread is prevented.

The best function of INF is its ability to modulate an immune response. Natural killer (NK) cells are uniquely energized by INFs. They also play regulatory roles for macrophages and T-lymphocytes and B-lymphocytes when the immune system is geared up to fight a viral infection. Because they can regulate cell functions and stimulate the immune system, they have certain anticancer properties. Research into these properties is ongoing, but with mixed results so far.

Common Viruses

The relationship between humans and the viral world is a complex and intimate one. There is no escaping our exposure to them. Often this relationship is symbiotic. At other times, viruses become pathogenic and manifest signs and symptoms of disease. Some of the more common viruses are discussed in this section. Emerging, re-emerging, and eradicated bacterial and viral diseases are discussed in a later section.

Herpes Viruses

Herpes virus infections are very common among the animal population. Approximately 100 strains have been identified, each belonging to the family *Herpesviridae*. The name is from the Greek Herpein, meaning "to creep," signifying chronic, recurring conditions. In 1950, Burnet and Buddingh proved that herpes simplex virus could cause a latent infection after the initial one. In fact, a common characteristic of the herpes virus is that, after initial infection, it remains **dormant** until conditions become appropriate for reactivation. Appropriate conditions typically involve internal triggers, such as reaction to stress or an immunocompromised condition combined with external triggers, such as overexposure to sunlight.

Eight strains of human herpes viruses have been identified. The herpes viruses discussed here include herpes simplex virus 1 (the cause of cold sores), herpes simplex virus 2 (the cause of genital herpes), Epstein-Barr virus (the cause of infectious mononucleosis), cytomegalovirus, and varicella zoster virus (the cause of chickenpox and shingles).

The family is subdivided into alpha, beta, and gamma classifications. Alpha herpes viruses include herpes simplex virus 1 (HSV-1), herpes simplex virus 2 (HSV-2), and varicella-zoster virus (VZV). Alpha herpes viruses exhibit a short reproductive cycle and variable host range. They establish themselves after initial infection within sensory nerve ganglia and remain dormant until a trigger releases them.

Beta herpes viruses include cytomegalovirus (CMV), human herpes virus type 6 (HHV-6), and human herpes virus type 7 (HHV-7). The beta herpes viruses exhibit a longer reproductive cycle and a restricted host range. They establish themselves after initial infection within white blood cells of various tissues of the body.

Gamma herpes viruses include Epstein-Barr virus (EBV) and human herpes virus type 8 (HHV-8). These viruses establish themselves within T-lymphocytes and B-lymphocytes.

Herpes Simplex Virus

Antibodies to herpes simplex virus (HSV) are found in virtually every adult's serum. Infection is believed to occur within the first few years of life. Infection by HSV typically occurs through breaks in the skin or mucous membranes and direct contact with lesions, as well as during intimate contact such as kissing or sexual intercourse. However, the virus can be shed in the absence of clinical lesions. HSV-1 is usually associated with oral and ocular lesions, whereas HSV-2 infects the genitals and anal regions.

Initial infection is typically asymptomatic, although minor vesicular lesions may be present. HSV-1 causes vesicles to erupt on the mucocutaneous junctions of the nose or mouth, and then enters sensory nerve endings and travels up the axon to establish itself in the ganglion of the trigeminal or fifth cranial nerve (CN V). HSV-2 causes vesicles to erupt around the genitals or anus and then retreat to the sacral ganglia. Recurrence with HSV-2 is far more common than HSV-1. Severity of the lesions from initial infections by HSV-1 and HSV-2 are typically worse than subsequent recurrences (see Figure 8-8).

Despite the tendencies for the viruses to develop in separate areas, HSV-1 can occur in genitalia and HSV-2 can occur in the oral area. The two viruses under the microscope appear nearly identical. More common is the social stigma attached to these viruses. HSV-1 is sometimes considered the "good virus" while HSV-2 is the "bad virus."

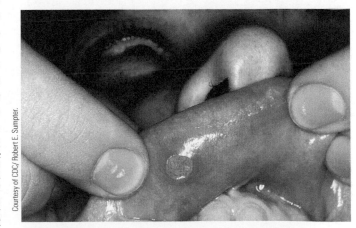

Courtesy of CDC/ Robert E. Sumpter.

Figure 8-8 Lesion on the interior of the upper lip due to the herpes simplex virus type-1 (HSV-1). Also known as a cold sore, this lesion is caused by the contagious, herpes simplex virus and should not be confused with a canker sore, which is not contagious.

HSV persists as a plasmid within the nucleus of the neuron for a lifetime and may remain in this dormant state for years. This retreat to the ganglion allows HSV to escape the immune response during initial infection. Reactivation causes the plasmid to begin rapid multiplication, and the new viral particles travel the length of the neural axon to infect the skin of the area supplied by the nerve.

Varicella-Zoster Virus

Infection by varicella-zoster virus (VZV) typically occurs during childhood, resulting in the disease commonly referred to as chickenpox. After multiplication at the inoculation sites (respiratory tract or conjunctiva), the virus enters the bloodstream and reticuloendothelial system. It finally manifests on the skin and mucosa as fluid-filled vesicles (see Figure 8-9).

After initial infection, the virus retreats into the sensory ganglia, reactivating when conditions are right (usually during immunosuppression). Like HSV, the virus travels the length of the axon to re-infect the skin supplied by the sensory nerve (usually the thoracic **dermatomes** or the area supplied by the trigeminal nerve). The vesicles that result are quite painful, and **neuralgia** can occur. This reinfection is commonly referred to as **shingles**. Therapy consists of a prescribed cycle of the antiviral medication, acyclovir available as a topical ointment (Zovirax) or oral medication (Valacyclovir). The best course of action is prevention by vaccination in older adults, although, in some cases, even younger adults can suffer outbreaks of shingles.

Cytomegalovirus

CMV can invade nearly every type of human cell and can become the cause of liver failure, retinal inflammation, and colitis. Females can easily pass the virus to a fetus during pregnancy. Cytomegalovirus is responsible for birth defects, including vision and hearing loss, seizures, and cerebral palsy.

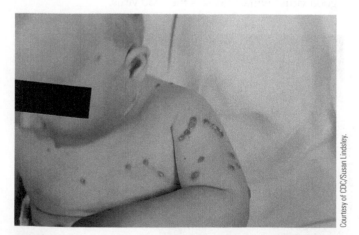

Figure 8-9 Image of infant whose upper torso displayed the characteristic "dewdrop or a rose petal" maculopapular lesions in various stages of development, i.e., Papules, vesicles, and crusts, dispersed in a region indicative of early onset of chickenpox, a disease caused by the varicella-zoster virus.

Approximately 1 in 150 live births in the United States results in these devastating effects. Felicia Goodrum, a researcher from the University of Arizona's College of Medicine, and their team received National Institutes of Health funding after they discovered a molecular switch that CMV uses in response to environmental conditions and cues to pull itself out of its dormant state and are seeking to find a drug that can inhibit the viral reactivation.

Cytomegalovirus infection is usually asymptomatic, rarely causing disease in healthy individuals. Most are infected within the first few years of life, and most adults have antibodies within serum. Transmission of the virus usually occurs through close contact (saliva secretions) or blood transfusion. Adult infection often resembles infectious mononucleosis.

Epstein-Barr Virus

It is estimated that 90 percent of the world's population has been infected with the Epstein-Barr virus (EBV), and is the virus that causes infectious mononucleosis (also known as glandular fever). There is an established connection between EBV infection and nasopharyngeal carcinoma and a high-grade B-cell lymphoma called Burkitt's lymphoma that occurs in equatorial Africa and New Guinea.

Infectious mononucleosis (IM) caused by EBV is usually acquired through close contact and an exchange of saliva. Because kissing is common among adolescents, they are the most frequently infected. Symptoms of infectious mononucleosis include **lymphadenopathy**, fever, malaise, splenomegaly (enlarged spleen), and hepatomegaly (enlarged liver).

The clinical diagnosis is made from the triad of fever, pharyngitis, and lymphadenopathy lasting 1 to 4 weeks. Tests for clinical confirmation include the Paul-Bunnell test (monospot). Most patients with acute IM make heterophile antibodies that agglutinate the red blood cells of sheep.

The virus persists within the B-lymphocytes in a plasmid (episomal) form, transforming the B-cell into a continuously dividing cell. A lymphoma (tumor of the lymphatic system) can result if the growth is not kept in check by the immune system. There is no clinical proof that latent EBV causes chronic fatigue syndrome, although many suspect that it is responsible.

There is no specific treatment for IM, other than treating the symptoms. **Steroids** are prescribed by some physicians to reduce swelling of the throat and tonsils. Enlarged spleens or livers should be closely monitored for potential rupture.

Human Herpes Virus 6 and 7

Human herpes virus 6 (HHV-6) was isolated in 1986 in the peripheral blood mononuclear cells of patients with lymphoreticular disorders. Physicians had long wondered what caused roseola infantum in infants, a febrile illness with a rash, and HHV-6 was confirmed as the culprit.

Human herpes virus 7 (HHV-7) is closely related to HHV-6 and was isolated from peripheral blood mononuclear cells. It is not known to cause any human diseases but could be a common co-factor for HHV-6.

Gastrointestinal Viruses

Viral infections of the gastrointestinal (GI) tract can be divided into two categories. Those that cause signs and symptoms in the GI tract are called enteropathogenic diseases. The enteropathogenic viruses include members of the *Caliciviridae* family: rotavirus, adenovirus, astrovirus, and norovirus. These viruses are typically single-stranded, non-enveloped, spherical or hexagonal shaped, and chemically icosahedral. Complications from viral gastroenteritis infections account for up to 2.2 million deaths annually worldwide. Adenoviruses are more commonly connected to respiratory illnesses.

Non-enteropathogenic diseases enter the body through the gastrointestinal tract but manifest in other body systems and organs. They include the enteroviruses discussed in the next section.

Rotavirus

Rotaviruses are non-enveloped, icosahedral, triple-layered particles with double-stranded RNA segments that form the complex circular shape (from the Latin word rota, meaning wheel) (see Figure 8-10). Rotaviruses are responsible for severe gastrointestinal infections of very young children. It is estimated that prior to the introduction and widespread use of vaccines, in the United States, 20 to 60 children died each year from complications including dehydration as a result of severe watery diarrhea, vomiting, and fever. Statistics for 2008 described more than 450,000 deaths worldwide in children younger than age 5.

Two vaccines were developed and distributed for infants in 2006. One of the vaccines is given in two doses at ages 2 and 4 months. The other is given in three doses at ages 2, 4, and 6 months in a similar manner to other routine childhood vaccinations. The CDC estimates that since the addition of rotavirus vaccination protocols for infants, 40,000 to 50,000 hospitalizations of infants and young children have been prevented. Adults may also contract rotaviruses, especially those

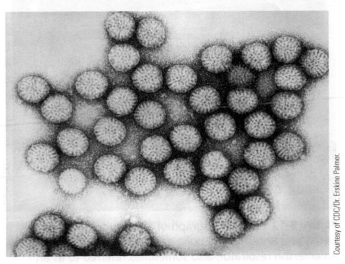

Figure 8-10 A transmission electron micrograph (TEM) reveals the ultrastructural morphology of a number of intact rotavirus double-shelled particles.

Courtesy of CDC/Dr. Erskine Palmer.

living in congregate living settings such as nursing homes or assisted living facilities; however, their symptoms are usually much less severe.

Norovirus

Noroviruses are non-enveloped, single-stranded RNA viruses responsible for acute gastroenteritis infections. They belong to the *Caliciviridae* family and include sapoviruses. Once described in 1929 as "the winter vomiting disease," it was previously called "Norwalk-like" virus after an outbreak in 1968 at a school in Norwalk, Ohio. Often described as the "stomach flu," the virus, unrelated to the respiratory influenza virus, is the most common cause of acute gastroenteritis and foodborne-disease outbreaks. Most norovirus outbreaks happen from November to April in the U.S. and in years when there is a new strain of the virus, there can be 50 percent more norovirus illness. Each year, the CDC reports that on average in the United States, norovirus causes:

- 900 deaths, mostly among adults aged 65 and older
- 109,000 hospitalizations
- 465,000 emergency department visits, mostly in young children
- 2,270,000 outpatient clinic visits annually, mostly in young children
- 19 to 21 million cases of vomiting and diarrhea illnesses

Astroviruses

Astroviruses are named for their characteristic star shapes. They are responsible for less severe gastroenteritis infections in younger populations. Astroviruses are the chief cause of acute diarrhea in immunocompromised patients.

Enteroviruses

The enteroviruses are part of the family *Picornaviridae* and the genus *Enterovirus*. They are very small viruses made up of ribonucleic acid (RNA) with a protein covering. The group includes rhinoviruses, polioviruses, coxsackieviruses, and echoviruses. In addition, there are 61 strains of pathogenic non-polio enteroviruses (see Figure 8-11).

Infection by members of this group of viruses can cause many different diseases that affect a variety of target organs: neurologic (polio, encephalitis, meningitis), respiratory (cold, flu, tonsillitis, pharyngitis), and cardiovascular (myocarditis).

Rhinovirus

One of the most common communicable infections in humans is termed the "common cold." The human **rhinoviruses**, types A, B, and C, belong to the *Picornaviridae* family and are found primarily in the upper respiratory tracts (mouth and nose); these cause the majority of colds. These viruses are some of the smallest, measuring on average only 30 nm.

The viral particles are easily spread by aerosol spray and by contact with inoculated surfaces. Symptoms include

laryngotracheobronchitis often called croup, bronchiolitis, and pneumonitis.

Mumps is a common acute disease seen primarily in children. The virus that causes mumps produces obvious salivary gland inflammation. The virus enters the body via the pharynx or conjunctiva and then spreads to the salivary glands or in some cases to the testes, ovaries, pancreas, and brain. The main characteristic of mumps is painful enlargement of the parotid glands (see Figure 8-15).

Measles is another acute disease seen primarily in children. The virus invades the lymphatic and respiratory systems via the oropharynx. Clinically, the virus produces respiratory symptoms during the initial **prodromal stage** (fever, cough) and a subsequent rash during the eruptive stage (red spots on the head and body).

Human Parainfluenza Viruses Human parainfluenza viruses (PIVs) are responsible for approximately 30 percent to 40 percent of acute lower respiratory tract infections in infants and children. The virus first grows in the ciliated epithelial tissues of the upper respiratory tract (nose and throat) and then spreads into the lungs. The most common diseases caused by these viruses are croup, bronchiolitis, and pneumonia. Types 1 and 2 are responsible for more severe lower respiratory tract infections, such as acute laryngotracheobronchitis (croup). Type 3 is the most virulent of the PIVs, causing increased morbidity and potential mortality. Types 4a and 4b are rarely isolated and, when diagnosed, tend to be the least virulent. The various parainfluenza viruses are found worldwide and are endemic to some areas and epidemic at relatively predictable times. The disease is transmitted via respiratory droplets (see Figure 8-16).

Respiratory Syncytial Virus Respiratory **syncytial** virus (RSV) is the causative pathogenic agent for most respiratory infections in infants. RSV is also the major cause of viral pneumonia and bronchiolitis in adults and children. The virus initiates as a local infection in the upper respiratory tract,

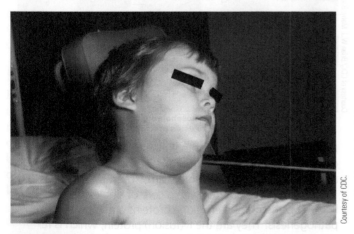

Figure 8-15 Child with a mumps infection and characteristic swollen neck region due to an enlargement of the salivary glands.

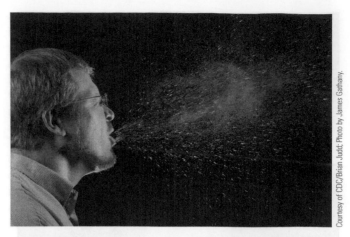

Figure 8-16 Respiratory droplet dispersal following a violent sneeze.

invading the ciliated epithelia of the nose, eye, and mouth, then moves into the lower respiratory tract to cause croup, pneumonia, or bronchiolitis. The lower respiratory infections are most often seen in infants. Premature infants are especially at risk. The virus is endemic worldwide, with yearly epidemics occurring. Currently there are no vaccinations for RSV; however, during the normal flu season months of autumn and early spring, young children at risk may be given monthly inhalation mist treatments with ribavirin, an antiviral medication.

Metapneumovirus The human metapneumovirus (hMPV) was first discovered in 2001. Found worldwide, it is a common pathogen responsible for upper and lower respiratory tract infections, primarily in infants and young children, and is a known trigger for asthma. Individuals who are immunocompromised, including those with lung transplants or chronic obstructive pulmonary disease (COPD), are also at increased risk for contracting hMPV. The seasonal nature of outbreaks for both RSV and hMPV may increase the chance for co-infections with both viral strains in susceptible patients.

Adenovirus

Adenoviruses are double-stranded DNA viruses with icosahedral capsids. The virion is non-enveloped, spherical, and approximately 70 to 90 nm in size. Adenoviruses cause **pharyngitis**, acute respiratory disease, pneumonia, pharyngoconjunctival fever, viral **conjunctivitis** (pink eye), genitourinary infections, and gastroenteritis. Transmission is through the fecal-oral route, direct contact (hand to eye), or respiratory aerosols.

The virus usually causes localized infection, but generalized infection occurs in immunocompromised populations. Many of the localized viral infections are easily spread among young children in day-cares and schools. Enteroviruses are responsible for a small percentage of acute respiratory childhood illnesses and a slightly larger percentage of infantile gastroenteritis.

Coronavirus

There are six types of coronaviruses that can infect humans. Named for the crown-like spikes on the surface of the virus, they are grouped into subcategories: alpha, beta, gamma, and delta. The two forms that had gained public notoriety in the past two decades were SARS (severe acute respiratory syndrome) and MERS (Middle East respiratory syndrome). SARS was first recognized in 2002 in China. It caused a worldwide outbreak of more than 8,000 cases and 774 deaths. According to the CDC, there have been no further detected cases of SARS since 2004.

In 2012, hundreds of people became ill with a coronavirus first detected in Saudi Arabia, and it was given the name Middle East respiratory syndrome. In 2015, over 16,000 people in South Korea were quarantined because of possible exposure to MERS. By mid-July when the outbreak tapered off, 186 cases had been confirmed with 36 fatalities. All of the individuals who contracted the illness were connected to countries around the Arabian Peninsula.

Coronaviruses in general cause symptoms similar to other upper respiratory infections, and most individuals will contract mild infections in their lifetimes; however, mainly the very young, older adults, and immunocompromised individuals are at increased risk for this family of viral pathogens (see Figure 8-17).

The pathogen first described as a novel coronavirus in late 2019 first described as 2019-nCoV then later designated as SARS-CoV-2. The virus, first recognized in the Wuhan province of China, spread rapidly in 2020 and was responsible for the COVID-19 pandemic which has infected over 340 million globally and 70 million in the U.S., resulting in a global death rate in early-2022 of over 5.5 million and 864,000 in the U.S. The resulting mutations of the original coronavirus responsible for COVID-19, including the highly transmissible 2021 delta and omicron variants,

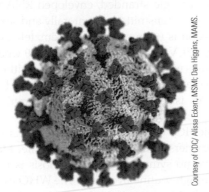

Courtesy of CDC/ Alissa Eckert, MSMI; Dan Higgins, MAMS.

Figure 8-17 Illustration created at the CDC shows ultrastructural morphology exhibited by coronaviruses. Note the spikes that adorn the outer surface of the virus, which impart the look of a corona surrounding the virion. A Novel Coronavirus, Named Severe Acute Respiratory Syndrome Coronavirus 2 (SARS-CoV-2), was identified as the cause of an outbreak of respiratory illness Named Coronavirus Disease 2019 (COVID-19).

caused additional surges in infection rates and deaths, including in children who were previously at less risk with the original virus, but subsequently at greater risk of serious infections due to the delayed availability of approved vaccines for children under 12 years of age.

Influenza A

Influenza viruses are divided into types A, B, and C. Types A and B cause seasonal outbreaks in human populations and are constantly mutating. Type C causes only mild upper respiratory symptoms and is not believed to cause epidemic outbreaks. This constant change requires a modified yearly vaccine. Occasionally, a completely new influenza virus appears for which there is no immunity or vaccine. This is called an antigenic shift and often results in local epidemics or global pandemics, the most devastating of which occurred in 1918 (called the Spanish flu) and killed 25 to 50 million people worldwide (700,000 Americans died), more deadly than the COVID-19 pandemic a century later. The agent responsible for this pandemic is now known as influenza A virus (H1N1).

Hippocrates was the first to describe the disease. The first documented influenza pandemic occurred in 1580, and since that time 31 such possible influenza pandemics have been documented, with three occurring in the past century (in 1918, 1957, and 1968). It is believed by scientists that the viruses responsible for these epidemics originated from animals (the 1918 epidemic is believed to have been caused by either birds or swine).

The WHO and CDC have adopted specifications and naming conventions for various strains of influenza viruses.

The components for this nomenclature include the following:

- The antigenic type (A, B, or C)
- Type of original host (avian, equine, or swine; however, if human, then no designation is made)
- Geographic origin (Taiwan, Hong Kong, etc.)
- Strain number
- Year of isolation (1918, 2009, etc.)
- The hemagglutinin and neuraminidase antigen description in parentheses for type A strains (H1N1), (H5N1), or (H3N2)

Examples provided from the CDC are:

- A/duck/Alberta/35/76 (H1N1) for a virus of duck origin
- A/Perth/16/2009 (H3N2) for a virus of human origin

The flu vaccines given annually include mixtures of A(H1N1), A(H3N2), and one or two influenza B strains. Each year the vaccine mixture is modified to include the previous year's strains, making it important for healthcare workers to keep up with the current vaccine stock each year to reduce the severity of symptoms if exposed.

Influenza causes a wide range of symptoms, including fever, cough, muscle aches, and chills. Most influenza infections are self-limiting and do not require hospitalization. As with many viral infections, the very young and old and the immunocompromised tend to have more severe symptoms and may require hospitalization.

Hepatitis Viruses

Hepatitis is an inflammation of the liver caused by viral, bacterial, or fungal infection. Inflammation of the liver can also be caused by toxins, alcohol, and autoimmune disorders. The disease was first described in the Babylonian Talmud in the fifth century. It was not until 1969 that the first hepatitis virus was isolated (hepatitis B). Hepatitis A was isolated in 1973, followed by C, D, and E. Although at least 20 viruses affect the human liver, this chapter only discusses A through E because the other viruses affect other organs. These other viruses include cytomegalovirus, mumps virus, and the yellow fever virus.

Hepatitis A Virus

Hepatitis A virus (HAV) is an RNA virus that is transmitted primarily by the fecal-oral route, although it is also found in semen and blood. As a member of the enterovirus group of picornaviruses (it is also known as enterovirus type 72), HAV contains a linear strand of RNA.

The illness caused by HAV usually begins with **jaundice**, fever, and weakness, preceded by flu-like symptoms and lymphadenopathy (see Figure 8-18). Relapses may occur after the initial infection for up to a year after the initial symptoms have subsided, but chronic infection by HAV does not occur.

Gammaglobulin is given after initial exposure. Vaccination is effective and required for all school children in the United States. Treatment includes rest, fluids, and avoidance of alcohol.

Hepatitis B Virus

Hepatitis B virus (HBV) contains a circular, partly double-stranded DNA genome. It is acquired parenterally (blood

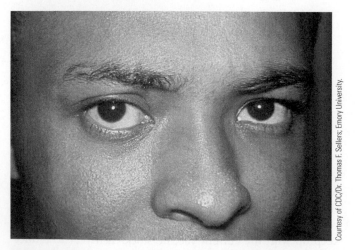

Figure 8-18 The viral disease Hepatitis A is manifested here as icterus, or jaundice of the conjunctivae and facial skin.

transfusions, contaminated needles) or sexually. As a blood-borne pathogen, HBV transmission has long been of concern in healthcare settings where sharps injuries from hollow-bore needle sticks, puncture from sharp surgical instruments or solid-bore suture needles, or inoculation into the eyes from blood splatter can present particular risk for healthcare workers in those critical care areas. The acute phase causes jaundice, weakness, fever, and nausea.

One in 20 HBV infections results in chronic hepatitis (defined as persistent hepatitis 6 months after the onset of the acute illness). Chronic HBV infection can be benign with normal liver tests or may be an aggressive inflammatory process that can lead to **cirrhosis** (hardening of the liver). HBV is also known to cause cancer of the liver.

There are two types of vaccines for HBV, one which involves three injections and is highly recommended for all operating room personnel. Another vaccine, Heplisav-B, a two-dose injection, was given FDA approval in 2020 for use in adults over age 18 who have not previously been vaccinated and those for whom incomplete immunity was demonstrated by blood titers. Acute exposure (needle stick) is managed with the HBV vaccine and hepatitis B high-titer immunoglobulin injection (HBIG). Interferon has also been approved for HBV infection treatment, administered daily for 4 months. Lamivudine is being used as a treatment for HBV and HIV infections; however, it may cause lactic acidosis, a serious condition affecting the liver.

Hepatitis C Virus

The Hepatitis C virus (HCV) was known as non-A, non-B hepatitis virus (NANBH) until 1989. It belongs to the family *Flaviviridae* and genus Hepacivirus. Other genera include Flavivirus and Pestivirus. Flavivirus diseases include yellow fever, Dengue fever, Japanese encephalitis and tick-borne encephalitis. Pestivirus diseases include bovine viral diarrhea and classic swine fever.

HCV is a single-stranded, enveloped RNA viral blood-borne pathogen transmitted parenterally and sexually. Mode of transmission is unknown in approximately 20 percent of cases. Acute HCV infection develops 6 to 10 weeks after exposure. Victims may have flu-like symptoms without jaundice. Because liver enzymes are usually not measured at that time, the infection is not typically detected until years after exposure.

Chronic HCV occurs in 50 percent to 60 percent of cases, and most carriers remain contagious for life. Many chronic carriers have no symptoms until diagnosis is made coincidentally through routine liver tests. The WHO estimated that approximately 3 percent of the human population (150–200 million people worldwide) are infected with HCV. Many develop aggressive hepatitis and eventual cirrhosis and liver failure, requiring transplantation. Diagnosis is confirmed by hepatitis C antibody blood test or liver biopsy to measure the severity of infection. The U.S. Preventive Services Task Force had published its recommendation for routine hepatitis C screening of adults from18 to 79 years of age born between

1945 and 1965. Those at elevated risk of exposure and possible infection include:

- Personal history of illicit drug use by injection or inhalation
- Abnormal liver function tests with no identifiable cause
- Children born to mothers with hepatitis C infection
- Healthcare workers and first responders with exposure events to blood
- Hemophilia patients treated with clotting factors prior to 1987
- Long-term dialysis patients
- Organ transplant or blood transfusion recipients received prior to 1992
- Intimate partners of known hepatitis C patients
- HIV-infected individuals
- Individuals who have served time in prison settings

Direct-acting antiviral drug treatments of HCV have been approved including sofosbuvir/velpatasvir (Epclusa®). These drugs alone or in combination do not depend on interferon or ribavirin, which were previously available treatments. Patients are advised that hepatitis B infections could be reactivated with the drug regimen resulting in potential for severe or fatal liver disease.

Hepatitis D Virus

Hepatitis D virus (HDV), also known as the delta virus, is an incomplete RNA virus that infects only those liver cells that are already infected with HBV. It takes advantage of the HBV enzymes for replication and the acquisition of a protein coat that allows it to survive outside of the liver. Structurally, HDV is unlike any of the other hepatitis viruses. It is uncommon in the United States. The virus is transmitted parenterally or sexually as a co-infection with HBV or to chronic HBV patients. Chronic carriers of HBV who are infected with HDV develop a superinfection that can be fatal. Neither interferon nor transplantation is effective for HDV. The hepatitis B vaccine prevents infections of HDV in individuals not already infected with HBV.

Hepatitis E Virus

Hepatitis E virus (HEV) is similar to HAV: Both are RNA viruses transmitted through the fecal-oral route and both cause acute, but not chronic, infection. HEV is believed to be the primary causative agent for hepatitis in countries with poor or marginal sanitation and contaminated water supplies. The illness is usually benign but can be fatal for pregnant women.

Human Immunodeficiency Virus

In 1981, researchers at the CDC came to the realization that a new epidemic called acquired immunodeficiency syndrome (AIDS) was spreading rapidly in the United States. The most noticeable characteristic of the new disease was vulnerability

of those infected to opportunistic infections and a profound decrease in their T-lymphocyte counts. It was also noted that infected homosexual males and intravenous drug users were developing a very rare type of skin cancer called Kaposi's sarcoma (see Figure 8-19).

In 1983, the virus that caused AIDS was isolated and given the name human immunodeficiency virus (HIV). By 1985, the chief routes of HIV transmission were identified: blood, sexual contact, and mother to child. The main target cells for the virus were identified as CD4 T-lymphocytes and macrophages and with that recognition, an antibody test was established.

It is believed that the virus began in African apes as simian immunodeficiency virus (SIV), and it most likely jumped species when the animals were hunted, slaughtered, and eaten. This exposure to the infected animal blood was most likely the original route of transmission and may have occurred as long ago as the late 1800s. As global travel increased, so did the new human form of the viral disease. Some researchers believe that HIV has been in the United States since the mid to late 1970s.

The CDC reports that, by 1997, HIV infection had become a pandemic, with 28 million infections worldwide. Eight million people infected with HIV developed AIDS at that time. By 2000, 36 million people were infected. To date, it is estimated that 39 million people have died from the disease and 35 million worldwide are living with the disease. The estimated HIV prevalence in adults 13 years of age and older in 2019 was nearly 1.2 million cases in the United States. Globally in 2020, there were approximately 38 million individuals living with HIV, nearly 2 million of which were children under age 15.

The leading known risk factors for HIV infection include male-to-male contact (69 percent) and injection drug use (7 percent) accounted for 76 percent of all cases in the United States in 2019. Heterosexual contact accounted for the remaining 23 percent. The age group with the highest number if new infections in the U.S. in 2019 was ages 25–34 years.

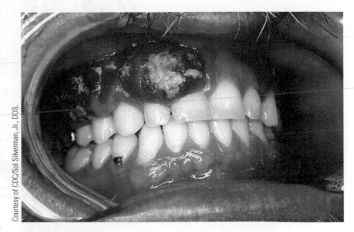

Courtesy of CDC/Sol Silverman, Jr., DDS.

Figure 8-19 HIV-positive patient presented with an intra-oral Kaposi's sarcoma lesion with an overlying candidiasis infection.

HIV belongs to a family of RNA viruses distinguished by possession of a viral reverse transcriptase that transcribes viral RNA into provirus DNA that is integrated into the host cell's genome. These so-called retroviruses are generally host-specific and are divided into two subfamilies: oncoretroviruses (with human T-cell lymphotropic virus, or HTLV) and lentiviruses (HIV) (see Figure 8-20).

Decades after the first cases of HIV and AIDS were diagnosed and researchers scrambled to find drug treatments to treat the diseases, anti-retroviral drugs have revolutionized treatment. The disease, at least in the United States, has become a manageable long-term chronic infection for which various pharmaceutical combinations have been developed for individual patient needs. There are one-a-day pills that contain combinations of anti-retrovirals. Currently, there are more than 30 approved, effective drugs used to treat patients and maintain their CD4 T-lymphocyte counts. The disease has no cure, but it can be managed and relatively good health can be maintained by those infected if healthy lifestyles and drug regimens are followed closely.

Viroids

Farmers in the 1920s began noticing their potato crops were being killed and deformed by an unknown pathogen. The process was eventually called potato spindle tuber disease (PSTD). In 1971, Dr. Theodor Diener, a plant pathologist with the US Department of Agriculture, discovered the cause of the potato disease. Measuring only one-eightieth the size of a normal virus, the potato spindle tuber **viroid** was determined to be the causative agent of the potato crop disease.

More recent studies by researchers have isolated more than 30 other species of viroids that cause diseases in food crops such as coconuts and tomatoes and in flower species of chrysanthemums and dahlias. The only recognized defense currently used against the spread of viroids to other plants is complete destruction of the entire crop.

Researchers found that viroids are little more than naked loops or short strands of RNA without protein coats. Their genetic material is composed of fewer than 400 nucleotides as compared to the typical influenza virus, which has approximately 14,000 nucleotides in its genetic material. Once inside the host cell, the viroid RNA invades the host cell's RNA strands, tricking it into making new copies. The RNA segment then breaks off and loops itself into a circular shape.

Viroids may represent the prehistoric ancestors of modern viruses in a similar fashion that archaea are to modern prokaryotes. However, it is impressive that in both cases, these microbial ancestors continue to exist and thrive in the modern world. Scientists acknowledge that there are likely many more species of viroids yet to be discovered in other life forms than just the few species of plants noted to fall victim to viroid pathogens.

Prion Diseases

One of the great challenges to scientists has been how to deal with diseases caused by non-living proteins. At least in the case

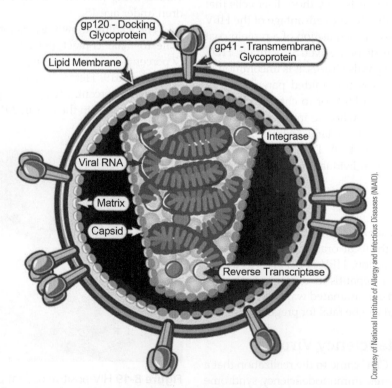

Figure 8-20 An illustration from National Institute of Allergy and Infectious Diseases (NIAID) that depicts the ultrastructural morphology of the human immunodeficiency virus (HIV).

of non-living viruses, the mechanisms by which they are able to replicate and transfer their genomes are fairly well understood. In the case of the lethal prion proteins, research is ongoing, but to date, no forms of treatment or potential cures have been discovered. The research continues to focus on the pathogenicity of these non-living agents and the diseases they cause.

Transmissible Spongiform Encephalopathy

Transmissible spongiform encephalopathies (TSEs) first discussed in Chapter 2 are a group of diseases found in both animals and humans that are caused by infectious agents found mainly in structures of the central nervous system, most commonly the brain. These agents called prions have no nucleic acids and no cellular structure. Researchers believe disease results from normal proteins called PrP^c, which develop abnormal folds thereby creating prions or PrP^{sc}. These proteins sit on the surface of neural tissues, such as the brain and spinal cord, and eventually destroy these tissues, creating holes and resulting in the eventual sponge-like appearance.

The purpose or physiologic function of the proteins that can become pathogenic prions is currently unknown. It is thought to be similar to proteins isolated in patients with Alzheimer's disease; however, no other correlations between the two have been definitively made.

There have been documented cases of familial transmission of Creutzfeldt-Jakob disease (CJD) from parent to offspring. These incidents are thought to comprise only approximately 10 percent of the known cases, with the other 90 percent being acquired from outside sources. Ingesting infected cattle is the main focus of research. Other ways in which these abnormal proteins are passed through iatrogenic transmission (medical or surgical care) include:

- the use of prion contaminated surgical instruments from previous CJD patients
- implantation of harvested human cadaver dura mater or corneal tissue from patients later found to have unrecognized CJD
- from invasive electrodes used on a patient after having been used on an affected individual
- after receiving injections of human growth hormone derived from the pituitary glands of human cadavers.

The CDC states that no known cases of iatrogenic transmission of CJD has occurred in the U.S. since 1976 and since more stringent protocols have been established to deal with contaminated surgical instrumentation. Surgical and sterile processing personnel must remain vigilant with prevention measures in any patients who have been identified as possible CJD or vCJD infections. Specific decontamination or disposal of potentially infected materials is discussed further in Chapter 21.

Animal TSE infections are called bovine (cattle) spongiform encephalopathy (mad cow disease), ovine (sheep) spongiform encephalopathy (scrapie), and chronic wasting disease (CWD) in North American hooved animals such as deer, elk, and moose (see Figure 8-21). The prion infections in humans are Creutzfeldt-Jakob disease (CJD) and variant Creutzfeldt-Jakob disease (vCJD), Gerstmann-Straussler-Scheinker syndrome, fatal familial insomnia, and kuru.

The CDC state on their website: "Classic CJD is a human prion disease. It is a neurodegenerative disorder with characteristic clinical and diagnostic features. This disease is rapidly progressive and always fatal. Infection with this disease leads to death usually within 1 year of onset of illness.

Creutzfeldt-Jakob disease (CJD) is a rapidly progressive, invariably fatal neurodegenerative disorder believed to be caused by an abnormal isoform of a cellular glycoprotein known as the prion protein. CJD occurs worldwide and the estimated annual incidence in many countries, including the United States, has been reported to be about one case per million population." Variant CJD (vCJD) is distinctly different from classic CJD in a number of ways, although both have long incubation periods before the onset of observable symptoms. Classic CJD and vCJD differences include:

- age of death in CJD is 68 years and in vCJD it is 28 years
- average duration of apparent illness is 4–5 month for CJD and 13–14 months for vCJD

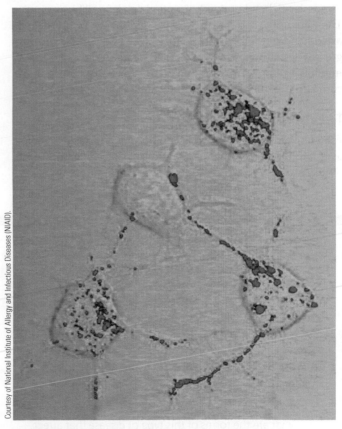

Courtesy of National Institute of Allergy and Infectious Diseases (NIAID).

Figure 8-21 Photomicrograph by National Institute of Allergy and Infectious Diseases (NIAID) of prion proteins stained in red.

- initial CJD symptoms are neurologic disorders or dementia and behavioral or psychiatric symptoms with generalized diffuse pains are initially seen in vCJD and delayed signs of dementia

- the absence of florid plaques (areas of erythema) in brain tissue in CJD and presence of large numbers in vCJD as well as other diagnostic protein markers.

A Texas patient who died of vCJD in 2014 was the fourth known case in the United States since the first case detected in 1996 in the United Kingdom. The patient had traveled extensively in Europe and the Middle East, most likely having contracted it overseas.

Researchers have determined there is a causal relationship between outbreaks in Europe of bovine spongiform encephalopathy and vCJD in that the agent responsible for the outbreak of prion disease in cows with BSE is the same agent responsible for vCJD in humans.

Gerstmann-Straussler-Scheinker Syndrome

Gerstmann-Straussler-Scheinker syndrome is an extremely rare neurodegenerative disease found in only a few families around the world. An estimated 85 percent of CJD cases are classified as sporadic infections. A much smaller proportion, 5–15 percent of affected individuals develop inherited mutations of the prion protein gene resulting in Gerstmann-Straussler-Scheinker syndrome and fatal familial insomnia. The rare inherited prion disease manifests symptoms of **ataxia** and **dementia** between the ages of 35 and 55. It progresses slowly, usually over 2 to 10 years. As with all transmissible spongiform encephalopathy diseases, there is no cure and treatment is geared toward alleviating symptoms.

Fatal Familial Insomnia

Fatal familial insomnia (FFI) is another prion disease classified as a rare disease by the National Institutes of Health (NIH). Similar to G-S-S, it is an autosomal dominant inherited disease that may be caused by mutations of the PRNP gene or "prion protein." Patients present with symptoms of increasing insomnia progressing to death within 9 months on average with no known treatment or cure available.

Kuru

Kuru was a rare disease that became an epidemic in a highlands region of New Guinea in the 1950s among the Fore tribe. As a funeral rite, family members were expected to consume the bodies, including the brains, of the deceased as a sign of respect and remembrance. The disease was highly contagious and easily transmitted through the practice of cannibalism, which was strongly discouraged by the government following the outbreak of kuru (Fore tribe word for shiver). As with most TSEs, the onset of symptoms could be in excess of several decades, but once symptoms appeared death would occur within 6 to 12 months. Once the practice had been discontinued and those infected had succumbed to the disease, kuru was considered eradicated.

MICRO NOTES

"Going Viral"

The expressions "going viral" and "computer virus" came about because of the actual nature of how viruses work. If a video goes "viral" on the Internet, it means it has spread very quickly in a relatively short period of time. Doesn't influenza spread like that in the fall and winter months? A computer virus is designed to be spread to many other "hosts" and either may cause massive damage to the new computer where it was downloaded or may lurk there for long periods until it is activated by a command or simple key stroke of the owner, and then "@%(*#&$%!" The same thing probably many people who get shingles or chicken pox might say.

 ## Under the Microscope

Dr. Yousef scheduled a craniotomy for biopsy of possible variant Creutzfeldt-Jakob disease (vCJD) in a patient with a history of having lived in the United Kingdom for 5 years prior to returning to the United States 10 years ago. The patient is no longer ambulatory due to loss of coordination and diffuse dysesthesia (pain). The current mental status of the patient is declining rapidly.

1. What is the term used for the general category of prion diseases?

2. What are the forms of this type of disease that affect animal species.

3. What is the significance of the patient having lived in the United Kingdom 10 years ago?

4. How do the two forms of CJD suspected in this patient compare and contrast?

5. How does CJD differ from pathogenic viruses or viroids in appearance and replication?

6. What is the typical course of the disease process and the overall prognosis for the patient?

CHAPTER 9

Microbial Disease Transmission

Learning Objectives

After completing the study of this chapter, you will be able to:

1. Define key terms.
2. Compare and contrast the three types of disease outbreak.
3. Describe various methods of disease transmission.
4. Discuss factors relating to pathogenicity.
5. Describe the non-specific host defenses in humans.
6. Apply critical thinking skills in relating chapter material to the surgical environment of care or broader global community.

Key Terms

Adherence	Eradicated	Host	Phagosome
Cytopathic effects	Fomites	Hydrolyze	Phlegm
Determinants	Helminths	Keratin	Sharps injuries
Disseminated	Homeostasis	Neurotransmitter	Surface receptors

The Big Picture

Standard Precautions are a set of practices healthcare workers use to prevent disease transmission between patients and themselves and to guard against potential cross-contamination of patients and the environment. One key factor in this process is the use of personal protective equipment or PPE that serve as dual-benefit barriers to protect patients from healthcare workers and vice versa. Another key factor is the human body's natural defense mechanisms against pathogenic bacterial or viral invaders.

During your examination of the topics in this chapter, consider the following:

1. What are common methods of disease transmission?

2. What are the portals of entry for pathogenic invasion of various body systems?

3. Which components of PPE are appropriate for protection of the portals of entry in patients and personnel in the surgical environment of care ?

4. What are examples of how patients could be infected by cross-contamination in the perioperative area?

5. What are the various natural defense mechanisms against pathogenic invasion and damage to human tissues and body systems?

Clinical Significance Topic

The past decade has seen several examples of public health and healthcare system crises. The 2014 Ebola outbreak in several western countries in Africa caused panic, due in part to the sensationalism by the news media. The COVID-19 pandemic which spread widely in 2020 and the years beyond 2020 exposed the fact that many healthcare workers are insufficiently trained to deal with unfamiliar disease outbreaks such as Ebola and overwhelming international and local public health crises that arise in a global viral pandemic. Physicians, nurses, aides, and volunteers in Africa, and eventually here in the United States, were exposed to and infected with the deadly Ebola virus, not because they were careless but rather for a number of reasons including: they were not fully trained on use of the PPE available; appropriate PPE was unavailable; or the response protocols for highly contagious infections were insufficient. The COVID-19 pandemic created a critical shortage of PPE in the U.S. and globally. The spotlight on the mistakes made and lack of preparation has exposed the holes in the disease prevention plans for healthcare institutions. In the future, healthcare worker skills competencies, disaster-planning implementation, and availability of sufficient stocks of appropriate PPE should be part of every hospital's infectious disease or general preparedness planning programs. Certified Surgical

Technologists (CSTs) and all healthcare providers should take personal responsibility as well for seeking out, practicing, and adhering to disaster training and preparation, even while keeping fingers crossed that they may never have to implement it.

Disease Transmission

Diseases that affect humans can come from nearly every member (eukaryotes, prokaryotes, viruses, viroids, and prions) of the various classification models: Two Empires, Three Kingdoms, Tree of Life, and others. Humans have a fundamental, intimate, and complicated relationship with the microbial world, both internally and externally. We rely on our individual microbiomes to maintain **homeostasis** and to break down foods into usable nutrient forms. Our bodies are taught how to coexist with the microbial world from the first encounter with the birth canal of our mothers, inoculating us with our first microbes. The majority of our total body weight is actually comprised of microbial cells. The preponderance of life forms on earth is microbial. It is unreasonable then, to consider the microbial world as our enemy, except when it actually does become just that—the enemy.

Research scientists have focused great attention on bacteria and other potential pathogenic organisms in the hopes of finding both cause and cure of disease. Only within the past half-century, the technology of electron microscopes allowed them to study the empire of tiny viruses and other non-living viroids and prions. Breakthroughs in science correlate with the technological advances in research tools, and innovations in applying the scientific method have opened new avenues for discovery.

Epidemiology

The World Health Organization (WHO) states, "Epidemiology is the study of the distribution and **determinants** of health-related states or events (including disease), and the application of this study to the control of diseases and other health problems. Various methods can be used to carry out epidemiological investigations: surveillance and descriptive studies can be used to study distribution; analytical studies are used to study determinants." They define these determinants as:

- Social and economic environment
  - Social status and income. Those individuals with higher incomes and social status have greater access to healthcare services and optimal living conditions.
  - Education. Lack of education is linked with poor health, increased stress levels, and reduced self-confidence.
  - Social support networks. Community and family support networks are linked to better healthcare.
  - Cultural beliefs and traditions. Cultural beliefs, traditions, and ritual behaviors all influence community attitudes toward healthcare.

- Physical environment
  - Access to safe drinking water and clean air.
  - Adequate shelter and living conditions.
  - Safe workplace environments and conditions.
  - Access to healthcare providers and facilities.

- Individual characteristics and behaviors
  - Gender. Males and females suffer different types of diseases or have differing responses to and outcomes of disease processes.
  - Genetics. Heredity and inherited traits play a substantial role in health and life expectancies.
  - Personal habits and coping mechanisms (smoking, drinking, exercise, diet) affect overall individual health.

Disease Outbreaks

Outbreaks of disease refer to groups or clusters of cases statistically above what would normally be expected in a given time period in a given location. The media frequently sensationalize reported outbreaks of local, national, or global significance, causing widespread panic. The public should be made aware of potential health risks; however, emphasis can and should be placed on accurate, factual, statistical data and provide valid, scientifically-developed recommended preventative and treatment options. In the field of epidemiology, an outbreak may represent incidents of endemic, epidemic, or pandemic disease cases (see Figure 9-1).

Endemic Disease

Diseases that are considered endemic are those that are constantly present in a region, community, or population but affect a relatively few number of people. The number of reported cases fluctuates, but the disease is never entirely **eradicated** (see Figure 9-2). The incidence of the disease at a particular time depends on the following factors:

1. Population behavior
2. Percentage of immune individuals
3. Environmental conditions
4. Source of infection
5. Virulence of the pathogen
6. Genetic susceptibility of individuals

Histoplasmosis, a fungal disease caused by *Histoplasma capsulatum*, is found around the world and is endemic to some parts of the United States. Minor infections may cause few symptoms, but some individuals will suffer with an acute respiratory illness that may become chronic in nature. It resembles tuberculosis but demonstrates a distinctive pattern on chest x-ray. **Disseminated** forms of the disease are often fatal (see Figure 9-3). Anti-fungal medications may be effective in treating less severe cases. *H. capsulatum* has been found in caves harboring bats, poultry coops, and bird roosts.

Epidemic Disease

An epidemic is defined as a disease that occurs with a greater than normal incidence of reported cases. Epidemic diseases

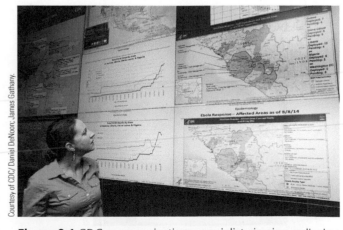

Courtesy of CDC/ Daniel DeNoon; James Gathany.

Figure 9-1 CDC communications specialist viewing a display of maps and graphs outlining current epidemiologic trends exhibited by the 2014 West African Ebola outbreak. The maps highlight those countries and their regions in which the virus had made its mark, while the graphs reveal the numbers of infected healthcare workers (HCWs) over time.

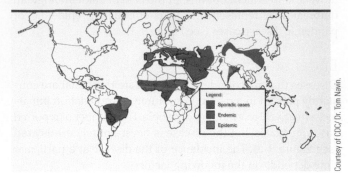

DISTRIBUTION OF VISCERAL LEISHMANIASIS, 1983

Courtesy of CDC/Dr. Tom Navin.

Figure 9-2 Map from 1983 showing global locations where leishmaniasis had been detected and, based on the legend, was classified as "sporadic" (dark red color), "endemic" (olive coloration), and "epidemic" (orange coloration).

typically reach a maximum and then rapidly decrease because the percentage of the population that is susceptible is eventually exhausted.

A population or community that has not been exposed to a particular pathogen will often experience an epidemic. For example, measles and other diseases were brought into the Native American tribes by European explorers and settlers, destroying many tribes who had no previous exposure to the pathogens that were unwittingly carried to their homelands by these newcomers.

Epidemics of typhoid fever, cholera, and dysentery are frequent in communities where sanitation practices are inadequate to prevent the spread of infection. Healthcare workers who travel to these communities are more susceptible to the local diseases because they never developed a natural immunity through exposure during childhood. Other important epidemic diseases of the past include: smallpox, bubonic plague, polio, diphtheria, scarlet fever, and vector-borne disease including malaria and leishmaniasis.

More recent concerning epidemics, as outlined by John G. Bartlett, M.D., of Johns Hopkins University School of Medicine, include: insect-borne diseases (West Nile virus, Lyme disease); fungal infections (blastomycosis, coccidioidomycosis); imported infections (malaria, Chikungunya); vaccine-preventable diseases (pertussis, measles, polio, meningitis); respiratory diseases (MERS, Influenza A H7N9 and H5N1); and food-borne infections (norovirus, cyclospora, and listeriosis).

Pandemic Disease

A pandemic outbreak of disease in current times is a worldwide event. Seen commonly as a result of a new strain of a viral infection, the spread of cases is quick and crosses national and international borders easily due to twenty-first century globalization. Travel by air, land, and sea allow infected individuals to cross-contaminate large groups of fellow passengers; from there, those newly infected go on to infect their families and communities, and thus starts to spread exponentially.

In centuries past, pandemics were large epidemic outbreaks that spread; however, with lower population numbers and larger physical distances between urban areas, they were mostly unable to reach the same numbers that pandemics of the past 100 years have been able to reach. The most notable pandemics of the past century are the influenza virus, commonly called the "Spanish Flu," of 1918, and the HIV-AIDS crisis, which began in the 1970s and continues currently. The largest pandemic of recent times, almost exactly a century after the 1918 influenza pandemic, is the recent unprecedented spread of the SARS-CoV-2 novel coronavirus responsible for the COVID-19 pandemic and the subsequent dangerous, highly-transmissible variant mutations of the original virus (see Figure 9-4). The public health crisis challenged scientists

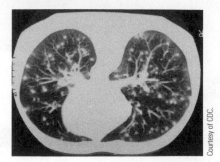

Courtesy of CDC.

Figure 9-3 A transaxial CT scan of a patient's thoracic cavity reveals evidence of a histoplasmosis infection, due to the fungal organism *Histoplasma capsulatum*, with the classic "snowstorm" appearance of both the left and right lung fields.

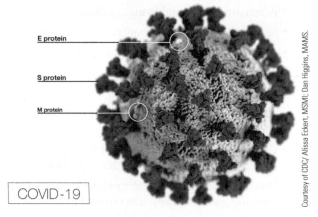

E protein

S protein

M protein

COVID-19

Courtesy of CDC/ Alissa Eckert, MSMI; Dan Higgins, MAMS.

Figure 9-4 CDC Illustration reveals ultrastructural morphology exhibited by coronaviruses. Note spikes on the outer surface of the virus which impart the look of a corona surrounding the virion when viewed with electron microscope and showing protein particles E, S, and M, also located on the outer surface. The novel coronavirus named severe acute respiratory syndrome coronavirus 2 (SARS-CoV-2), was the cause of an outbreak of respiratory illness first detected in Wuhan, China in 2019 and has been named coronavirus disease 2019 (COVID-19).

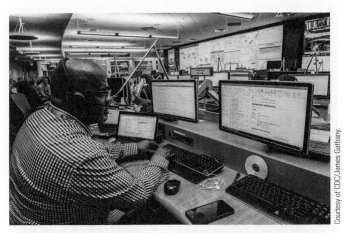

Courtesy of CDC/James Gathany.

Figure 9-5 Centers for Disease Control and prevention (CDC) activated its emergency operations center (EOC) to assist public health partners in responding to the coronavirus disease 2019 (COVID-19) outbreak first identified in Wuhan, China.

and healthcare workers to try to manage the incredible speed and spread of the disease (see Figure 9-5).

Pathogens

A pathogen is anything that is capable of causing disease. As discussed, most microbes are non-pathogenic; however, even those that typically do no harm can become the cause of disease if the conditions change and they gain access to tissues where they do not belong. Some microbes, however, are extremely dangerous under any circumstances and can infect plants, animals, humans, and even other microbes (see Table 9-1).

The ability of a microbe to invade the host and cause disease is called virulence. The terms virulence and pathogenicity (the ability of a microbe to cause disease) are often used in the same context, but this is not completely accurate. Virulence actually refers to the degree of pathogenicity and the severity of the disease process. Accordingly, some pathogenic microbes are more virulent than others. An infectious disease is the result of invasion by and growth of a pathogenic microbial colony. A communicable disease is one that can be transmitted from person to person, and a contagious disease is a communicable disease that can be relatively easily transmitted. The enhancement of transmissibility was seen in the COVID-19 pandemic with the development of the delta- and omicron-variants which occurred approximately a year after the original SARS-CoV-2 virus spread globally and an adequate vaccination program was delayed due to widespread misinformation and politicization of the public health response.

Virulence most often increases in pathogens as they are transmitted from human to human. This explains why virulence increases during an epidemic and it explains the increase of virulence of pathogens in hospitals, where there is

Table 9-1 Common Bacteria and Related Diseases

Bacteria	Disease
Staphylococcus aureus (Gram+)	Skin and wound infections, pneumonia, and food poisoning
Staphylococcus epidermidis (Gram+)	Wound and nosocomial infections
Streptococcus pyogenes (group A strep) (Gram+)	Acute pharyngitis (sore throat)
Streptococcus pneumoniae (Gram+)	Pneumonia
Enterococci (Gram+)	Nosocomial infections
Escherichia coli or *E. coli* (Gram−)	Urinary tract infections and sepsis
Neisseria species (Gram−)	Meningitis and gonorrhea
Haemophilus influenzae (Gram−)	Sinusitis, pneumonia, and otitis media
Salmonella species (Gram−)	Typhoid fever and food poisoning
Shigella species (Gram−)	Dysentery
Legionella (Gram−)	Pneumonia (Legionnaire's disease)
Bacillus species (Gram+)	Anthrax, endocarditis, food poisoning, and septicemia
Vibrio species (Gram−)	Cholera

the opportunity for the pathogen to invade a continuously changing population of susceptible hosts (patients and potentially even healthcare workers).

Virulence factors are molecular substances that pathogenic microbial organisms secrete. The end goals of these factors are:

- Colonization within a host (specific tissues, organs, or cellular adhesion)
- Obtaining nutritional support and/or reproductive avenues from the host
- Evasion of the host's immune system responses
- Suppression of the host's immune system responses
- Entry and exit pathways into host cells

Pathogens cause disease by gaining access to the host through several portals of entry. Pathogens may adhere to or penetrate through tissues to cause damage. Some pathogens can cause disease through accumulation of cellular waste products. The following sections discuss pathogen reservoirs, portals of entry, and the myriad ways that microbes can cause disease.

Pathogen Reservoirs

Reservoirs of pathogens, also referred to as reservoirs of infection, are the sources or holding areas for pathogens. Potential pathogens can survive in these portals until they can be transferred to the host, where they can multiply and cause disease. Reservoirs may be living hosts or inanimate objects, called **fomites**.

Living hosts include humans, animals (such as cattle, cats, dogs, and rodents), plants, and insects. Humans are exposed to pathogens by direct contact with other humans, animals, or insects through touch, bites, or the consumption of the meat of infected animals. The most significant source of human infections is through contact with other humans, primarily because many of the human pathogens are species-specific, meaning that they can cause disease in only one species. The term "zoonosis" refers to diseases that are transmissible to humans by animals such as cows, cats, horses, and pigs.

Arthropod vectors include mosquitoes, flies, fleas, and ticks (see Figure 9-6). Insects, such as the anopheles mosquito, can transmit a species of *Plasmodium* that is responsible for causing malaria. Also, the tsetse fly can carry trypanosomes that cause African sleeping sickness.

The following are definitions of the categories of disease carriers:

1. Human carriers are individuals who carry the pathogen but are asymptomatic. They can, however, unknowingly transmit the pathogen to others who then develop the disease. Human papilloma virus (HPV) is a common human carrier pathogen that passes back and forth between sexual partners. Several strains of HPV are known to cause dysplasia, which can lead to cervical cancer in females. Condyloma, also known as genital warts, is a sexually transmitted disease that can infect both male and female genitalia (see Figure 9-7).

2. Incubatory carriers are capable of transmitting the pathogen during the incubation period of an infectious

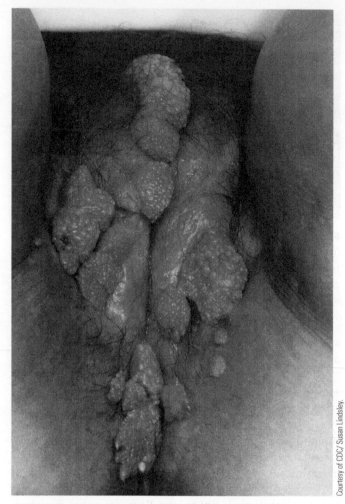

Courtesy of CDC/ Susan Lindsley.

Figure 9-7 A female patient's perineum revealing numbers of cutaneous outgrowths of *Condylomata acuminata* (venereal warts) caused by human papilloma virus (HPV) infection in the vaginal labia and perianal region.

disease. Human immunodeficiency virus (HIV) is one of the most well-known pathogens that has a long incubation period.

3. Convalescent carriers harbor a pathogen and can transmit it while recovering from the disease. The recovery period is referred to as the convalescence period. Cholera has a long convalescence period in which the person can carry the microorganism for many months.

4. Active carriers have recovered from the disease but harbor the pathogen indefinitely.

5. Passive carriers harbor the pathogen without ever having had the disease. Human carriers are responsible for the spread of staphylococcal infections, hepatitis, dysentery, and sexually transmitted diseases (STDs). One of the most famous cases of a passive carrier causing disease in others was Mary Mallon, better known as Typhoid Mary.

Inanimate reservoirs include air, soil, food, fluids (such as water and milk), and fomites. Fomites include hospital bedding

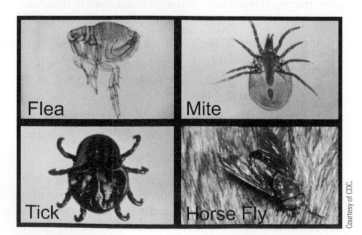

Courtesy of CDC.

Figure 9-6 These four arthropods, a flea, mite, tick, and a horse fly, are often the source of many vector-borne infectious diseases.

and equipment, such as bedpans and tables. The skin and respiratory and intestinal tract secretions of patients and healthcare workers easily contaminate fomites within hospitals and other healthcare settings.

Methods of Transmission

Microorganisms can be transmitted from an infected person to a non-infected person in the following ways:

1. Direct contact with an infected person:
   a. Touching: An infected person does not practice good hand-washing techniques and touches another person. Example: hospital *Staphylococcus* infections in newborn nurseries caused by healthcare workers.
   b. Sneezing: Infected persons do not cover their noses or mouths when sneezing or coughing and the air droplets contain viruses or bacteria.
   c. Secretion contact: Examples include kissing and sexual intercourse, during which STDs such as gonorrhea, syphilis, herpes, HPV, and chlamydia are transferred between partners.
   d. Blood and body fluid contact: A non-infected person who has a cut or scratch can come into contact with the blood of an infected person and become infected. Examples of diseases easily passed through blood and body fluid contact are hepatitis B (HBV) and hepatitis C (HCV), and HIV. Injection drug users who share needles are also easily infected. Surgery personnel have to be aware of the dangers of **sharps injuries**. Research has shown that the surgical team is at higher risk for contracting HBV than HIV.

2. Indirect contact: An infected individual can contaminate a fomite, food, or something else with which the non-infected person comes into contact.
   a. Fomites, such as hospital bedding, equipment, and supplies
   b. Food prepared by an infected person (Hepatitis A (HAV) can be transmitted to consumers by employees who do not wash their hands after using the restroom.)

3. Contact with carriers (see previous section—reservoirs)

4. Contact with animal or insect carriers (see previous section—reservoirs)

Portals of Entry

The portals of entry into a host are skin, parenteral routes, and mucous membranes. The following sections discuss each of the portals (see Table 9-2).

Skin

The skin or integumentary system is the largest organ system of the body and the first line of defense against external pathogens. Most microbes cannot penetrate intact, undamaged skin. However, the sweat glands and hair pores of the skin may serve as portals of entry. Additionally, some fungi can grow on the skin or in subungual spaces (under nails) and cause infections. The larvae of the hookworm can actually penetrate the skin to become embedded in the deeper layers.

Table 9-2 Portals of Entry with Examples of Related Microorganisms and Diseases

Portal of Entry	Microorganism	Microorganism Type	Disease Produced
Skin	*Staphylococcus aureus*	Bacterium	Impetigo
	Papilloma virus	Virus	Warts
	Tricophyton	Fungus	Ringworm
Wound	*Clostridium tetani*	Bacterium	Tetanus
	Rabies virus	Virus	Rabies
Respiratory tract	*Bordetella pertussis*	Bacterium	Whooping cough
	Influenza virus	Virus	Influenza
	Blastomyces dermatitidis	Fungus	Blastomycosis
Gastrointestinal tract	*Clostridium difficile*	Bacterium	Diarrheal illnesses (often accompanied by pseudomembranous colitis)
	Polio virus	Virus	Polio
	Giardia lamblia (*G. duodenalis*)	Protozoan	Giardiasis
Genitourinary tract	*Treponema pallidum*	Bacteria	Syphilis
	Herpes simplex virus type II	Virus	Genital herpes
	Candida albicans	Fungus	Vaginitis

Parenteral Route

Once the skin barrier has been compromised (through a wound, injection, cuts, or bites), the parenteral route (referring to tissues beneath the skin) for microbial invasion is established. The pathogens can then directly invade the underlying tissues of the skin and possibly penetrate further into the mucous membranes.

Mucous Membranes

A layer of mucous membranes lines the respiratory tract, gastrointestinal tract, genitourinary tract, and conjunctiva of the eyes. Many pathogens gain entrance to the body by penetrating these membranes. Most of the pathogens penetrate the mucous membranes of the gastrointestinal and respiratory tracts.

The respiratory tract is the easiest route of penetration. Pathogens enter through the nose and mouth as airborne microbes on dust particles and moisture droplets. Examples of diseases that are caused by pathogens that gain entrance through the respiratory tract include the common cold, influenza, COVID-19, pneumonia, measles, tuberculosis, smallpox, and Hanta virus.

Pathogens gain entrance to the gastrointestinal tract through contaminated water and food or by the fecal-oral route from poor hand hygiene. Most microbes are destroyed by the hydrochloric acid formed in the stomach or by bile that is used for the digestive process in the small intestine. Microbes that can survive these substances are usually pathogens that are eliminated through feces to be transmitted to other hosts via contaminated water, food, or fingers. Examples of diseases that gastrointestinal microbes can cause include hepatitis A, dysentery, cholera, typhoid fever, and giardiasis.

The pathogens that enter through the genitourinary tract are usually sexually contracted. Some microbes that cause STDs can enter through intact mucous membranes, but others require some type of wound such as a cut or opening caused by a hypodermic needle. Common examples of STDs are HIV, chlamydia, herpes, syphilis, and gonorrhea.

Selective Portals of Entry

Many pathogens have a preferred route of entry and in many instances cannot cause disease unless the preferred route is used. For example, *Salmonella typhi*, the bacteria responsible for typhoid fever, will cause the disease when it enters the body through swallowing, but when placed on the surface of the skin no symptoms will occur. However, *Yersinia pestis*, the bacteria that causes plague, can use various portals of entry to produce the disease.

Attachment to Host Tissues

After pathogens have entered a host, they will attach to the tissues of the host. This is called **adherence** and it is a necessary event for the process of pathogenicity and effective disease transmission. The attachment between the host and pathogen is achieved by adhesins located on the surface of the pathogen. Adhesins are molecules that bind to specific **surface receptors** on the cells of the host tissues. Adhesins are usually located on the pathogen's glycocalyx or other types of microbial structures, such as fimbriae.

Most adhesins are composed of glycoproteins or lipoproteins, and the receptors are usually sugars. Adhesins vary in structure and the different cells of the host will have different receptors that also vary in structure. This is important for scientists researching methods of preventing or controlling infections. A means for controlling the disease is available if the receptors, adhesins, or both can be altered, and adherence can be inhibited.

The bacterium *Streptococcus mutans* is a pathogen that contributes to tooth decay by adhering to teeth by its glycocalyx. It produces an enzyme called glucosyltransferase that converts glucose into a polysaccharide called dextran, which then forms the glycocalyx. Disease-causing strains of *Escherichia coli* have adhesins on fimbriae that are specific to certain kinds of receptors on the cells of the host, particularly in specific areas of the small intestine. *Treponema pallidum*, the pathogen that causes syphilis, uses the end of its cell, which is shaped like a hook to attach to the host cells (see Figure 9-8).

Contributing Factors for Bacterial Invasion

To cause disease, the majority of pathogens must penetrate the host's tissues. The following are factors that aid the bacteria in penetrating the host defenses.

Enzymes

The virulence of bacteria is aided by the production of exoenzymes. The enzymes have various actions, such as lysing (destruction by enzymatic digestion) cells and dissolving blood clots and intercellular substances. Some medical microbiologists use the term invasins for the cellular surface proteins (enzymes) that promote the ability for pathogens to invade tissues. These invasins damage host tissues in a localized area and can be difficult to distinguish from exotoxins.

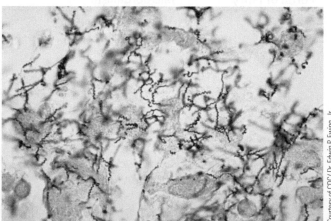

Courtesy of CDC/ Dr. Edwin P. Ewing, Jr.

Figure 9-8 Prepared using the modified steiner silver stain method, this photomicrograph revealed the presence of *Treponema pallidum* Spirochetes, in this testicular tissue sample, harvested from an experimentally infected rabbit. *T. pallidum* is the cause for syphilis.

Some bacteria produce leukocidin, a substance that lyses macrophages, phagocytes, neutrophils, and leukocytes. The leukocidin produced by streptococci has a double action: the enzyme breaks down the lysosomes in leukocytes, causing the death of the cell, and the enzymes released from the destroyed lysosomes damage other intracellular structures.

Coagulases are responsible for coagulating the fibrinogen in blood. Fibrinogen, a plasma protein produced by the liver, is converted into a coagulase when it combines with thrombin, forming fibrin for the stabilization of a blood clot. The fibrin clot can protect bacteria from phagocytosis and other defensive actions of the host. Coagulases are commercially produced for therapeutic use by individuals with bleeding disorders and are given preoperatively when the individual requires surgery.

Hyaluronidase is a bacterial enzyme that destroys hyaluronic acid, the substance that is responsible for holding the cells of connective tissue together. This action aids in the spread of the microorganisms from their original area of infection. Hyaluronidase is produced by some species of *Clostridium*, the microorganism responsible for gas gangrene, a dangerous infection of wounds seen by many operating room personnel. Hyaluronidase has therapeutic uses as well. It can be mixed with a local anesthetic to break down tissue after injection, aiding the spread of the local anesthetic drug through the tissues. It is also used as an injection to dissolve the connective tissue called zonules that hold the lens of the eye in place to facilitate the removal of the lens during cataract surgery.

Kinases lyse fibrin and dissolve clots formed by the body to wall off an infection. Streptokinase is produced by *Streptococcus pyogenes*, and staphylokinase is produced by *Staphylococcus aureus*. By lysing the fibrin clot, kinases enable the pathogens to invade and spread through the body. Streptokinase is commercially produced for injection into the body to dissolve blood clot(s) called a thrombus (plural, thrombi) for patients who are experiencing a heart attack due to obstructed coronary arteries.

Another important bacterial exoenzyme is hemolysin, which causes the lysis of erythrocytes. Bacteria produce different types of hemolysin that vary in the type of lytic reactions they cause. Staphylococci and streptococci produce hemolysins. Streptolysin S (SLS) destroys the albumin in blood serum and can also lyse phagocytic leukocytes. *Clostridium perfringens* produces hemolysin that allows for tissue destruction. *C. perfringens* also produces the enzyme collagenase, which breaks down collagen, the protein found in tendons, bones, and cartilage. *C. perfringens* (a primary cause of gas gangrene) is able to penetrate deep into the tissues of the body by secreting collagenase and hyaluronidase.

Bacterial Capsules

As previously discussed, some bacteria synthesize glycocalyx that forms a capsule around the cell wall. This increases the virulence of the bacterial species because the capsule inhibits phagocytosis by preventing phagocytic cells from attaching to the bacterium. Some types of bacteria whose virulence is increased by the presence of a capsule include *Haemophilus influenzae*, *Bacillus anthracis*, and *Klebsiella pneumoniae* (see Figure 9-9).

Cell Wall Chemical Substances

The cell walls of some bacteria have chemical substances that increase virulence. For example, the cell wall of *Mycobacterium tuberculosis* contains chemical waxes that resist the digestive process of phagocytes.

Additionally, *S. pyogenes* synthesizes an acid-resistant and heat-resistant protein called M protein, which is located in the cell wall and on fimbriae. The protein guides the attachment of the bacterial cell to host epithelial cells and aids in resisting leukocyte phagocytosis. The human body can produce an antibody specific for destroying M protein.

Pathogenic Damage Methods

Pathogens damage host cells using three methods: direct damage, production of toxins, and immune reactions. The first two mechanisms are discussed next. The third method is discussed in later sections.

Direct Damage

If a pathogen survives the host's defenses and attaches to the **host** cells, it can invade the other tissues of the body. The pathogen is now free to metabolize, multiply, and kill other cells. As previously discussed, the bacteria can produce exoenzymes that aid in penetrating the cells or penetrate with the use of fimbriae. The penetration itself damages the host cell; however, most bacteria damage the host cell by producing toxins.

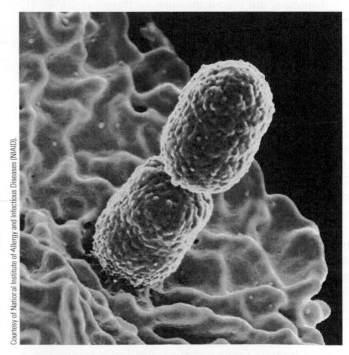

Courtesy of National Institute of Allergy and Infectious Diseases (NIAID).

Figure 9-9 Produced by NIAID, this digitally colorized scanning electron micrograph depicts two mustard-colored, rod-shaped, carbapenem-resistant *Klebsiella pneumoniae* bacteria interacting with a green-colored human neutrophil.

Toxins

Some microbes can produce toxins that are dangerous to the host cells and tissues. The ability of microbes to produce toxins is called toxigenicity. When released, blood and lymph fluid transport the toxins that can cause serious and occasionally fatal results. The production of toxic products by pathogens is probably the most determining factor of their pathogenicity. The effects of toxins include fever, mild to severe diarrhea, shock, and multiple organ-system failures. Toxins can destroy blood vessels and cause nervous system disorders. Two types of toxins are produced: exotoxins and endotoxins.

Toxemia is the medical term used to describe the presence of toxins in the bloodstream. Systemic toxemia, also known as blood poisoning, is the most serious form and occurs when the toxin has been transported throughout the body. Toxemia in pregnancy (also known as preeclampsia) refers to a syndrome characterized by hypertension, diffuse edema, and protein in the urine, and may be a precursor to dangerous seizures (eclampsia). The specific causes for toxemia in pregnancy are unknown, but they may be linked to immune responses to fetal development as well as other conditions. It is not, however, otherwise related to bloodstream toxemia.

Exotoxins The majority of bacteria that produce exotoxins are Gram-positive. Exotoxins are proteins, many of which are enzymes produced inside the bacterial cell. The genes for most exotoxins are transported on plasmids or bacterial phages. Exotoxins are effective in producing disease because they are soluble in body fluids and can easily diffuse into the bloodstream for rapid systemic distribution.

Exotoxins are placed into one of three categories: (1) neurotoxins, which interrupt normal nerve impulse transmission; (2) enterotoxins, which affect the epithelial cells that line the gastrointestinal tract; and (3) cytotoxins, which destroy host cells or affect their normal functioning.

Exotoxins are some of the most dangerous substances produced by bacteria. Typically, only very small amounts are needed to produce the disease, and it is the toxin that is responsible for the signs and symptoms of disease, not the bacteria itself. *Clostridioides difficile* (formerly called *Clostridium difficile*), commonly referred to as C-diff, produces two exotoxins (A and B) and is responsible for antibiotic-associated diarrhea (AAD). The CDC categorizes 80 percent of the cases of *C. difficile* as healthcare-associated infections (HAIs).

The human body can produce antibodies called antitoxins, which provide immunity. When exotoxins are altered or made harmless by heat, iodine, or other chemicals, they can stimulate the body to produce the antitoxin. Harmless exotoxins, called toxoids, can be used as vaccines to induce antitoxin production to produce immunity to certain diseases. Diphtheria is one example of a disease in which immunity is induced by toxoid injection.

The bacteria *Corynebacterium diphtheriae* synthesizes a toxin when it is invaded by a phage. The toxin is classified as a cytotoxin that prevents protein synthesis in eukaryotic cells. Its biophysical action is as follows:

1. The protein toxin is composed of two polypeptides called A (active) and B (binding). Only polypeptide A causes disease signs and symptoms, but B is required for A to enter the host cell.

2. Polypeptide B binds the protein to the surface receptors on the host cell so that the entire protein can penetrate the plasma membrane and enter the cytoplasm.

3. Polypeptide A can then exert its action on the host cell by preventing protein synthesis and destroying the cell.

The bacteria *Vibrio cholerae*, responsible for cholera, produces a toxin called cholera toxin that acts in the same manner as the diphtheria toxin, except the cholera toxin binds to the plasma membrane of the epithelial cells that line the small intestine. The result is the discharge of large amounts of fluid by the epithelial cells, causing severe diarrhea. Individuals can quickly become dehydrated due to the loss of fluid and electrolytes.

An example of a neurotoxin is the botulinum toxin produced by *Clostridium botulinum*. This neurotoxin exerts its effect at the neuromuscular junction to prevent the transmission of nerve cells to the muscle. The toxin binds to the nerve cell and prevents the **neurotransmitter** acetylcholine from being released to travel across the junction. The infected individual experiences muscle paralysis that leads to respiratory failure because the muscles of respiration cannot expand and contract.

Endotoxins There are key differences between exotoxins and endotoxins. The majority of bacteria that contain an endotoxin are Gram-negative, and the toxins are a component of the outer portion of the cell wall. Endotoxins are lipopolysaccharides, but exotoxins are proteins. Gram-negative bacteria have a membrane that surrounds the peptidoglycan cell wall, which contains lipopolysaccharides (LPSs). The lipid part of the LPS comprises the endotoxin (see Figure 9-10).

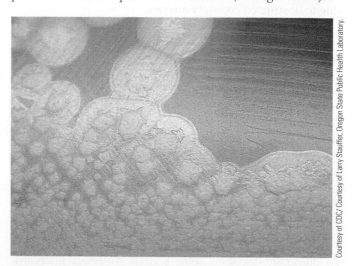

Courtesy of CDC/ Courtesy of Larry Stauffer, Oregon State Public Health Laboratory.

Figure 9-10 Laboratory growth medium of egg yolk agar Inoculated with *Clostridium botulinum* bacteria and incubated for 72 hours. Note the presence of the lipase reaction, which manifests as a shiny margin that surrounds each colony.

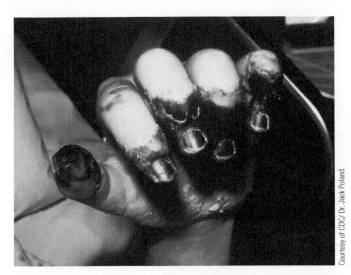

Courtesy of CDC/ Dr. Jack Poland.

Figure 9-11 Gangrene of the left hand, causing necrosis of the distal fingers and thumb from abnormal coagulation within the blood vessels of his digits caused by the presence of systemically disseminated plague bacteria, *Yersinia pestis*, otherwise known as septicemia.

When the bacteria die and the cell wall is lysed, the endotoxin is released to exert its effect. No matter what the species of bacteria, all endotoxins produce the same signs and symptoms, including fever, muscle and bone joint aches, chills, and, in severe cases, shock that could lead to death.

Septicemia, the systemic distribution of an endotoxin, can lead to a severe life-threatening complication called disseminated intravascular coagulation (DIC). The endotoxin causes the overstimulation of coagulating proteins, which causes systemic intravascular clotting, preventing blood from reaching tissues and resulting in tissue necrosis.

Examples of bacteria that produce endotoxins include *Neisseria meningitidis*, the agent that causes meningococcal meningitis, and *Proteus* spp., the agents that cause most urinary tract infections (UTIs). *Yersinia pestis* responsible for the disease commonly called the plague produces septicemia responsible for abnormal coagulation of capillary blood flow and necrosis of the digits (see Figure 9-11). Endotoxins do not induce the body to produce an antitoxin that is effective against it. Antibiotics are available to fight against the bacteria that produce endotoxins.

Pathogenicity of Viruses

Viruses have several methods for avoidance of the host's defenses, allowing for virus reproduction that results in the death of the host cell. When the virus penetrates the cell, it is protected from the natural immune system of the body.

Methods of Entry

Viruses gain entry into a cell by attaching to matching receptor sites on the target host cell. After the virus attachment site contacts the receptor site, chemicals imitating those needed

by the cell trick the cell into giving the virus access to its interior. As discussed in Chapter 8, viruses are not considered true living organisms. They contain either RNA or DNA (but not both) and cannot synthesize the materials needed to remain viable and grow in numbers. They must be able to penetrate and take over the host cell's metabolism machinery and genetic material to reproduce.

The virus that causes AIDS (HIV) actually hides its attachment sites so the body's immune system does not recognize the virus as being dangerous, allowing the virus to attack the immune system. HIV is cell-specific just as other viruses are, meaning that it only attacks specific cells, namely the cells in the immune system, which are called T-lymphocytes. T-lymphocytes have receptor sites for which the HIV attachment sites have an affinity for contact (see Figure 9-12).

Cytopathic Effects of Viral Infection

The effects of viruses on the host cells are called **cytopathic effects** (CPEs), and they are often used as a means of diagnosing a viral infection. CPEs that cause cell death are called cytocidal effects, and those that cause cell damage (but not cell death) are called non-cytocidal effects.

CPEs produced by viruses include granules called inclusion bodies, which are found in the nucleus or cytoplasm of infected cells. The bodies vary in shape, size, and laboratory staining. Inclusion bodies are categorized as either acidophilic (stain with an acid stain) or basophilic (stain with a basic stain). Inclusion bodies aid in the identification of the virus that causes the infection. Examples include the Negri bodies that are present in the cytoplasm of nerve cells infected with the rabies virus. Diagnostic inclusion bodies are also found in the herpes and smallpox viruses (see Figure 9-13).

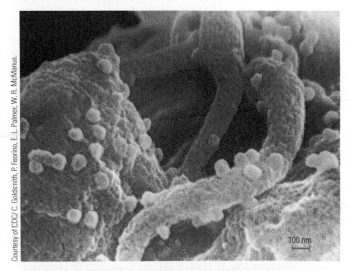

Courtesy of CDC/ C. Goldsmith, P. Feorino, E. L. Palmer, W. R. McManus.

100 nm

Figure 9-12 Digitally colorized scanning electron microscopic (SEM) image shows the green, spherical, human immunodeficiency virus (HIV-1) virions with human lymphocytes and some of their extended pseudopodia.

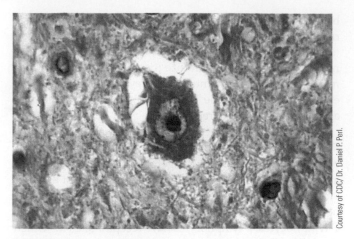

Courtesy of CDC/Dr. Daniel P. Perl.

Figure 9-13 Stained brain tissue specimen with histopathologic changes associated with rabies encephalitis by the presence of Negri bodies, which are cellular inclusions found most frequently in the pyramidal cells of the cerebellum.

Viruses can cause the cell's lysosomes to release enzymes that damage or destroy the host cell's intracellular structures, resulting in the death of the cell. Viruses can also disrupt various other activities of the cell, causing cell death, such as stopping cellular mitosis.

Viruses can either damage or cause changes to the chromosomes of the host cell. The result is either a mutation in the chromosomes of the cell or cell death due to the destruction of the chromosomes.

Some viral infections can cause antigenic changes on the surface of the infected host cell. These antigenic changes trigger the body's own immune system to destroy the cell with antibodies.

When normal cells of any type that are grown on a Petri dish come into contact with other cells, cell growth will cease in recognition of the fact that continued growth will result in cell death. This is called contact inhibition. Cancer-causing viruses called transforming viruses alter host cells so that they become abnormally shaped cells whose growth is unregulated because they no longer recognize contact inhibition. This explains the abnormal, uninhibited growth of a cancerous tumor.

Non-specific Host Defenses

Previous sections of this chapter present the impression that pathogenic bacteria and viruses have the unlimited ability to invade and infect the human body. If this were the case and microbes did not encounter host resistance, then humans would be constantly sick and dying in great numbers because of disease. Fortunately, this does not occur thanks to various defenses presented by the host. These defenses either keep microbes out of the body completely or, once inside, trap and destroy them. The body's defensive ability is called resistance and the lack of resistance is called susceptibility.

In this section, we discuss non-specific host defenses, which refer to the defenses that protect the body against any type of pathogen, no matter the species. Non-specific defenses include the skin, mucous membranes, phagocytes, inflammation, and fever. Specific defenses refer to systems that fight against particular pathogens.

Skin

The two layers of the skin, the outer epidermis and inner dermis, are composed in such a way to provide a barrier that is rarely penetrated by most microbes as long as it remains intact. The dermis is a thick layer of tough connective tissue. The epidermis is thinner, but the epithelial cells are closely knit with little to no space between the cells. The very top layer of the epidermis is dead epithelial cells and is covered by a protein called **keratin**. However, fungi can **hydrolyze** keratin, resulting in the fungal infection called athlete's foot.

The sebaceous glands are located in the skin and produce sebum. Sebum prevents the hair from drying out and also forms a thin protective layer on the surface of the skin. A component of sebum is unsaturated fatty acids that inhibit the growth of some pathogenic bacteria and fungi. The fatty acids also cause the skin pH to be between 3 and 5 (acidic), which probably aids in inhibiting the growth of microbes.

The sweat glands, also located in the skin, are responsible for perspiration. Perspiration helps keep body temperature normal by cooling evaporation, eliminating some body wastes, and washing away microbes from the skin surface. Perspiration has lysozymes, which are enzymes that can break down Gram-positive bacterial cell walls. Lysozymes are also components of tears, saliva, and certain tissue fluids.

Mucous Membranes

Mucous membranes line the respiratory, gastrointestinal, and genitourinary tracts. Specialized epithelial cells, called goblet cells, line the membrane and secrete mucus. Some pathogens survive and even thrive because of the moist environment provided by the mucus. When a sufficient number of the microbes are present, they invade the host. An example of such a pathogen *is Treponema pallidum*, the pathogen responsible for the sexually transmitted disease syphilis.

However, the mucus can also catch microbes and not allow them to penetrate further into the respiratory or gastrointestinal tracts. Another mechanism found in the respiratory tract is the cilia. The cilia line the tract and move in a synchronous, wave-like motion, moving inhaled dust, debris, and microbes forward to the pharynx to be expelled by the host through sneezing or coughing of **phlegm**.

The mucous membrane lining of the genitourinary tract is flushed out by the flow of urine. The flushing action prevents microbial stasis and consequent colonization in the tract.

The stomach contains glands that produce highly acidic gastric juices. The pH is approximately 1.2–3.0 and consists of hydrochloric acid and mucus. The high acid level usually assures that microbes cannot survive. Exceptions include the toxins produced by *C. botulinum* and *S. aureus* that survive the gastric juices. Another important exception is *Helicobacter pylori*, which survives by neutralizing the acid and allowing it to grow. *H. pylori* has been discovered to be a major contributor to the cause of stomach and duodenal ulcers.

Phagocytes

Phagocytosis is the second line of defense put forth by the human body. Phagocytosis is the process of surrounding and ingesting another microbe or foreign particle. The cells responsible for this action are called phagocytes, all of which are leukocytes (white blood cells); however, not all leukocytes are phagocytes. The five types of white blood cells (WBCs) or leukocytes in human blood are:

- Basophils
- Eosinophils
- Lymphocytes (T-cells and B-cells)
- Monocytes
- Neutrophils (bands are young neutrophils)

When an infection in the human body occurs, the number of leukocytes increases. If a patient presents with signs and symptoms that indicate they are suffering from appendicitis, then blood will be drawn from the patient and the surgeon will most likely order a complete blood count (CBC) with differential to be completed by the laboratory. Normal WBC counts are 4,500 to 10,000 per microliter (µL).

To provide more specific diagnoses, a differential blood count may be ordered. The differential count determines the percentages of the five types of WBCs, and physicians can gain insight into potential disease processes based on these differential counts.

There are two categories of leukocytes: granulocytes and agranulocytes. When placed under a light microscope after staining, large granules can be seen in the cytoplasm of granulocytes. Based on how the granules stain, granulocytes are placed into three categories:

- Neutrophils that stain with a mixture of acidic and base dyes and are colored a light lilac
- Eosinophils that are dyed with eosin, an acidic dye, and stain red or orange
- Basophils that are stained with methylene blue and, therefore, stain a bluish color. The function of basophils is not fully understood, but they are important in the process of inflammation that will be discussed later (see Figure 9-14).

Neutrophils are motile and effective phagocytes that are active in the beginning stages of an infection. They leave the bloodstream to enter the infected area and begin the process of destroying the invading microbes.

Eosinophils can also leave the bloodstream, but their major role is the production of toxic proteins to fight parasites, such as **helminths**. The eosinophils attach to the surface of parasites and secrete peroxide ions that kill them. During an infection by a parasitic worm, the number of eosinophils greatly increases.

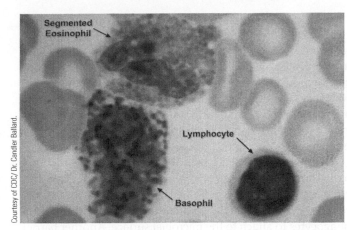

Courtesy of CDC / Dr. Candler Ballard.

Figure 9-14 Photomicrograph of a blood smear with numbers of biconcave red blood cells (RBCs), or erythrocytes, and three types of white blood cells (WBCs), or leukocytes: a segmented eosinophil granulocyte (top) with its multilobular nucleus, a basophil granulocyte (bottom), and a small lymphocyte with its proportionally large nucleus.

Agranulocytes do have granules in the cytoplasm; however, they cannot be seen with the light microscope after staining. The two types of agranulocytes are monocytes and lymphocytes. Monocytes do not become phagocytic until they exit the bloodstream and enter the body's tissues, where they mature into macrophages. The increase in macrophages and lymphocytes within the lymph nodes causes them to swell during an infection. As the blood and lymph fluid travel through body organs that contain macrophages, the microbes are removed by phagocytosis. Lymphocytes are not phagocytes but are important in the specific defense of the body called the immune response.

As previously mentioned, macrophages develop from monocytes during the inflammatory response to an infection. There are two types of macrophages. Those that exit the bloodstream and travel to the infected region are called wandering macrophages, and those that remain in tissues and body organs to trap foreign material are called fixed macrophages or histiocytes.

Macrophages are located in the tissues of the reticuloendothelial system (RES). This non-specific system refers to the collection of phagocytic cells (including macrophages) that line the sinusoids of the spleen, lymph nodes, bone marrow, intestines, liver (Kupffer cells), and brain (microglia). The main function of the RES is removal and destruction of foreign debris and microbes, excess cellular secretions, dead leukocytes, erythrocytes, and body tissue.

Phagocytosis The granulocytes, particularly the neutrophils, are most active during the initial stages of a bacterial infection. In the later stages, the macrophages become the most dominant phagocyte, destroying the remaining living and dead bacteria. During fungal and viral infections, macrophages are the most dominant phagocyte during all stages of the infection.

The process of phagocytosis is divided into four parts: chemotaxis, adherence, ingestion, and digestion. Chemotaxis refers to the attraction of phagocytes to microbes that is due to chemicals from injured tissue cells, peptides, and other microbial products. Motile bacteria contain receptors in the cell wall that sense the chemical stimuli and once detected, the information is transmitted to the flagella. If the signal is favorable, the bacteria will move toward the chemical stimulus (see Figure 9-15).

The phagocyte attaches to the microbe by first adhering to its surface. Adherence can either take place in a fairly simple manner or be difficult. Some bacteria, such as *S. pyogenes*, contain a protein called M protein that makes it difficult for phagocytes to attach to the microbial surface. Another barrier is slippery mucoid capsules that surround bacteria, as occurs with *H. influenzae* type B.

Antibody molecules secrete a serum protein that can coat a bacterial cell and promote the attachment of phagocytes to the pathogen. The process of coating is called opsonization and the antibody molecules are referred to as opsonins.

After the phagocyte is able to adhere to the pathogen, the process of ingestion can begin. The phagocyte extends pseudopods or "false feet" that surround the microbe. The pseudopod's sides meet to completely surround the pathogen, and the resulting sac is called a **phagosome**.

The last step of the process is digestion. The phagosome releases itself from the plasma membrane and enters the cytoplasm. As previously discussed, the cytoplasm contains lysosomes that contain enzymes. When the phagosome and lysosomes make contact, they from a single structure called a phagolysosome. The enzymes are now able to destroy the bacteria. This digestive process is called degranulation because the granules in the granulocytes are used and decrease in number. After the bacteria have been digested, the phagolysosome is called a residual body, and the leftover contents

cannot be digested. The residual body moves through the cytoplasm to the edge of the phagocyte and releases the wastes to the outside of the cell.

Complement

Complement is a group of 25–30 enzymatic serum proteins found in blood plasma that constitute the "complement system." The name is derived from the fact that they complement the action of antibodies in immune and allergic reactions. The complements circulate in the plasma in an inactive form until needed in the antibody–antigen reaction that is a part of the second line of defense. Complement is a nonspecific defense mechanism because it binds to different antigen–antibody immune complexes. Once it binds to the complex, the complement cascade is activated and performs the following functions:

- Increases the inflammatory response
- Attaches to the antibody to assist in the lysis of the antigen
- Aids in neutralizing the toxins of some types of microbes
- Attracts phagocytes (chemotaxis) to the region

Iron

The virulence of bacteria is increased when free iron is present. Many pathogenic bacteria use iron for the synthesis of exotoxins. Leukocytes produce interleukin-1 (IL-1), which, among other functions that are later discussed, stimulates the liver to store iron, thereby depriving the pathogen of necessary free iron.

Iron is tightly bound to iron transport proteins in the body called transferrin, ferritin, and lactoferrin. This deprives pathogens of the needed iron supply. However, some pathogens obtain the iron needed for survival by producing and releasing their own iron-binding proteins called siderophores. The iron binds to the siderophores and the pathogen takes up the siderophores to gain the iron. *Neisseria meningitidis*, the microbe responsible for causing meningitis, has receptors on the cell surface that bind directly to the iron transport proteins. The cell can then take up the proteins along with the attached iron atoms.

Inflammation

A defensive response to a bodily injury is called inflammation. The four signs of inflammation are pain, heat, redness, and swelling (edema). Pain is due to tissue nerve damage, pressure exerted by edema, or toxins; heat and redness, also associated with inflammation, are caused by an increase in blood flow to the affected area; and swelling (edema) is due to a build-up of fluid in the surrounding tissue spaces (see Figure 9-16).

Inflammation is a necessary and beneficial response of the body. It is responsible for three primary processes:

1. Destroying the invasive substance and removing it and any products produced by the substance.

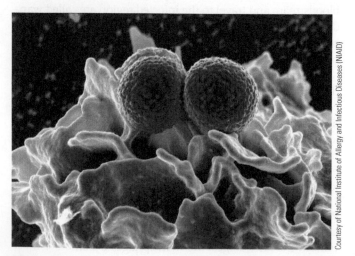

Courtesy of National Institute of Allergy and Infectious Diseases (NIAID)

Figure 9-15 SEM Image of two blue-colored, spherical, methicillin-resistant, *Staphylococcus aureus* (MRSA) bacteria in the process of being phagocytized by an un-colored, human white blood cell (WBC).

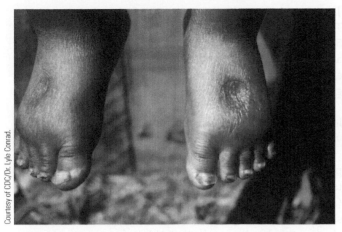

Figure 9-16 A Nigerian child with swollen feet, also known as "pedal edema," due to kwashiorkor, a disease caused by severe dietary protein deficiency.

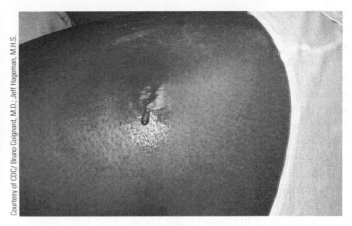

Figure 9-17 Cutaneous abscess caused by methicillin-resistant *Staphylococcus aureus* (MRSA) bacteria on the hip which had begun to spontaneously drain, releasing its purulent contents.

2. Limiting the extent of the infection by "walling off" the substance and the by-products. For example, if an individual has a brief episode of appendicitis and the appendix bursts, the patient will not immediately exhibit signs of inflammation and infection. This is due to the formation of an abscess that has been walled off. This wall is the body's attempt to isolate the infection by forming a connective tissue wall that inhibits the ability of the pathogens to penetrate deeper into the surrounding tissue.

3. Repairing and/or replacing damaged tissue.

Vasodilation The process of inflammation occurs in three stages: vasodilation, phagocyte migration, and tissue repair. Vasodilation refers to the dilation, or increase in diameter, of blood vessels, which aids in increasing the blood flow to the damaged area. Vasodilation also increases the permeability of the blood vessels, allowing host defensive agents that normally travel in the bloodstream to pass through the vessel wall and enter the damaged tissue. Three primary chemicals that are released by damaged cells are responsible for vasodilation: histamine, kinins, and prostaglandins.

Histamine is found in mast cells located in connective tissue, platelet cells, and basophils. Histamine is released from the injured cells that contain it and has a direct effect on the blood vessels. Kinins are found in plasma, the liquid, straw-colored portion of blood. Kinins cause vasodilation and an increase in the permeability of blood vessels. They also play a part in chemotaxis by attracting neutrophils to the damaged tissue. Prostaglandins are also released by damaged cells. They increase the action of histamine and kinins and aid phagocytes as they travel through the blood vessel walls.

Vasodilation also allows the quick delivery of blood-clotting substances to the injured area through permeability. The blood clot that forms in the area of damage inhibits microbes and/or toxins from spreading throughout the body. The result is the formation of an abscess. Abscesses (pus accumulations) are a combination of body fluids and dead cells that tend to collect in a cavity (see Figure 9-17). Pathogens that cause abscess formation

are called pyogenic bacteria and include staphylococci, which typically produce yellowish-green pus. *Pseudomonas aeruginosa* produces a bluish exudate, which is caused by the pigment pyocyanin produced by the bacteria.

Phagocyte Migration As neutrophils and monocytes travel to the area of injury, they attach to the inner endothelial lining of the blood vessels. Once the blood vessels dilate, the phagocytes are able to leave the vessels by passing through the endothelial cells to the injured tissue. The phagocytes can begin the process of eliminating the pathogens.

Tissue Repair The last stage of inflammation is tissue repair, in which the tissue replaces the damaged or destroyed cells. Repair actually begins during the first phase of inflammation but obviously cannot be complete until all pathogens and other substances have been removed and are no longer causing tissue damage.

The extent to which tissue can regenerate itself depends on the type of tissue. For example, skin can easily regenerate depending on the amount of damage. The liver can also regenerate, but not as easily. However, cardiac tissue cannot regenerate. When an individual has a severe cardiac infarction, a large amount of cardiac tissue can be damaged and the person will be incapacitated.

Fever

The last non-specific host defense discussed in this chapter is fever. Inflammation is an example of a response to a local area of injury. Fever, an abnormally elevated body temperature, is an example of a systemic reaction. A frequent cause of fever is a viral or bacterial invasion.

The hypothalamus is a portion of the diencephalon of the brain forming the floor and part of the lateral wall of the third ventricle. Its somatic functions include sleep, appetite, and temperature. The development of a fever occurs in the following steps. First, when phagocytes ingest bacteria, lipopolysaccharides located in the cell wall are released, inducing the phagocytes to release interleukin-1 (IL-1) inflammatory cytokines.

Second, the presence of IL-1 tells the hypothalamus to release prostaglandins, which elevate the temperature, thereby causing fever.

For example, as the body is invaded by a pathogenic bacterium, the body temperature rises. The physiological response is shivering and an increased rate of metabolism, all of which contribute to an increasing body temperature. Even though the temperature is higher, a person experiences chills and the skin is cold and clammy. Until IL-1 is eliminated, the elevated body temperature will continue.

As the infection is brought under control within the body, vasodilation and sweating begin. These are two heat-losing processes that signify that the body temperature is falling. This phase of the fever is called crisis.

Fever is a defensive mechanism, but only up to a certain point because IL-1 increases the production of T-lymphocytes. A moderate fever is beneficial because only a few bacteria can survive the temperature and usually for only a short period of time. Also, the elevated body temperature increases the effect of interferons. The action of interferons is not completely understood as related to fever, but it is believed that interferons decrease the amount of iron, thereby inhibiting the growth of microbes. However, fever that is unchecked can be debilitating and life-threatening if not controlled.

Interferons

Interferons are proteins that are produced when leukocytes, T-lymphocytes, and fibroblasts are infected. They enter the host's surrounding cells and inhibit the synthesis of proteins that viruses need for multiplication. Hence, they "interfere" with viral replication. Interferon is a highly potent natural antiviral agent that results in inhibition of the spread of infection that allows other host defenses to fight the disease more effectively.

Interferons are not pathogen-specific, but effective against a variety of pathogens and not just the pathogen that stimulated their production. However, interferons are species-specific, meaning that they are effective only in the species of animal that produced them.

There are three classifications of interferons: alpha, beta, and gamma. Alpha and gamma interferons are produced by T-cell lymphocytes; beta interferon is produced by fibroblasts. There are many different types of interferons: 13 alphas, 5 betas, and an unknown number of gamma interferons. The alpha and beta interferons are the most powerful. Interferons are not classified according to function, but rather by their genetic and chemical make-up.

Interferons perform other functions besides fighting viral infections. They also regulate cell motility and division, activate macrophages, and reject transplanted tissue.

Cells that have been infected by a virus are stimulated to produce interferons. The interferons exit from the cell and enter healthy cells, causing them to produce antiviral proteins (AVPs). AVPs are enzymes that interfere with protein synthesis and inhibit the spread of the viral infection. Most types of viruses stimulate the production of interferon.

Recently, interferons were thought to be highly effective agents in the fight against viral diseases and cancer. Large amounts of interferon were produced using recombinant DNA technology. Unfortunately, the results were disappointing. The interferon was highly toxic and ineffective against many cancers and viral diseases. Instances of effective uses include treatment of rare leukemias and some chronic viral infections, such as herpes and hepatitis.

MICRO NOTES

"What's in a Name?"

In microbiology, adhesins are molecules that bind to specific surface receptors on the cells of the host tissues. They should not be confused with the adhesions that surgeons encounter in surgical procedures which involve a patient's tissues that have been previously operated on and subsequently adhere to one another. This abnormal sticking together is secondary to a previous inflammatory response, either in normal healing or from infected tissues. Both terms relate to the ability of surfaces to attach and hold together firmly.

 ## Under the Microscope

A patient was brought to the operating room in 2021 for a laparoscopy procedure for suspected ruptured ectopic pregnancy. The patient was given a screening COVID-19 test and found to be positive. The surgeon states the procedure is an emergent situation and cannot be postponed.

1. What type of disease outbreak includes COVID-19 infection?

2. Which type of pathogen does this patient have and what is the method of transmission and portal of entry?

3. Which portals of entry will the surgeon access to perform the required surgical procedure?

4. Which portals of entry will the anesthesia provider access in administration of medications and maintenance of the airway?

5. Which non-specific host defenses are likely already reacting to this patient's infection and ruptured fallopian tube?

6. Which types of non-specific host defenses will respond to the invasion of the patient's abdomen in performing the laparoscopic procedure?

CHAPTER 10

Parasites and Vectors

Learning Objectives

After completing the study of this chapter, you will be able to:

1. Define key terms.
2. Compare and contrast the various human parasites.
3. Describe various methods of parasitic disease transmission.
4. Discuss the survival mechanisms used by parasites.
5. Describe the "neglected" diseases that are making a resurgence in the United States and foreign countries.
6. Apply critical thinking skills in relating chapter material to the surgical environment of care or broader global community.

Key Terms

Abscess	Cysticercosis	Hydroceles	Peristome
Aerosolized	Dehydration	Krill	Phlebovirus
Anticoagulant	Dysentery	Lymphatic system	Pollinators
Bubonic plague	Ectoparasites	Malabsorption	Symbiont
Cestodes	Encephalitis	Oocysts	Trematodes
Commensals	Entomologists	Opportunistic	Vectors
Comorbidities	Erythrocytic schizogony	Parasitology	
Contractile vacuoles	Exoskeleton	Pellicle	
Cyst	Filariasis	Peristalsis	

The Big Picture

Surgical technologists may not encounter parasitic infections very often in the operating room. If they should ever decide to participate in foreign medical mission or humanitarian work in developing countries, however, they may have to take preventative measures to reduce their risk of infection. During your examination of the topics in this chapter, consider the following:

1. Which parasites might require surgical removal in the operating room?

2. What are the various types of vectors of parasitic disease?

3. Which geographic regions have frequent outbreaks of parasitic infections?

4. What are the routes of transmission for most parasites?

Clinical Significance Topic

Surgical technologists and other surgical team members sometimes choose to participate in volunteerism such as medical mission service, typically in foreign and developing countries. This extremely fulfilling gift of service allows practitioners to bring back unforgettable memories, stories, and photos of their experiences. The potential downside of these opportunities is the potential for exposure to parasitic infection from various sources such as arthropod vectors (mosquitoes, ticks, fleas, etc.), contaminated water sources, or food prepared under suboptimal sanitary conditions. Healthcare volunteers should be sure to research all recommended vaccines and prophylactic medication regimens and bring insect repellents and protective clothing with them to prevent bringing back lasting parasitic reminders of their trips. Awareness and prevention can be the best travel insurance these selfless caregivers have.

Table 10-1 **Common Parasites and Their Mechanism of Transmission and Related Disease or Condition**

Parasite	Route of Transmission	Specimen for Testing	Disease or Condition
Giardia lamblia	Drinking or eating contaminated feces	Feces	Severe diarrhea
Entamoeba histolytica	Drinking or eating contaminated food or water	Feces	Amoebic dysentery
Hookworm	Soil larvae can penetrate bare feet	Feces	Iron deficiency/ anemia
Pinworm	Ingestion of infected food, or soiled bedding or clothing; common in children	Feces	Anal itching
Plasmodium	Bite of infected mosquito	Blood	Malaria

Overview of Parasitology

The study of invertebrates that are human pathogens is called **parasitology**. The environmental conditions discussed for other infectious diseases also apply to the development of a parasitic disease. Parasitic diseases are detected through the same methods of microscopic examination and laboratory methods. The routes of pathogenic disease transmission determine the types of specimens collected for testing (see Table 10-1).

Types of Human Parasites

A parasite is an organism that lives on, with, or in another organism as one member of a symbiotic relationship in which the invading **symbiont** (parasite) takes up residence and extracts its nourishment from and at the expense of the other member of the relationship referred to as the host, sometimes even killing the very host that sustains it. These parasites can be single-cell eukaryotes (protozoa), prokaryotic species of, *Rickettsia*, helminths, arthropods, and **ectoparasites**.

Protozoa

In the Five Kingdom classification system of organisms, protozoa come under the heading of Protista (single-cell eukaryotes). Under the Three Domains system, they are included in Eukarya. The Two Empires system categorizes protozoa as Cellular. Unlike prokaryotic bacteria, protozoa possess one or more nuclei and specialized cellular structures, including organelles called vacuoles. Vacuoles digest nutrients and mitochondria, the principal source of energy for most eukaryotic microbes. Protozoa are heterotrophic microbes, using organic and inorganic environmental materials as food sources.

Protozoan, the singular form, is derived from Greek and means "first animal." More than 60,000 species of protozoa have been identified by scientists. Multicellular plants and animals play host to more than 10,000 species of parasitic protozoa. Many species are normal gut flora in insects and animals, helping to break down food into usable nutrients. Protozoa feed on bacteria, other protozoa, organic waste from other organisms, and some types of fungi.

These microscopic single-cell organisms range in size from 5 µm to 500 µm and can have an incredible variety of shapes. They all require moisture to grow and reproduce and are especially abundant in polluted waters; however, they also thrive in soil and stores of decaying organic waste (see Figure 10-1).

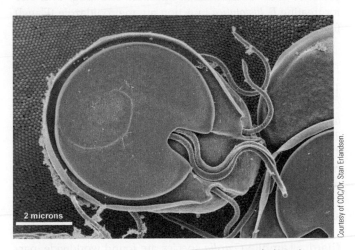

Figure 10-1 This scanning electron micrograph (SEM) revealed the ventral surface of a *Giardia muris* trophozoite that had settled atop the mucosal surface of a rat's intestine. The *Giardia's* ventral adhesive disk resembles a suction cup. The edge of the suction cup, called the ventrolateral flange, partially encircles the adhesive disk and is absent posteriorly where a ventral pair of flagella emerges from above, dorsal to the disk. *Giardia muris* has four pairs of flagella that are responsible for the organism's motility. The adhesive disk facilitates adherence to the intestinal surface.

Courtesy of CDC/Dr. Stan Erlandsen.

Protozoa may live in colonies or singly, have unprotected, thin cell walls, or be covered in protective scales or shells. When faced with hostile conditions and lack of moisture, some species of protozoa become dormant. They create a covering called a **cyst** and break out of it when the environment is more suitable. Similar to other single-cell organisms, most protozoa reproduce asexually by simple binary cell division, creating two identical daughter cells. For those that reproduce sexually, they conjugate by opening channels between two similar protozoa and exchange gametes (DNA-containing organelles), creating new protozoa with traits from both parent cells. They are able to reproduce within human tissues.

Protozoa typically found in human intestinal tracts may be transmitted to other hosts via the fecal-oral route (ingestion of contaminated food or water; from person-to-person). Parasitic protozoa that live in human blood or tissues can also be transmitted by bites from arthropods such as mosquitoes, ticks, and flies. Pathogenic protozoa are classified by their modes of motility (how they move) or method of transmission:

- Amoebas—also known as Sarcodina—a subphylum of phylum Sarcomastigophora; utilize temporary pseudopods for movement. Example: *Acanthamoeba* species (spp.)

- Flagellates—also known as Mastigophora; have one or more whip-like structures that propel them in undulating motions. Example: *Giardia* spp.

- Ciliates—also known as Ciliophora; have hair-like structures (cilia) similar to flagellates; however, cilia are shorter and more numerous. Example: *Balantidium coli*

- Sporozoans—also known as Apicomplexa; are either non-motile in the adult state or very slow-moving. Example: *Plasmodium* spp.

- Microsporidia—obligate intracellular parasites; form protective spore coats and utilize polar tubules to inject infective sporoplasm into host cells. Example: *Enterocytozoön bieneusi*

Intestinal Protozoa

Amoebas, flagellates, and ciliates are classifications of parasitic protozoa responsible for common intestinal diseases. The **vectors** for these diseases are humans and the route of transmission is typically the fecal-oral route and spread in overcrowded, poor, or developing areas with poor sanitation systems and sub-optimal hygiene practices.

Amoeba

The life cycle of the amoeba is divided into two stages: (1) trophozoite, which is the metabolically active, motile, reproducing stage and (2) cyst, which is the dormant, infective stage. Reproduction is by binary fission in which the trophozoite splits into two daughter organisms (see Figure 10-2). As long as the environmental conditions are favorable, the

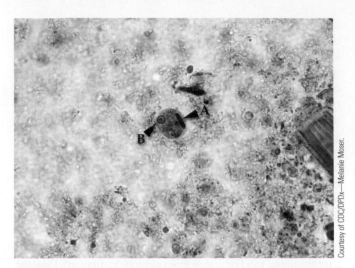

Courtesy of CDC/DPDx—Melanie Moser.

Figure 10-2 Photomicrograph depicted a cyst of the single-celled parasite, *Entamoeba histolytica*. Stained blue, the cyst, in the center, in the highly infective phase life cycle phase as it matures, the organism is extremely resilient to the elements due to the protective cyst wall and is able to survive from days to weeks in the external environment. Note the presence of an elongated, blunt ended chromatoid body within the cyst "A", and a well-defined nucleus "B", with its centrally-situated karyosome.

amoeba remains in the trophozoite stage, but the trophozoite is not infectious. As soon as conditions become difficult or unfavorable, such as a decrease in the amount of moisture or temperature ranges outside those required for growth and survival, the cyst form develops to become more resistant to the harsher conditions. Motility is achieved by extension of a pseudopod (false foot).

Entamoeba Histolytica *Entamoeba histolytica* causes the disease amebiasis, also known as amebic **dysentery**. It was first described in 1875, when it was discovered in the feces of a Russian male with severe dysentery. Further scientific discoveries concerning the organism, including pathogenic characteristics, were made in 1913.

The cyst and trophozoite forms of *E. histolytica* are found in fecal specimens of infected patients. Trophozoites will be seen in fresh stool specimens. After the stool is exposed to the environment for a period of time, the infectious cysts will be found. Trophozoites will also be found in the GI tract.

Entamoeba histolytica infections occur when cysts are ingested in feces-contaminated water or food. Person-to-person transmission can occur through anal intercourse and is seen most frequently in males who have sex with males. The use of human feces for fertilizer also contributes to the spread of infection because the feces in the soil enter the water supply during rainy conditions. Asymptomatic carriers typically contribute more to the spread of the disease than symptomatic persons. The feces of carriers contain infective cysts, whereas the feces of symptomatic individuals contain the non-infectious trophozoites.

Following ingestion of contaminated food or water, the cysts produce trophozoites, which are released in the small intestine. The trophozoites produce a cytotoxin that is responsible for damage to the mucosal tissue of the intestines and allows the organism to invade the internal tissues of the body. The cytotoxin creates flask-shaped lesions in the intestinal mucosa, producing inflammation, hemorrhage (bloody diarrhea), and the ability of opportunistic pathogens such as *Escherichia coli* to cause a secondary infection due to the microbial population imbalance created. The symptoms of a primary infection include abdominal cramps and pain, bloody diarrhea that also contains mucus, and amebic dysentery with accompanying weight loss. Individuals with these symptoms should be monitored for likely **dehydration**.

Secondary infection occurs when *E. histolytica* enters the bloodstream or **lymphatic system** to invade body organs. This is referred to as extraintestinal amebiasis and occurs in only a small percentage of infections. Trophozoites are associated with extraintestinal amebiasis. The most commonly infected organ is the liver, but infections of the pulmonary, cardiovascular, and central nervous systems can occur. The liver is most often involved because trophozoites in the blood are removed as they pass through the organ. The right lobe is most commonly infected. **Abscess** formation can occur along with hepatomegaly (pathogenic enlargement of the liver).

Diagnosis is based on examination of fecal specimens that will contain trophozoites and cysts. Specimens obtained by aspiration during a sigmoidoscopy procedure can also be examined. Extraintestinal amebiasis is difficult to diagnose in comparison to intestinal amebiasis. The presence of antibodies is most likely the best diagnostic aid for determining the presence of an extraintestinal infection. The drugs of choice for treating *E. histolytica* infection are metronidazole (Flagyl) followed by iodoquinol.

Flagellates

The flagellates that are clinically significant to humans are *Giardia lamblia*, *Trichomonas vaginalis*, and *Dientamoeba fragilis*. *Giardia lamblia* has the trophozoite and cyst stage, whereas *Trichomonas* and *Dientamoeba* only have a trophozoite stage. The name flagellates indicates that the organisms achieve motility by means of one or more flagella. Flagellates are surrounded by a semi-rigid, thin film called a **pellicle** that provides a more definite shape as compared to the less defined shape of the amoeba.

Giardia Lamblia *Giardia* species are found worldwide, particularly outdoors in wilderness areas that include mountain streams and lakes. The organism has four pairs of flagella that propel it in a rapid, twisting motion. The anterior end of the cell is broad and round in shape, and the posterior end tapers to a point. The species is carried in the feces of beavers and other warm-blooded animals. The water is contaminated by feces and the *Giardia* organism is ingested, causing the disease giardiasis. Individuals who live in mountain regions and tourists are always reminded not to drink the water of mountain streams and lakes. *Giardia* is also acquired by person-to-person spread by the fecal-oral route or oral-anal route. The cysts are resistant to chlorine used in water treatment plants, so the water treatment should include filtration and treatment with a variety of chemicals (see Figure 10-3).

Infection with *G. lamblia* begins with the ingestion of cysts. Cysts and trophozoites are found in the feces of infected patients. After ingestion, each cyst releases two trophozoites in the duodenum and jejunum, and the organism reproduces by binary fission. The trophozoites attach to the villi of the intestine by means of a ventrally located sucking disk. The sucking disk prevents the organism from being removed by the **peristalsis** of the small intestine. For this reason, trophozoites are usually not passed in the feces, except in watery diarrhea. The sucking disk also absorbs contents of the intestine and some epithelial cells, thereby meeting the nutritional needs of the organism. Inflammation of the intestinal mucosa occurs, but tissue destruction and necrosis do not occur as found with *E. histolytica* infections. Additionally, spread of *G. lamblia* to other parts of the body is rare.

Giardia lamblia infection results in an asymptomatic carrier or symptomatic disease. The incubation period before symptomatic disease develops is 1–4 weeks, with an average of 10 days. The symptoms range from mild diarrhea to the more severe **malabsorption** syndrome. The onset of symptoms is sudden, characterized by the following: foul-smelling, watery diarrhea; abdominal cramps and pain; flatulence; and steatorrhea (excess fat or oily discharge in the feces). Blood

and mucus are not present, attesting to the absence of intestinal mucosal tissue destruction. The infected individual will typically spontaneously recover in 10–14 days.

Diagnosis is made by examination of the patient's stools. Multiple specimens may have to be obtained because many organisms may be present in the stool specimen one day but none will be detected the next day. One stool specimen per day for 3 days should be obtained for laboratory examination. Specimens can also be obtained by duodenoscopy aspiration or tissue biopsy of the upper part of the small intestine.

Dientamoeba Fragilis *Dientamoeba fragilis* was initially classified as an ameoba, but the internal structures of the trophozoite reflect characteristics of the flagellates. The organism only occurs as a trophozoite with no cyst stage occurring in its life cycle. *D. fragilis* is found worldwide. Transmission of the organism is not well-understood. One theory is that the organism resides in the eggs of the pinworm *Enterobius vermicularis*. An individual becomes infected by ingesting the eggs. A large number of individuals infected with the pinworm also are diagnosed with infection by *D. fragilis*. This suggests that a connection exists between the pinworm and *D. fragilis*. Transmissions by fecal-oral and oral-anal routes have not been definitely established.

The majority of infected individuals are asymptomatic, and the organism colonizes in the cecum and upper colon. Symptomatic patients experience abdominal cramps and pain, episodes of diarrhea, weight loss, and flatulence. Irritation of the mucosal tissue of the colon occurs, but tissue damage is not present. Laboratory diagnosis is made by microscopic examination of stool specimens. Multiple stool specimens are necessary because as mentioned previously, a large number of organisms may be present in one specimen but absent in others.

Ciliates

The ciliates are the most complex protozoans with cyst and trophozoite stages in their life cycle. *Balantidium coli* is the only ciliate that is pathogenic to humans.

Balantidium Coli The outside of the *B. coli* cell is covered by cilia that provide motility. It has an opening or mouth called a cytostome located at the posterior end of the cell, food vacuoles, two **contractile vacuoles**, and two nuclei involved in the reproductive process. The life cycle of *B. coli* involves ingestion of infectious cysts, release of trophozoites, and invasion of the mucosal lining of the terminal ileum, cecum, and colon. The trophozoites reproduce by conjugation followed by binary fission in the lumen or wall of the colon.

B. coli is distributed worldwide, with human infection occurring primarily in tropical regions. However, the incidence of infections in humans is low. Swine are the primary source of infection; monkeys are less often the source. Transmission is by the fecal-oral route, with infection occurring by the ingestion of contaminated water or food. Outbreaks of the disease, called balantidiasis, have been associated with contamination of the water supply by pig feces. Food handlers

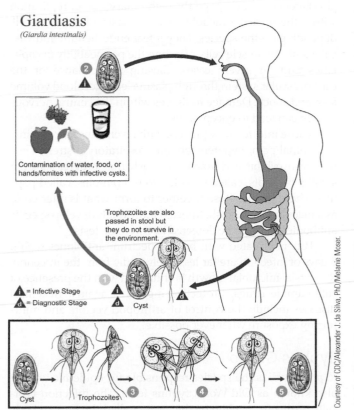

Giardiasis
(Giardia intestinalis)

Contamination of water, food, or hands/fomites with infective cysts.

Trophozoites are also passed in stool but they do not survive in the environment.

⚠ = Infective Stage
d = Diagnostic Stage

Cyst

Cyst   Trophozoites

Courtesy of CDC/Alexander J. da Silva, PhD/Melanie Moser.

Figure 10-3 Illustration of the life cycle of *Giardia lamblia*, the causal agent of giardiasis.

who do not practice good hygiene have also been implicated in outbreaks.

Asymptomatic carriers and symptomatic disease both occur with *B. coli*. Symptomatic disease is characterized by abdominal pain, abdominal cramps, abdominal tenderness, nausea, and watery stools with blood and pus present. *B. coli* produces proteolytic enzymes and cytotoxic substances that aid in tissue destruction and invasion, including ulceration of the mucosal tissue. This accounts for the presence of blood and pus in the stools of the infected patient. Extraintestinal invasion is very rare.

Laboratory diagnosis is made by microscopic examination of a stool specimen to confirm the presence of trophozoites and cysts. The trophozoite is large and covered with cilia, and the macronucleus is easily seen. The cyst is smaller and only has a single nucleus (see Figure 10-4).

Rickettsia

Rickettsia are very small Gram-negative pleomorphic coccobacilli approximately 0.8–2.0 μm in length, an intermediate size between viruses and bacteria. They are obligate intracellular parasites that can only replicate within the eukaryotic cell of the host because they require a rich cytoplasm to stabilize a highly permeable cell membrane. They have typical bacterial cell walls and occur singly, in pairs, or in strands. Only one species, *R. prowazekii*, has flagellae. They are nonmotile and do not form spores. Identification through culturing and staining is difficult because the organisms only weakly absorb the counter stain, safranin. Special staining techniques, namely Macchiavello, Castaneda, and Giemsa stains, are utilized.

Rickettsiaceae species were named for the man who discovered them, American pathologist Howard Taylor Ricketts, who died of typhus in 1910 while studying the disease. The genus *Rickettsia* is generally divided into three groups: typhus, spotted fever, and scrub typhus. This genus is responsible for diseases such as Rocky Mountain spotted fever, epidemic typhus, Brill-Zinsser disease, and scrub typhus.

Species include the following: *Rickettsia prowazekii*, the causative pathogenic parasite for epidemic typhus; *Rickettsia typhi*, the pathogen responsible for murine (endemic) typhus; *Rickettsia rickettsii*, the causative pathogen for spotted fever; *Rochalimaea quintana*, the pathogen for trench fever; and *Coxiella burnetii*, the causative parasite for Q fever. A mild disease, known as rickettsial pox, is caused by *Rickettsia akarii*. *R. typhi* and *R. prowazekii* replicate in the cytoplasm of the host cell, whereas *R. rickettsii* replicates within the nucleus.

Transmission and Diagnosis

Transmission to humans is through the bites of infected ticks or mites as the organisms gain access to saliva glands, and by the feces of infected lice or fleas as the organisms multiply in the gastrointestinal tract of the arthropod vectors, and are passed through their feces to the human host. Once in the bloodstream, the organisms spread to targeted cells and begin direct cellular damage through binary fission replication within the nucleus, vacuole, or protoplasm of the host cell, depending on the species. They infect endothelium and vascular smooth muscle cells, affecting the permeability of capillaries and, in severe cases, causing the collapse of the cardiovascular system through plasma leakage, blood volume loss, and shock. Damage to tissues within the central nervous system can lead to encephalitis.

Those infected may present with fever, nausea, vomiting, abdominal pain, hypotension, and respiratory distress. They may also exhibit a characteristic rash that progresses from small pink spots, called macules, to red pimples, called papules. These papules fuse together to form what is referred to as a maculopapular rash. Infected individuals develop specific antibodies that can be detected by serologic tests.

Patients treated with broad-spectrum antibiotics within 5 days of infection are far less likely to die from the infection. Rickettsial microbial growth is enhanced with the presence of sulfonamide drugs. Protective measures against rickettsial diseases include the control of arthropod vectors and minimizing exposure whenever possible.

Typhus Group

R. prowazekii is the species responsible for epidemic typhus, also known as Old World typhus fever. The infection typically results from a bite by the vector called the human body louse (*Pediculus humanus*) or from feces of the lice (plural of louse) that make their way into a skin scratch or abrasion.

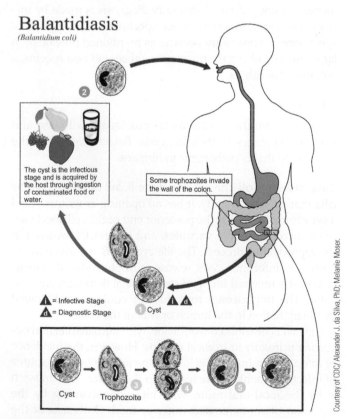

Balantidiasis
(Balantidium coli)

The cyst is the infectious stage and is acquired by the host through ingestion of contaminated food or water.

Some trophozoites invade the wall of the colon.

i = Infective Stage
d = Diagnostic Stage

Cyst

Cyst   Trophozoite

Courtesy of CDC/ Alexander J. da Silva, PhD; Melanie Moser.

Figure 10-4 Illustration of the life cycle of the parasite, *Balantidium coli*, the causal agent of balantidiasis.

After 10 to 14 days, a sudden onset of fever and severe headache occur. Fever typically increases to 104°F and may last up to 2 weeks. At approximately the fourth day of symptoms, a rash of pink spots appears on all parts of the body except the face, hands, and feet. Chills and delirium from the high fever, malaise, vomiting, and shock may soon follow. Untreated, the mortality rate can reach 30 percent.

Reactivation of an old typhus infection is referred to as Brill-Zinsser disease, also known as benign typhus. *R. prowazekii* can remain dormant in the lymph nodes for many years; however, with stress it can manifest again with milder symptoms.

Endemic (murine) typhus is caused by *R. typhi*, which is transmitted by fleas from infected rats or mice. Symptoms are similar to those of epidemic typhus but are usually much milder. Mortality rates are approximately 5 percent.

Scrub Typhus Group

Scrub typhus is caused by *Orientia tsutsugamushi*, which is transmitted by a mite that lives on rodents. Symptoms are similar to those of epidemic typhus with the addition of a red nodule that turns into a black scab (eschar) at the site of the bite. Left untreated, mortality may reach 40 percent. Scrub typhus is typically found in areas of Japan, Southeast Asia, and the Southwest Pacific.

Spotted Fever Group

Rocky Mountain spotted fever is caused by *R. rickettsii*, which is transmitted by the American dog tick (*Dermacentor variabilis*), and other tick species. Reservoirs include rabbits, birds, rodents, and dogs. It is most commonly seen in the southeastern and south central United States and is actually rare in the Rocky Mountains. At least 17 other species are responsible for diseases within the spotted fever category found worldwide.

Rocky Mountain spotted fever is characterized by symptoms that appear 2 weeks after infection and include a sudden onset of high fever, severe headache, fatigue, muscle pain, chills, and rash. The rash begins on the extremities, may spread to the soles of the feet and palms of the hands, and then spreads to the rest of the body (see Figure 10-5).

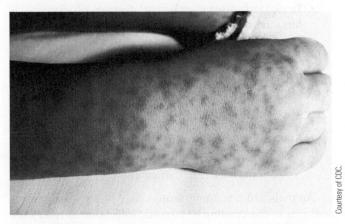

Courtesy of CDC.

Figure 10-5 Rash caused by Rocky Mountain spotted fever.

Metazoa

Metazoa, sometimes called metazoans, are multicellular organisms classified as Kingdom Animalia, Domain Eukaryote, or Empire Cellular. Metazoa are motile and comprise cells that differentiate into a variety of tissues and organs, often including digestive tracts lined with specialized cells. Parasitic metazoa include helminths (worms), ectoparasites, and arthropods.

Helminths

Helminths, from the Greek word for worms, are large, multicellular organisms that are visible to the naked eye in their adult forms. Similar to protozoa, they may be free-living or parasitic. Commonly named for their body shapes, the three categories of human parasitic helminths are:

- Flatworms (platyhelminths)—including flukes (trematodes) and tapeworms (cestodes)
- Roundworms (nematodes)—larval and adult forms can reside in the GI tract, blood, lymphatic system, and subcutaneous tissue
- Thorny-headed worms (acanthocephalans)—thought to be intermediate between cestodes and nematodes

The tapeworm species *Taenia* are ingested by humans eating undercooked or raw contaminated pork or beef (see Figure 10-6). *Schistosoma mansoni* is a well-known blood fluke that uses snails as an intermediate host.

Ectoparasites

Ectoparasites live on the surface of its host or within its skin layer, but not in internal tissues. Fleas, ticks, mites, mosquitoes, and lice are examples of ectoparasites. Mosquitoes can be broadly classified as ectoparasites because of their requirement for blood to survive; however, they do not reside in or on humans. Arthropods are examples of ectoparasites.

Arthropods

Arthropods are members of the phylum Arthropoda, the largest phylum in the animal kingdom. They range in size from giant crustaceans such as king crab to the tiny marine **krill** abundant in oceans. These organisms have segmented bodies covered with protective **exoskeletons** and jointed appendages. Out of the approximately 1 million species of arthropods, most are insects. Different species of arthropods have adapted to become marine or terrestrial inhabitants. In the plant kingdom, arthropods can be valuable **pollinators** or fatal parasitic predators.

Arthropods bite, sting, and infest humans, but rarely secrete harmful toxins. Their medical significance in the infection process is their role as disease-carrying vectors (see Figure 10-7).

Vectors

In parasitology, a vector is defined as an organism that does not directly cause disease, but rather spreads pathogenic

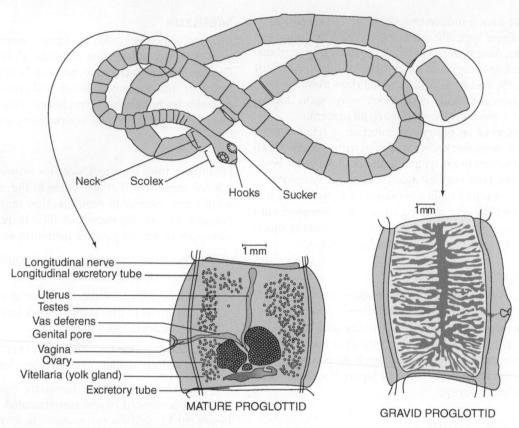

Neck   Scolex   Hooks   Sucker

1mm

Longitudinal nerve
Longitudinal excretory tube
Uterus
Testes
Vas deferens
Genital pore
Vagina
Ovary
Vitellaria (yolk gland)
Excretory tube
MATURE PROGLOTTID

1mm

GRAVID PROGLOTTID

Figure 10-6 General anatomy of an adult tapeworm.

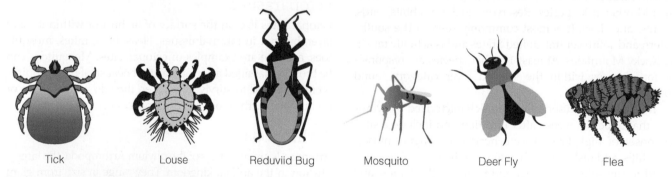

Tick   Louse   Reduviid Bug   Mosquito   Deer Fly   Flea

Figure 10-7 Examples of arthropod vectors.

organisms from one host to another. In molecular biology, a vector is a plasmid or virus that carries foreign genetic material into a host cell. In both definitions, there is a host and an organism (large or small) that transmits a foreign substance into a host, thereby infecting the host cell. The invading pathogen may elicit little reaction or produce potentially catastrophic results for the host.

Examples of vectors and the diseases they spread include:

- Mosquitoes: malaria, yellow fever, Dengue fever, West Nile fever, chikungunya, lymphatic filariasis, Japanese **encephalitis**
- Tsetse flies: African sleeping sickness (human African trypanosomiasis or HAT)
- Fleas: **bubonic plague**

- Ticks: Lyme disease, rickettsial diseases (Rocky Mountain spotted fever), tularemia
- Lice (body louse): typhus
- Triatomine ("kissing") bugs: Chagas disease (American trypanosomiasis)
- Phlebotomine sand flies: leishmaniasis
- Black flies: onchocerciasis (river blindness)
- Aquatic snails: schistosomiasis
- Food products: campylobacteriosis, botulism, hepatitis A, salmonellosis, *E. coli*, shigellosis

Animals, wild or domesticated, may be unwitting intermediaries in the creation of parasitic infections as reservoirs for microbial stowaways. Parasites from animals can be

Table 10-2 **Host–Parasite Relationships**

Host	Description
Final host	Host in which the parasite lives for its entire life cycle, including sexual maturity and reproduction.
Intermediate host	Hosts in which parasites reside at an immature stage. A parasitic life cycle may include one or more intermediate hosts.
Reservoir host	Parasites reside on this type of host to be transmitted to humans or other animals. For example, beavers serve as a reservoir for *Giardia lamblia*. When the infected beavers defecate into mountain water, the *G. lamblia* cysts can then be ingested by humans who drink the water.

transferred to humans through their feces or consumed in undercooked meat. Table 10-2 describes the three types of host–parasite relationships.

Vector-Borne Diseases

Pathogens transmitted by vectors cause significant human, animal, and plant disease and are studied by epidemiologists, microbiologists, zoologists, **entomologists**, infectious disease specialists, veterinarians, and public health researchers. Vectors are rarely adversely affected by and, in some cases, have come to rely and depend on the parasites or bacteria they transport from host to host. Researchers are challenged with trying to predict vector behavior. Changes in local climate conditions, urban sprawl, political conflicts, and microbial mutations are factors that scientists must factor into their findings, but over which they have little control. Many of the vector-borne diseases, especially those carried by mosquitoes, are found in tropical and sub-tropical climates (see Figure 10-8). Other

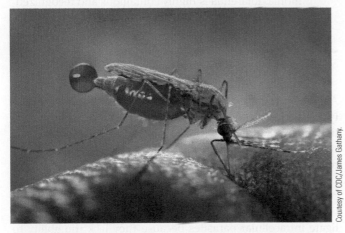

Figure 10-8 Lateral view of a feeding female *Anopheles gambiae* mosquito obtaining its blood meal through its sharp, needle-like labrum, which it had inserted into its human host. Note the red color of the labrum, as it was filled with blood, and the bright red abdomen that had become enlarged due to its blood meal contents. You can also see a droplet of blood that was being expelled from the distal tip of its abdomen. *A. gambiae* is a known vector for the parasitic disease malaria.

Courtesy of CDC/James Gathany.

arthropod vectors, including ticks, mites, flies, and fleas, are found in most climates and geographic locations.

The Division of Vector-Borne Diseases (DVBD) is a specialized group of scientists from the United States and around the world commissioned by the CDC to study the incredibly diverse nature of disease transmitted by vectors. Their research labs are located in Atlanta, Georgia; Puerto Rico; and Fort Collins, Colorado.

Some of the vector-borne viral diseases currently being investigated include the following:

- Chikungunya: a virus carried by the *Aedes aegypti* and *Aedes albopictus* species of mosquitoes in mainly tropical areas. Symptoms are similar to Dengue fever and affected individuals may actually suffer from simultaneous infection. Chikungunya has been found in the islands of the Caribbean in recent years.

- Dengue Fever: virus endemic in Puerto Rico and other tropical and sub-tropical nations. Dengue is discussed more in this chapter in the section on neglected tropical diseases.

- Eastern Equine Encephalitis Virus: carried by mosquitoes. Rare in humans, but a few cases per year occur in the United States, mainly in Atlantic and Gulf coast states. Symptoms may not manifest in mild cases; however, in severe cases there is a 33 percent mortality rate and survivors suffer significant brain damage.

- Heartland Virus: **phlebovirus** first described in 2012. Several cases were found in Tennessee and Missouri in 2014. Thought to be transmitted by bites from mosquitoes, ticks, or sandflies. Diffuse malaise symptoms occur. Patients were hospitalized, with one fatality.

- Japanese Encephalitis: virus carried by mosquitoes found mainly in Asia and Western Pacific nations. Found only in the United States in travelers. One in four cases is fatal, but it is a vaccine-preventable disease.

- La Crosse Encephalitis: mosquito-carried virus found in upper mid-western, south-eastern, and mid-Atlantic states in the United States. Most severe cases occur in children younger than 16 years of age. Symptoms range from none to severe headaches, seizures, and coma, and it may be fatal.

- Powassan Virus: carried by ticks and found mainly in the northeast and Great Lakes states. Approximately 180 cases have been reported in the United States over the past 12 years. Neurological symptoms require hospitalization and respiratory support. Long-term neurological deficits may occur in more severe cases.

- St. Louis Encephalitis: mosquito-borne virus found mainly in central and eastern United States. Neurological symptoms range from mild to severe. Severe cases are more likely in older adults.

- West Nile Virus: mosquito-borne virus found in increasing areas of the United States. Most will suffer no symptoms; however, 1 percent of individuals may develop serious, sometimes fatal neurologic illness.

- Yellow Fever: viral infection carried by mosquitoes. Rare in the United States. Mainly found in travelers to endemic countries (South America and Africa).

- Zika: viral infection carried by mosquitoes and transmitted between intimate partners, from mother to fetus, and potentially through blood transfusion. Zika may cause significant birth defects including microcephaly (abnormally small head/brain size) and possible Guillain-Barré syndrome, a nervous system disorder (see Figure 10-9).

The bacterial vector-borne diseases under investigation by the DVBD include the following:

- Anaplasmosis (*Anaplasma phagocytophilium*): black-legged tick-borne disease that causes a variety of flu-like symptoms that can progress to respiratory difficulty, hemorrhage, kidney failure, and neurological involvement. Fatal in less than 1 percent of cases. Of concern is the potential for transmission of *A. phagocytophilium* in blood donation from asymptomatic infected individuals.

- *Bartonella* infections: Cat scratch disease (*Bartonella henselae*), trench fever (*Bartonella quintana*), and Carrión's disease (*Bartonella bacilliformis*). Symptoms commonly seen include fever, lymph node inflammation, rash, papules or pustules, and headaches. In severe cases it may progress to encephalitis or subacute endocarditis.

- Ehrlichiosis infections: include *Ehrlichia chaffeensis* and *Ehrlichia ewingii*, which are tick-borne diseases with clinical features similar to anaplasmosis. Potentially transmitted in donated blood products and organs.

- Lyme Disease (*Borrelia burgdorferi*): tick-borne spirochete infection that causes symptoms of fever, fatigue, headache, and characteristic rash patterns. Without treatment, symptoms can involve joints, heart, and central nervous system. *Borrelia* is discussed in later sections.

- Plague (*Yersinia pestis*): transmitted by fleas on rodents. Plague was responsible for millions of deaths during the Middle Ages in Europe. Localized outbreaks continue to occur in Asia and Africa and occasionally in the United States, mainly in the western states; however, antibiotic therapy is able to treat the illness.

- Rocky Mountain Spotted Fever (*Rickettsia rickettsia*): transmitted by several species of ticks in North and South America. Severe and potentially fatal if not treated within first 5 days of infection. *Rickettsia* diseases are discussed in detail in subsequent sections.

- Southern Tick-Associated Rash Illness (STARI): similar to Lyme disease; carried by the lone star tick species (*Amblyomma americanum*). The bacteria responsible are unknown; however, researchers have ruled out *Borrelia* as a causative bacterium. The lone-star tick is found in nearly half of the United States, concentrated in the eastern half from the Great Lakes south-eastward, although they have been reported even as far north as Maine.

- Tick-Borne Relapsing Fever: caused by *Borrelia*. Two types of relapsing fever have been identified: tick-borne, which is found in the western United States and associated with rustic settings (mountain cabins, camping), and louse-borne, which is associated with infected lice spreading in refugee camps of conflict areas of developing countries.

- Tularemia (*Francisella tularensis*): bacterium found naturally in rodents, rabbits, and hares; spread by bites of ticks, flies, or other insects, handling of animal carcasses, inhalation of **aerosolized** bacteria, or ingestion of contaminated food or water. Symptoms can progress to respiratory difficulty and potentially fatal pneumonia. Tularemia is highly contagious and recognized as a potential biological weapon in aerosolized form.

Host–Parasite Relationships

As has been discussed in prior chapters, organisms of every type establish relationships with other organisms. These relationships may be beneficial to one or both, and they may cause harm to one of them. The various types of microbial relationships are reviewed and summarized in Table 10-3.

Parasites may be obligate or **opportunistic**. Obligate parasites depend on different hosts to sustain them through their stages of development and reproduction. Viruses are obligate intracellular parasites because they lack the ability to reproduce without a host cell. Eukaryotic protozoa can be free-living or seize opportunities to invade and overrun other cells, turning them into pathogenic hosts.

Infection with a parasite does not always result in damage or disease to the host. Some parasites are actually **commensals**. Chronic, asymptomatic infections are important to the parasite because the carriers are responsible for transmitting the parasite to other hosts, thereby continuing the life cycle.

Why Zika is Risky for Some People

Zika infection during pregnancy can microcephaly and other birth defects. Microcephaly is a birth defect in which a baby's head is smaller than expected when compared to babies of the same sex and age. There have also been increased reports of Guillain-Barré syndrome, an uncommon sickness of the nervous system, in areas affected by Zika.

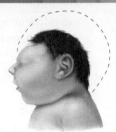

Microcephaly

How to Prevent Zika

There is no vaccine to prevent Zika. The best way to prevent diseases spread by mosquitoes is to protect yourself and your family from mosquito bites and from getting Zika through sex.. **Here's how:**

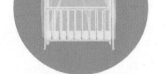

- Wear long-sleeved shirts and long pants.
- Stay in places with air conditioning and window and door screens to keep mosquitoes outside.
- Take steps to control mosquitoes inside and outside your home.
- Treat your clothing and gear with permethrin or buy pre-treated items.
- Use Environmental Protection Agency (EPA)-registered insect repellents. Always follow the product label instructions.
- When used as directed, these insect repellents are proven safe and effective even for pregnant and breastfeeding women.
  - Do not use insect repellents on babies younger than 2 months old.
    - Mosquito netting can be used to cover babies younger than 2 months old in carriers, strollers, or cribs to protect them from mosquito bites.
  - Do not use products containing oil of lemon eucalyptus or para-menthane-diol on children younger than 3 years old.
- Sleep under a mosquito bed net if air conditioned or screened rooms are not available or if sleeping outdoors.
  - Prevent sexual transmission of Zika by using condoms or not having sex.

What to Do if You Have Zika

There is no specific medicine to treat Zika. Treat the symptoms:

- Get plenty of rest.
- Drink fluids to prevent dehydration.
- Take medicine such as acetaminophen to reduce fever and pain.
- Do not take aspirin or other non-steroidal anti-inflammatory drugs.
- If you are taking medicine for another medical condition, talk to your healthcare provider before taking additional medication.

To help prevent others from getting sick, strictly follow steps to prevent mosquito bites during the first week of illness.

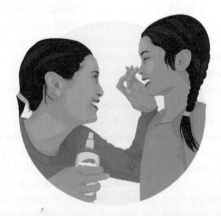

www.cdc.gov/zika

Second page of infographic image available at: https://www.cdc.gov/zika/pdfs/fs-zika-basics.pdf

Figure 10-9 Zika basics.

Table 10-3 Microbial Relationships

Relationship	Description	Microbial example
Symbiosis	Two different organisms live together in close association, usually in mutually beneficial relationship.	*Escherichia coli* living in the intestine of humans
Mutualism	Both organisms benefit from the relationship.	Protozoa live in the intestine of termites, allowing termites to digest the wood that is eaten; termite provides food for protozoa.
Commensalism	One organism benefits while the host neither benefits nor is harmed.	Indigenous microflora of humans are provided nutrients, but the human host neither benefits nor is harmed.
Parasitism	Organism benefits at the expense of the host organism, thereby harming the host organism.	Tapeworms in the intestine of a human host
Ectoparasites	Parasites that live on the outside of the body; referred to as an infestation	Mites, lice, ticks
Endoparasites	Parasites that live on the inside of the body; referred to as an infection	Helminths, parasitic protozoans
Facultative parasites	Referred to as an opportunistic pathogen; capable of living on host independently	The microspora *E. bieneusi*
Incidental parasite	Infects a species that is not the normal host	*Dipylidium caninum*, tapeworm that usually infects dogs and cats but humans have been known to acquire the tapeworm.

More commonly, parasitic infections are responsible for damaging effects to the host and can impair human organ functions. Helminths cause mechanical damage. Tapeworms use hooks to attach to the GI tract of humans and the hooks, especially if the infestation is severe, can cause significant damage to the tissue by tearing of the intestine. Tapeworms also use vitamin B12, depriving the host and leading to anemia. A protozoan, such as *G. lamblia*, has a sucker on the underside of its body that is used to attach itself to the host. The parasite can then feed by highjacking the nutrients from the host, resulting in difficulty absorbing nutrients, a condition called giardiasis, which is one in a class of malabsorption syndromes (see Figure 10-10).

Nematodes can cause bowel obstruction due to the large numbers that crowd the GI tract. The most common nematode responsible for obstruction is *Ascaris,* creating a condition called ascariasis. Ascariasis is caused by *Ascaris lumbricoides* and is diagnosed by the presence of large adult worms (as long as 1 foot) that emerge from the anus (see Figure 10-11). These adult worms have small teeth that can chew through the intestinal wall, allowing entry into the abdominal cavity. Once diagnosed, ascariasis can be treated with antiparasitic drugs such as albendazole or mebendazole; however, large infestations that cause bowel obstructions require surgical resection.

Some species of parasites can cause host tissue damage due to excretions that are toxic to the host. Two examples of damaging excretions are the **anticoagulant** excretion of hookworms and enzymes of *Entamoeba.*

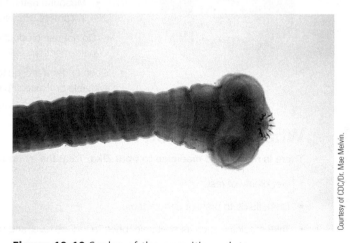

Courtesy of CDC/Dr. Mae Melvin.

Figure 10-10 Scolex of the parasitic pork tape worm, *Taenia solium.*

Survival Mechanisms

The nutritional requirement of parasites is not complex and requires using the available organic nutrients. Amoebae (plural of amoeba) and other protozoa use the processes of phagocytosis or pinocytosis of soluble material. The engulfed material is then enclosed in digestive vacuoles. The flagellates and ciliates ingest their food via an area called the **peristome** or cytostome. The

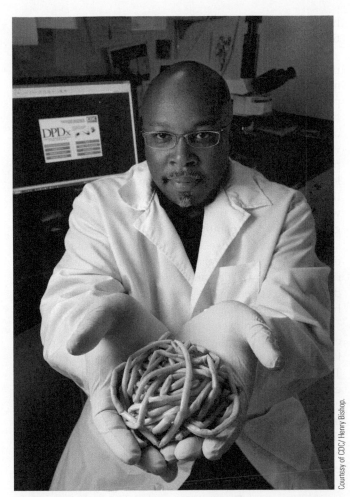

Figure 10-11 CDC/ National Center for Emerging and Zoonotic Infectious Diseases (NCZVED)/Division of Parasitic Diseases (DPDx) laboratory technician holding a mass of *Ascaris lumbricoides* worms, which had been passed by a child in Kenya, Africa. This nematode parasitizes the human small intestine and is spread from human-to-human by the fecal-oral route.

microsporidia ingest nutrients by simple diffusion and the particles are then enclosed in vacuoles. The undigested nutrient particles and waste are eliminated from the cell by expelling the material at the cell surface. Respiration in the majority of parasitic protozoa is by facultative anaerobic processes.

Parasitic organisms have evolved and adapted in ways that have allowed them to create facultative parasitic relationships. The changes over time may have involved morphologic and physiologic changes allowing the parasite to resist enzymatic attacks by the host and enhance attachment to the host tissues. For example, tapeworms do not have a digestive system. One theory is that when tapeworms first invaded the GI tract of hosts, possibly by accidental ingestion, they adapted by eliminating body systems they no longer needed because the host provided the substitute. Without a digestive system the tapeworm relies on the pre-digested food from the GI tract of the host.

Survival of parasitic protozoa in the harsh environmental conditions of the host is aided by cyst development. The

unfavorable conditions include low oxygen, exposure to the acidic secretions of the GI tract, and internal high osmotic pressure. The parasitic protozoan develops into a cyst that is less metabolically active, thereby requiring fewer nutritional requirements. The cell wall of the cyst is thick, protecting it from the enzymes and other substances of the host. The cyst form also facilitates the transmission of the organism from host to host in harsh external environmental conditions.

Endoparasites survive due to the complex ability to evade the host's immune system and respond to attacks by continuously changing their surface antigens.

Helminths survive by producing a large number of resilient eggs. This increases the odds that the next generation of parasitic organisms will survive. Asexual reproduction at the larval stage of parasites within intermediate hosts also increases the chances of the organisms gaining access to the next intermediate or final host.

Reproductive Methods

The methods of reproduction by parasites have evolved over time because of the difficult task of finding suitable hosts. This reproductive evolution has aided in ensuring that the parasites survive and continue to exist. Asexual and sexual reproductions have been observed in helminths and protozoa.

Asexual Reproduction

There are three methods of asexual reproduction by parasites: (1) mitotic fission; (2) schizogony; and (3) budding. The first two methods are the most common. Mitotic fission is commonly seen in protozoa. Mitotic fission produces two daughter cells. *Trichomonas vaginalis* is an example of a protozoan that reproduces by mitotic fission.

Schizogony refers to multiple fission. During this type of reproduction, the nucleus is divided several times by mitotic fission and the cytoplasm is distributed among the daughter cells. *Plasmodium* divides by **erythrocytic schizogony**, which gives rise to merozoites. The red blood cell eventually ruptures, freeing the merozoites, which then infects additional erythrocytes (see Figure 10-12).

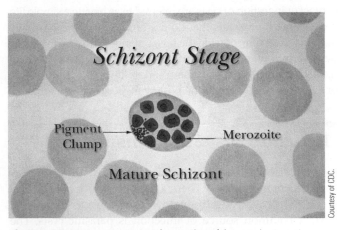

Figure 10-12 A mature erythrocytic schizont during the *plasmodium* spp. life cycle.

A few helminths are able to asexually reproduce by budding. Budding enables the number of worms to significantly increase in a host that may have only consumed a single egg. This ensures survivability within the host. Tapeworms in the larval stage reproduce by budding.

Sexual Reproduction

Some protozoans reproduce by conjugation, producing gametocytes. The majority of helminths reproduce by cross-fertilization and self-fertilization. Sexual reproduction is more efficient than asexual reproduction and provides the ability to genetically adapt to changing environments, increasing the chances of survival of the species.

During conjugation, two parasites fuse and exchange their genetic material. The organisms separate and continue the cycle of reproducing by conjugation with others. An example of conjugation is *Plasmodium*. Gametocytes are produced and fuse in the human host and then are ingested by the *Anopheles* mosquito as it feeds on the host. The sexual cycle of *Plasmodium* finishes inside the mosquito.

The majority of **trematodes** and **cestodes** are hermaphrodites, which means that the organism contains both female and male reproductive organs. The parasites either self-fertilize or cross-fertilize with another of its kind.

Life Cycles of Parasites

There are two types of parasitic life cycles: complex life cycle and simple life cycle. Both types of life cycles occur in species of protozoans and helminths.

Complex Life Cycle

Parasites that rely on one or more intermediate hosts and a final host are said to have a complex life cycle. This further complicates the ability of the parasite to survive and reproduce. In addition to the need for intermediate hosts, some parasites can only mature in a particular environment in which the intermediate hosts are available.

Simple Life Cycle

Parasites with a single host that are transmitted by either direct contact or ingestion of cysts are referred to as having a simple life cycle. Some protozoans that do not produce a cyst can usually live for a short time outside the host but must find a host quickly, by either direct contact or transmission by a vector, or they will die. In many parasites that have a simple life cycle, cysts, oocysts, or eggs are transmitted to the host by the fecal-oral route.

Parasitic Disease Transmission

Parasitic disease is transmitted in similar ways that other organisms are transmitted. There must be a source of infection, a method of reaching the pathway or transmission, and a host. A common source of infection is parasitic cysts. The source of infection for parasitic helminths is eggs or larvae. The routes of transmission that are discussed are ingestion of contaminated food or water, direct contact with an infected host, transfer of the parasite by a vector, respiratory inhalation, and trans-placental infection.

Ingestion of contaminated food and water are two of the most common methods of transmitting disease to humans and animals, particularly in developing nations with poor sanitary systems and poor hygiene practices. Food handlers with poor hygiene habits, in developed or developing countries, contaminate food. Feces-contaminated water is another primary means of transmission. Some parts of the world still use human feces for fertilization, allowing fecal contamination of the water supply, transmitting bacterial and parasitic diseases to humans downstream who share and use the contaminated water for daily hygiene and food preparation.

Direct contact between people cannot be avoided in areas of overcrowding. Transmission also occurs in prisons, factories, businesses, and daycare centers. Disease transmission by direct contact often involves the fecal-oral route due to poor hygiene practices or lack of proper routine hand washing.

Arthropods transmit parasites mechanically or biologically. Arthropods act as a mechanical vector when the parasite is attached to the arthropod, such as on the outside of the body. The parasite can then rub off and be deposited onto the host or exposed food. Some arthropods defecate on the host following completion of their blood meal. The parasitic microbe is carried in the feces of the vector and when the host rubs its skin where the parasite has been deposited, the host unknowingly transfers the fecal material into the bite site, providing the parasite a percutaneous passageway to deeper tissues.

When the arthropod serves as a biological vector, it is an intermediate host. The parasite can then be injected into a human host through the bite of the arthropod vector. Two common parasitic protozoa transmitted in this manner are *Plasmodium*, the cause of malaria carried by the *Anopheles* mosquito, and *Trypanosoma*, the cause of African sleeping sickness carried by the tsetse fly. The *Anopheles* mosquito transmits *Plasmodium* into the bloodstream of the host, where it infects large numbers of erythrocytes or red blood cells (RBCs). The erythrocytes rupture and release toxic compounds.

Respiratory infections occur when parasitic eggs become airborne. The human host develops an infection when the eggs are inhaled. Trans-placental infection is uncommon, but pregnant females are warned to eliminate exposure to cat feces in litter boxes. The pregnant woman may inhale **oocysts** from cat feces or ingest them if deposited onto undercooked pork or beef that contains the cysts. The cysts are *Toxoplasma gondii*. The parasite has the ability to cross the placental barrier and infect the nervous system of the fetus, causing fetal demise (see Figure 10-13).

Malaria

Malaria is the most common parasitic infection in humans worldwide. The World Health Organization (WHO) estimates that 229 million cases of malaria occurred in 2019, and 409,000 people died from the parasitic infection. There are nearly 2,000 cases of malaria diagnosed in the United States annually, mostly in individuals who have traveled to areas

liberated into the blood stream, infected hosts manifest symptoms of high fever, chills, and shaking.

Mosquitoes of the *Anopheles* species are the vectors for transmission of the four major species of *Plasmodium* that infect humans: *P. falciparum*, *P. malariae*, *P. ovale*, and *P. vivax*. When the mosquito vector feeds from the infected host, the gametocytes rapidly produce gametes that mate within the mosquito. The resulting oocysts eventually rupture and release sporozoites into the salivary glands of the mosquito, awaiting the next blood meal and access to a new human host. The mosquito vector suffers no ill effects from the parasitic passengers.

Malaria infections can be categorized as uncomplicated or severe (complicated). Some infections produce few if any symptoms. As the symptoms of uncomplicated malaria are similar to those of influenza, infected individuals living in areas where malaria is rare or eradicated fail to identify the actual infective process. In the United States, those who have traveled to endemic countries in the previous 1 to 3 weeks should consider the possibility of malarial infection and seek medical care. Some of the species of *Plasmodium* may remain dormant in the human host's liver and cause relapses, even years after the first onset of symptoms.

In severe cases, when infected erythrocytes gain access to cerebral blood vessels, it causes a syndrome called cerebral malaria presenting with behavioral changes, seizures, or even coma. Cerebral malaria has a high mortality rate. Other clinical manifestations of severe malaria include acute respiratory distress syndrome (ARDS), severe hypoglycemia, hypotension with cardiovascular collapse, kidney failure, and metabolic acidosis (see Figure 10-14).

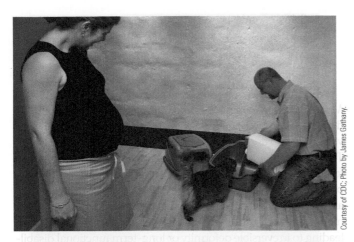

Figure 10-13 Pregnant women and immunocompromised individuals should avoid contact with cat litter and feces due to potential for exposure to *Toxoplasma gondii*, the etiologic agent responsible for the parasitic disease toxoplasmosis.

Courtesy of CDC; Photo by James Gathany.

with large rates of infection. Large-scale intervention and treatment programs have cut the death rate of malaria by 44 percent between 2010 and 2019. The disease is most prevalent in poor countries in the tropics or subtropics. Young children, pregnant women, the elderly, and the immunocompromised are at highest risk for severe infections.

Pathogenic *Plasmodium* species invade human liver cells and erythrocytes (red blood cells). As they reproduce, the cells rupture and the released daughter cells (merozoites) spread and infect other surrounding cells. Once these specialized male and female reproductive cells called gametocytes are

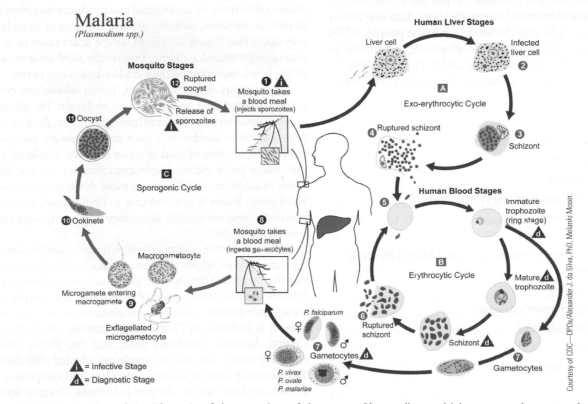

Figure 10-14 Illustration of the life cycle of the parasites of the genus *Plasmodium*, which are causal agents of malaria.

Courtesy of CDC—DPDx/Alexander J. da Silva, PhD, Melanie Moser.

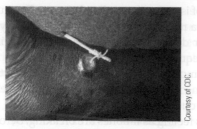

Figure 10-17 Close view of a patient's left ankle, shows method used to extract a guinea worm from one of the leg veins. Dracunculiasis, more commonly known as guinea worm disease, is a preventable infection caused by the parasite *Dracunculus medinensis*.

overs years. Alveolar echinococcosis (AE) disease is caused by infection with the larval stage of *Echinococcus multilocularis*, a smaller tapeworm found in foxes, coyotes, and dogs with small rodents as intermediate hosts. AE in animals in endemic areas are relatively common. AE cases in humans are rare but more severe than CE, causing parasitic tumors in the liver, lungs, brain, and other organs which can be fatal if untreated. AE is found globally and is prevalent in the northern parts of Europe, Asia, and North America. Treatment for both types of parasitic disease include a "wait-and-see" approach for asymptomatic small cysts in CE to radical surgery to remove the cystic lesions in AE. Intermediate treatment options include anti-parasitic medications and chemotherapy for extended periods.

Parasitic flukes of the species *Fasciola hepatica*, also called the common liver fluke or sheep liver fluke, and its cousin, *Fasciola gigantica*, are the cause of the disease called fascioliasis. The parasite is found in 2 million people living in more than 70 countries around the world with *F. hepatica* seen in all continents except Antarctica. The highest rates of infection are seen mainly in areas where sheep and other cattle graze including the highlands of Peru and Bolivia where the disease is considered hyperendemic. Water is contaminated with larvae that have matured in an aquatic snail that serves as an intermediate host. The mature larvae are then ingested by humans who eat raw watercress or other uncooked water plants. Transmission can also occur through consumption of undercooked sheep or goat liver. The larvae bore through the human intestinal wall into the abdominal cavity and into the liver or bile ducts where they become mature flukes and produce eggs. Cases of fascioliasis have been documented in the United States and Europe. The drug of choice is triclabendazole. The drug is given by mouth, usually in two doses.

Human African Trypanosomiasis, called a sleeping sickness, is a parasitic infection caused by *Trypanosoma brucei* that is found in different areas of the African continent. Three significant species named for the specific regions in which they were first identified (African from *T. brucei*, East African from *T. brucei rhodesiense*, and West African from *T. brucei gambiense*) are transmitted to humans through bites of infected tsetse flies of the *Glossina* species. In the first stage of the infective process, the parasite circulates in the blood of the human host, causing diffuse symptoms of fever, headache, and muscle and joint pains, and it may cause lymphatic inflammation near the bite site. In the second stage, it invades the central nervous system and produces neurologic symptoms such as personality changes, confusion, and sleepiness, and, left untreated, it can progress to partial paralysis and eventual coma and death. The East African disease progresses the most quickly; there is only a matter of months from bite to death. The West African strain takes more time, up to 6 or 7 years, with 3 years being the average time before death. In 2017–2018, fewer than 2,000 cases were reported to the WHO, down from the more than 10,000 cases per year for the 50 years prior to 2009. The recommended drug for first stage *T. b. gambiense* infection is pentamidine and is available by prescription in the United States. Other drugs for treatment of African trypanosomiasis are not commercially available in the United States, and must be obtained from the CDC. On average, approximately one person per year in the United States contracts the disease, usually after having visited Africa on sightseeing or safari trips.

Phlebotomine sand flies spread the disease leishmaniasis, which is caused by the parasites of the 20 species of the genus *Leishmania*. Found on every continent except Australia and Antarctica according to the CDC, Old World (defined as the Eastern hemisphere) leishmaniasis is found in parts of Asia, the Middle East, Africa (mainly in the tropical region and North Africa), and southern Europe. Infections referred to as New World leishmaniasis (defined as the Western hemisphere), are found in parts of Mexico, Central America, and South America, excluding Chile and Uruguay (see Figure 10-18).

There have been cases reported in the United States in Oklahoma and Texas. Cutaneous leishmaniasis affects 700,000 to 1.2 million people, resulting in skin lesions of varying severity, size, and location. Visceral leishmaniasis affects 100,000 to 400,000 and can cause life-threatening symptoms involving the liver, spleen, and bone marrow.

Leprosy, also known as Hansen's disease, is an infection caused by bacteria called *Mycobacterium leprae*. These bacteria

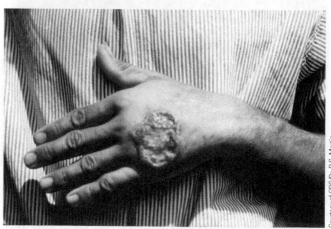

Figure 10-18 Central American adult with skin ulcer due to leishmaniasis.

grow very slowly, possibly taking up to 20 years to develop signs of the infection. Reported cases include approximately 150 people in the United States and 250,000 around the world. Leprosy has been present in the human population since ancient times and was feared as a highly contagious, devastating disease leaving affected individuals stigmatized, isolated, and shunned. Researchers have found that transmission does not easily occur and the *M. leprae* bacterial infection is easily treatable once recognized. *Mycobacterium leprae* is discussed further in Chapter 14.

The CDC estimates that 120 million people are currently infected with lymphatic **filariasis** and more than 1 billion are at risk throughout 73 countries. Mosquitoes are the vectors for transmitting the microscopic nematodes that cause lymphedema of the extremities, breasts, or testicles. *Wuchereria bancrofti*, *Brugia malayi*, and *Brugia timori* are the three species identified as causative parasite species that can live in the blood and lymph systems of human hosts for years. Mosquitoes acquire the parasites from the human host and transmit them to another host with its subsequent feedings. Most people will demonstrate no signs or symptoms of infection; however, some may have serious and debilitating swelling from decreased lymphatic drainage. Men may suffer painful and in some cases extreme **hydroceles** of the scrotum (see Figure 10-19). The skin of swollen extremities may harden, a condition called elephantiasis (see Figure 10-20).

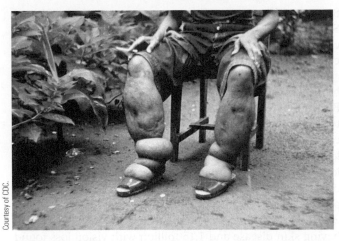

Figure 10-20 Elephantiasis of leg due to filariasis in Luzon, Philippines.

In some cultures, people with visible manifestations of filariasis are shunned and made outcasts. Diethylcarbamazine (DEC) has been used for years as treatment of lymphatic filariasis. It should not be given to patients with other filarial diseases such as onchocerciasis.

Mycetoma is a disease caused by bacteria and fungi found in soil and water that enter the body through a break in the skin. Signs of infection are firm, painless, debilitating subcutaneous masses that eventually invade underlying bone (see Figure 10-21). Mycetoma can be caused by actinobacteria such as *Nocardia brasiliensis* or fungal species. Researchers have documented 17,607 cases between 1950 and 2017 although the actual number of cases is likely much higher. Mycetoma affects poorer people of all ages in rural, dry climate, equatorial regions of Africa, Latin America, and Asia who have limited access to healthcare. Fewer than

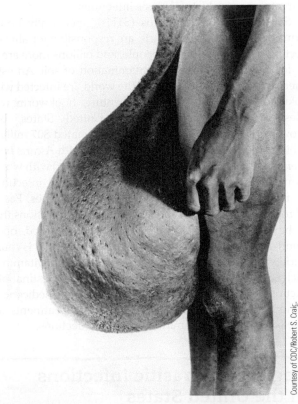

Figure 10-19 Patient presented with massive edema of the penis and scrotum, which had been due to a filarial infection caused by an invasive nematode worm of the superfamily, *Filarioidea*.

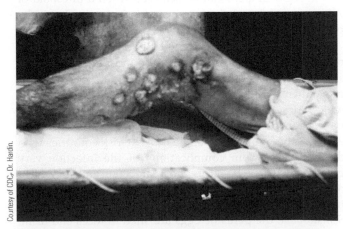

Figure 10-21 Right leg of patient with numerous cutaneous lesions of a disease process known as actinomycosis, or mycetoma, a slowly progressive, destructive infection of the cutaneous and subcutaneous tissues, fascia, and can progress to a point where it can affect bone as well, caused by the Gram-positive, fungus-like aerobic bacteria of the order *Actinomycetales*.

80 cases of mycetoma have been reported in the United States between 1890 and 2020 and travelers to affected areas are unlikely to get mycetoma. *Actinobacteria* are discussed further in Chapter 14.

Onchocerciasis, also known as river blindness, is caused by the larvae of microfilarial worms, *Onchocerca volvulus*. Black flies are the vectors for transmission from human host to human host. The microscopic worms embed in the skin, causing intense itching and skin lesions called lizard or leopard skin. If the worms migrate in blood to the eyes, then loss of vision called river blindness occurs. Multiple bites over extended periods of time are typically required to cause physical signs of infection. In 2017 there were at least 20.9 million people infected worldwide with 14.6 million having skin disease and 1.15 million with vision loss found primarily in 31 sub-Saharan African countries. Infections are also found in a few areas of South America and Yemen in the Middle East. Four countries in Central America have been verified by the WHO as free from onchocerciasis: Colombia, Ecuador, Mexico, and Guatemala. Insecticides are effective in killing the populations of black fly vectors. Medications are available for treatment and a yearly vaccine can prevent infection.

Rabies is a preventable viral disease most often transmitted through the bite of a rabid animal. Each year, rabies causes approximately 59,000 deaths worldwide. The rabies virus infects the central nervous system of mammals, ultimately causing brain dysfunction and death. Most reported rabies cases occur in wild animals including bats, raccoons, skunks, and foxes; however, any mammal can get rabies with dog rabies remaining common in many countries without widespread vaccination programs. Exposure to rabid dogs causes over 90 percent of human rabies infections and 99 percent of human rabies deaths. Medical care after potential exposure and before symptoms is critical. Control of rabies in regional areas can be achieved when a threshold of 70 percent of dogs being vaccinated is maintained, thereby preventing human deaths.

Schistosomiasis, also called Bilharzia or snail fever, ranks second only to malaria as the most common parasitic disease. An estimated 236.6 million people required preventive treatment for schistosomiasis in 2019, out of which more than 105.4 million people were reported to have been treated. Estimates published by the WHO in 2019 for the number of people in 74 at-risk countries who die each year from complications of the infection vary greatly (24,000–200,000 in the year 2000) and may have decreased due to prevention campaigns and enhanced treatment regimens. Caused by various species of *Schistosoma*, the parasitic eggs are shed in feces and urine of infected humans into freshwater areas where certain types of snails live and become infected with the parasite. Inside the snails, the parasites mature, reproduce, and leave the snails, contaminating the water. The mature parasitic worms floating in the freshwater penetrate the skin of humans who enter the water. Once inside, the worms

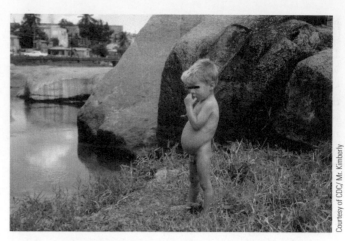

Courtesy of CDC/ Mr. Kimberly

Figure 10-22 Young Puerto Rican boy with distended belly due to the human pathogenic parasite of the genus, *Schistosoma*, causing the disease schistosomiasis, also known as bilharzia.

take up residence in the host's blood vessels and tissues (see Figure 10-22). While the worms themselves do not cause symptoms, the host's immune responses cause inflammation to try to fight the foreign invaders. If the eggs produced by the parasites cannot be passed from the gastrointestinal or genitourinary tracts, they may cause blockage and scarring. Praziquantel is the medication prescribed for treatment of schistosomiasis infections.

Soil-transmitted helminths (STHs), specifically hookworms, whipworms, and ascaris, are responsible for already infecting more than 1 billion people, and billions more are at risk for exposure from fecal contamination of soil. An estimated 576–740 million people in the world are infected with hookworm. Until the early 20th century, hookworm was widespread in the south-eastern United States, but is now nearly eliminated. Globally, an estimated 807 million 1.2 billion people in the world are infected with *Ascaris lumbricoides* and 604–795 million people are infected with whipworm. Better sanitation practices have reduced infections that now are mainly found in developing countries. Fecal-oral routes of transmission are responsible for infections that can be a result of poor hygiene, undercooked food, open wounds, or unwashed fruits and vegetables. The STHs cause a variety of clinical signs, including malnutrition, vitamin A deficiency, delayed development, anemia, and intestinal obstructions or prolapse (see Figure 10-23). The medications albendazole and mebendazole are effective treatments for these parasitic soil-transmitted helminth infections.

Neglected Parasitic Infections in the United States

Parasitic diseases are rampant around the world and are often most prevalent in developing countries. The population

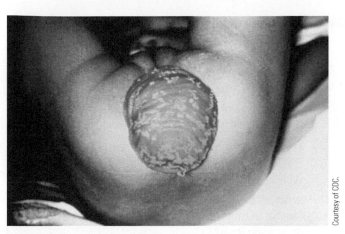

Figure 10-23 Rectal prolapse in a female child due to a parasitic *Trichuris trichiura* infestation. The rectum has lost its intestinal support due to this nematode invasion and protruded from the anal opening. Note the numbers of worms atop the rectal mucosal lining.

of the United States may not be affected by many of these infections; however, we are not immune to certain parasites and healthcare providers must be aware and not rule out possible relatively uncommon causes in patients who present for treatment. The CDC has identified what it calls neglected parasitic infections in the United States. These are:

- Chagas disease: see previous section on neglected tropical diseases.
- Cyclosporiasis: parasitic infection caused by single-celled *Cyclospora cayetanensis*. Foodborne outbreaks of cyclosporiasis in the U.S. have been linked to various types of imported fresh produce. Intestinal infection symptoms include diarrhea, loss of appetite, weight loss, stomach cramps/pain, gas or bloating, nausea, and fatigue. Other flu-like symptoms of vomiting, body aches, headache, and fever may also occur. Diagnosis is made with stool sample and fluids and antibiotics are given for treatment.
- Cysticercosis: see previous section on neglected tropical diseases.
- Toxocariasis: also known as roundworm disease; caused by *Toxocara canis* in dogs and less commonly by *Toxocara cati* from cats. Ingestion of larvae shed in feces of dogs and cats either in soil or in undercooked meat is the route of transmission. Once in the body, larvae circulate in blood and can develop into symptoms of fever, cough, inflammation of the liver, or eye problems. Toxoplasmosis: caused by the protozoan *Toxoplasma gondii*. In the United States, nearly 11 percent of people older than age 6 have been exposed to the parasite. It is believed that worldwide, up to 60 percent of the human population has been infected. It is one of the most common food-borne parasitic infections from eating undercooked meat (pork, lamb, venison) or inadequate cleaning of food preparation surfaces and utensils. Pregnant women can transmit the parasite to their fetuses with potentially devastating neurological or ophthalmological consequences. Pregnant women are advised not to handle cat litter box contents to prevent the possibility of fecal-oral transmission of shed larvae. Less commonly, parasitic infection can occur through transplanted organs or blood products or to laboratory personnel.

- Trichomoniasis: also referred to as "trich," caused by the parasitic protozoan *Trichomonas vaginalis*. It is the only flagellate that is a parasite of the urogenital system. Motility is achieved by four flagella and an undulating membrane that begins at the anterior end of the organism and extends approximately halfway up the cell. The cell displays a jerky motion. The anterior end of the cell is rounded and the posterior end tapers to a point. *Trichomonas vaginalis* does not form cysts and only lives as a trophozoite. It is a common, curable sexually transmitted disease. In 2018 in the United States, an estimated 2.6 million people were infected. Typically, only one in three develop symptoms. Trichomoniasis can increase the risk of getting or spreading HIV. Pregnant women are at risk for pre-term labor or low-birth-weight fetuses. Re-infection is possible without treatment of all infected sexual partners. Oral antibiotic treatment is effective in treating infection.

MICRO NOTES

"You're Bugging Me!"

A number of scientists have proposed that Charles Darwin may have suffered for years with Chagas disease. Darwin, the scientist who first proposed the theory of evolution, traveled extensively in the mid-1800s to South America, the Galapagos Islands, and Africa over the course of 5 years. He kept records of his travels and research and documented insect bites he suffered along the way. Although he died in 1882 at the age 73 of a heart attack, the list of symptoms that plagued him after his voyage and until his death bear strong resemblance to Chagas, which is caused by the parasitic protozoan *Trypanosoma cruzi*. *T. cruzi* is known to be carried by a number of insect species found in South America.

Under the Microscope

Darius, a CST working in Labor and Delivery, finished setting up for a Cesarean section delivery and went to help the circulating nurse bring the patient back to the OR. The young female patient was tearful because she was told the parasite she had been infected with may have also infected her fetus, causing it to be 8 weeks premature. The patient had traveled to Central America early in the pregnancy and her spouse was deployed overseas and she had not had any help with house cleaning and pet care chores.

1. Which parasites could cause premature birth or congenital disease?

2. By which type of vector and transmission route could the patient have been infected?

3. What might the significance of foreign travels and home pet-care circumstances represent?

4. What could the impact be for the neonate as it develops?

5. What are survival mechanisms used by parasites capable of causing impact to a pregnant female or the developing fetus?

CHAPTER 11

Mycology

Learning Objectives

After completing the study of this chapter, you will be able to:

1. Define key terms.
2. Compare and contrast the different forms of fungal organisms.
3. Describe routes of transmission in fungal disease.
4. Discuss the ways fungal species can be beneficial to humans.
5. Describe the infections in humans caused by yeasts.
6. Apply critical thinking skills in relating chapter material to the surgical environment of care or broader global community.

Key Terms

Annelides	Chlamydoconidia	Leavening	Septate
Arthroconidia	Chlorophyll	Mycelium	Sinonasal
Aseptate	Conidia	Onychomycosis	Sporangiospores
Bioremediation	Conidiophores	Phialide	Sterols
Blastoconidium	Hallucinations	Rheumatism	Zygospores
Candidemia	Hyphae	Rhinocerebral	

The Big Picture

Fungi are fascinating microbes that seem to enjoy masquerading as plants. The majority of infections they cause are in individuals who are immunocompromised and unable to defend against pathogens. In some cases, opportunistic fungi find ways to cause infection in healthy persons as well.

During your examination of the topics in this chapter, consider the following:

1. Which infections are potentially life-threatening to those without adequate immune defenses?

2. Which opportunistic fungal organisms are potential pathogens in healthy individuals who share public spaces?

3. In which ways can some common forms of fungi be beneficial to humans?

4. What type of pathogenic mutation has made treating fungal infections more difficult?

Clinical Significance Topic

Patients may develop healthcare-associated fungal or yeast infections. Healthcare workers may carry fungal infections under fingernails from use of artificial nails, tips, or wraps. For that reason, these cosmetic devices are prohibited for surgical technologists who will be scrubbing and donning sterile surgical attire. Nurses working with neonates or other critically ill patients should also refrain from wearing artificial nails after documentation of infections transmitted from caregivers to patients. Various types of prokaryotic bacteria may appear along with eukaryotic microbial pathogens, so prevention of contamination by either source is imperative.

Overview of Mycology

Mycology is the study of fungi. These microorganisms, which can also be considered macro-organisms, are multicellular eukaryotes that are listed as fungi and include yeasts, mushrooms, and molds. Fungi are important in nature and the human food industry. Scientists theorize that there are actually more than a million species of fungi on earth. These incredibly diverse microbes are thought to have originated approximately 900 million years ago on land, although they adapted to life in salt and freshwater environments as well. They are more prevalent in hot or warm climates such as the tropics but have been found in much colder parts of the planet. Researchers estimate that approximately 85 percent

of plants form symbiotic relationships with fungi. Very few (400 or so) of the 100,000 plus identified species of fungi are human pathogens.

Fungi are heterotrophs that release enzymes to break down organic matter into absorbable forms. They do not require sunlight and are often found and grow best in dark areas. They are consumers of dead and decaying organic matter and expert recyclers of carbon and nitrogen. Most species of fungi are aerobic; however, yeasts perform an anaerobic process called fermentation that is used by humans to make wine and beer and makes yeast breads rise.

Penicillin, the first antibiotic discovered, was produced from a mold called *Penicillium notatum*. Penicillin G, now a commonly used antibiotic, is produced from the blue-green fungal mold strains of the *Penicillium* species including both the original *P. notatum* and *P. chrysogenum* (see Figure 11-1). A type of yeast used for thousands of

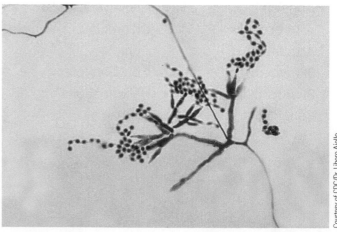

Figure 11-1 This micrograph depicts multiple conidia-laden conidiophores and phialides of a *Penicillium marneffei* fungal organism.

years, *Saccharomyces cerevisiae*, also known as brewer's or baker's yeast, is one of the most studied eukaryotic microbes. The first written historical accounts of fermentation of alcohol dates back 6,000 years in Mesopotamia. Egyptian records depict the use of yeast in the **leavening** of bread as far back as 5,000 years ago.

Mushrooms are fungi that grow well in dark areas or underground. They are often mistaken as plants because of the appearance of their cell structure; however, with no **chlorophyll**, they are unable to produce their own energy from light the way plant cells do. Mushrooms are important staples of many cultural diets; however, numerous varieties produce toxins capable of causing **hallucinations** or even fatal reactions. Certain species of mushrooms have been studied and used for their **bioremediation** properties of absorbing contaminants from soil, including septic tank contents, radioactive waste, and oil spills. They also show potential promise as insecticides and cancer treatments.

Fungal Pathogens

Fungal diseases are called mycoses (singular, mycosis). The mycoses are classified according to the tissue of the human body that is affected (see Table 11-1).

Most fungal infections are superficial and not life-threatening. Individuals who are immunocompromised, such as those with HIV/AIDS, organ recipients, or those undergoing cancer treatment, are at the highest risk for opportunistic infections that change from minor, superficial irritations to serious, deep tissue or systemic infestations (see Figure 11-2). The primary reservoirs of fungi are organic soil and animals. Either the hosts contact the fungi while outside and inhale spores or the spores enter through a wound in the skin. Humans are also reservoirs of certain opportunistic yeasts.

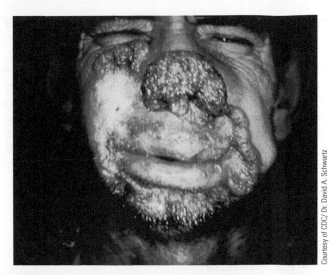

Figure 11-2 Face of a patient with nodular lesions caused by a blastomycosis fungal infection caused by *Blastomyces dermatitidis*.

Courtesy of CDC/ Dr. David A. Schwartz

Characteristics of Fungi

The cell membrane of a fungus is composed of lipids called **sterols**. As mentioned previously, compared to plants, the cell walls of fungi are composed of polysaccharides but do not contain chlorophyll. Fungi are either unicellular, such as yeasts, or multicellular, such as molds.

Molds are made up of long filaments called **hyphae**. The hyphae are either **aseptate** or septate. **Septate** hyphae are divided into sections or separate cells by walls called septa (singular: septum). Hyphae that do not have septa are aseptate and the cytoplasm is not divided into individual cells. The hyphae grow by branching out and growing longer to form a mass of hyphae called **mycelium**.

Yeasts have round cells. Yeasts reproduce by budding, whereby a protuberance called a **blastoconidium** is created by the parent cell (see Figure 11-3). Some yeast species

Table 11-1 Common Fungal Diseases and Causative Agents

Fungi	Disease/Condition
Tinea species	Dermatomycosis (ringworm skin infection)
Candida	Candidiasis, vaginal infections, thrush (white throat)
Histoplasma capsulatum	Histoplasmosis chronic lung infection
Aspergillus	Systemic infections in immunocompromised patients

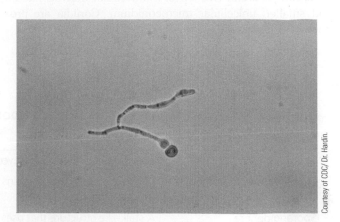

Figure 11-3 Ultrastructural morphology of the fungus, *Candida albicans* showing a germ tube formation and outgrowth of the *C. Albicans* spore can be seen with the budding yeast cell.

Courtesy of CDC/ Dr. Hardin.

produce buds that grow longer and are similar to the hyphae of molds called pseudohyphae (false hyphae).

The morphology of fungi is not fixed because some species are dimorphic which means that a few fungi live either as a mold or as a yeast, depending on the growth conditions. When the fungi grow in tissue at body temperature, they are seen as unicellular yeast. When grown at room temperature or when specimens are taken from the soil or dust, they grow in the saprophytic form as a mold with hyphae and spores. Dimorphic fungi include the following species:

- *Histoplasma capsulatum*
- *Blastomyces dermatitidis*
- *Coccidioides immitis*
- *Paracoccidioides brasiliensis*
- *Candida albicans*

Reproductive Methods

Fungi reproduce either sexually or asexually by producing spores. A true spore is formed by either asexual cleavage or sexual meiosis. However, species of fungi can only produce one kind of sexual spore.

Asexual Reproduction

There are two types of asexual spores: sporangiospore and conidiospore. These spores are important for identification and classification in the laboratory. Sporangiospores are true spores formed by cleavage from a sporangium (plural, sporangia). The sporangium is supported by branches that are specialized hyphae structures called sporangiophores (see Table 11-2). Sporangiospores are produced only by the class of fungi called *Zygomycetes*. *Chlamydospores* are asexual spores with thick walls formed by rounding and enlargement within a hyphal segment. *Candida albicans* produces chlamydospores (see Figure 11-4).

Conidia (singular, conidium) are produced by most of the fungi. Conidia are not true spores because they are not formed by conjugation or cleavage. Conidia produced by the same fungus are of two types: multicellular macroconidium and smaller, unicellular microconidium. Conidia are produced in the following ways:

- Directly from the hyphae

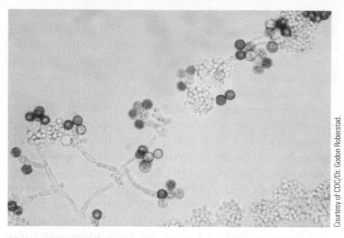
Courtesy of CDC/Dr. Godon Roberstad.

Figure 11-4 Image of chlamydospores, the reproductive, thick-walled structures of the fungus *Candida albicans*.

- Directly from yeast cells
- By specialized cells called **conidiophores**

Conidiophores are small branches that support the conidia. Other supporting structures include the following:

1. **Annelides:** a cell that produces conidia by growing longer, ending in a tapered tip
2. **Arthroconidia:** square-like conidia formed by a modified hyphal cell
3. **Chlamydoconidia:** round, large conidia with a thick wall formed at the end, sides, or inside the hyphae
4. **Phialide:** a cell that produces conidia but does not grow longer as the conidia are formed and released

See Table 11-3 for representative asexual conidiospores.

Sexual Reproduction

Most fungi asexually reproduce, but sexual spores can be produced. The production of sexual spores requires the mating of two different strains of the fungus. This is rarely seen in the laboratory; however, some fungi will produce sexual spores in culture. There are three types of sexual spores: ascospores, basidiospores, and zygospores.

Table 11-2 Structures Associated with Sporangiospore Production

Structure	Description
Sporangiospore	Asexual spore of the zygomycete produced by cleavage from a sporangium
Sporangium (pl. sporangia)	Saclike structure that contains sporangiospores, from which they are produced by cleavage from the membrane
Sporangiophore	A stalk-like structure that rises from the hyphae and from which the sporangium arises by swelling at the tip
Columella	A swollen portion of the sporangiophore that extends into the sporangium

Table 11-3   **Commonly Observed Conidia**

Type of Spore	How Formed	Diagram
Arthroconidium	Modification of hyphal cell	
Blastoconidium	A bud coming off a parent cell	
Chlamydoconidium	Round, thick-walled, structures formed at the end, sides, or within the strand of a hypha or pseudohypha	
Macroconidium	The larger of two conidia, formed by the same fungus, generally multicellular	
Microconidium	Smaller of two conidia formed by the same fungus, generally unicellular	

Classification

The type of spore produced is used for the classification of fungi. Table 11-4 lists the four phyla and classes with characteristics.

Zygomycetes species produce the sexual **zygospores**; however, this has never been observed in laboratory specimens. *Zygomycetes* organisms are identified by two characteristics that are not seen in other fungi:

- Form asexual **sporangiospores**
- Produce aseptate hyphae

Treatment

Anyone can acquire a fungal infection. Superficial infections of cuticle nail beds, the soles of feet (athlete's foot), and vaginal yeast infections can affect healthy individuals and can be effectively treated with anti-fungal medications. Systemic fungal infections are much more serious and may present unique challenges, especially if they have developed anti-fungal resistance.

Treatment of systemic fungal diseases has been difficult due to the limited number of drugs available. The problem with anti-fungal agents is their high level of toxicity in humans. Fungal cells are similar to human cells; therefore, the drugs that affect fungi also affect human cells, causing severe toxic reactions. Newer anti-fungal agents such as fluconazole and others in the azole class are relatively effective, but the patient must still be monitored for toxic reactions. Their mechanisms of action range from altering the fungal cell membrane to interfering with lipid membrane synthesis.

Opportunistic Fungal Infections

Fungal microbes, pathogenic and non-pathogenic, exist everywhere that other microbes do. Most individuals suffer no

Table 11-4   **Fungal Phyla and Classes**

Phylum	Class	Asexual Spore	Sexual Spore	Type of Hyphae
Zygomycota	Zygomycetes	Sporangiospore	Zygospore	Aseptate
Ascomycota	Ascomycetes	Conidium	Ascospore	Septate
Basidiomycota	Basidiomycetes	Conidium	Basidiospore	Septate
Deuteromycota (fungi imperfecti): produce no sexual spore	—	Conidium	None	Septate

effects of that exposure; however, those most likely to show signs and symptoms are those who are immunocompromised due to corticosteroid treatment, chemotherapy regimens, HIV/AIDS, diabetes, chronic antibiotic therapy, or any process that leaves them vulnerable to opportunistic infections.

Opportunistic fungal infections are relatively common in HIV/AIDS patients and the number of reported fungal infections has increased. Immunosuppressive and corticosteroid drugs depress the T-cell immune system.

Patients who have undergone organ transplant surgery are given immunosuppressive drug therapy preoperatively and postoperatively, elevating their risk for developing a fungal infection. Malignancies, particularly leukemia and lymphoma, form cells that destroy the lymph nodes and bone marrow, where T-cells are normally produced.

Antibiotics are a factor in the development of fungal infections, particularly yeast infections, when the yeast is part of the normal microbiome (flora) of the body. The yeast is present in low numbers, and their numbers are kept from increasing by the bacteria that are also part of the normal microbiome. When antibiotics are administered to treat an infection, they can have the adverse effect of lowering the normal bacterial count, allowing the fungi not affected by the antibiotic to multiply in number. As the antibiotic therapy is discontinued, the fungi should be brought under control and into balance by the rebound of the resident bacteria.

Many opportunistic fungi are saprophytes in nature. These fungi are not dimorphic, meaning they exhibit no change in morphology between the saprophytic and parasitic form. Fungi are molds in nature but change to the hyphal form when they cause an infection. Yeast remains in yeast form when it is responsible for an infection.

Aspergillosis

Aspergillosis is a term that refers to a number of infections caused by species in the genus *Aspergillus*. There are several species in the genus, but the most common opportunistic species that have been encountered in infections are *A. flavus*, *A. fumigatus*, and *A. niger*. *Aspergillus* is a mold that produces septate hyphae. It is frequently seen as a bread mold and as a contaminant in air conditioning units. It is not part of the normal microbiome of humans.

In the laboratory, *Aspergillus* produces conidiophores from hyphae. The conidiophores develop a swollen end called a vesicle. Phialides are produced by the vesicles and **conidia** are then produced from the phialides (see Figure 11-5).

Infections by *Aspergillus* occur most commonly in the respiratory tract as airborne conidia are inhaled through the nose into the lungs. Following inhalation, a severe bronchial infection might occur and, in the immunocompromised patient, most likely develop into pneumonia. Pneumonia infections from *Aspergillus* are severe, characterized by the destruction of lung tissue and necrosis. Tissue biopsies reveal a large number of hyphae growing within the necrotic lung tissue.

Aspergillus has an affinity for blood vessels, with serious consequences. Upon invasion, the organism obstructs the

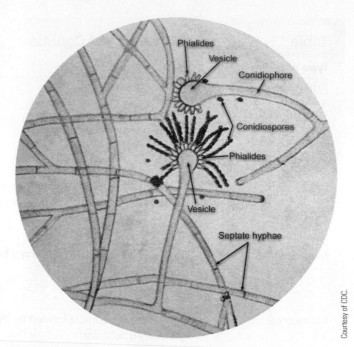

Figure 11-5 This illustration depicts the ultrastructural details found in the common mold *Aspergillus*, including the organism's septate hyphae, conidiophores, which support the apparatus responsible for the development of the organism's asexual conidiospores (i.e., vesicle and phialides).

blood flow. The decrease in blood flow to tissue and organs can cause ischemic damage and necrosis, which can also lead to diminished organ function. Entry into the vascular system also allows the organism to spread to other regions of the body, causing systemic infection.

Conidia can become established in the nasal passages and sinuses, causing a **sinonasal** infection. At few instances, the organism will destroy the nasal sinus bones and bone segments at the base of the cranium, allowing access by the organism into the brain. Infection of the brain can also occur due to intravascular dissemination of the organism. The brain infections can lead to abscesses or meningitis. Disseminated infections frequently affect the liver, heart, and kidney. These infections are very difficult to treat and have a high mortality rate.

Aspergilloma is a complication that is the result of colonization of an existing cavity in the lung by *Aspergillus*. For example, a patient may have cavities that healed from a tuberculosis infection. The patient inhales *Aspergillus* spores that become lodged in the cavity. The spores develop into hyphae that grow into a large mass referred to as a fungus ball, or aspergilloma (see Figure 11-6). The mass of hyphae do not invade the lung tissue but can cause bleeding.

Direct laboratory examination of clinical specimens is important in the diagnosis of aspergillosis. The observance of hyphae in the clinical specimen confirms that the organism is *Aspergillus*. Specimens can be examined by wet preparations or stained specimens.

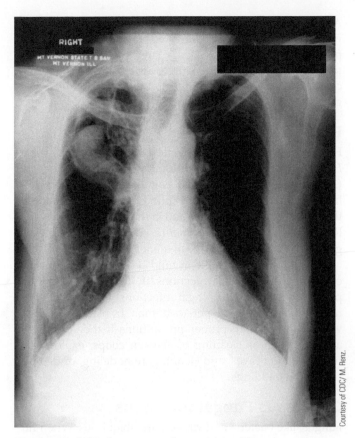

Courtesy of CDC/ M. Renz.

Figure 11-6 AP chest x-ray of a patient with pulmonary histoplasmosis. Note the presence of a radiolucency in the patient's right upper lobe, which was diagnosed as a probable aspergilloma or fungus ball.

Mucormycosis

Mucormycosis is an uncommon infection caused by a group of fungi called *Mucoromycotina*, previously called *Zygomycota*. These fungi are typically found in the soil and in association with decaying organic matter, compost piles, or rotting wood. The organism grows rapidly, producing thick colonies.

Rhizopus arrhizus is the most commonly identified pathogen in mucormycosis infections. Less frequent causes of infection include *Lichtheimia (Absidia) corymbifera*, *Apophysomyces elegans*, *Cunninghamella bertholletiae*, *Rhizomucor pusillus*, and *Saksenaea vasiformis*. All cause similar diseases in humans, including infections of the lungs, sinuses, eyes, and face, and rarely in the central nervous system. The diagnostic and treatment approaches for all of the fungal strains are similar.

There are no vaccines for fungal infections. Inhalation of spores is the most common mechanism of infection; however, mucormycosis cannot be transmitted from person to person. Preventing direct exposure to the pathogenic reservoirs (rotting or decayed wood and leaf piles) by wearing face masks, protective clothing, and gloves is advised.

Healthy individuals rarely develop mucormycosis. Those individuals affected typically have risk factors including cancer, transplanted organs, uncontrolled or poorly controlled diabetes mellitus, neutropenia (low white blood cell count), or significant skin trauma. In infections of diabetes mellitus patients, the blood sugar level is not the contributing factor to development of the infection, but rather ketoacidosis (accumulation of ketone bodies in the blood, resulting in metabolic acidosis) is a risk factor for developing mucormycosis.

Pulmonary mucormycosis occurs more often in patients with blood cancers or severe neutropenia, or in those who have been on prolonged steroid treatment. The symptoms include fever, cough, chest pain, and dyspnea (shortness of breath). Pathogenic access to the blood vessels of the pulmonary system (angioinvasion) results in tissue necrosis and possible cavitation (formation of empty spaces) with hemoptysis (coughing up blood).

Rhinocerebral mucormycosis is commonly seen in cancer patients with neutropenia, hematopoietic stem cell transplant (HSCT) recipients, and patients with diabetic ketoacidosis. Symptoms may include unilateral (one-sided) facial swelling, fever, headaches, sinus congestion or pain, and serosanguinous (bloody) nasal discharge. If the infection is left untreated and spreads, ptosis (drooping eyelid), proptosis (eye dislocation), loss of extraocular muscle function, and vision disturbance may occur with drainage of black pus from the eyes. Black lesions of necrotic tissue may appear on the hard palate of the mouth or in the nasal cavities (see Figure 11-7).

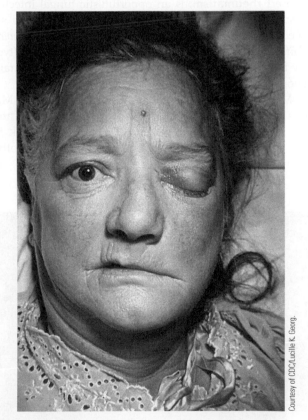

Courtesy of CDC/Lucille K. Georg.

Figure 11-7 This patient presented with a rhinocerebral zygomycotic infection of her face due to *Rhizopus arrhizus* fungal organisms. Note the left eye proptosis with accompanying ptosis of the upper lid and generalized swelling and erythema.

Primary skin (cutaneous) infection results in acute inflammation with pus and abscess formation, leading to necrosis (tissue death). Secondary cutaneous infection may occur if the pathogen spreads into the blood (hematogenously disseminated infection). The lesions begin as reddened (erythematous), hardened, and painful cellulitis patches that become blackened ulcers.

Gastrointestinal mucormycosis is a rare infection seen in severely malnourished individuals and transplant recipients. The fungal spores are thought to be ingested, and the most commonly affected organs are the stomach, colon, and ileum.

Disseminated mucormycosis infections may become secondary to any of the infections described; however, they are most likely to occur in patients with pulmonary infections and neutropenia. The most common site of secondary infection is the brain; however, secondary necrotic lesions have also been found in the spleen, heart, and other organs. Clinical signs in patients with brain involvement include lethargy and changes in mental status.

Coccidioidomycosis

Species of the fungus *Coccidioides* are found in the soil of dry, arid regions of the southwest United States, Mexico, and Central and South America (see Figure 11-8). Coccidioidomycosis, also called valley fever, San Joaquin Valley fever, or desert **rheumatism**, is an opportunistic fungal infection transmitted by inhalation of microscopic spores from soil kicked up by blowing winds and dust storms. *Coccidioides immitis* (found in California) and *Coccidioides posadasii* (typically found outside of California) are the recognized strains responsible for coccidioidomycosis infections.

Most individuals show no signs of clinical disease. Mild cases cause symptoms similar to influenza infections. Those with weakened immune systems are at elevated risk for more serious clinical signs and symptoms similar to other systemic fungal infections. Pregnant women, Filipinos, and African-Americans have statistically elevated risk factors as well. Initial exposure typically gives relative immunity from further infection and relapses are uncommon. Person-to-person transmission is only possible in extremely rare cases of exposure to open, infected wounds or infected organs transplanted to a new host.

Histoplasmosis

Histoplasmosis, a fungal infection caused by the species *Histoplasma capsulatum*, is found in the soil around the world (Africa, Asia, Australia, and Central and South America); however, it is most commonly found in the United States in the central and eastern states and in the Ohio and Mississippi River valleys. Soil environments contaminated with bat guano and bird droppings have higher levels of *Histoplasma*.

Symptoms are flu-like in mild cases and are similar to other systemic fungal infections if disseminated. House pets are susceptible to fungal infections; however, there is no recognized risk of pet-to-human transmission. Individuals should take proper precautions if they engage in activities such as cleaning of chicken coops, exploring of bat-populated caves, and cleaning, remodeling, or demolition of old buildings.

Cutaneous Fungal Infections

Fungus, like bacteria and viruses, are ubiquitous. When humans have weakened immune responses, systemic fungal infections from opportunistic pathogens can occur. Breaks in the skin surfaces of even healthy individuals provide access points for various strains of fungi, including yeasts and molds, which result in potentially chronic irritation and rashes (see Figure 11-9). Anti-fungal medications may be effective in treating these common outbreaks; however, awareness of exposure potential and use of protective clothing and gloves or avoidance of contaminated areas may prevent transmission.

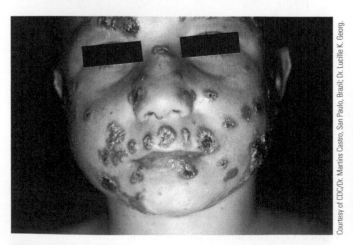

Figure 11-8 Brazilian child's face displaying the mycotic infection paracoccidioidomycosis. Also known as "Brazilian blastomycosis," this disease is caused by the fungus *Paracoccidioides brasiliensis*.

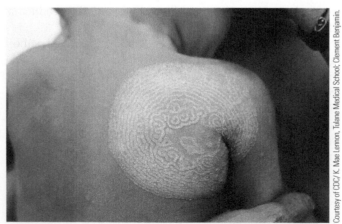

Figure 11-9 A child in New Guinea, with early cutaneous manifestations of tinea imbricata, also known as tokelau, involves the superficial layers of skin and caused by the fungal organism, *Trichophyton concentricum*, cultured from samples taken from this lesion.

Fungal Nail Infections

Onychomycosis, also known as tinea unguium, is the term for common fungal infections of the fingernails or toenails that can cause the nail to become discolored, thick, and more likely to crack and break. Infections are more common in toenails than in fingernails and are rarely painful unless severe and deforming (see Figure 11-10).

Fungal nail infections are often chronic conditions, lasting months to years. They are difficult to cure and may require prescription anti-fungal pills taken by mouth. In severe cases, the infected nail may require complete excision. Preventative measures include the following:

- Keep nails clean, dry, and relatively short
- Do not share nail clippers/scissors with others
- Do not walk barefoot in public showers or locker rooms
- Insist on properly trained, licensed nail salon personnel and sterilized instruments or bring your own
- Avoid wearing artificial nails or wraps
- Do not bite or chew nails, hangnails, or cuticles

Dermatophytosis

Fungal infections of the skin (cutaneous) layers are clinically known as tinea or dermatophytosis. Forty different species from the *Trichophyton*, *Microsporum*, and *Epidermophyton* genera are responsible for a wide variety of fungal skin infections (see Figure 11-11). These infections, also commonly called "ringworm," can affect different anatomical regions:

- Feet—tinea pedis, also commonly known as "athlete's foot"
- Scalp—tinea capitis
- Groin or inner thighs—tinea cruris, also known as "jock itch"
- Beard area of face—tinea barbae
- Hands—tinea manuum
- Extremities and other body parts—tinea corporis

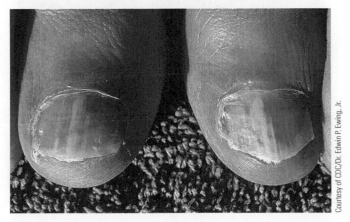

Figure 11-10 Onychomycosis due to *Trichophyton rubrum* on right and left great toe.

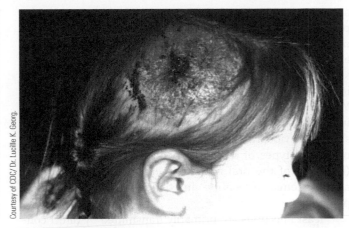

Figure 11-11 A patient's scalp with an erythematous, crusty, infected lesion known commonly as a kerion, ringworm, or tinea capitis caused by the dermatophytic fungal organism *Trichophyton verrucosum*.

Modes of transmission of dermatophytosis include person-to-person, animal-to-human, and contaminated public environmental surfaces. People are advised to not share clothing, bedding, or personal hygiene products with someone with known fungal infections.

Pets (cats and dogs) as well as pigs, horses, sheep, goats, and cows can acquire cutaneous fungal infections and pass them to humans. Infected areas in these animals may have loss of hair and reddened, circular or irregular, scaly patches. The lesions may or may not cause itching. Infected animals should be taken for veterinary care.

Tinea pedis and tinea cruris can be effectively treated with over-the-counter creams, powders, or ointments. Tinea capitis requires oral prescription anti-fungal medication for treatment, which may take up to 3 months. Topical preparations are ineffective with scalp infections.

Characteristics of Yeasts

In the past, the two yeast species that have been of pathogenic significance were *Candida albicans* and *Cryptococcus neoformans*. However, as with fungi, all species of yeast are now considered opportunistic pathogens that can cause life-threatening infections in immunocompromised patients. The spectrum of infections ranges from superficial infections to systemic life-threatening infections. In the laboratory, the identification of the various species now depends on knowledge of the morphology, culture, and biochemical aspects of the organism.

Yeasts are unicellular and reproduce asexually by the process called blastoconidia formation (budding) or fission. They are classified as *Ascomycetes* or *Deuteromycetes*. Yeasts are found worldwide and some species are part of the normal microbiome of the body. They are found in soil and water and on the skins of many vegetables and fruits. Yeasts are important in the food industry because they are responsible for the fermentation processes in the production of alcohol products and breads. *Saccharomyces cerevisiae*, under anaerobic conditions, ferments sugar to alcohol. Under aerobic conditions, this yeast breaks down simple sugars into carbon dioxide and water, so it is important in the fermentation process of bread making. Yeasts are also a source of nutrition to humans by providing many types of vitamins and proteins. However, as stated previously, some species of yeast are the cause of several types of diseases, including meningitis, thrush (infection of the oral mucous membrane by *C. albicans*), and systemic infections in the immunocompromised patient.

Yeast infections are primarily transmitted by direct contact and aerosols. The common site of entry is the respiratory tract. Other infections are due to the ability of yeasts that are part of the normal microflora to multiply and cause infection. As previously mentioned, cases of yeast infections have increased and species have been increasingly isolated from clinical specimens taken from patients who are undergoing chemotherapy or intentional immunosuppression, or in HIV/AIDS patients.

Candida

More than 20 species of *Candida* yeasts are human pathogens, with *Candida albicans* being the most common. *C. glabrata*, *C. kefyr*, *C. parapsilosis*, and *C. tropicalis* are other species isolated from the mucosal surfaces of the GI tract, rectal region, oral cavity, and vagina. An important morphologic feature of the genus *Candida* is that they multiply by forming septate hyphae, blastospores, and pseudohyphae. The exception is *C. glabrata*, which is identified in urinary tract infections and systemic infections in immunocompromised patients and which produces only yeast cells.

The range of infections caused by species in the genus *Candida* include the following: localized, self-limiting diseases of the skin and nails; mucosal surface infections of the mouth, esophagus, bronchi, and vagina; and multiple organ systemic disease. Skin infections are common in obese patients with skin folds such as inframammary areas or abdominal panniculus. The warm, sweat-moistened areas create opportune environments for proliferation of yeast cells which infect dermal layers and result in erythema and may progress to open sores. Diagnosis of the disease is by microscopic observation and laboratory culture (see Figure 11-12).

The infection candidiasis is caused by *C. albicans*. It is a part of the normal human microbiome of the mouth and esophagus, vagina, and intestinal tract. It produces pseudohyphae, but not a capsule, a factor that differentiates the species from *C. neoformans* in the laboratory. *C. albicans* has been identified as the cause of several types of opportunistic infections.

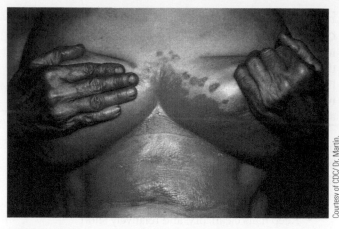

Figure 11-12 Female patient's breasts lifted upward, exposing her upper abdomen and inframammary area with a skin rash and erythema known as candidiasis, or moniliasis, caused by the fungal organism *Candida albicans*.

Thrush

Oral candidiasis, otherwise known as "thrush," is an uncommon disease of healthy adults. It is more commonly seen in infants younger than age 1 month (5–7 percent), older adults, and in immunocompromised individuals (9–31 percent in HIV/AIDS patients and 20 percent in cancer patients). Characterized by white patches or plaques of the tongue and mucous membranes of the mouth, oral candidiasis can cause difficulty swallowing and cracking at the corners of the mouth (angular cheilitis) (see Figure 11-13).

Strict oral hygiene should be followed by at-risk individuals. Patients who use inhaled corticosteroids should rinse their mouths with water following the use of inhalers. Chemotherapy patients may be advised to rinse with chlorhexidine mouthwash. Anti-fungals may be prescribed for severe infections. These may be topical, oral, or a combination based on the disease and the health status of the individual.

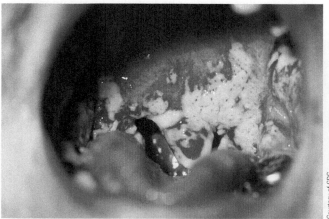

Figure 11-13 Oral thrush, *Candida albicans*.

Genital Yeast Infection

Genital or vulvovaginal candidiasis is also called a "yeast infection." It occurs when there is overgrowth of the normal population of yeast secondary to changes in the acidity or hormone levels in the vagina. Considered common, an estimated 75 percent of all adult females have had at least one vaginal yeast infection in their lifetime, frequently following antibiotic therapy for unrelated illness. Pregnancy and diabetes increase the risk for candidiasis infection.

Females with vaginal candidiasis experience genital itching, burning, and sometimes a "cottage cheese-like" vaginal discharge. Although it is much less common, males with genital candidiasis may experience an itchy rash on the penis. Antifungal creams or suppositories may be prescribed or available over-the-counter; however, it is important for an accurate diagnosis of the fungal pathogen to be obtained prior to use of medications to prevent development of resistant disease.

Invasive Candidiasis

Bloodstream fungal infections from *Candida* are rare in healthy individuals; however, those predisposed to opportunistic pathogens are at risk for systemic **candidemia**. If unrecognized and untreated, then candidemia can spread to most organs of the body and result in multiple organ failure and death. The Centers for Disease Control and Prevention list candidemia as the fourth most common bloodstream infection in the United States. At risk individuals include:

- Patients in intensive care or critical care units
- Premature or very low-birth-weight babies
- Post-operative patients
- Patients with central venous access lines
- HIV/AIDS patients

Rates of occurrence are 8 to 10 cases out of 100,000 people who acquire invasive candidiasis. Infants younger than 1 month and weighing less than 1,000 grams (2.2 pounds) have a 5 percent to 20 percent rate of infection. Diagnosis is made through blood cultures. Treatment with intravenous anti-fungal medications may follow for several weeks before clearance of bloodstream infection. Healthcare workers must use strict hand hygiene procedures to prevent transmission of fungal infections to vulnerable patients.

Cryptococcus

Cryptococcosis, also called European blastomycosis, is an infection caused by one of several yeast species of the genus *Cryptococcus*. The focus of this discussion is *C. neoformans*, the primary pathogen of this genus.

Cryptococcus neoformans has cells that vary in size, so it is referred to as a pleomorphic yeast. Each cell can produce one or more buds that detach to become a new yeast cell. The characteristic feature is the polysaccharide capsule that surrounds the yeast cell. No other yeasts produce a capsule, so recognition as *C. neoformans* is definitive. The presence of a capsule is also the key to the pathogenicity of *C. neoformans*.

The site of entry is the respiratory tract, causing primary lung infections. The infection may be asymptomatic or produce symptoms that are comparable to other lung infections. The pulmonary infection can be detected by an x-ray with a solitary pulmonary nodule observed that mimics carcinoma. Accurate clinical diagnosis of lung infection with *C. neoformans* is done by identifying the organism in a clinical specimen.

C. neoformans can spread to other organs of the body, particularly the central nervous system. It is the leading cause of fungal-caused meningitis. It is recognized as an important cause of morbidity and mortality in HIV/AIDS patients and organ transplant recipients.

Cryptococcal meningitis is the most frequent type of infection, but infection of the brain tissue (encephalitis) can occur. The infection is caused by the spread of yeast from the lungs to the meninges surrounding the brain. Cryptococcal meningitis is a chronic infection with the following symptoms: chronic headache, altering states of consciousness, and fever and rigidity of the neck muscles that lasts for several weeks. Diagnosis is achieved by performing a spinal tap, which withdraws cerebrospinal fluid (CSF) for examination in the laboratory. Recovery depends on the health of the patient prior to infection. Immunocompromised patients typically experience a longer period of infection with elevated symptoms.

Pulmonary cryptococcosis is usually a self-limiting disease. However, surgical excision of a nodule identified on chest x-ray may be performed, providing a clinical specimen for laboratory analysis and treatment. Disseminated cryptococcosis is fatal if untreated.

Anti-fungal Resistance

Antibiotic resistance is a topic of great concern and is frequently discussed in medical journals and infectious disease symposia. The focus is now turning toward a similar problem of increasing and emerging anti-fungal resistance. Fungal infections, once considered relatively rare, are becoming more prominent, mainly in immunocompromised patients, but increasingly in the general population. Fungal infections, often difficult to treat, can become invasive and systemic, with resulting substantial morbidity and mortality rates.

Candida fungal infections are of primary concern for anti-fungal resistance against first-line and second-line anti-fungal drugs such as fluconazole and echinocandins (anidulafungin, caspofungin, and micafungin) (see Figure 11-14). *C. glabrata*, the species most often found to be resistant to fluconazole, has been treated with echinocandins; however, new forms of echinocandin-resistant *C. glabrata* are emerging. Treatment of these multi-drug-resistant fungal pathogens becomes extremely expensive and therapies may be toxic to already compromised patients.

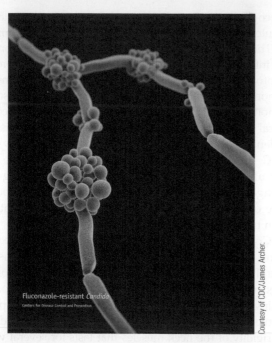

Fluconazole-resistant *Candida*
Centers for Disease Control and Prevention

Courtesy of CDC/James Archer.

Figure 11-14 3D computer image of fluconazole-resistant species of *Candida* based on scanning electron micrographic imagery.

Aspergillus species are also developing resistance to azole-type anti-fungal medications. Researchers are studying the potential collateral effects of industrial food growth and processing with anti-fungals for crop protection.

MICRO NOTES

"A Giant Fungus Among Us"

In 1998, forestry scientists working in the Blue Mountains of eastern Oregon discovered a type of fungus commonly called a honey mushroom or, scientifically, *Armillaria ostoyae*. It turns out that it covers a 3.5-mile area or, in other words, the size of 1,665 football fields. It is considered the largest living single organism in the world. It is estimated to be at least 2,400 years old, but it may actually be up to 8,000 years old. It has caused the death of thousands of trees in the area, where it grows among the roots and trunks of trees and reaches as far down as 10 feet with its fungal rhizomorphs that spread down, up, and across areas looking for food (trees). Scientists took samples of the fungus from different areas for DNA testing and found that they were virtually identical, verifying that it was one "humongous fungus" indeed!

 ## Under the Microscope

Dr. Chen is an ENT specialist who is examining a patient in the hospital emergency department and notes that the patient's facial and sinus bones are severely necrotic and the orbit of one eye has collapsed. Dr. Chen suspects a type of fungal infection and schedules biopsies for that day.

1. What type of fungal infection does Dr. Chen think the patient has?

2. Which types of common fungal organisms can become opportunistic pathogens capable of causing serious infection in humans?

3. How might this patient have become infected?

4. What types of treatment might be required if the diagnosis is confirmed?

5. Is this type of infection an emergency situation?

CHAPTER 12

Gram-Positive Cocci

Learning Objectives

After completing the study of this chapter, you will be able to:

1. Define key terms.
2. Compare and contrast the different forms of Gram-positive cocci.
3. Describe the staphylococcal pathogens and the diseases they cause.
4. Describe the streptococcal pathogens and the diseases they cause.
5. Discuss the morphological characteristics of the Viridans Group and Enterococci.
6. Apply critical thinking skills in relating chapter material to the surgical environment of care or broader global community.

Key Terms

Boils	Exudate	Impetigo	Splenomegaly
Bullous	Furunculosis	Invasins	Subdural effusion
Carbuncles	Glomerulonephritis	Myringotomy	Ventilators
Cytokines	Gram-variable	Non-Bullous	
Debilitation	Hydrocephalus	Otitis media	
Endocarditis	Hyperbaric oxygen	Pustules	

The Big Picture

Staphylococci and streptococci are among the most common sources of infection for our patients in healthcare settings and termed healthcare-associated infections (HAIs); however, some strains have become more prevalent in community-acquired infections. These organisms, found everywhere, cause problems from minor skin irritations to fatal necrosis. During your examination of the topics in this chapter, consider the following:

1. What are the common characteristics of Gram-positive cocci?

2. Which types of infections are typically mild and which have the ability to cause life-threatening illness?

3. What are ways in which individuals can reduce the potential for infection from this microbial pathogen?

4. Which well-known bacteria are capable of mutating into new strains with concerning properties?

Clinical Significance Topic

Each time a surgical incision or percutaneous puncture is made with a scalpel, trocar, or other sharp device, the layers of skin are opened and the deeper tissues beneath are exposed to the outside environment. A routine surgical technique is to isolate the initial scalpel used, also known as the "skin knife" somewhere on the back table to designate it as contaminated. When a scalpel is needed for internal tissue dissection, the surgeon should be given a new "deep knife." The normal microbial population of the epidermal layer of our skin includes numerous bacteria, including *Staphylococcus aureus* and *S. epidermidis*. Although many different bacteria may be identified in surgical site infections (SSIs), a high percentage are colonized with these common staphylococci. The surgical routine of separating the scalpels and not allowing skin microbes to gain access to sterile deep tissues from those on the surface and in the subdermal layer of the skin is considered a standard practice and an example of proper sterile technique.

Focus Groups

The incredible variety of microbes and their classification criteria have been broadly outlined in preceding chapters. In this and subsequent chapters, the focus is narrowed, and specific classes of bacteria are more closely examined. The general descriptions of microbial properties (aerobic vs. anaerobic or facultative; Gram-positive vs. Gram-negative) are used to group similar types of organisms for ease of discussion.

Review of Morphology and Staining

As discussed in Chapter 4, cell shape is one method of classifying bacteria. The three primary groups are cocci (round or spherical), spirilla (coiled), and bacilli (rod-shaped). The microbial cells are arranged in groups due to the cells remaining attached to each other after division. Paired cocci are called diplococci. Streptococci are arranged in chain formations. The sarcinae are the cocci arranged in a cuboidal structure. Cocci arranged in clusters are referred to as staphylococci and are spherical in shape.

Gram staining is a valuable method of determining the characteristics of bacterial cell membranes or walls. The laboratory method differentiates bacteria and fungi (including yeasts and molds) into one of two groups: Gram-positive or Gram-negative. The color of the bacteria at the end of the staining procedure, either purple or red, depends on the chemical composition and thickness of the bacterial cell walls. Gram-positive organisms will appear dark blue or purple from the retained crystal violet dye. Gram-negative organisms will lose the purple color during the rinsing stage and take on the color of the safranin counterstain, thereby appearing pink or red (see Figure 12-1).

Not unexpectedly and with an understanding of the nearly infinite possibilities for variation in the microbial world, there are exceptions to the Gram stain study results. Some species of bacteria are able to demonstrate positive results under certain conditions and negative results under

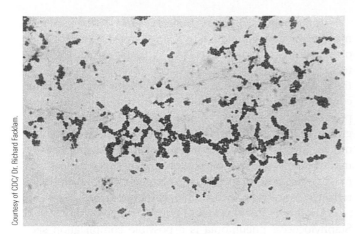

Courtesy of CDC/ Dr. Richard Facklam.

Figure 12-1 Under 250x magnification, presence of numerous, spherical (cocci), Gram-positive, *Staphylococcus aureus* bacteria.

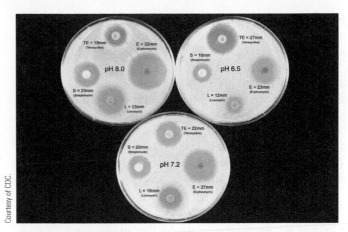

Courtesy of CDC.

Figure 12-2 This set of three petri dish culture plates contained agar inoculated with a culture composed of *Staphylococcus* sp. bacteria. On top of the growth medium in different pH levels, antibiotic-impregnated disks are placed for an antibiotic sensitivity test.

others. These species are considered **Gram-variable** and reflect the differences in cell wall and lipid layers.

Another possible reason for ambiguous results on Gram staining studies is human error. Laboratory technicians with less experience may potentially skew test results by over-rinsing, exposing samples to stains for time periods that are too short or too long, or misinterpreting staining results in final analysis documentation. Competency training and monitoring of personnel as well as standardization of testing procedures may help ensure validity of all routine laboratory studies, including Gram staining.

Occasionally, a Gram-negative result is stated as "no organism seen." This refers to the absence of bacteria or numbers too few to be observed under the microscope. Gram staining is performed as a preliminary study that assists medical practitioners in choosing whether to prescribe antibiotics and, if so, which type. In cases of severe illness, urgency is required and decisions regarding drug therapy can be made relatively safely based on bacterial appearance. However, more targeted, and effective therapy can be achieved only through the results of the second half of the culture and sensitivity laboratory test. The limitation of culture and sensitivity testing is the time factor involved with allowing the bacteria to grow or die based on the culturing technique and observing all of the results.

Sensitivity is determined by culturing bacteria on treated agar plates or with specialized suspensions. The ability to inhibit growth of the colony of bacteria demonstrates sensitivity to the specific drug to which it was exposed. In cases of antibiotic-resistant bacteria, growth is seen even when exposed to traditionally effective chemical formulations (see Figure 12-2). Antimicrobial resistance and antibiotic resistance are discussed further in later sections.

Oxygen Requirements

Bacteria can be additionally classified by their response to oxygen in the surrounding environment, as outlined in

Chapter 4. Broadly speaking, bacteria that grow well in the presence of oxygen are considered aerobic. Those that die in oxygen environments are classified as anaerobic. Some bacteria have developed the ability to adapt to various oxygen levels, and those organisms are considered facultative or aerotolerant. Even though culture and sensitivity tests may be needed for definitive identification of bacterial typing, generalizations may be made for some bacterial species. Abscesses found deep in body tissues would most likely be caused by anaerobic organisms due to the lack of oxygen in their micro-environment. Bacteria typically found on the surface of the skin would be expected to be aerobic due to the constant exposure to ambient air. Those able to adapt to various tissue types and oxygen concentrations are termed facultative. Aerotolerant bacteria prefer to live without oxygen but are able to tolerate low levels to survive.

In this chapter, we examine bacteria that are commonly responsible for healthcare-associated infections (HAIs) and surgical site infections (SSIs). However, the classification of these bacterial pathogens may vary in the literature due to the ability of the various species to adapt to changes in their environments for survival. Gram-positive, round or spherical, facultative anaerobes include species of *Staphylococcus*, *Streptococcus*, Viridans group, and *Enterococcus*.

Staphylococci

One of the most common species of Gram-positive, facultative anaerobic organisms is the species *Staphylococcus*. The name comes from the Greek words staphylo, meaning a cluster of grapes, and kokkos, meaning round berries. These perfectly describe the appearance of growing *Staphylococcus* colonies. Two particular types of organisms frequently responsible for surgical site infections (SSIs) and healthcare-associated infections (HAIs) are *S. aureus* and *S. epidermidis*.

To distinguish the two organisms in the laboratory, additional observations are made of the cultures. Colonies of the microbes produce a different color on culture that contains blood. *S. aureus* is yellow and *S. epidermidis* is white.

Two other tests routinely performed to isolate bacterial species from one another are the catalase and coagulase tests. These laboratory studies can be reviewed in Chapter 3 in the section on specialized laboratory analyses.

Staphylococcus aureus

S. aureus is a facultative anaerobe that grows aerobically on the skin's surface and anaerobically in the pores of the skin. It primarily colonizes the nasal passages in 15 to 40 percent of individuals. The microbe, also an opportunistic pathogen, is strong enough to resist the low moisture, temperature extremes, and high salt content of the skin, but rapidly multiplies in moist areas, such as the mucous membranes of the nose, axillary region, and around the anus.

The major sources of energy for *S. aureus* are carbohydrates and amino acids. It is a chemo-organotroph, acquiring energy from aerobic respiration; however, during anaerobic conditions, lactic acid fermentation is the energy source. It can grow in a temperature range of 10°C to 45°C (50°F–113°F), with an optimum temperature between 30°C and 37°C (86°F–98.6°F). The pH range of growth is 4.2 to 9.3, with the optimum range of 7.0 to 7.5.

A number of virulence determinants (factors) contribute to the pathogenicity of *S. aureus* in humans. These factors include:

- Surface proteins that enhance bacterial colonization
- **Invasins** (leukocidin, hyaluronidase, kinase), which facilitate the spread of bacteria
- Protein capsule, which protects against phagocytes
- Catalase positive
- Coagulase positive
- Secretion of toxins (leukotoxin, hemolysin), which lyse human cell walls
- Acquired antibiotic and antimicrobial resistance

S. aureus is a commonly isolated pathogen identified in numerous infections, ranging from superficial skin infections (**boils, carbuncles, impetigo**, scalded skin syndrome) and serious cases of food poisoning to life-threatening internal organ and skeletal involvement (endocarditis, osteomyelitis, necrotizing fasciitis), respiratory disease (sinusitis, pneumonia), bloodstream infections (bacteremia, toxic shock syndrome), and postoperative surgical site infections. In healthy individuals with intact immune systems and host defenses, infections typically remain localized and controlled at the site of entry. The entry site can be a normal hair follicle or, more commonly, a break in the skin such as a traumatic wound or surgical skin incision.

Intraoperatively, suture materials and other materials may become contaminated by *S. aureus*, resident microflora of the patient's dermal layers, or by other breaks in sterile technique, giving the organism access to the deep internal tissue layers of the body. Serious infections can arise after contamination of surgical wounds involving implantation of prosthetic devices, e.g., total joint components, vascular grafts, mesh grafts, breast implants, indwelling catheters, and others. In many cases, the implanted material must be removed to fully treat the infected wound, because the bacteria may create a **biofilm** layer over the implant that prevents bacterial clearance even with antibiotic treatment.

Another frequent portal of entry is the respiratory tract. Staphylococcal pneumonia is a possible complication secondary to influenza infection or in patients with underlying lung disease or who are placed on mechanical **ventilators**.

Staphylococcus epidermidis

S. epidermidis is immediately distinguished from *S. aureus* in a laboratory culture by its white color. Additionally, *S. epidermidis* is coagulase-negative, whereas *S. aureus* is coagulase-positive. The most common site for *S. epidermidis* to reside is, as its name suggests, on the skin, but it can be found around the eye or in the ear and mouth, and it is considered a commensal organism that is part of the normal microbiome of the nose. It is a frequent cause of intravenous catheter, urinary, and prosthetic device infections, as well as subacute bacterial **endocarditis** in the presence of implanted intracardiac prosthesis (see Figure 12-3).

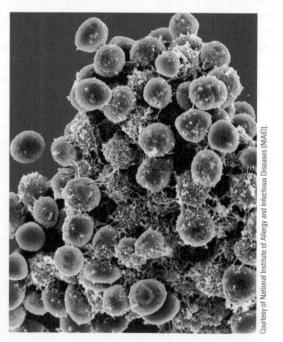

Figure 12-3 Digitally colored scanning electron micrograph image from niaid depicts a clump of green-colored *Staphylococcus epidermidis* bacteria enmeshed in purple-colored filamentous extracellular matrix.

Courtesy of National Institute of Allergy and Infectious Diseases (NIAID).

When artificial heart valves are implanted, endocarditis is a recognized possible complication. *S. epidermidis* can be introduced into deeper tissues at the time of surgery. The clinical signs and symptoms often do not develop for up to 1 year after the surgical procedure. The infection commonly occurs where the valve is sutured to the heart tissue. An abscess forms, leading to separation of the valve from the tissue at the suture line. This causes mechanical failure. Antibiotic treatment and surgical intervention to replace the damaged valve are initiated promptly.

The 2011 "Guidelines for the Prevention of Intravascular Catheter-Related Infections" prepared by the Centers for Disease Control and Prevention estimated that 250,000 bloodstream infections occur in hospitals in the United States, 80,000 of which occur in intensive care units (ICUs). The CDC's National Healthcare Safety Network (CDC NHSN) found that from 2015 to 2019, there was a 31 percent decline in central-line–associated bloodstream infections (CLABSIs). Researchers have been studying the impact of the coronavirus disease 19 (COVID-19) pandemic, theorizing that HAIs in hospitals may have increased due to the exponential increase in hospitalizations and long-term ventilator and central line use.

Microbial pathogens most often associated with this category of HAIs include the coagulase-negative staphylococci (CoNS), including *S. epidermidis*, *S. aureus*, *Enterococcus*, and *Candida* spp. These serious infections are due to the use of indwelling catheters left in place for long periods of time for percutaneous tube feeding purposes, vascular access, and management of critically ill patients. *S. epidermidis* produces an extracellular polymeric substance consisting mainly of an exopolysaccharide that forms a microbial biofilm. The biofilm adheres to the catheters and shunts and protects the bacterial cells from antibiotics and phagocytosis.

Infections of artificial joints from CoNS staphylococci may result in mechanical failure of the total joint prostheses. Treatments include antibiotic therapy and possible replacement of the prosthetic devices. The potential for reinfection when an artificial joint is replaced is very high. Patients with severe surgical site infections may not tolerate secondary surgical replacement and may have to undergo permanent fusion of the joint.

Staphylococcus lugdunensis

Staphylococcus lugdunensis, first identified in 1988, is a relatively uncommon, although virulent, coagulase-negative staphylococcus (CoNS). Its characteristics are very similar to, and it is often mistaken for *S. aureus*. *S. lugdunensis* is believed to be part of the normal skin microflora of the human perineal region. Toxic shock syndrome, osteomyelitis, septic arthritis, and postoperative endopthalmitis have been attributed to *S. lugdunensis* as at least one of several colonizing organisms. *S. lugdunensis* has been identified in serious and potentially fatal cases of endocarditis complicated by heart failure, and it has caught the attention of researchers and epidemiologists. In some studies, mortality rates for these cases of endocarditis appear higher when compared with other CoNS. Depending on the laboratory methods used, identification may be difficult and actual rates of incidence may be under-recognized.

Staphylococcal Diseases

Infections and diseases caused by *Staphylococcus* species are extremely common in humans. These vary widely in their frequency and severity and represent a category of concerning pathogens developing increasing antibiotic resistance and mechanisms of transmission. These concerns are discussed in detail in later chapters.

Folliculitis, Furunculosis, and Carbuncles

Folliculitis is an infection of the hair follicle that causes the development of **pustules**. Folliculitis can lead to the development of **furunculosis** and boils (also known as carbuncles). The severity of the infection determines the prognosis. The most common cause of the infection is coagulase-positive *S. aureus*. Patients are predisposed to the infection due to an infected wound, **debilitation**, diabetes, alcoholism, tight clothes that cause friction, and chafing of the skin.

Folliculitis is marked by pustules that appear in a hair follicle on the face of men with beards (sycosis barbae), eyelids (styes), and scalp, arms, and legs of children (see Figure 12-4). When folliculitis progresses to furunculosis, hard, painful pus-filled nodules appear that enlarge until they rupture, discharging the pus. After the nodule ruptures, the pain usually disappears. If the staphylococcal infection persists, then severely painful carbuncles develop. These are deep abscesses that drain through multiple openings onto the skin surface. The patient may develop a fever in conjunction with the localized inflammatory response.

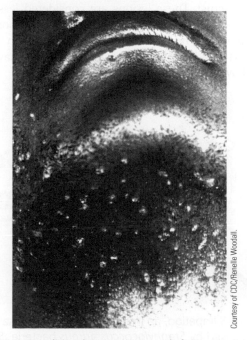

Courtesy of CDC/Renelle Woodall.

Figure 12-4 Condition known as pseudofolliculitis barbae (PFB). This condition occurs in areas of the body where hair is shaved.

The characteristic skin lesions and culture of the exudate that reveal the presence of *S. aureus* confirm the preliminary diagnosis. A complete blood count (CBC) would likely reveal an elevated white blood cell count. Treatment involves systemic antibiotics and instructions given to the patient for cleansing and dressing of the wound. In some cases of furunculosis that do not drain on their own, surgical incision and drainage (I&D) of the lesions may be required. Healthcare providers should advise patients not to scratch or attempt to rupture a boil on their own because this can contribute to spread of the lesions.

Impetigo

Impetigo is a superficial skin infection that occurs in non-bullous and bullous forms. Coagulase-positive *S. aureus* and group A-type *Streptococcus pyogenes* are causative agents in impetigo infections. Diagnosis is made through testing of the **exudate** and isolating the microbial species present. Impetigo most commonly occurs on the face and around the nose, although bullous lesions can be found over all areas of the body. Common impetigo, also called impetiginous dermatitis, is a secondary disease acquired after skin trauma or primary disease.

Non-bullous impetigo, also known as impetigo contagiosa, is a highly contagious communicable infection that begins with small red macules that turn into pus-filled vesicles in a short period of time (see Figure 12-5). When the vesicles break open, a thick honey-colored crust forms from the exudate. Non-bullous impetigo is a self-limiting infection that typically resolves within 2 weeks. Approximately 70 percent of impetigo infections are of the **non-bullous** form.

Bullous impetigo can occur in intact skin and is almost always due to *S. aureus*. In **bullous** impetigo, the vesicle is thin-walled and ruptures, secreting an exudate that forms a thin, clear crust. These lesions are considered less contagious than the non-bullous form. Infants are more commonly affected; however, bullous impetigo can also be diagnosed in older children and adults. Lesions may be distributed over the entire body.

Large areas of skin loss may result from sloughing caused by the endotoxins released into the dermal tissues. Ecthyma, a possible complication of bullous impetigo, is a deep ulcerative infection that may produce associated lymphadenitis (see Figure 12-6).

Scalded Skin Syndrome

Staphylococcal scalded skin syndrome (SSSS) is a severe disorder recognized by peeling of the skin and epidermal erythema, leaving weepy areas that have a scalded, burned appearance. Infants and children younger than age 5 years are most commonly affected. An exfoliative toxin produced by strains of *S. aureus* is responsible for the separation of the dermal and epidermal layers of the skin. However, the mechanism of how the toxin causes the separation is unknown. Laboratory evidence has shown that the toxin has protease activity, indicating that specific proteins that maintain the epidermis may be the target of the toxin.

Treatment consists of intravenous antibiotic therapy along with fluid replacement to prevent possible dehydration due to extensive tissue involvement. Strict aseptic technique must be followed to prevent introduction of a secondary systemic infection because the body's first line of defense (the skin) is compromised. The affected areas are left uncovered or loosely covered to prevent sloughing of the skin. Prognosis for full recovery is favorable. Scaled skin syndrome is characterized by three stages:

1. Erythema: Erythema is observable around the mouth and spreads to the entire body. Nikolsky's sign, sloughing of the skin when friction is manually applied, appears.

2. Exfoliation: In the localized form of the disease, superficial peeling and crusting occur and spread is minimal. The more severe form is characterized by large bullae that erupt and spread to cover the entire body. When the bullae erupt, sections of skin are denuded.

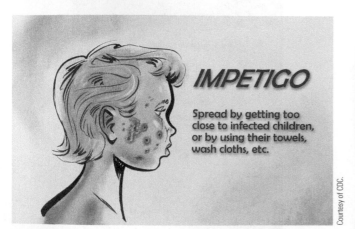

Figure 12-5 Impetigo, an inflammatory skin disease usually caused by *Staphylococcus aureus* bacteria. Sometimes group a *Streptococcus* sp. Can rapidly spread from close contact, such as children in a childcare facility or school.

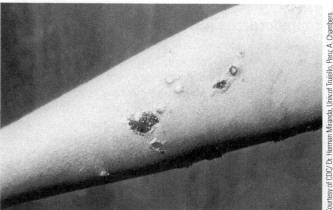

Figure 12-6 Streptococcal impetigo lesions on the volar surface of the left forearm also commonly caused by *Staphylococcus aureus* bacteria.

3. Desquamation: The affected areas become dry and soft and powdery scales form. Normal skin grows back to cover the scales within 5 to 7 days (see Figure 12-7).

Food Poisoning

Staphylococcal food poisoning is the most frequently reported type in the United States, with *S. aureus* being the most frequently isolated causative agent. Only strains that can produce the heat-resistant protein enterotoxin cause food poisoning. The gastroenteritis caused by the bacteria produces abdominal cramping, diarrhea, chills, and vomiting. The symptoms may begin in as little as 30 minutes after ingestion because the toxin is already present in the food; however, usually appear within 1 to 6 hours. Food poisoning is rarely fatal, but cases of mortality among older adults, infants, and debilitated individuals have been reported.

The bacteria rapidly multiply in the food and also produce a potent enterotoxin. Because enterotoxin-producing *S. aureus* exists on the skin of the hands and mucous membranes of most individuals, it can be transferred to the food product by a food handler. Once formed, the heat-resistant toxin cannot be destroyed by cooking and the food misleadingly looks and smells normal. Uncooked homemade foods contaminated by the food preparer or inoculated surfaces have the highest potential for disease transmission. Food poisoning is also frequently the result of improper food handling or storage. The foods most often infected are eggs, mayonnaise, dairy products, potato salad, and ham.

Gastrointestinal infections are not spread person-to-person and group outbreaks occur only if the same food is eaten by affected individuals. Signs and symptoms, including nausea, vomiting, abdominal cramping, and diarrhea, usually will clear in a few days. Antibiotics are ineffective against the endotoxin and are not prescribed for staphylococcal GI infections; therefore, prevention is the key. In severe cases of dehydration, an infected person may need IV fluids and electrolyte supportive therapy. Strict hand-washing techniques should be followed and refrigeration of food at 5°C (41°F) will prevent growth of the bacteria and the subsequent production of the enterotoxin.

Toxic Shock Syndrome

Strains of *S. aureus* produce an exotoxin called toxic shock syndrome–associated toxin (TSST). The toxin is a super-antigen responsible for producing the disease toxic shock syndrome (TSS). A similar infection called toxic shock-like syndrome (TSLS) is caused by streptococcal bacteria.

Anyone can become infected with TSS; however, it was first identified as a public health concern in 1978 in cases involving menstruating females who used super-absorbent vaginal tampons frequently or for prolonged time periods. As the bacteria multiply, they produce TSST, which is absorbed into the bloodstream, producing serious systemic infections. The super-antigen toxin stimulates T-cells non-specifically, without the normal antigenic recognition. As many as one in five T-cells is activated, as compared to the normal antigen activation, which is 1 in 10,000. **Cytokines** are released in very large amounts, causing the symptoms of TSS, which include:

- High body temperature: 102°F to 105°F (39°C–41°C)
- GI symptoms (nausea, vomiting, diarrhea)
- Bright red skin rash that can occur over most of the body that looks like a sunburn (see Figure 12-8)
- Skin peeling occurs approximately 1 to 2 weeks after onset of rash, particularly on the palms and soles of feet

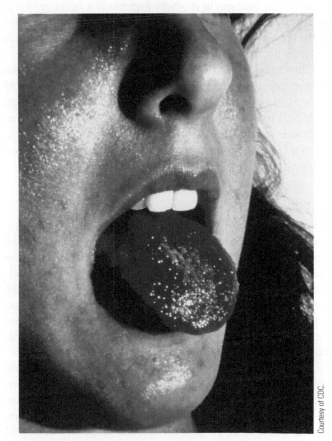

Figure 12-8 Patient with a condition referred to as strawberry tongue associated with toxic shock syndrome (TSS) caused by *Staphylococcus aureus*.

Courtesy of CDC.

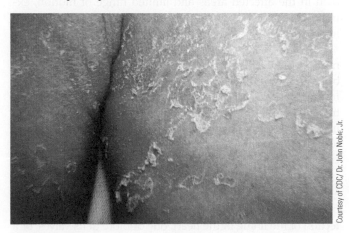

Courtesy of CDC/Dr. John Noble, Jr.

Figure 12-7 Desquamation, also known as sloughing of the skin.

- Neurological symptoms (headache, confusion, seizures)
- Muscle fatigue and general malaise
- Tachycardia (rapid heart rate)
- Tachypnea (rapid breathing)
- Hypotension (low blood pressure)
- Organ (commonly kidney or liver) failure

In later stages, if left untreated, the patient's blood pressure will dramatically decrease, and the patient will go into shock. With prompt treatment by IV fluids and antibiotics, the patient should recover; however, 30 percent of patients may experience recurrence of the infection.

Those at risk include individuals who have had any type of staphylococcal infection, including pneumonia, wound infection, extensive burns, or abscess. Recent childbirth and use of any packing materials (including vaginal or nasal tampons) are also recognized risk factors for toxic shock syndrome.

In cases involving menstrual tampon use, the toxin-producing strains are part of the normal microbiome of the vagina, and too few to cause disease. However, the use of tampons creates the chance for the toxin to enter the body in three ways: (1) inserting the tampon can cause injury to the vaginal wall tissue, providing an opening for the bacteria; (2) blood-soaked tampons provide an ideal moist environment for the bacteria to multiply and reach a number that is sufficient to cause disease; and (3) the longer a tampon is left in the vagina, the greater the chances for bacterial growth and infection to occur.

Toxic shock syndrome is considered a statistically rare disease process. The last reporting date in the year 1999 showed 113 cases in the United States. It is reported that, on average, 1 to 2 people in 100,000 will experience TSS per year. Prognosis statistics vary from a 5 to 15 percent mortality rate up to a 50 percent mortality rate in severe toxic shock cases resulting in multiple organ failure.

Osteomyelitis

Osteomyelitis is a chronic bone marrow and bone infection most frequently caused by the invasion of *S. aureus*, but it can be caused by other types of organisms. The infection occurs at one site of the body, such as a surgical site, but travels by the bloodstream to the bone. In children the long bones (particularly the femur) are usually affected, and in adults the vertebrae and pelvis are most commonly affected. Infections in children are usually acute and respond better to treatment than chronic infections suffered by adults (see Figure 12-9).

Indirect causes of infection include dental, bladder, and respiratory infections. Direct causes are the result of trauma, such as penetrating wounds, open fractures, and surgical procedures. Overall osteomyelitis risk factors include diabetes, injection drug use, peripheral vascular disease, rheumatoid arthritis, prolonged steroid use, HIV/AIDS, sickle-cell disease, hemodialysis treatments, and alcoholism. Two in 10,000 suffer osteomyelitis annually.

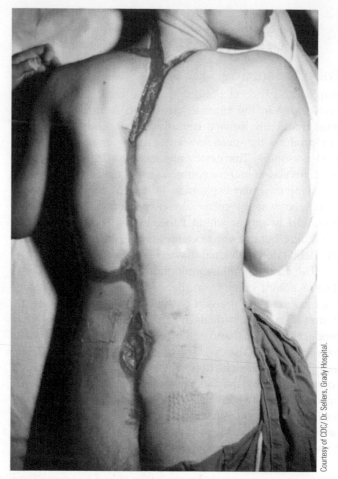

Courtesy of CDC/ Dr. Sellers, Grady Hospital.

Figure 12-9 Patient in a prone position which exposed her back, and the bacterial cutaneous lesion that ran the length of her spine as a result of a *Staphylococcus* sp. infection involving entire spinal column.

Individuals with osteomyelitis experience persistent pain that increases in severity over the course of the infection. They also have fever and tenderness in the area of bone that is infected. Pus is often present in affected tissues. Due to pain in the affected areas and limited range of motion, extreme care should be taken, and gentleness used in positioning of the extremity.

The radiographic diagnostic procedures used to diagnose osteomyelitis include tomography and radionuclide bone scanning. A bone biopsy with culture may be performed. The treatment is aggressive, with high dosages of intravenous antibiotics and strict bed rest. In cases of chronic infection, surgical removal of necrotic bone must be performed. Chronic osteomyelitis can persist for years with reoccurrences and remissions, despite antibiotic treatment.

Infective Endocarditis

Infective endocarditis is a bacterial (rarely may be fungal) infection of the lining of the heart, one or more of its valves, or a septal defect. The heart valves may be native valves or prosthetic implants. Valvular insufficiency is a primary effect of infective endocarditis, leading to congestive heart failure and myocardial abscesses. Left untreated, it is a fatal infection.

Endocarditis is separated into three broad types: native valve endocarditis or NVE (acute or subacute); prosthetic valve endocarditis or PVE (early or late); and intravenous drug abuse endocarditis or IVDA.

Acute NVE cases are typically diagnosed in otherwise healthy individuals with no valvular disease. It is an aggressive, rapidly progressing infection usually caused by *S. aureus* or the group B species of *Streptococcus*. The bacteria travel from the initial site of infection via the bloodstream to the heart valves, and after arrival they quickly start destroying the heart valve tissue. If left untreated, death results in a matter of days to just a few weeks.

Early PVE cases occur within 60 days of implantation and are usually caused by coagulase-negative staphylococci (CoNS), Gram-negative bacilli, and fungal *Candida* species. Late PVE are more than 60 days from implantation and usually are caused by staphylococci, alpha-hemolytic streptococci, and enterococci. *S. aureus* is now considered the most common cause of both early and late PVE as well as IVDA infections. Infective endocarditis from *S. aureus* has a 30 to 40 percent mortality rate.

The normal tissue of the valves has a smooth surface and is a light red color. The bacterial infection creates a rough, reddened surface that is easily seen on visual inspection during surgery or pathological examination. The inflammation causes the valve opening to narrow and malfunction. The infection can also affect the endocardium and pericardium of the heart (see Figure 12-10).

Symptoms experienced by the patient include heart murmur, chronic fever, **splenomegaly**, and embolism. Treatment must be prompt and includes the intravenous administration of antibiotics specific to the infecting pathogen. If the heart valves are seriously damaged, then the patient must undergo heart valve replacement surgery. Approximately 15 to 25 percent of IE patients require surgical intervention along with antibiotic infusions.

Streptococci

Similar to staphylococci, streptococci are Gram-positive, facultative anaerobes that are found in many tissues of the human body. Other general characteristics of streptococci include nonmotility; non-spore-forming; occurring in pairs or chains; and catalase-negative. *Streptococcus* species are divided into broad classes based on their hemolysis characteristics. Streptococci are further classified on the basis of colony morphology and biochemical reactions. The type of hemolytic reaction on blood agar has long been used for classification purposes. The three classifications are alpha, beta, and gamma (see Figure 12-11).

Species of streptococci in the alpha (α) class (including the viridans and *S. pneumoniae*) cause some destruction of erythrocytes (red blood cells). The beta (β) streptococci are much more destructive in their hemolysis with the complete lysis of red blood cells surrounding the colony of bacteria on the culture plate. The beta (β) streptococci also produce toxins that affect blood clotting factors and white blood cells. Non-hemolytic colonies are designated gamma (γ) hemolytic and do not affect red blood cells (see Figure 12-12).

In the 1930s, a scientist named Rebecca Lancefield originated a classification system based on 18 group-specific antigens. This system, called the Lancefield groups, further separates the beta hemolytic streptococci into lettered groups (A, B, C, D, F, and G). With the advances in serologic methods, several types of streptococci have been shown to have several group antigens. Group A streptococci are beta (β) hemolytic. Group B streptococci can be alpha (α), beta (β), or gamma (γ) hemolytic. The majority of *Streptococcus pneumoniae* are α hemolytic but can cause β hemolysis in anaerobic conditions. Groups A and D can be transmitted to humans via food.

Although Lancefield grouping is helpful in classifying bacteria based on hemolysis potential, it is imprecise and the molecular taxonomies have improved the classification and identification processes. The Lancefield groups can be subdivided into large and small colony-forming groups. The "pyogenic" groups are large colonies with multiple virulence factors.

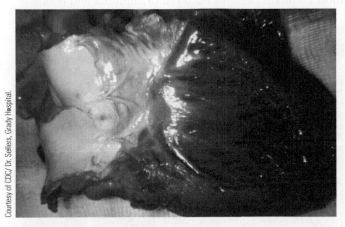

Figure 12-10 Human heart opened to expose the heart's interior, highlighting the organ's left ventricle, and aortic valve from a patient who had died from bacterial endocarditis.

Courtesy of CDC/ Dr. Sellers, Grady Hospital.

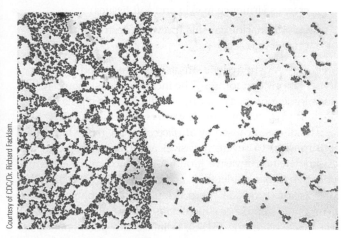

Courtesy of CDC/ Dr. Richard Facklam.

Figure 12-11 A photomicrograph of *Streptococcus mutans* bacteria using gram stain technique.

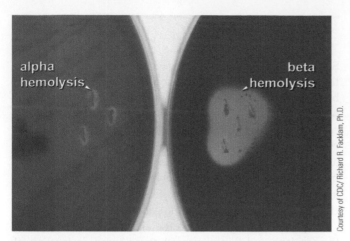

Courtesy of CDC/ Richard R. Facklam, Ph.D.

Figure 12-12 Petri dishes filled with soy agar containing sheep's blood. The plate on the left had been stabbed and streaked with an inoculum containing *Streptococcus mitis*, an alpha-hemolytic bacterial member of the viridans group. The right plate was stabbed with an inoculum containing group a *Streptococcus pyogenes* (gas), a typical beta-hemolytic bacteria.

The definitive identification of streptococci relies on the serologic reactivity of cell wall polysaccharide antigens. The cell wall structure of group A streptococci is one of the most well-researched. The cell wall is composed of peptidoglycan. Unlike *Staphylococcus*, all streptococci lack the enzyme catalase. Non–group A streptococci strains do not have definite virulence factors, whereas group A streptococci have several virulence factors, including:

- Lipoteichoic acid, a strongly acidic polymer in the cell wall, and M protein that aids in the bacterial attachment to the host
- Toxins, such as pyrogenic toxin (the cause of the rash in scarlet fever)
- Streptokinase (an enzyme that dissolves blood clots)
- Streptolysins (toxins that destroy phagocytes)
- Hyaluronic acid capsule (protective capsule that increases virulence in skin and soft tissues)
- Polysaccharide capsule (prevents destruction by phagocystosis)

Group A β-hemolytic streptococci are spread by respiratory secretions and fomites. The incidences of skin and respiratory infections peak during childhood. Infections can be transmitted by asymptomatic carriers.

The diseases caused by *Streptococcus* spp. range from mild (non-invasive) to severe (invasive) and chronic. Some of the well-known non-invasive group A streptococcal diseases include strep throat, scarlet fever, and impetigo. Severe acute invasive diseases include necrotizing fasciitis, pneumococcal pneumonia, streptococcal meningitis, bacteremia, streptococcal toxic shock syndrome (STSS), cellulitis, and puerperal sepsis. Chronic diseases, termed non-suppurative (not pus forming) sequelae, include rheumatic fever and post-streptococcal

glomerulonephritis. These chronic diseases occur weeks to months after an untreated streptococcal infection in other areas of the body (e.g., strep throat or impetigo).

Group B streptococci are normal vaginal microflora but are closely monitored in pregnant women due to the potential for transfer to an infant during vaginal delivery. Colonization by group B streptococci in a neonate can cause life-threatening infection and possible serious, lifelong neurological deficits. The human body utilizes a number of immune responses to defend against streptococcal infections. Natural and acquired immunity are discussed in a later chapter.

Diagnoses are based on cultures from clinical specimens. Serologic methods are used to detect group A and group B antigens. The bacitracin sensitivity test differentiates group A from other β-hemolytic streptococci. Acute glomerulonephritis and acute rheumatic fever are identified by anti-streptococcal antibody titers. Treatment consists of appropriate antibiotic therapy and prophylactic vaccines are available for some species while others are being investigated.

Streptococcal Pathogens and Diseases

Scientific focus has primarily been on two group B streptococcal species that are the cause of severe infections: *S. pyogenes* and *S. pneumoniae*. Additional species have been receiving increased attention including, *Streptococcus agalactiae* and *S. viridans*, as well as enterococci, previously classified as group D streptococci.

Streptococcus pneumoniae

Streptococcus pneumoniae is a Gram-positive, facultative anaerobe that is an opportunistic pathogen located in the eye, ear, mouth, and nose, most predominantly in the upper respiratory tract. The cells are round and occur in pairs (diplococci) (see Figure 12-13). A strain of *S. pneumoniae* is the most common cause of bacterial pneumonia and is one of

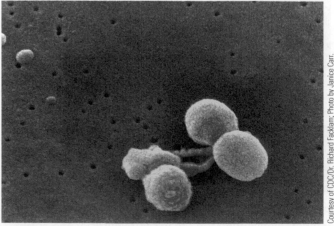

Courtesy of CDC/Dr. Richard Facklam; Photo by Janice Carr.

Figure 12-13 Scanning electron micrograph image of *Streptococcus pneumoniae*.

three of the most common causes of bacterial meningitis. According to the CDC, each year in the United States *S. pneumoniae* is responsible for:

- Approximately 400,000 cases of pneumococcal pneumonia (30 percent of all adult community-acquired pneumonias)

- 3,000 cases of pneumococcal meningitis (13–19 percent of all bacterial meningitis infections)

- 28 to 55 percent of the 20 million cases of otitis media are pneumococcal

- Approximately 12,000 cases of bacteremia with a fatality rate of 15 to 60 percent, most pronounced in older adults.

Pneumococcal meningitis and sepsis (bacteremia) killed approximately 3,500 people in the United States in 2018 according to the CDC. Worldwide, pneumococcal disease kills a half million children younger than 5 years of age according to the World Health Organization (WHO). Other major fatal pneumococcal diseases are pneumonia and meningitis. For children in developing countries who contract *S. pneumoniae*, 40 to 70 percent will die or suffer disabling effects.

Anyone can become infected with pneumococcal bacteria; however, individuals with the highest risk factors are:

- Children younger than age 2 years

- Adults older than age 65 years

- Children in daycare and adults in nursing homes or long-term care facilities

- Children or adults between 19 and 64 years of age who are immunocompromised due to HIV/AIDS, sickle cell anemia, cancer, chronic heart or lung disease, and damaged or missing spleen

- Children or adults with cochlear implants or cerebrospinal (CSF) leaks

- Adults with chronic conditions such as asthma, diabetes, heart, liver, or lung disease, and alcoholism

- Children of American Indian, Alaskan Native, or African American ethnicity

The pneumonia-causing strain is recognized by a capsule that is mucoid and shiny in appearance (see Figure 12-14). A non-encapsulated strain is distinguished by a dry and pitted capsule that is a frequent cause of pneumonia in children and the elderly. The encapsulated form is more virulent. Penicillin-resistant strains of *S. pneumoniae* are increasing in prevalence in the general population.

Streptococci may be distinguished from other bacterial species by their response to certain chemicals on culture plates. Sensitivity to optochin, a chemical that inhibits pneumococci, provides a presumptive identification of α-hemolytic streptococci such as *S. pneumoniae*. Another laboratory study, the Neufeld-Quellung test, aids in identification of *S. pneumoniae* when a type-specific antibody causes

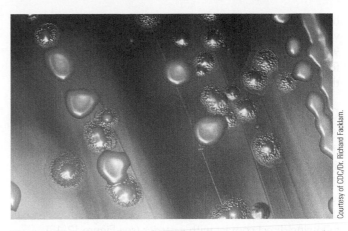

Figure 12-14 Doughnut-shaped *Streptococcus pneumoniae* bacterial colonies.

Courtesy of CDC/Dr. Richard Facklam.

the cell capsule to enlarge. Currently, 92 pneumococcal serotypes have been identified. Other identifying features are negative catalase test and solubility in bile salts.

Pneumococcal Pneumonia

Pneumonia caused by *S. pneumoniae* is called pneumococcal pneumonia. The infectious process of pneumococcal pneumonia begins when the patient is infected by inhaling respiratory droplets containing bacteria that were exhaled by another person nearby. This is the most common way the disease is transmitted. The pneumococci multiply in the lungs, beginning the inflammatory response. The alveoli become filled with fluid from surrounding lung tissue, erythrocytes, and neutrophils. The disease is not a result of bacterial toxins, but rather results from the ability of the bacterial cells to cause a severe inflammatory response.

The number of strains that are displaying drug resistance is increasing. Many of these strains have become highly virulent and resistant to multiple types of antibiotics, including vancomycin. One type of protection has been the development of a vaccine. Two vaccines have been developed for individuals with specific risk factors.

Children younger than age 2 years are at high risk for serious pneumococcal disease. A pneumococcal conjugate vaccine called PCV13 or Prevnar® protects against 13 serotypes of pneumococcal bacteria. Following the initiation of routine vaccination protocols for infants and toddlers younger than age 2, the rates of pneumonia, bacteremia, and meningitis decreased significantly in the United States. Some children older than age 2 with specific risk factors may also benefit from PCV13. Adults older than age 65 are also at elevated risk and vaccination is recommended for this age group. Immunocompromised adults older than age 19 years may also be given a single dose for protection. Refer to the previous section for the list of risk factors.

Pneumovax® or PPSV23 (23-valent pneumococcal polysaccharide vaccine) is recommended for all adults older than age 65 and for adults between the ages of 19 and 64 who have asthma or smoke. Individuals older than age 2 years with high risk factors may be given the PPSV23 vaccine. The vaccine contains polysaccharide antigens of the 23 out of 92 known capsular serotypes. These 23 serotypes account for 90 percent of all bacterial pneumococcal infections in the United States.

Otitis Media

S. pneumoniae is responsible for a large percentage of ear infections, called **otitis media**. It most commonly occurs in children ages 1 to 8 years. The bacterial cells secrete exotoxins that are the cause of the infection. The ear infection is usually in conjunction with, or subsequent to, a common cold or nasal or throat infection. Additionally, otitis media infection can occur following direct contact with a carrier (see Figure 12-15).

The treatment is appropriate antibiotic therapy. For patients with chronic otitis media, a **myringotomy** procedure may be performed. This minor surgical procedure performed under general anesthesia involves making a small puncture incision in the tympanic membrane (ear drum) and placement of a very small tube that allows for drainage of pus and relieves pressure and pain. Frequently, the treatment is done for both ears and is scheduled as a bilateral myringotomy tube (BMT) procedure.

Pneumococcal Meningitis

The brain and spinal cord are protected by bone and three membranes called the meninges. There is no normal microflora of the nervous system; therefore, the cerebrospinal fluid is considered sterile. Microbial pathogens gain access to the central nervous system (CNS) through trauma, such as fractures and surgery, via the vascular or lymphatic systems, or along the nerves of the peripheral nervous system (PNS).

A serious infection of the three membranes is called meningitis. The three major causes of bacterial meningitis are *Haemophilus influenzae* (the primary cause in children), *Neisseria meningitidis* (the primary cause in adolescents), and *Streptococcus pneumoniae* (the primary cause in older adults). Pneumococcal meningitis is the major cause of bacterial meningitis in neonates from *S. agalactiae* and this is discussed in Chapter 17.

The early clinical symptoms of meningitis are similar to a cold. As the infection progresses, symptoms include severe chronic headache, fever, pain, and stiffness of the neck and back.

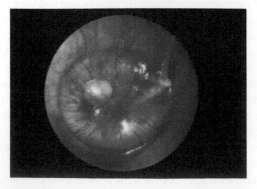

Figure 12-15 Acute otitis media with bulging eardrum.

Symptoms can quickly progress to neurological signs, including confusion, restlessness, dizziness, convulsions, coma, and death if left untreated.

Definitive diagnosis is made by culture of the cerebrospinal fluid obtained by lumbar puncture (spinal tap). The type of bacterial pathogen that is causing the infection determines the antibiotic therapy. Even with antibiotic treatment, approximately 20 percent of patients die and 25 to 50 percent will suffer severe CNS complications, including brain damage, seizures, **hydrocephalus**, **subdural effusion**, or hearing loss.

Streptococcus pyogenes

Streptococcus pyogenes is part of group A, β-hemolytic streptococci that cause strep throat, rheumatic fever, scarlet fever, and the so-called flesh-eating disease, necrotizing fasciitis. The bacterial cells occur in chains. The microbes are commensals that become opportunistic pathogens commonly found on the skin, in the eyes and ear, and in the respiratory tract. It is estimated that 5 to 15 percent of the world population harbor *S. pyogenes*, most often in the respiratory tract, without showing signs of disease. During the winter and spring months, up to 20 percent of children may be asymptomatic carriers of group A *Streptococcus*.

S. pyogenes bacteria have cell envelopes (includes the cell membrane, cell wall, and glycocalyx) that contain an antigenic protein called protein M which aids in protection from host phagocytes and helps the cell adhere to pharyngeal cells. Other virulence factors of *S. pyogenes* include:

- Hyaluronic acid capsule: inhibits phagocytosis because the acid is chemically similar to the host connective tissue. This allows the bacterial cells to "hide" their own antigens and not be recognized as antigenic by the host

- Exotoxins: erythrogenic toxin that causes the rash in scarlet fever and systemic toxic shock syndrome

- Enzymes: streptokinase, streptodornase, and hyaluronidase

The fluorescent antibody technique is often used for the identification of *S. pyogenes*. Fluorescent dyes, called fluorochromes, glow when viewed with an ultraviolet microscope. The dye attaches to the antibodies in the patient's serum, which then adheres to the pathogen.

Early in the 20th century, many females died from puerperal fever due to *S. pyogenes*. With the advent of antibiotics, puerperal fever and erysipelas, a severe form of cellulitis accompanied by a high fever and systemic toxicity, are no longer common (see Figure 12-16). Researchers have studied the phenomenon of excess mortality following influenza infection. They have found that serious secondary bacterial infections that take advantage of debilitated, immunocompromised individuals dramatically increase morbidity and mortality rates following influenza outbreaks. During the influenza pandemic of 1918–1919, it is believed that the secondary infections caused by *S. pneumoniae* and

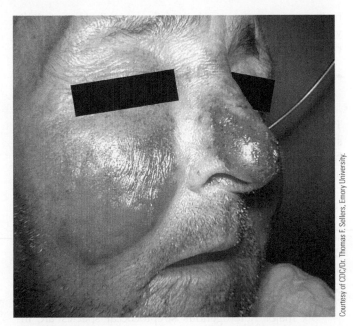

Figure 12-16 Facial erysipelas from *Streptococcus*, also called cellulitis.

S. pyogenes were responsible for up to 90 percent of the deaths of infected soldiers. Even in more recent history, during the 2009 "swine flu" (H1N1) pandemic, 29 percent of the deaths were attributed to secondary bacterial pneumonia infections. *S. pyogenes* was the causative bacterial pathogen in 27 percent of those deaths according to research experts. The ongoing COVID-19 pandemic and development of hyper-transmissible variants such as delta and omicron prevents definitive analysis of impact of secondary infections. The vast global numbers of individuals requiring ventilator assistance and the extensive range of systemic effects of the SARS-Co-V-2 viral infection will presumably result in a broad variety of secondary infection sequelae.

Although its role is not fully understood, *S. pyogenes* has been linked to pediatric neuropsychiatric disorders such as obsessive-compulsive disorder (OCD) and Tourette's syndrome. *Streptococcus pyogenes* has experienced a resurgence in attention due to the rapidly progressive diseases it can cause including necrotizing fasciitis. Its success as a major pathogen is owed to its ability to rapidly colonize, multiply, and spread in the host while evading phagocytosis and the immune system.

Streptococcal Pharyngitis

Streptococcus pyogenes is the leading cause of strep throat, or acute pharyngitis, accounting for 5 to 10 percent of cases in adults and 15 to 30 percent of pediatric cases. It is an acute bacterial infection of the throat that causes fever, chronic pain, difficulty swallowing, and inflammation of the tonsils and pharynx. Upon examination, the patient's pharynx (throat) reveals white patches of pus on the pharyngeal epithelium. Each year as many as 1.8 million individuals in the United States suffer streptococcal pharyngitis (see Figure 12-17).

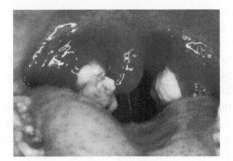

Figure 12-17 Streptococcal pharyngitis.

Scarlet Fever

Scarlet fever, also known as scarletina, is most commonly associated with strep throat; however, cases have been documented following streptococcal skin infections. The *S. pyogenes* strain that causes streptococcal pharyngitis produces an erythrogenic pyrogenic toxin called *S. pyogenes* exotoxin (SPE). The degree and severity of symptoms are dependent upon the immunity status of the individual and virulence of the toxin-producing strain in the population. Approximately 1 in 10 individuals (10 percent) will develop scarlet fever following strep throat. After age 10 years, approximately 80 percent of children develop immunity to the bacterial toxin.

Signs of scarlet fever are a fever in excess of 101°F (38.3°C), a sandpaper-like red rash of the skin, and a rash of the tongue resembling the texture of a strawberry, similar to that seen in toxic shock syndrome. Later in the course of the disease, the upper membrane layer is shed, leaving the tongue bright red and swollen. Eventually the skin also peels off, much like sunburned skin.

Necrotizing Fasciitis

Necrotizing fasciitis, otherwise known as the "flesh-eating" bacteria, has been dramatized in recent years by the news media. The bacteria are a strong invasive strain that involves infection of the fascia and may penetrate into the underlying muscle. They produce an enzyme called protease that destroys proteins and aids the bacterial cells in their invasion of epithelial cells. The strain also produces the pyrogenic toxin that is the cause of streptococcal toxic shock syndrome (STSS). When viewed with a microscope, the cell surface is mucoid, indicating that it has a thick capsule with a large amount of M protein.

The portal of entry for the opportunistic pathogen is usually a break in the skin (e.g., cut, scrape, burn, incision, or insect bite). These breaks can be extremely minor and easily dismissed. Symptoms similar to muscle strains may begin hours after the injury. Inflammatory signs of pain, redness, heat, and swelling may be observed; however, the intense level of pain the infected individual experiences may not seem to correlate with the outwardly visible signs and therefore can be misdiagnosed by healthcare providers. This potential delay in accurate diagnosis and onset of prompt antibiotic therapy may result in devastating results. In severe and rapidly progressing infections, surgical debridement (removal of infected or dead tissue) and even amputation may be necessary. **Hyperbaric oxygen** therapy may be initiated to preserve tissue.

Group A streptococcal strains are the most frequent cause of necrotizing fasciitis; however, other pathogens can also produce the debilitating disease. The other causative bacteria include *E. coli*, *S. aureus*, *Klebsiella*, *Clostridium*, and *Aeromonas hydrophila*. Various insects, including recluse spiders, cause extensive and progressive tissue destruction similar to bacterial necrotizing fasciitis due to toxic venoms (see Figure 12-18). As part of its Emerging Infection Program (EIP), the CDC reports approximately 650 to 800 cases each year of group A streptococcal necrotizing fasciitis, with 25 to 30 percent of those cases being fatal. These numbers may be due to under-reporting; however, the trend does not appear to be increasing in frequency.

Streptococcus agalactiae

Better known as a group B streptococcus (GBS), *S. agalactiae* is part of the normal microbiome of the vagina, GI tract, and upper respiratory system. *S. agalactiae* was initially listed as a dangerous puerperal fever-causing pathogen. Sepsis in neonates is rare and usually seen following prolonged periods of amniotic membrane rupture. Infection in the neonate can occur in utero, during birth, or during the first few weeks of life. There are two categories of infection: early-onset disease, which is an infection occurring in neonates younger than age 7 days, and late-onset disease, which occurs in infants 7 days to 3 months old.

Females are predisposed to UTIs during pregnancy and immediately after giving birth. The infection is not typically dangerous because a majority of females who are pregnant are in good health. The symptoms are irritating, but the prognosis is excellent. Secondary complications are rare.

S. agalactiae infection is relatively rare in healthy adults and, nearly always, an underlying condition such as diabetes,

malignancy, or congestive heart failure contributes to an individual's susceptibility. The types of infections caused, and the risk factors are similar to those of *S. pneumoniae*.

Viridans Group Streptococci

The group of streptococci currently named viridans group streptococci (VGS), also sometimes referred to as gamma (γ) hemolytic, demonstrates a lack of hemolysis on blood agar plates. As a group, they are catalase-negative. When cultured in the laboratory, early bacterial colonies are easily mistaken for *S. pneumoniae*. However, as the colony matures, *S. pneumoniae* groups develop a depression in the center, the so-called doughnut appearance. The viridans colonies remain dome-shaped (see Figure 12-19). Viridans streptococci are also optochin-resistant on culture. The name given to the group is based on the Latin word for green (viridis), which is how they appear on blood agar plates.

Six major heterogenous streptococcal species are included in the viridans group. These are *S. mutans*, *S. salivarius*, *S. anginosus*, *S. mitis*, *S. sanguinis*, and *S. bovis*. The group *S. mutans* are most known as commensals in the human mouth, which become opportunistic pathogens in dental disease or procedures. Half of all bacterial endocarditis infections are from *S. mutans*. Several of the other species are generally found in animals; however, isolates have been identified in immunocompromised patients.

Enterococci

Previously, taxonomists had created a streptococcal group D; however, these 17 species have been reclassified under the genus *Enterococcus*. These bacteria are Gram-positive, facultative

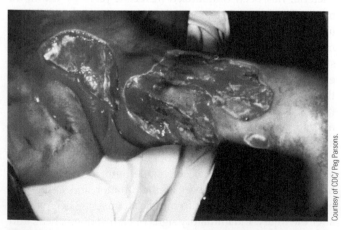

Figure 12-18 Patient with tissue necrosis of the lower abdominopelvic and upper thigh skin and underlying musculofascial layers. Wound appearance is similar to that of bacterial necrotizing fasciitis, however, in this case, the infection was secondary to a bite by a Chilean recluse spider 41 days prior to the photo.

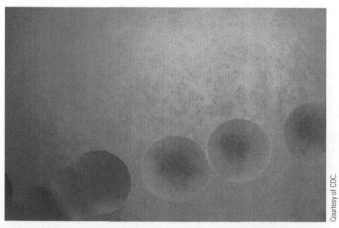

Figure 12-19 Petri dish filled with soy agar medium containing sheep's blood and *Streptococcus anginosus* bacteria, a Gram-positive viridans group of streptococci (VGS) with characteristic color changes, including a hazy, faded, indistinct region surrounding each colony in which only some of the red blood cells (RBCs) were destroyed, or hemolyzed.

Courtesy of CDC/ Peg Parsons.

Courtesy of CDC.

anaerobes that are usually either α-hemolytic or γ-hemolytic. *Enterococcus faecalis* and *Enterococcus faecium* are the most prevalent species cultured from humans (90 percent of isolates of the genus *Enterococcus*) (see Figure 12-20). The species within this group have numerous intrinsic antibiotic resistance mechanisms and are proficient at acquiring new resistance genes or mutations by conjugation (bacterial mating). *E. faecium* is responsible for the majority of vancomycin-resistant enterococci (VRE) infections, a serious class of healthcare-associated infections (HAIs).

Enterococci are commensals in the gastrointestinal tract of humans. As opportunistic pathogens, they are frequently responsible for urinary tract infections as well as intra-abdominal infections, bacteremia resulting in meningitis, and endocarditis. An infectious diseases specialist should be consulted in cases of serious infections caused by *Enterococcus* species, particularly when multi-resistant strains are isolated.

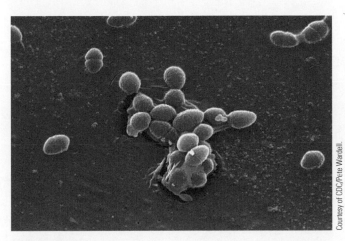

Courtesy of CDC/Pete Wardell.

Figure 12-20 This digitally colorized scanning electron micrograph image depicts large numbers of Gram-positive *Enterococcus faecalis* sp. Bacteria.

MICRO NOTES

"The Mighty Microbe"

"An incredible strain of bacteria called *Deinococcus radiodurans* has been included in the *Guinness Book of World Records* with the label of "world's toughest bacterium." The name of the bacterium indicates that it is a coccus (berry-shaped) that has the ability to withstand radiation (radiodurans). In fact, *D. radiodurans* can survive exposure to radiation thousands of times greater than would be fatal to humans. It can suffer cell damage, but it is able to repair itself and keep going. Scientists are intrigued by the fact that it can be found in such diverse places on the planet, but none that requires its incredible talent of survival, and are seeking ways to use *D. radiodurans* in bioremediation projects involving radioactive waste.

Under the Microscope

Jonathan, a surgical technology student in clinical rotations, was given the assignments for the next day: to be in the ENT room and scrub and write a case analysis paper for several bilateral myringotomy tube (BMT) cases incorporating the probable history and diagnosis as well as the procedural steps. The following questions would be helpful in that research.

1. In what age group would the patients most likely be included?

2. What types of infections would the histories of patients having this type of procedure most likely include?

3. Which body system and anatomy is involved in this diagnosis and where will the incisions be made?

4. Which types of bacteria typically cause conditions that require the surgical intervention by an ear, nose, and throat (ENT) surgeon?

5. What are other types of non-ENT-related infections would be caused by the bacterial groups in this chapter?

CHAPTER 13

Gram-Positive Bacilli

Learning Objectives

After completing the study of this chapter, you will be able to:

1. Define key terms.
2. Compare and contrast the different forms of Gram-positive bacilli.
3. Describe the *Bacillus* pathogens and the diseases they cause.
4. Describe the *Clostridium* pathogens and the diseases they cause.
5. Discuss the role of pathogenic bacteria in bioterrorism.
6. Apply critical thinking skills in relating chapter material to the surgical environment of care or broader global community.

Key Terms

Bactericidal	Endospore	Non-hemolytic	Sporulates
Bacteriocins	Fasciitis	Opisthotonos	Vegetative
Cellulitis	Gastroenteritis	Peritonitis	Ventriculoatrial
Emetic	Hemolysin	Septicemia	Ventriculoperitoneal
Endophthalmitis	Iatrogenic	Shock	
Endosome	Indigenous flora	Spastic paralysis	

The Big Picture

*C*lostridioides difficile and other potentially life-threatening infections have become a concerning problem for healthcare settings such as hospitals and long-term care facilities as well as the food industry. Many pathogenic microbes can be spread by similar mechanisms. During your examination of the topics in this chapter, consider the following:

1. Which patient populations are at increased risk for serious healthcare-associated infections (HAIs)?

2. What are routine practices that everyone, including healthcare providers, can take to minimize transmission of disease?

3. How can food-borne infections by Gram-positive bacilli be prevented?

4. Which characteristics of these types of bacteria make them extremely virulent and difficult to kill?

Clinical Significance Topic

Bacteria have developed fascinating survival tactics. *Geobacillus stearothermophilus* is a rod-shaped, spore-forming bacteria, that as its name indicates, loves steam. It is considered one of the extremophiles, bacteria that grow best in extreme environments. *G. stearothermophilus* (formerly called *Bacillus stearothermophilus*) was isolated in steam vents of Yellowstone National Park. In the hospital, these bacteria are used as biological indicators (BIs) for steam sterilizers that run from 250°F to 270°F. The challenge for steam sterilizers is to kill the measured population of *G. stearothermophilus* in a test ampule or strip. When the sterilized BI has been incubated and shown to have no growth, the sterilizer is considered to be working properly and the instruments processed by this method are considered sterile.

Overview of Bacilli

Chapter 4 discussed the various ways the species of bacteria are classified: based on their shape, oxygen requirements, staining results, and motility. Bacilli are rod-shaped bacteria that are Gram-positive on staining; however, some species will become Gram-negative in their mature form and therefore may be listed in the literature as Gram-variable. Most species are catalase-positive.

Bacilli are found in soil samples around the world and also in animal intestinal tracts. They are saprophytes, which mean they use dead and decaying organic material as food. They utilize oxygen in varying amounts and are classified as either aerobic or facultative anaerobic. Individual bacterial cells are often motile with the aid of appendages called flagella. Estimates of the number of known species of bacilli vary from 40 to 295; however, only a very few have clinical significance in humans as pathogens (*Bacillus anthracis* and *B. cereus*), for use in scientific research and as monitors in sterilization processes (*B. subtilis* and *G. stearothermophilus*), or in the production of antibiotics such as bacitracin and polymyxin (*B. subtilis* and *B. polymyxa*).

The family *Bacillaceae* comprise the **endospore**-forming bacteria, a key virulence factor that allows the bacterial cells to survive in the soil or under adverse environmental conditions for potentially unlimited time periods. Once conditions are again favorable, the bacteria revert to a **vegetative** state and begin reproduction and colony growth (see Figure 13-1).

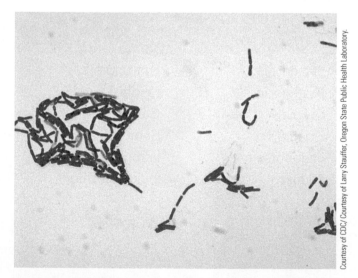

Courtesy of CDC/ Courtesy of Larry Stauffer, Oregon State Public Health Laboratory.

Figure 13-1 1000x Magnification and using the malachite green spore staining technique, the green-stained endospores are visible among the red-colored, *Bacillus anthracis* bacteria.

Bacillus anthracis

B. anthracis has been causing disease in humans for centuries. It was the first species of bacteria proven to be directly responsible for causing disease in humans. As discussed in Chapter 1, Robert Koch grew the bacteria in laboratory culture in 1877, showing its ability to form spores, and injected the cells into animals to produce the anthrax disease (see Figure 13-2).

The bacteria are viewed as single or paired in clinical specimens and as long chains in laboratory cultures. Two other virulence factors besides spore-forming ability are:

1. Antiphagocytic polypeptide capsule that blocks leukocytes and prevents phagocytosis
2. Anthrax toxin that consists of three components:
   a. A protective antigen: induces protective antitoxic antibodies
   b. An edema factor: necessary for the edema (swelling)-producing activity of the toxin
   c. A lethal factor: contributes to host death by oxygen depletion, shock, respiratory and/or cardiac failure, and increased vascular permeability

The three toxic components are individually ineffective; however, when they are combined, they are lethal. The capsule is non-toxic; however, it protects the cell from the **bactericidal** effects of serum and against engulfment by host phagocytes. The capsule is most important during the early course of infection, but during the later stages it plays a less significant role because the anthrax toxin is the dominant disease factor (see Figure 13-3).

Anthrax in Humans

Humans are infected by exposure to contaminated animals or their products or by direct exposure to bacterial cells by alternative means such as biological weapons. The disease itself is

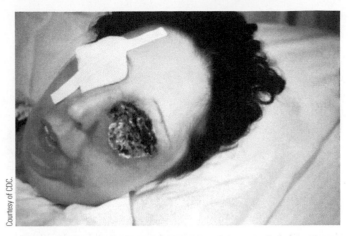

Figure 13-3 Female patient is shown here on day 24 of a *Bacillus anthracis* infection involving her left eye.

Courtesy of CDC.

acquired by inhalation, ingestion, or inoculation. The majority of infections result from the spores that are contained in contaminated soil or infected animal products, such as hides or hair, entering through exposed skin. Inhalation anthrax, also known as wool-sorters disease, results from breathing in the spores. The name wool-sorters disease originates from the former high number of individuals who became infected when processing the hair of infected goats and sheep. Rare person-to-person transmission has been documented in cases of cutaneous anthrax through contact with infected lesions. Otherwise, anthrax is not considered transmissible and quarantine of patients is unnecessary; however, contact precautions should be observed if open lesions are present.

Anthrax is commonly found in agricultural regions of Central and South America, sub-Saharan Africa, central and southwestern Asia, southern and Eastern Europe, and the islands of the Caribbean. Outbreaks in wild or domestic animals in the United States are rare, largely due to the success of widespread cattle vaccination programs.

Routes of Anthrax Transmission

Anthrax can gain entrance into the human body in one or more of four ways: cutaneous, inhalation, GI tract, or injection. As mentioned previously, anthrax spores can get into the skin, usually through a cut or scrape, resulting in cutaneous anthrax. This happens through handling of infected animals or their wool, hides, or hair. Cutaneous anthrax affects the skin and tissue around the site of infection and is most often seen on the head, neck, forearms, and hands (see Figure 13-4). It begins as a painless bump at the site of inoculation 1 to 7 days after exposure. It progresses to a painless ulcer approximately 1 to 3 cm in diameter with a necrotic center. Cutaneous anthrax infections are rarely fatal with initiation of medical treatment.

Inhalation anthrax may be contracted by workers in industrial wool processing plants, slaughterhouses, or animal tanneries. They may breathe in the spores when working with contaminated animals. Inhalation anthrax spores multiply rapidly in the thoracic lymph nodes and then spread

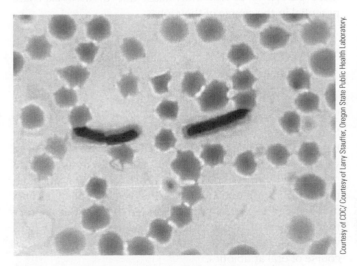

Figure 13-2 Photomicrograph of the ultrastructural morphology depicted by Gram-positive *Bacillus anthracis* bacteria.

Courtesy of CDC/ Courtesy of Larry Stauffer, Oregon State Public Health Laboratory.

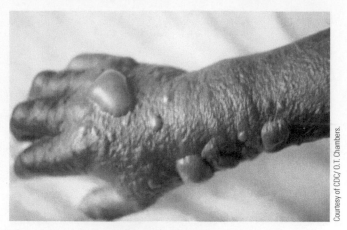

Courtesy of CDC/ O.T. Chambers.

Figure 13-4 Dorsal view of right forearm and hand with a cluster of boils, or carbuncles, primarily on the hand and wrist from a cutaneous anthrax infection caused by the bacterium *Bacillus anthracis*.

throughout the rest of the body in lymph fluid. Inhalation anthrax is the most lethal form of the disease. Onset of symptoms usually occurs within 7 days after exposure but may not present for up to 2 months. It is a pulmonary disease that leads to respiratory failure and systemic shock. The mortality rate is high (45 percent), even when treatment and intensive supportive measures have been initiated early in the course of the disease. Without proper prompt treatment, only 10 percent to 15 percent of infected individuals survive (see Figure 13-5).

Gastrointestinal anthrax infection can occur following ingestion of uncooked or undercooked meat from infected animals. The bacterial spores can penetrate mucosal tissues

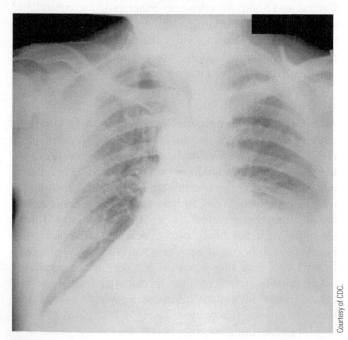

Courtesy of CDC.

Figure 13-5 PA view chest x-ray on the 4th day of a case of inhalation anthrax, caused by the bacterium, *Bacillus anthracis*. Note the radiographic characteristics of widened mediastinum and pleural effusion.

along the pharynx, esophagus, stomach, or intestines. Rarely have any cases of GI anthrax been reported in the United States. With treatment, 60 percent of individuals survive the infection; however, without treatment, more than half of the cases are fatal.

A newly recognized form of anthrax infection has not yet been seen in the United States, but injection anthrax has been documented in Europe. Injection of heroin by individuals with substance use disorder transfers bacterial spores through infected needles and directly into deep tissues or blood vessels.

Diagnosis and Treatment

B. anthracis is easily detected by observation with the use of a microscope. The cultures are obtained from skin lesions, blood, or respiratory secretions or by measuring specific antibodies in the blood of suspected infected individuals. Colonies that are grown in the laboratory are **non-hemolytic** and adherent, and they grow rapidly. Cultures and biochemical tests are used to definitively identify the characteristics of *B. anthracis*, including appearance of chains of bacilli, sticky adherence of bacteria, absence of hemolysis, and lack of motility.

Treatment with appropriate antibiotics is effective if administered before the onset of lymphatic spread or **septicemia**. Due to the ability of spores to delay activation for up to 60 days, individuals exposed to anthrax may require antibiotic therapy for 60 days after exposure. Ciprofloxacin and doxycycline are two of the antibiotics used to prevent anthrax.

Prevention

Preventative control of the disease among animals is essential. Animals should be vaccinated in endemic areas and carcasses of dead, anthrax-infected animals should be properly incinerated.

In humans, vaccination is available, prior to exposure, for three groups of at-risk individuals due to their exposure potential in the course of their jobs:

- Laboratory workers who may be exposed to anthrax
- Veterinarians who may treat potentially infected animals
- Certain members of the US Armed Forces

The anthrax vaccine adsorbed (AVA) is a licensed vaccine that provides protection against cutaneous and inhalation types of anthrax in adults between 18 and 65 years of age. The vaccine is given in five intramuscular injections over 18 months. After that, annual boosters are required to maintain prophylactic immunity. The vaccine has not been recommended for the general public except in the event of a bioterrorism incident. If that were to occur, then exposed individuals would be given three injections over 4 weeks and a 60-day course of oral antibiotics.

Spores can be killed by steam or gas sterilization or incineration. The spores can also be destroyed by boiling at 100°C for 30 minutes. The vegetative (non-endospore) cells can be killed by 0.05 percent hypochlorite solution (1 table-spoon of bleach per gallon of water).

Bioterrorism and Anthrax

The unfortunate reality of this century is that the potential for bioterrorism attacks is real and ever-present. Agencies such as the CDC have plans and protocols in place to work closely with local health agencies in the event that an attack is made, possibly involving large numbers of people. Due to the pathogenicity of anthrax in humans, animals, and plants, anthrax is a likely choice for a biological weapon based on the following criteria recognized by the CDC:

- Anthrax spores are found in nature or can be pro-duced in a lab, and they can survive for a long time, even in harsh environments.

- Anthrax makes a good weapon because it can be released discretely. The undetectable microscopic spores could be put into powders, sprays, food, and water.

- Anthrax has been used as a biological weapon before. In 2001, powdered anthrax spores were deliberately put into letters that were mailed to members of the US Congress and the television media via US mail. Twenty-two people, including 12 mail handlers, were infected with anthrax, and 5 people died from their infections.

Inhalation anthrax, the deadliest form, could potentially be distributed in large population areas without detection. Until large numbers of affected individuals seek medical attention, the incident might go unnoticed. Delay in treatment of any form of anthrax greatly increases the potential for fatality.

Emergency Preparedness

The CDC recommends that families should not panic, but rather should consider preparing emergency kits for any potential natural or man-made disasters. In the event of a bioterrorism attack with anthrax, public health departments would set up large-scale response facilities called points of dispensing (PODs) for the distribution of antibiotics to those exposed. Individuals should bring information with them pertaining to their medical history, medications being taken, and allergies. Once antibiotics have been prescribed, it is important for individuals to continue to take them as directed until finished, even if it seems like a long course.

Recognition of the signs and symptoms of inhalation anthrax will help those who were possibly exposed to decide when to seek medical treatment. These signs and symptoms are:

- Fever, chills, cough
- Shortness of breath
- Chest pain or discomfort
- Headache
- Nausea, vomiting, abdominal cramps
- Exhaustion and body aches
- Drenching sweat

Bacillus cereus

Most *Bacillus* species are considered opportunistic pathogens that have a low level of virulence; however, the other species that is clearly a pathogen is *B. cereus*. It is known to be the cause of ocular infections, IV catheter sepsis, and gastroenteritis. Like *B. anthracis*, it is commonly found in the soil and is a Gram-positive, facultative anaerobic organism that is motile, spore-forming, and hemolytic-positive.

Gastroenteritis infections from *B. cereus* are characterized by an **emetic** toxin that causes vomiting and three enterotoxins that are cytotoxic and cause severe diarrhea. Symptoms resemble those from other forms of food poisoning (*S. aureus*, *Clostridium perfringens*). The infection usually runs its course in 24 hours. The bacteria are transferred to prepared foods and multiply rapidly at room temperature. The spores make destruction difficult, even with heating of contaminated food.

B. cereus has been reported in a number of cases of severe **endophthalmitis**. There are two forms of the infection: exogenous, which results from external trauma to the eye, and endogenous, which results from bacteria gaining access to the posterior chamber of the eye through the blood supply. Seventy percent of the cases reported resulted in total loss of vision due to enucleation (surgical removal) or evisceration (rupture of membranes) of the infected eye.

Some researchers have started to examine the possibility of many more cases of *B. cereus* causing serious, non-intestinal, invasive systemic disease. Two metal workers from different cities in Texas suffered fatal cases of pneumonia and sepsis caused by *B. cereus* in 2007. More focus will likely be given to *B. cereus* in the future because it is a more pathogenic bacterial species than previously believed.

The other infections caused by *B. cereus* and *B. subtilis* include central nervous system infections acquired after the insertion of **ventriculoperitoneal** or **ventriculoatrial** shunts that are used to treat hydrocephalus and endocarditis acquired after the insertion of intravascular catheters.

Diagnosis and Treatment

B. cereus and the other *Bacillus* species are easily grown in the laboratory. To confirm food poisoning, the food should be cultured. Isolation of the microbe from the patient is difficult and not attempted due to the high rate of fecal contamination. The diarrheal toxin can be detected using an animal model (e.g., rabbit ileal loop). The emetic toxin is only detected when the microbe is grown on media prepared with rice, confirming that rice is the most common food contaminated with *B. cereus*. *B. cereus* is easily detected in specimens taken from individuals who have an infection in the eye or a catheter.

Gastroenteritis has such a fast course of symptoms that treatment is focused on preventing dehydration. Food poisoning is best prevented by the proper refrigeration and cooking of food. Temperatures less than 212°F (100°C) can allow some of the spores to survive the cooking process and spread bacterial contamination.

Listeria Species

Listeria is a genus that consists of six species, although *Listeria monocytogenes* and *L. ivanovii* are the only species that cause disease in humans. *Listeria* is a Gram-positive, non-spore-forming, catalase-positive, facultative anaerobe that causes food poisoning, meningitis, and bacteremia. The microbe is motile at room temperature but not at 37°C (98.6°F), which is a useful characteristic for identification purposes. *Listeria* is found in soil samples around the world. More than 40 species of wild and domesticated mammals, 17 species of birds, and up to 10 percent of humans are known to be reservoirs of *Listeria* with no expression of disease (see Figure 13-6).

Listeria monocytogenes is an intracellular pathogen that grows in macrophages and epithelial cells. In laboratory cultures it grows in fibroblasts. The bacterial cells produce the **hemolysin** listeriolysin O. The hemolysin is needed for the bacterium to be released from the host cell. The process of growth occurs in the following manner:

- The *Listeria* cell binds to specific surface receptors on the macrophage or epithelial cell, causing phagocytosis. The bacterium enters the cell in an **endosome**.

- Before the endosome attaches to lysosomes and is killed by the enzymes, listeriolysin dissolves the endosome membrane.

- The bacterium then replicates and moves to the surface of the cell.

- Two pseudopods develop, one for the release of the new bacterium and the other for transfer of the bacterial cell to another macrophage or epithelial cell to begin the process again.

Gram-stain preparations of cerebrospinal fluid (CSF) may not reveal *Listeria* microbes. This is due to the fact that they are present in very low concentrations as compared to other meningitis-causing bacteria that are readily present. *Listeria* readily grows on most kinds of laboratory culture and is observed as round colonies after 1 or 2 days of incubation. The bacterial cell's motility is also used for identification purposes when cells are grown in a liquid medium or semisolid agar.

It is relatively uncommon for the organism to cause disease in healthy humans, and it is known to cause disease in people who are immunocompromised or over age 65 and pregnant females. Laboratory studies are only performed in cases with a strong suspicion of *Listeria* infection, and definitive diagnosis is made when bacteria are isolated in cultures of blood, CSF, or amniotic fluid samples.

Listeriosis

Listeria monocytogenes is the cause of a common food-borne disease called listeriosis. Listeriosis is the third leading cause of death from food poisoning, according to the CDC. One of the most effective means of reducing bacterial contamination is proper hand washing (see Figure 13-7). Annually in the United States, 1,600 individuals are infected with *Listeria* and 260 die. Ninety percent of those who show symptoms are from the at-risk group (older adults, pregnant females, and patients who are immunocompromised), and approximately 20 percent suffer fatal complications of the illness. Individuals older than age 65 years account for 58 percent of listeriosis cases and are four-times more likely than the general public to become infected. Meningitis is the most common form of *Listeria* infection in adults. *Listeria*-caused meningitis should always be suspected in organ transplant patients, patients with cancer, or pregnant females. Bacteremia is relatively asymptomatic, with the patient presenting with general flu-like symptoms of chills, muscle aches, and possibly high fever.

Pregnant females account for 14 percent of listeriosis cases. They are 10-times more likely to become infected with *Listeria* than the general public and may suffer miscarriage

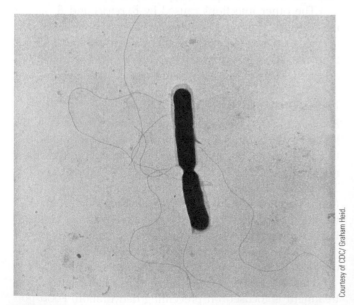

Figure 13-6 TEM image of the ultrastructural details of a *Listeria* sp. bacterium, including the presence of peritrichous flagella on the cell wall. Note that the bacterium was in the process of replicating by way of cell division.

Courtesy of CDC/ Graham Heid.

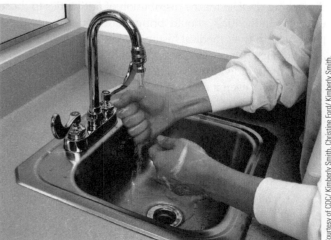

Figure 13-7 Image of proper handwashing as an effective way to prevent disease transmission.

Courtesy of CDC/ Kimberly Smith, Christine Ford/ Kimberly Smith.

due to listeriosis. Transmission can also be from mother to fetus, resulting in bacteremia, meningitis, or death in the immediate perinatal period. Hispanic pregnant females are 24-times more likely to become infected, possibly due to the higher likelihood of consumption of unpasteurized milk or contaminated pasteurized soft cheeses such as queso fresco. Because the onset of symptoms may be delayed following ingestion of contaminated food, causation may be missed. The two forms of perinatal infections are:

- Early-onset disease: bacterial cells are transferred to the fetus by the mother across the placenta or when the amniotic membranes rupture at the time of birth. This happens when the mother eats contaminated food while pregnant.

- Late-onset disease: acquired during or soon after birth.

Early-onset disease is medically known as granulomatosis infantiseptica. It is a severe disease that has a high mortality rate. Often spontaneous abortion in the second or third trimester or stillbirth will occur after infection. If the baby is born, then the infection is characterized by the formation of abscesses and granulomas in many of the body organs. Late-onset disease usually occurs 2 to 3 weeks after birth, and the infant will have either meningitis or meningo-encephalitis with septicemia. The signs and symptoms of *Listeria* meningitis are the same as those caused by other organisms (such as *Streptococcus*), so these other organisms must be excluded as the causative pathogen.

Patients who are immunocompromised are those individuals with cancer or undergoing cancer chemotherapy, those using chronic steroids for rheumatoid arthritis, anti-rejection drugs for organ transplant recipients, or other conditions, those with chronic or acute kidney or liver disease, and those living with HIV/AIDS.

Outbreaks of Listeriosis

Listeriosis usually peaks during the warmer months of the year, even though occasional cases are seen throughout the year. Studies have shown that the majority of listeriosis cases are food-borne. In comparison to other food-borne diseases, *L. monocytogenes* infections have the highest mortality rate. The microbe can grow in a wide pH range as well as in cold temperatures. Even with refrigeration, the bacterial cells are not affected and will continue to slowly multiply in the contaminated food, which attests to the strength of the non-spore-forming bacterium (see Figure 13-8).

Vegetables become contaminated from the soil or manure that is used as fertilizer. Animals will carry the bacteria and are asymptomatic but contaminate the food of origin, such as the meat or dairy products from cows. *Listeria* is killed by proper pasteurization when processing milk and by adequate heating procedures when preparing ready-to-eat processed meats. Recent past decades have seen foodborne listeriosis outbreaks in the United States involving caramel apples, mung bean sprouts, cheese and cream products, and cantaloupes.

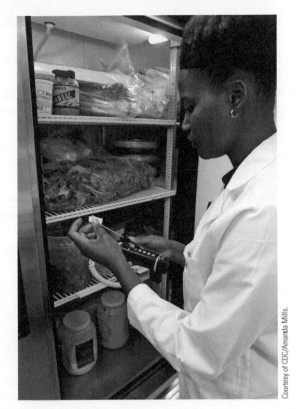

Figure 13-8 Health inspector taking thermal readings of refrigerated foods.

Prevention and Treatment

The United States Food and Drug Administration (FDA) and the CDC have reporting and surveillance programs in place for many types of diseases, including listeriosis. Additionally, they provide numerous online resources for the public to learn how to prevent food-borne illnesses (see Figure 13-9). Some of these strategies for the general public include:

- Rinse all raw produce (even those that will be peeled).
- Scrub firm produce (melons, cucumbers, squash).
- Dry the rinsed or scrubbed produce with clean paper towels.

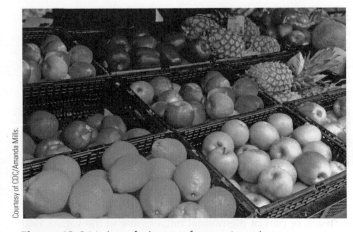

Figure 13-9 Various fruits at a farmers' market.

- Separate uncooked foods from cooked foods to prevent cross-contamination.
- Keep kitchen surfaces clean, especially after preparation of raw meats.
- Keep refrigerator surfaces and bins clean. *L. monocytogenes* can grow in refrigerators if not kept at or below 40° F (4.4°C) and the freezer compartment below 32°F (0° C).
- Cook meat and poultry to proper internal temperatures.
- Store prepared, pre-cooked foods properly. Special attention should be given to deli meats and cheeses and leftovers.
- Choose safe foods; do not drink unpasteurized milk or eat unpasteurized cheeses.

Additional precautions for at-risk individuals include:

- Avoid processed deli meats and store-prepared deli salads. Only eat hot dogs or sausages that have been heated to an internal temperature of 165°F (74°C) just prior to eating.
- Only eat soft cheeses that have been made with pasteurized milk. Be aware that some soft Mexican-style cheeses (queso fresco) may state they are made with pasteurized milk but have been shown to be contaminated with *Listeria* during production.
- Avoid refrigerated smoked seafood. Canned seafood and seafood cooked to proper temperature immediately before eating are considered safe.

Appropriate antibiotic therapy is used to treat *L. monocytogenes* infections. Individuals listed as high-risk are advised to avoid eating raw animal foods, cheeses, and unwashed raw vegetables. When infection occurs during pregnancy, antibiotics are immediately given to the pregnant female to prevent infection of the fetus. A vaccine is not available.

Lactobacillus

Lactobacillus is an important genus of lactic acid–producing, Gram-positive, rod-shaped, non-spore-forming bacteria that are considered facultative anaerobic or strictly anaerobic. *Lactobacillus* species are capable of growing in the presence of oxygen, but due to inefficient metabolism they grow poorly. However, the growth of other microbes is inhibited by the production of lactic acid, allowing the *Lactobacillus* to grow. Because it only produces lactic acid, it is referred to as homolactic. The lactic acid is produced from simple carbohydrates. Lactic acid production can spoil food; however, the process is important in the food industry in producing pickles from cucumbers, sauerkraut from cabbage, and yogurt from milk.

In humans, the species in the genus *Lactobacillus* are commensals, or part of the normal microbiome of the vagina, oral cavity, and intestinal tract. In the female, the normal vaginal microflora is influenced by the level of sex hormones. Within a few weeks after birth, the female infant's vagina has a population of lactobacilli. The lactobacilli are able to grow due to the transfer of estrogens from maternal to fetal blood, causing glycogen to be established in the cells that line the vagina. Lactobacilli convert the glycogen to lactic acid, and the pH level in the vagina becomes acidic. This provides an environment for acid-tolerant normal microflora to grow in the vagina.

As the estrogens decrease, other bacteria, such as *Corynebacterium*, become part of the normal microbial population. The result is a neutral pH until puberty. With the onset of puberty, the estrogen levels increase again, glycogen increases as it interacts with the lactobacilli, and the vagina once again becomes acidic. In the adult female, oral contraceptives, spermicides, and pregnancy increase glycogen. The normal resident microbes are destroyed during antibiotic therapy, upsetting the homeostasis of the vaginal microbiome. This imbalance can lead to vaginitis or urinary tract infections.

Researchers, including Martin Blaser, MD, theorize that the *Lactobacillus* species in a pregnant female's vagina plays a key role in establishing the first microbial population in the newborn as the fetus passes through the vaginal vault, becoming covered with lactobacilli. As the newborn is handed to its mother and allowed to nurse for the first time, the lactobacilli on the newborn's skin is transferred to the mother's breast and then swallowed by the infant with the colostrum (first milk produced after childbirth). The lactobacilli and other lactic acid–producing bacterial species then break down lactose, the predominant sugar found in milk, for use as energy by the infant and ensures that bacteria in the newborn's intestinal tract include species that can digest milk. These species have antibiotic properties that prevent dangerous bacteria from colonizing the newborn's gastrointestinal tract.

Dr. Blaser and other researchers express concern of the increase in rates of Cesarean section deliveries and the potential long-term effects on neonatal health. Scientists who studied the microbial populations of infants following both vaginal and C-section deliveries found that in the C-section group, lactobacilli were missing and bacteria normally found on skin and in the environment (*Staphylococcus, Corynebacterium, and Propionibacterium*) were present instead.

Additional studies of the behavior of vaginal microflora have revealed that some of the *Lactobacillus* species, specifically *L. jensenii* and *L. crispatus*, produce **bacteriocins** that may inhibit HIV. Bacteriocins are proteinaceous toxins produced by some species of bacteria that are protective defenses that inhibit growth of similar types of bacteria. These studies also established a relationship between a reduced number of these species in the vagina and transmission of HIV during sexual intercourse.

Nearly every species of commensal bacteria can become opportunistic pathogens if given access to sterile tissues. The systemic disease that *Lactobacillus* is associated with is endocarditis. Antibiotic resistance may be a concerning factor in treatment of endocarditis caused by *Lactobacillus*. If the damage to the heart valve is extensive, the patient must undergo heart valve replacement surgery.

Clostridium Species

The genus *Clostridium* includes all anaerobic, Gram-positive bacilli that produce endospores. The majority of members are strictly anaerobic; however, some species are aerotolerant. More than 100 species have been discovered. The microorganisms are widespread, found in water, soil, sewage, and often are part of the **indigenous flora** in the gastrointestinal tracts of animals and humans. Most species are harmless, but those that are well-known opportunistic human pathogens cause serious, often fatal diseases, including:

- Gas gangrene: *Clostridium perfringens, C novyi, C. septicum, C. histolyticum, C. sordellii*
- Botulism: *Clostridium barati, C. botulinum, C. butyricum*
- Tetanus: *Clostridium tetani*
- Colitis: *Clostridioides difficile (previously Clostridium difficile)*

The virulence factors that make *Clostridium* bacteria powerful pathogens include: protection from harsh environmental conditions by formation of spores; production of toxins, including enterotoxins and neurotoxins; and rapid growth periods in low-oxygen or no-oxygen areas.

Clostridium perfringens

C. perfringens can cause the severe and life-threatening gas gangrene infection. It is one of the few non-motile clostridia, although it rapidly grows on laboratory culture. The organism produces four lethal toxins, alpha, beta, epsilon, and iota toxins, which are used to subdivide it into five types (A, B, C, D, and E). *C. perfringens* type A is the cause of most human infections. Type A *C. perfringens* is a common inhabitant of the GI tract of humans and animals and is also found in soil and water that has been contaminated with feces. This habitat accounts for many of the infections suffered by humans who experience a traumatic injury that is contaminated by soil and/or water. Types B, C, D, and E do not survive in the soil and primarily colonize the GI tract of animals and, in rare cases, humans. Type A is the cause of gas gangrene, food poisoning, and soft tissue infections. Type C causes necrotizing enteritis.

Toxins

C. perfringens can cause a wide spectrum of diseases, with one of the most serious being myonecrosis (muscle tissue destruction), which has a high mortality rate even with rapid medical attention. The pathogenicity of the species is associated with the 12 toxins and enzymes it produces, some of which are minor and others lethal. The major toxins are discussed in the order of their lethality and importance.

Alpha toxin is produced by all types of *C. perfringens*; however, type A produces the largest quantities of the toxin. Lecithinase, a phospholipase enzyme, lyses erythrocytes, platelets, endothelial cells, and leukocytes. The toxin is responsible for increased vascular permeability with massive hemolysis, bleeding, myonecrosis, bradycardia (slow heart rate), hypotension, and hepatic toxicity.

Beta toxin causes necrosis in the small intestine and induces hypertension by causing the release of catecholamines. Epsilon toxin is activated by trypsin and increases the vascular permeability of the gastrointestinal wall. Iota toxin aids in increasing vascular permeability and necrotic activity.

Enterotoxin is a protein produced within the colon and released during spore formation. It is produced primarily by type A *C. perfringens*. It enters the cell membranes of the ileum and jejunum, altering the membranes and disrupting ion transport. To produce the enterotoxin, many cells from contaminated food must be ingested. Antibodies are found in individuals previously exposed to enterotoxin, but they do not confer any type of protection.

Diseases of *C. perfringens*

Myonecrosis, better known as gas gangrene, is a well-known and serious infection that shows the ability of the entire spectrum of damaging toxins. The prognosis is poor, with a reported mortality rate of 40 percent to 100 percent. The organism is introduced into the tissue by traumatic injury or surgery. The patient experiences the following signs and symptoms:

- Fever, profuse perspiration
- Pain and swelling of tissues
- Anxiety and increased heart rate
- Vomiting and jaundice
- Pale skin that turns gray, brownish-red, or black
- Air under the skin with crackling noise when touched
- Blisters with foul-smelling discharge

Pathological examinations of affected muscle reveal necrotic tissue and gas located in the tissue due to the metabolic activity of the dividing bacteria, thereby the name gas gangrene. The toxins, as previously discussed, cause extensive hemolysis and hemorrhaging (see Figure 13-10).

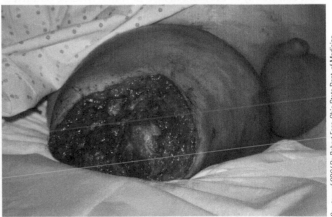

Courtesy of CDC/ Dr. Robert Fass, Ohio State Dept. of Medicine

Figure 13-10 Right thigh of a patient who had a re-amputation on the leg at a higher level than the initial excision due to development of gas gangrene in the tissues more proximal than the level of the initial amputation.

C. perfringens and *C. septicum* are also causative agents that cause **cellulitis**, a less serious disease process, and **fasciitis**, another serious and debilitating disease. Fasciitis rapidly progresses, much like gas gangrene; however, the tissue layer involved is the fascial layer that covers skeletal muscle and produces the characteristic gas.

C. perfringens is the third highest cause of food-borne disease and is responsible for nearly 1 million cases per year. Type A *C. perfringens* is responsible for causing the infection. The infection is the result of ingesting contaminated meats that contain a large number of the microbial cells. Enterotoxin is produced after the spores germinate in tissues and stimulates the release of cytokines from lymphocytes. The infected individual will have abdominal cramps and diarrhea without fever, nausea, or vomiting. The infection typically resolves within 24 hours and antibiotic therapy is not necessary. Refrigerating food prevents the production of enterotoxin and reheating also destroys the toxin.

Necrotizing enteritis is a rare infection that occurs in the jejunum, but it has devastating effects and a high mortality rate of 50 percent. Type C *C. perfringens* is responsible for causing the infection and produces the beta toxin. Upon pathological examination of the tissue of the jejunum, widespread necrosis of the tissue is found. The patient experiences severe abdominal pain, bloody diarrhea, **shock**, and **peritonitis** due to the escape of microbes through the necrotic intestinal tissue and into the peritoneal cavity.

Clostridium botulinum

Clostridium botulinum are Gram-positive, rod-shaped, spore-forming, mainly anaerobic bacteria that are subdivided into four groups, I, II, III, and IV, based on the toxin that is produced. The strains of types I and II are the cause of most human diseases. Seven botulinum toxins, A through G, have been described. Toxins A, B, E, and F are associated with human infections. The A toxin contains the neurotoxin subunit, and the B toxin contains a non-toxic subunit that protects the neurotoxin from being destroyed by gastric acids. *C. botulinum* is found worldwide, most commonly in the soil but also in water. Disease outbreaks in the United States are uncommon.

Botulinum Toxins

Botulinum toxin is similar to the tetanus toxin, except that it targets the cholinergic nerves. It blocks the release of the neurotransmitter acetylcholine at the synaptic junction. As with the tetanus toxin, the patient recovers when the nerve endings regenerate. *C. botulinum* also produces a binary toxin that consists of two components that increase vascular permeability.

Botulism

Botulism is a serious muscle-paralyzing disease caused by the toxic effects of the bacterium *C. botulinum*. *Clostridium butyricum* and *Clostridium baratii* have also been isolated in cases of botulism. There are five types of botulism: food-borne, wound, infant, adult intestinal toxemia, and **iatrogenic**.

On average, there are 145 cases reported each year according to the CDC. Food-borne botulism (15 percent of reported cases) is caused by the ingestion of canned foods contaminated by type A and type B toxins. Wound botulism (20 percent of reported cases) is considered relatively rare. Infant botulism (65 percent of reported cases) is the most frequent infection and is associated with the consumption of contaminated foods, particularly honey; however, botulism spores are found almost everywhere and infants can also be infected from environmental sources. Adult intestinal toxemia botulism and iatrogenic botulism are considered very rare.

In food-borne botulism, a rare but serious infection, symptoms manifest within 6 hours to 10 days, typically between 12 and 36 hours after ingestion of infected food. Signs of the paralysis caused by botulism toxins include:

- Abdominal cramping and constipation
- Double or blurred vision; drooping eyelids
- Dry mouth, slurred speech, and trouble swallowing
- Bilateral flaccid muscle weakness that progresses from the shoulder and neck level down toward torso and lower extremities
- Diaphragmatic paralysis causes individuals to stop breathing and requires mechanical ventilator assistance until function returns

Respiratory paralysis occurs because of the aggressiveness of the neurotoxin that irreversibly binds to the cholinergic nerves and blocks the neurotransmitters. Patients on ventilators may require supportive care for weeks to months (possibly even 1 year or more) before diaphragmatic function is regained. No fever is present throughout the course of the infection. Food-borne botulism is not spread from person to person.

Food-borne botulism may be prevented by practicing proper food handling and storage, especially in cases of home canning. Additionally, foods should be properly heated to kill bacterial contaminants and promptly refrigerated at adequate temperatures to prevent colonization in foods. Commercially canned foods should be examined for signs of possible botulism: leaking, bulging, rusting, or badly dented cans; cracked jars; jars with loose or bulging lids; foul odor; or any container that spurts liquid when opening. Resources are available through county health departments, the Centers for Disease Control and Prevention, and the US Food and Drug Administration.

Wound botulism, as indicated, is relatively rare. The name indicates that *C. botulinum* is introduced into a traumatic wound either by contaminated soil that enters through fissures in the skin or during the perioperative period (see Figure 13-11). The clinical signs and symptoms are similar to food-borne botulism, except the incubation period is longer and there may be no abdominal symptoms. The CDC states that most wound botulism cases are associated with injection of black-tar heroin, especially in California.

Infant botulism was first described in 1976 and is currently considered the most common form of botulism in the United States. Typically, infants between 1 and 6 months of age are affected. Infants lack the full spectrum of indigenous intes-

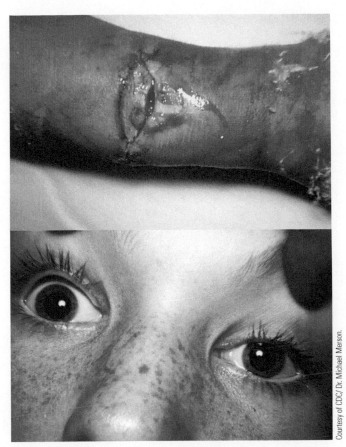

Figure 13-11-Top. Volar view of the arm of a 14 year-old patient who had a penetrating wound due to a compound fracture of the right ulna and radius just proximal to the wrist, and although treated, developed wound botulism. **Bottom.** same patient's eyes showing bilateral pupillary dilation due to the systemic dissemination of the botulinum toxin.

tinal or "gut" microflora, as previously discussed, and are at risk for developing an infection because *C. botulinum* microbes do not have to compete for establishment within the GI tract. Symptoms include droopy eyes, weak cry, poor sucking reflex, constipation, lethargy, flaccid paralysis (also called "floppy baby syndrome"), and, ultimately, respiratory failure. If any of these cascading symptoms are observed in an infant, immediate medical attention should be sought (see Figure 13-12).

Prevention of infant botulism is focused on avoiding foods that may contain the *C. botulinum* spores, which then grow in the intestinal tract and release the deadly toxins. Honey has been found to be the most common cause; however, corn syrups and peanut butter may also be potential sources. It is recommended that honey should not be given to infants younger than age 1 year. Numerous environmental surfaces may contain spores of *C. botulinum*, increasing exposure potential.

Adult intestinal toxemia botulism is a very rare infection that results from intestinal colonization. It is basically an adult form of infant botulism. Between 2006 and 2008, there were five cases of adult intestinal toxemia botulism reported in Ontario, Canada. Two patients were believed to have ingested contaminated carrot juice. In two cases, the patients

had a history of Crohn's disease and bowel surgeries in the distant past. One of the patients had ingested contaminated peanut butter. Researchers theorized that pre-existing bowel disease may be an elevated risk factor.

Iatrogenic botulism occurs as a complication of therapeutic botulinum A toxin. Patients may be injected with Botox® for treatment of muscle spasticity including cervical dystonia or bladder spasticity, chronic migraine headaches, hyperhidrosis (excessive sweating), or for cosmetic facial skin wrinkle treatment. Iatrogenic infections may be as a result of doses higher than recommended or vascular uptake of the injected toxin.

Clostridium tetani

The spores of the organism, *Clostridium tetani*, are easy to identify: They are rounded at the end of the cell and then a rod extends from the spore, forming what looks like a chicken or turkey drumstick (see Figure 13-13). In the laboratory, *C. tetani* is difficult to grow due to its extreme sensitivity to any level of oxygen and a low level of metabolic activity.

C. tetani is widespread; it is found in the soil and colonizes the GI tracts of humans and animals. As mentioned, the microorganism is extremely susceptible to oxygen, but it rapidly **sporulates** to survive in nature. In the United States, disease has been rare since the development of the tetanus vaccination. Since the mid-1970s, an average of 50–100 cases have been reported annually in the United States and in 2018, 23 cases were reported with no deaths. Most individuals are familiar with the vaccination that is usually given any time a person "steps on a rusty nail" or receives some type of penetrating injury with a "dirty" item. However, in other parts of

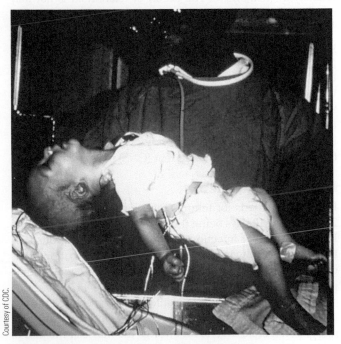

Figure 13-12 Infant with "floppy baby syndrome" signs of infant botulism.

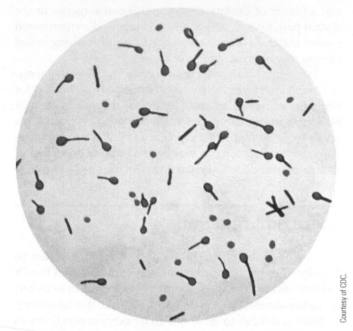

Figure 13-13 Illustration depicts a photomicrographic view of methylene blue spore–stained *Clostridium tetani* bacteria.

Courtesy of CDC.

the world, especially developing countries where the tetanus vaccine is not as readily available, the mortality rate can be high, with many deaths occurring in neonates. Cases in the United States are often a result of missed vaccinations or failure to get booster vaccinations every 10 years.

Tetanus Toxins

C. tetani produces two toxins: tetanospasmin (neurotoxin) and tetanolysin (hemolysin). The action of tetanolysin is not fully understood and has not been revealed in the laboratory. Tetanospasmin is produced during the bacterial stationary phase of growth and released upon cell lysis. It is the agent causing the primary clinical signs and symptoms of a tetanus infection. It acts by blocking neurotransmitters at the inhibiting synapse, thus causing constant excitatory synaptic activity known as **spastic paralysis**. In contrast to *C. botulinum*, it does not affect the transmission of acetylcholine. Once the toxin has bound, it is irreversible and recovery depends on the regeneration of axonal terminals of central nervous system (CNS) neurons.

Diseases of *C. tetani*

Incubation periods for tetanus infections are between 3 and 21 days, with 10 days being the average. As a general rule, the farther the site of infection is from the central nervous system, the longer the incubation time. Shorter incubation times correlate with increased severity of the disease, higher complication rates, and fatality.

The most common form of infection is generalized tetanus (80 percent of cases). Trismus, also known as lockjaw is the most recognized manifestation and involves the masseter muscles of the face. The characteristic "smile" that results from the constant contraction of the masseter muscles is called risus sardonicus or

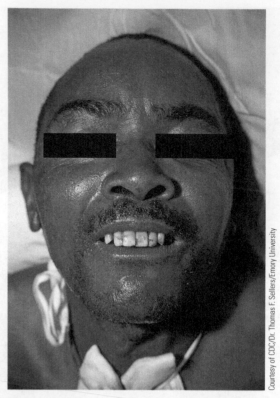

Courtesy of CDC/Dr. Thomas F. Sellers/Emory University

Figure 13-14 Facial tetany: note the contraction of the masseter and neck muscles.

rictus grin (see Figure 13-14). Other characteristic signs of tetanus are sweating, restlessness, and chronic back spasm and arching referred to as **opisthotonos** (see Figure 13-15). As the disease progresses, the autonomic nervous system is involved and the signs include profound sweating that can lead to dehydration, alternating hypertension and hypotension, and cardiac arrhythmias. The fatality rate for generalized tetanus is 10 to 20 percent.

A less severe form of tetanus is localized tetanus, in which the infection remains localized to the muscles at the site of infection. The localized tetanus is typically mild; however, cases of conversion to generalized tetanus have been reported.

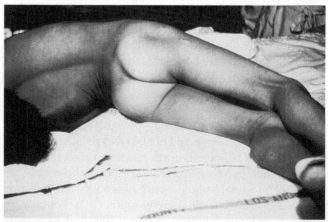

Courtesy of CDC.

Figure 13-15 Adult with advanced case of tetanus experiencing severe back spasm known as opisthotonos due to *Clostridium tetani* exotoxin.

The rarest and most life-threatening type of tetanus is cephalic tetanus. The primary site of infection is the head or face and has been associated with otitis media infections. Unlike generalized and localized tetanus, cephalic tetanus results in flaccid cranial nerve palsies (paralyses) rather than spasm. Spasm of the jaw muscles may also be present. Incubation is short (1–2 days). Cephalic tetanus can also become generalized.

Neonatal tetanus (tetanus neonatorum) is a deadly infection of the umbilical stump of an infant. After the umbilicus falls off, it may become infected and the disease then becomes generalized. Incubation is typically 4 to 14 days, with 7 days being the average. The mortality rate is close to 100 percent and infants that do survive often have developmental complications (see Figure 13-16).

Treatment and Prevention

Tetanus is a medical emergency requiring hospitalization, immediate treatment with human tetanus immunoglobulin, a tetanus toxoid booster, anti-spasm medications, aggressive wound care, and antibiotics. Tetanus antitoxin (of equine origin) in a single large dose should be given intravenously if immunoglobulin is not available. Mechanical ventilation and medications to control autonomic nervous system instability may be required in generalized tetanus cases. An adequate airway may be established by tracheostomy or nasotracheal intubation. Subsequently, mechanically assisted respiration may be required. Sedatives and muscle relaxants may be used to control muscle spasms.

A tetanus vaccine has been available for many years. In cases of active tetanus infection, a vaccination is given concurrently with supportive treatment. Prophylactically, a series of three doses is given (Tdap) with the recommendation that a booster shot should be given every 10 years thereafter to maintain immunity.

Clostridioides difficile

Clostridioides difficile, until recently called *Clostridium difficile*, is a Gram-positive, rod-shaped, anaerobic, spore-forming bacillus that has gotten the attention of public health departments and national organizations such as the Joint Commission and CDC because of the predominance of outbreaks being healthcare-associated infections (HAIs). The name was given to *C. difficile* in the 1930s because of the difficulty microbiologists had in isolating it in culture (see Figure 13-17). More recently, it is often referred to as "*C. diff.*"

C. difficile is found in soil, like many other species of bacteria, and is also a commensal in the human gastrointestinal tract. The opportunistic pathogen has multiple virulence factors that make it very difficult to treat. It is resistant to heat and stomach acids. In the intestinal tract, it secretes toxins that damage the colon, causing severe, long-lasting diarrheal disease (see Figure 13-18).

The factor that makes the infection an HAI is that in nearly all cases, patients have a history of frequent, long-term use of antibiotic treatments. The antibiotics given are ineffective against the *C. difficile* bacteria. In killing off resident microbial species, the pathogenic and toxic *C. difficile* colonies proliferate unchallenged by competing and defending resident organisms. Compounding the problem is the fact that patients are typically in the healthcare setting due to other health problems for which the antibiotic therapy may have been initiated and the transmission has been linked to poor hand hygiene of healthcare workers (HCWs). *C. difficile* is shed in feces and able to survive in its spore state on environmental surfaces for long periods. Any inanimate surface (fomite) can become a temporary reservoir for *C. difficile* bacterial spores. Direct contact of the patient with contaminated surfaces or indirect contact from hands of others who have touched contaminated items or surfaces transfers the bacteria to at-risk patients. The fecal-oral route of transmission is also a common and efficient method of infection.

Symptoms of *C. difficile* include fever, abdominal pain and tenderness, nausea, loss of appetite, and frequent watery diarrheal stools (3 or more per day for 3 or more days). Older adults, infants, and immunocompromised patients are at high risk for dehydration due to the loss of fluids and electrolytes in diarrheal stools. In severe cases of colonic injury, patients may undergo colon resection to remove infected and necrotic sections of bowel.

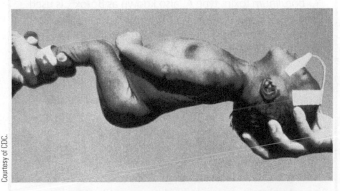

Figure 13-16 Neonate displaying bodily rigidity produced by *Clostridium tetani* exotoxin, called "neonatal tetanus."

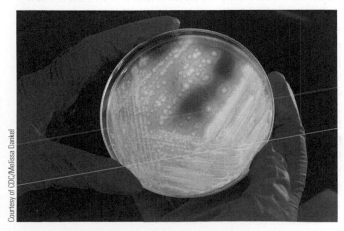

Figure 13-17 Culture plate illuminated with uv irradiation shows *Clostridium difficile* bacterial colonies that emitted a yellow-green, fluorescent glow.

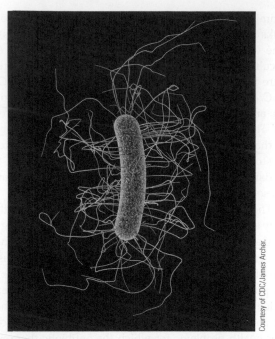

Courtesy of CDC/James Archer.

Figure 13-18 Ultrastructural morphology exhibited by a single Gram-positive *Clostridioides difficile* bacillus.

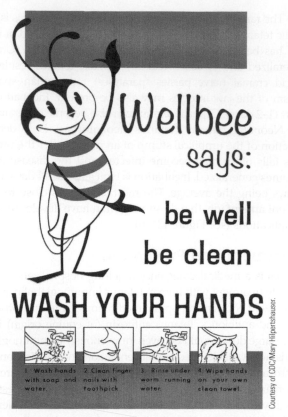

Courtesy of CDC/Mary Hilpertshauser.

Figure 13-19 This 1964 poster features the CDC's national symbol of public health "Wellbee," who was reminding the public to "be well, be clean, and WASH YOUR HANDS."

Treatment and Prevention

Discontinuation of antibiotics for other infections should be ordered if possible. Appropriate antibiotics for the *C. difficile* infection are ordered, although it may seem counterintuitive to prescribe more antibiotics when the problem was caused by the inappropriate use of other antibiotics. In approximately 20 percent of cases, the *C. difficile* infection returns following treatment, potentially again and again. Antibiotics of increasing strength are given for subsequent infections. It is an unfortunate realization that reinfections may be from bacteria that have developed increased resistance after each new course of treatment.

Experimental therapy involving "fecal transplantation" of uninfected feces from healthy individuals to debilitated *C. difficile* patients has shown great promise. The normal commensal bacterial species that have been killed off in the infected patient are replaced by the healthy donor's fecal microbial population, eliminating the overgrowth of *C. difficile*. Research surveillance of these treatments is ongoing and may become a standard treatment modality in the future.

Prevention of *C. difficile* is the goal. Patients and their families must learn to be their own advocates and demand that healthcare workers properly disinfect their hands by routine proper hand washing or with effective antimicrobial skin foams or gels prior to each interaction with a patient. Healthcare workers must be vigilant in maintaining proper aseptic techniques to prevent cross-contamination between patients (see Figure 13-19).

Patients must take prescribed medications, especially antibiotics, for the complete course and only as directed by their physicians. They should not seek antibiotics from multiple providers for illnesses that may not even be responsive to antibiotic therapy.

Physicians should practice restraint with regard to prescribing antibiotics, waiting until definitive culture and sensitivity results have been obtained so that antibiotics appropriate to the infection in question can be prescribed, reducing the increasing progression of antibiotic resistance.

MICRO NOTES

"Raising Eyebrows—or Not"

C. botulinum toxin, type A, also known as Botox®, is used in small doses as treatment of spasmodic torticollis, also known as cervical dystonia. The condition of severe spasm of the muscles of the neck and shoulders is a neurological disorder. The purified botulinum toxin is injected into muscles to provide relief by temporarily paralyzing the affected muscles. Botox® is also a popular cosmetic treatment for facial lines caused by natural aging. Injection into the muscles of the face relaxes the muscles and decreases the appearance of "laugh lines" or "crow's feet." Botox® has also been used for treatment of migraine headaches, hyperhidrosis (excessive sweating), and overactive bladder symptoms.

Under the Microscope

Jamal recently started moonlighting at a wound care center run by the hospital where he works and realized that the 70-year-old patient he was helping prepare for hyperbaric oxygen therapy was a diabetic who had also been undergoing chemotherapy for prostate cancer and recently had undergone a below-knee amputation (BKA) for gas gangrene in which Jamal was the CST.

1. Which types of microbes can cause gas gangrene?

2. How might the patient's diabetes and chemotherapy regimen have impacted the infectious process in his lower extremity?

3. What types of microbial characteristics contribute to the virulence of pathogenic microorganisms covered in this chapter?

4. What are preventative measures or treatments for infections caused by Gram-positive bacilli that this patient and others have available?

CHAPTER 14

Actinobacteria

Learning Objectives

After completing the study of this chapter, you will be able to:

1. Define key terms.
2. Compare and contrast the different genera of *Actinobacteria*.
3. Describe the *Corynebacterium* pathogens and the diseases they cause.
4. Describe the *Mycobacterium* pathogens and the diseases they cause.
5. Discuss the implications of drug resistance in tuberculosis.
6. Apply critical thinking skills in relating chapter material to the surgical environment of care or broader global community.

Key Terms

Filaments	Granulocytopenia	Mantoux test	Polyneuropathy
Fistula	Granuloma	Myocarditis	Pseudomembrane
Geosmins	Hypersensitivity	Papule	Trivalent
Granules	Lethargy	Pleomorphic	Ulcer

The Big Picture

The *Actinobacteria* microbes have often been misclassified and misnamed over time. The diseases they cause, however, have been responsible for human suffering for millennia. Ironically, some of the species studied have also led to development of antibiotics effective against other microbial pathogens. During your examination of the topics in this chapter, consider the following:

1. Which characteristics of these types of bacteria have caused the confusion in classification and naming?

2. Which types of systemic and local infections do the *Actinobacteria* species cause?

3. How widespread are the infections caused by these pathogens?

4. What are the challenges of treating tuberculosis infections in the United States and globally?

Clinical Significance Topic

The *Actinobacteria* species, *Streptomyces*, has been very good to the pharmaceutical industry and even better for those suffering numerous bacterial, fungal, and parasitic infections. In addition to anti-infective medications, *Streptomyces* isolates have also been used to develop anti-cancer agents. Surgical technology students studying antibiotics in pharmacology will certainly recognize the names streptomycin, tetracycline, neomycin, and chloramphenicol, and the anti-fungals nystatin and amphotericin B. This often mislabeled and misidentified family of bacteria has the same potential for becoming a pathogen as most bacteria. The study of its pathogenicity toward competing bacterial strains has given researchers insights into the most effective ways to combat bacteria by using the defense tactics of one of their own kind.

Class: Actinobacteria

The Class *Actinobacteria* is a group of Gram-positive bacteria with a high G+C (guanine and cytosine) ratio. Species belonging to this large group comprise a sizeable portion of common soil microbial life. They are crucial to the carbon cycle in nature, aiding in the decomposition of organic materials and replenishment of organic nutrients to soil. A number of species in this class are also commensals in human microbiomes. As with most types of bacteria, the majority of *Actinobacteria* play no significant role in humans; however, of those that do, several are significant pathogens.

Structurally, these bacteria have varied shapes, sizes, and characteristics. Some are aerobic while others are facultative anaerobes. Many have unique filamentous hyphae that resemble the mycelia of eukaryotic fungal organisms. This has contributed to confusion among scientists in the past who have assigned taxonomic names that imply classification as fungi with "myco" as part of the name. Species of *Mycobacterium* are bacteria that resemble fungi were named as part of that misclassification. Scientists have sequenced the genomes of 44 species of *Actinobacteria*.

Actinomyces

The genus *Actinomyces* comprises species of Gram-positive, microaerophilic to facultative anaerobic, non-spore-forming, filamentous rods. They belong to the class *Actinobacteria*. Commensal to the mouth, nose, and throat of animals and humans, these bacteria have a distinct "dust bunny" appearance when growing as **filaments**. *Actinomyces* bacteria are often misidentified as fungi because of their appearance. *Actinomyces israelii* is the normally non-pathogenic species associated with the upper aerodigestive tracts of humans that becomes pathogenic after dental procedures or abscess formation. There is discussion in the literature that proposes that *Actinomyces* may serve as a co-pathogen with other species of bacteria and that, as an individual entity, it is not an opportunistic pathogen (see Figure 14-1).

Actinomycosis

Actinomyces bovis was first isolated in 1877 as the causative agent of actinomycosis in cattle, a condition called "lumpy jaw" because of the suppurative (pus-forming) destruction of cattle jaw bones and soft tissues. The name of the disease actinomycosis, which occurs in both animals and humans, incorrectly implies that the infection is fungal. Actinomycosis is a bacterial infection, not fungal. Due to its normal presence in the mouth, nose, and throat, actinomycosis infections most commonly appear in the face and neck. The bacterial lesions create chronic swelling, suppuration, and the formation of an abscess sinus, **fistula**, or **granuloma**. The infection can penetrate multiple tissue planes. The sinus tracts can heal and become reinfected

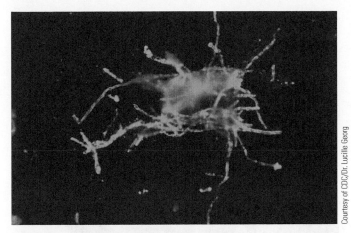

Figure 14-1 A photomicrograph of *Actinomyces israelii* under ultraviolet light, from a tonsillar infection with visible clump of the characteristic rod-shaped bacteria arranged in their common filamentous morphology and "dust bunny" appearance.

multiple times (see Figure 14-2). Actinomycosis is most commonly seen in immunosuppressed patients. The disease is not transmissible from human to human.

In rare cases, the infection can occur in the chest (pulmonary actinomycosis), abdomen, pelvis, or the brain. Pelvic infections of actinomycosis have developed after abscess formation around implanted intrauterine devices (IUDs). Infections in the thoracic cavity, abdomen, pelvis, and brain are often mistaken for tumors on diagnostic imaging studies. A definitive diagnosis cannot be made until the lesions are excised, examined by pathologists, and tissue cultures are obtained. Treatment with antibiotics may be prolonged (6–12 months) due to the tendency of the infection to recur multiple times and spread through adjacent tissues.

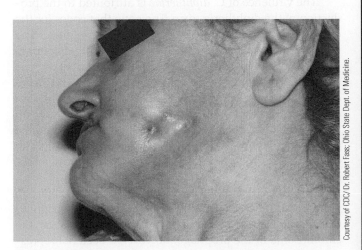

Figure 14-2 Facial fistula of the left cheek due to actinomycosis (mycetoma) infection caused by the Gram-positive, fungus-like aerobic bacteria of the order *Actinomycetales* which a slowly progressive, destructive infection of the cutaneous and subcutaneous tissues, fascia, and can progress to affect bone as well.

Corynebacterium Species

The genus *Corynebacterium* is composed of species that are non-spore-forming, Gram-positive, club-shaped or V-shaped bacilli, and either aerobic or facultative anaerobic. The microbes are generally non-motile, catalase-positive, and ferment carbohydrates that produce lactic acid. Two groups are included in the genus, *Corynebacterium diphtheriae* and all other non-diphtherial species of *Corynebacterium* referred to collectively as the diphtheroids. They normally colonize the skin, GI and GU tracts, and upper respiratory tract; however, a number of species have been identified that cause disease or are opportunistic pathogens.

Corynebacterium diphtheriae

Corynebacterium diphtheriae is a **pleomorphic** bacillus. When stained with methylene blue, it has observable **granules**. However, because many species have these same granules, it cannot be used purely for identification purposes. Another characteristic is that just after cell division, it exhibits a jerking motion that arranges the cells into patterns that have been described as resembling Chinese letters (see Figure 14-3).

Three strains of *C. diphtheriae* are gravis, intermedius, and mitis. All produce the diphtheria toxin and colonize the upper respiratory tract. The difference in virulence is due to their differing growth rates and quantity and rate of toxin production. The faster growing strains probably allow the organism to use the local iron supply more rapidly, allowing for the increased and rapid production of the diphtheria toxin. Gravis is the most virulent strain, having a generation time of 60 minutes, for intermedius it is 100 minutes, and for mitis it is 180 minutes.

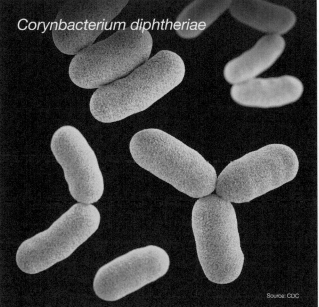

Corynbacterium diphtheriae

Source: CDC

Figure 14-3 3-D computer image of a group of Gram-positive, *Corynebacterium diphtheriae* bacteria.

Corynebacterium diphtheriae has been studied extensively, starting with Hippocrates in the fourth century. Due to well-established functions and actions of the species, effective methods of treatment and prevention have been developed. The study of *C. diphtheriae* parallels the advancements in medical microbiology as well as the understanding of the mechanisms of bacterial exotoxins.

Diphtheria

Corynebacterium diphtheriae is the causative bacterial agent for the disease known as diphtheria. Two types of the disease affect humans. Respiratory diphtheria is transmitted mainly through droplets from coughs and sneezes of infected carriers. A much less common type of diphtheria is the cutaneous form, which can be transmitted by direct contact with skin lesions. Once contact occurs, the organism is free to colonize the skin and gains access to the subcutaneous tissue when the integrity of the skin has been compromised, such as an abrasion or cut. A **papule** first develops and then progresses to an **ulcer** that is characterized by a grayish-colored membrane covering (see Figure 14-4). Infection can also occur indirectly by contact with contaminated objects.

Respiratory diphtheria is further described by the specific area most affected:

- Anterior nasal diphtheria
- Pharyngeal and tonsillar diphtheria
- Laryngeal diphtheria

Once the *C. diphtheriae* bacteria invade the respiratory tract, they produce toxins in tissues that cause fever, sore throat, weakness, and swollen lymph nodes in the neck (see Figure 14-5). A local lesion develops and necrotic injury to the epithelial cells occurs. Blood plasma leaks into the area of injury and a fibrin network forms, mixed with rapidly producing *C. diphtheriae* cells. A thick gray bacterial **pseudomembrane** develops from the fibrin network a few days after initial infection, which covers and coats upper respiratory tract structures, making breathing difficult. The

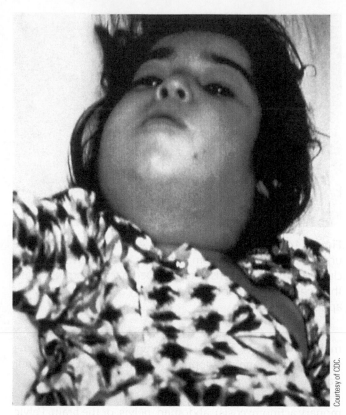

Figure 14-5 This child with diphtheria presented with a characteristic swollen neck, sometimes referred to as "bull neck."

pseudomembrane, composed of bacteria, dead cells, plasma cells, and lymphocytes, firmly adheres to tissues and is difficult to remove without causing bleeding of the underlying tissue.

The virulence of *C. diphtheriae* is attributed to the production of the diphtheria toxin. The gene that codes for the exotoxin is introduced by a lysogenic bacteriophage. The receptor site for the toxin is a heparin-binding epidermal growth factor that is present on the surface of eukaryotic cells that are abundantly located in the heart and nerve cells. This may explain why patients with severe diphtheria display cardiac and neurologic symptoms. When the toxin is released, it attaches to the host cell and enters the host cell by engulfment. It then moves into the cytoplasm and the toxin halts the production of protein, thereby destroying the cell.

Iron is an important factor in the organism's ability to produce diphtheria toxin. The gene, as mentioned previously, that codes for exotoxin production occurs on the chromosome of the prophage, however, a bacterial repressor protein controls the expression of this gene. The bacterial repressor is activated by iron, which demonstrates how the amount of iron in the bloodstream influences the production of toxin. Large amounts of toxin are rapidly produced by the lysogenic bacteria when the host has a condition of iron deficiency.

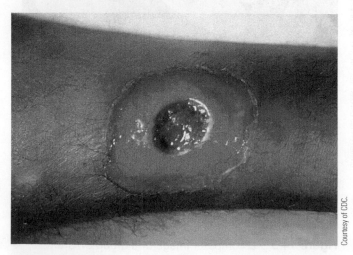

Figure 14-4 Diphtheria skin lesion on the leg.

Treatment and Prevention

The primary treatment that must be given as early as possible is the administration of the diphtheria antitoxin to neutralize the toxin before the pseudomembrane becomes established. Once the toxin enters a cell, it is irreversible and cell death occurs. Appropriate antibiotics are also given to eliminate the bacterial cells and further rid the body of the toxin. Respiratory support is provided to ensure a patent airway. The patient is placed in isolation to prevent spread to non-infected persons, and complete bed rest is required.

The disease process lasts approximately 7 to 10 days. Patients who recover will clear the dislodged membrane through expectoration (coughing up and spitting out). Complications of diphtheria include: airway obstruction; respiratory failure or pneumonia; **myocarditis**; paralysis, **polyneuropathy**; coma; and death. With appropriate treatment, 10 percent of patients may die from diphtheria. Without treatment, there is a 50 percent death rate.

Diphtheria vaccination in the United States began in the 1920s. In 1921, 206,000 cases were reported, with 15,520 deaths. Infants receive a **trivalent** vaccine that contains the tetanus toxoid, diphtheria toxoid, and pertussis vaccine (Tdap). Blood serum titers are currently used to determine individual immunity to various diseases, including diphtheria. This can be performed prior to deciding whether to administer booster doses.

Diphtheria Outbreaks

Once the diphtheria vaccine became widely available in the 1940s, reported cases declined to about 19,000 by 1945. From 1996 through 2018, 14 cases of diphtheria were reported in the United States, however, in 2018 more than 16,000 cases of diphtheria in other countries were reported to the WHO. Despite the availability of effective vaccines, booster doses should be given every 10 years to maintain immunity. Without that, and with some parents opting out of vaccinations of all kinds for their children, diphtheria is an ever-present pathogenic threat to public health everywhere.

Other *Corynebacterium* Species

Other *Corynebacterium* are part of the indigenous microflora and rarely cause disease in healthy humans. *Corynebacterium jeikeium*, also known as *Group JK Corynebacterium*, is well-known in the medical community as an opportunistic pathogen in immunocompromised patients, especially those who have an indwelling intravascular catheter. Carriers are uncommon; however, it has been shown that as many as 40 percent of hospitalized persons can be colonized. Consequently, risk factors for acquiring the disease include long-term hospitalizations, chemotherapy, and **granulocytopenia**. *Corynebacterium jeikeium* is very resistant to antibiotics. A person receiving antibiotic therapy during hospitalization is susceptible to the organism colonizing the skin and possibility of entering the body through the IV catheter and causing disease, primarily in the immunocompromised patient.

Corynebacterium urealyticum is another rare organism, but it must be considered in infections of the urinary tract. This species produces urease, an enzyme that catalyzes the decomposition of urine to ammonia and carbon dioxide. This can lead to the formation of calculi (stones) in the kidney, ureter, and bladder, potentially requiring surgical removal. Treatment for both of these species can be difficult due to their resistance to most antibiotics.

Mycobacterium Species

The family *Mycobacteriaceae*, a member of the class *Actinobacteria*, is distinguished from other bacteria by the unique structure of the cell wall. This distinction serves to separate this family from other prokaryotes. The cell wall contains a high quantity of lipids, including waxes. The waxes are composed of mycolic acids (fatty acids). This accounts for the microbes being Gram-variable, meaning that they do not consistently stain purple or red. To identify mycobacteria, a special acid-fast stain must be used. The acid-fast stain involves the use of acid and heat to remove the stain-resistant barrier. The microbes do not decolorize after rinsing with an acid, hence the name acid-fast. The acid-fast mycobacteria are seen under the microscope as red organisms from the penetration of the red dye against a blue or green background in a sputum specimen obtained from a patient suspected to have TB. *Mycobacteriaceae* organisms are straight or slightly curved. They may have filaments or branches that grow outward from the cell. They are non-motile and non–spore-forming (see Figure 14-6).

The genus *Mycobacterium* includes saprophytes, obligate parasites, and other types for which the nutritional requirements vary. Saprophytes can easily grow in simple laboratory media with uncomplicated nutritional needs. Other types of *Mycobacterium* require specific media with acids or albumin. The genus is aerobic, allowing the microbes to grow in a

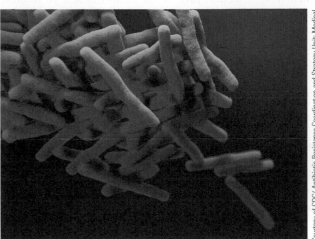

Courtesy of CDC/ Antibiotic Resistance Coordination and Strategy Unit; Medical Illustrators: Alissa Eckert; James Archer.

Figure 14-6 Illustration of drug-resistant, rod-shaped *Mycobacterium tuberculosis* bacteria.

variety of environmental areas. Species are found in the soil and in warm-blooded and cold-blooded animals such as humans, turtles, fish, snakes, and frogs.

The genus *Mycobacterium* includes species that are indigenous microflora, opportunistic pathogens, and true pathogens to humans. The skin and respiratory system are most commonly involved in infections. Patients who are immunosuppressed are at risk for developing infections caused by opportunistic pathogens including *Mycobacterium*. Species are responsible for causing diseases such as leprosy, tuberculosis (TB), and non-TB respiratory infection. Specimens of the microorganism are obtained from skin lesions, lymph nodes, eyes, and lungs.

Mycobacterium tuberculosis

As previously mentioned, the tubercle bacillus is a rod-shaped obligate aerobe distinguished by its waxy cell wall that influences the slow growth and unique staining properties of the cell. The waxy wall protects the cells against the lytic enzymes of the macrophages that engulf and try to ingest them.

Mycobacterium tuberculosis cells favor an environment high in oxygen concentration, so the organism tends to infect the upper lobes of the lungs. However, it still grows slowly even in optimal growth conditions, with a doubling time of 20 hours, as compared to 20 minutes, for *Escherichia coli*. The slow growth means that identification in the laboratory can potentially take up to 6 weeks. The progression of the disease is slow as well, with the exception of individuals whose immune system is compromised.

Tuberculosis has been described and given various names throughout the centuries. In 1882, Robert Koch discovered *M. tuberculosis*. Eight years later he developed tuberculin prepared from dead tubercle bacterial cells. This served as the basis for the development of the tuberculin skin test used today as a diagnostic tool.

One-fourth of the world's population is infected with tuberculosis. It is the leading infectious disease killer, with a worldwide infection rate of 1.7 billion cases, 10 million new cases per year, and 1.4 million deaths annually according to the CDC in 2021. In the United States in 2019, 8,916 cases of TB were reported. With the discovery of antibiotics, particularly streptomycin, in the United States, the number of TB cases significantly declined during the twentieth century.

Tuberculosis

Tuberculosis is a highly contagious disease that is spread person to person by droplets that contain the bacterial cells. When an infected person speaks, coughs, or sneezes, the aerosolized droplets can be inhaled by individuals in close proximity. The health status of the person inhaling the droplets may be the determining factor for whether an infection occurs. In healthcare settings, airborne precautions are used to minimize exposure. Patients with active tuberculosis disease may be isolated in negative-pressure, filtered-air rooms to prevent spread of airborne contaminants to areas outside the isolation room.

Not everyone who is exposed to TB acquires the disease and not everyone infected shows symptoms. The two distinguishing classes of TB are latent TB infection and TB disease. Individuals who have been exposed to and who have inhaled TB bacteria but show no signs of symptoms of the active disease have latent TB. They are not contagious to others. If, however, their immune system becomes compromised, then the dormant TB inside them may activate and transition to TB disease. TB disease is active, contagious, and produces symptoms including:

- Fever, chills, and night sweats
- Loss of appetite and weight loss
- Generalized weakness or fatigue
- Severe cough that lasts more than 3 weeks
- Coughing up blood in sputum

Disease Progression

The progress of TB follows two paths: primary tuberculosis and reinfection. Lesions characterize primary TB in the initial stage of the disease, followed by the acute exudative stage that rapidly spreads via the lymphatic system. The lesions typically heal with some scarring. The lesions will occur in the lower lobes of the lungs.

Reinfection TB is the chronic form characterized by lesions that secrete exudative fluid. Reinfection usually occurs due to tubercle cells that survived the primary TB infection. Lesions from reinfection usually establish themselves in the apex of the lungs, and new ones keep forming downward toward the lower lobes (see Figure 14-7).

When the contaminated aerosol droplets from an infected individual are inhaled by an uninfected person, the bacterial cells travel through the respiratory system to become established in the bronchioles or alveoli. The tubercle

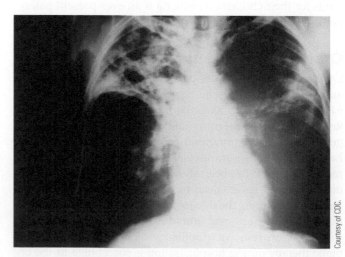

Figure 14-7 AP x-ray showing advanced tuberculosis; note the presence of bilateral pulmonary infiltrate and "caving formation" in the right apical region.

cells can then multiply with minimal to no resistance by the host. Macrophages engulf some of the bacterial cells, but they remain viable and multiply within the macrophage. Once the macrophage engulfs the tubercle cell, a phagosome develops, allowing the cells to multiply. They burst from the macrophage, destroying it in the process.

The lesions that occur in the lungs are of two types: exudative or productive. Exudative lesions are caused by the inflammatory response of the host's body. The lesions contain a liquid exudate composed of monocytes and neutrophils. The lesion continues to progress and either causes necrosis of the lung tissue, heals, or develops into a tubercle (a small, rounded nodule). Productive lesions do not have an exudate but consist of cells that are formed around the bacilli. This collection of cells is called a granuloma. The center of the granuloma is composed of a large number of cells surrounded by lymphocytes, monocytes, and fibroblasts. The inner part of the tubercle eventually becomes calcified and the outer part is a fibrous capsule called a Ghon complex. The Ghon complex can survive for many years or will eventually die.

The collection of specimens is critically important to identify and diagnose the presence of tubercle bacillus. The types of specimen collected include:

- Sputum (most common type of specimen)
- Bronchial washings and lung tissue samples
- Urine
- Cerebrospinal fluid (CSF)
- Bone marrow

Mis-diagnosis of TB

Statistics for 2020 demonstrated an unexpected additional decrease in TB cases due to several possible factors related to the COVID-19 pandemic. A decrease in immigration and travel is considered by researchers as a possible factor, however those changes cannot fully explain the decrease. Mitigation strategies implemented for reducing the spread of COVID-19, including wearing of masks, social distancing, and lockdowns might have also reduced the TB infection rate. A concern was raised that TB infections may have been overlooked or mis-diagnosed based on the predominant public health concerns of COVID-19 infection and the reluctance of many with early symptoms to seek healthcare during the pandemic. In cases of negative testing for SARS-CoV-2 and known risk factors for TB including being born in or having lived in a country with high TB incidence, living in a congregate setting (homeless shelter, nursing home, or a correctional facility), or being immune suppressed, healthcare providers have been advised to consider ordering rapid TB diagnostic tests such as sputum microscopy or nucleic acid amplification tests so patients with TB disease can commence appropriate antibiotic therapy.

TB Skin Testing

Mycobacterium tuberculosis induces a **hypersensitivity** reaction. The reaction is detected by skin tests using protein antigens from filtrates of tubercle bacillus cultures. The response is due to activated macrophages responding to the presence of *M. tuberculosis* cells and vascular permeability contributing to the reddened, swollen area at the site of antigen injection. A positive reaction occurs by fully developing in 48 to 72 hours; therefore, the skin must be examined during this time frame so the test results can be appropriately interpreted. The most accurate skin test is the **Mantoux test**. The test involves the intradermal injection of antigen purified protein derivative (PPD) within the epidermal layer (see Figure 14-8).

A positive reaction indicates that a person has a latent TB infection, active TB disease, or has been previously vaccinated. An individual who tests positive is subsequently scheduled for a chest x-ray, clinical examination, and collection of a specimen, most likely sputum (see Figure 14-9).

A negative reaction indicates the person has never been infected, or possibly that he or she is in the early stages of infection, when a reaction to the skin test does not yet register.

TB Blood Testing

Interferon-Gamma Release Assays (IGRAs) are whole-blood tests used for diagnosis of *Mycobacterium tuberculosis* infection. The two types of FDA-approved IGRAs available are QuantiFERON®-TB Gold In-Tube test (QFT-GIT) and T-SPOT® TB test (T-Spot). The tests are unable to differentiate latent tuberculosis infection from tuberculosis disease. The IGRAs work by measuring the immune reactivity to *M. tuberculosis*. Individuals who have been infected with *M. tuberculosis* will have white blood cells that release interferon-gamma (IFN-g) when mixed with antigens derived from *M. tuberculosis*.

Treatment and Vaccination

Often individuals who have been infected for the first time will not be diagnosed, and the infection heals without treatment. The drugs that are most effective against TB are

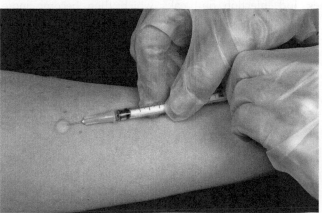

Figure 14-8 Mantoux tuberculin skin test that will cause a 6-mm to 10-mm wheal (a raised area of skin) to form at the injection site.

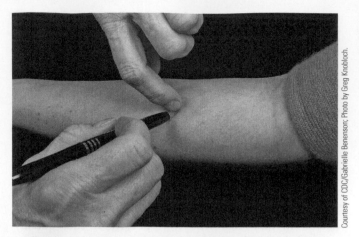

Courtesy of CDC/Gabrielle Benenson; Photo by Greg Knobloch.

Figure 14-9 Marking widest areas of induration (hard, dense, raised formation) for accurate measurement of the positive Mantoux tuberculin skin test reaction.

rifampin, ethambutol, isoniazid, and pyrazinamide. A combination of at least two of the drugs may be used to prevent *M. tuberculosis* from developing resistance.

The vaccine Bacille Calmette-Guerin (BCG) was developed and first administered starting in 1921. PPD was developed in 1934 as the diagnostic agent for tuberculosis. BCG vaccination provides partial protection, but the duration is unknown and is not considered a reliable vaccination. The live vaccine is made from an attenuated strain of the closely related *Mycobacterium bovis*. Mass vaccinations are only implemented when the risk of infection and number of negative skin tests are high. In the United States, BCG vaccination is not routine because it interferes with the PPD skin test that is most commonly used for diagnosis.

Drug-Resistant TB

Tuberculosis bacteria can become resistant to the standard drugs used to treat the disease. This resistance factor means that the drug can no longer kill the bacteria. Additionally, the strains of *M. tuberculosis* that have developed resistance pass on the genes for drug resistance to subsequent bacterial colonies and infection outbreaks which then become more difficult to manage. Misuse or mismanagement of drug treatment is typically the primary reason for development of resistance (see Figure 14-10). Examples of misuse include:

- Individuals do not complete the full course of drug treatment
- Prescribing the wrong treatment, wrong dose, or wrong duration of treatment
- Supply of drugs not available
- Drugs are of poor quality

Drug resistance is most likely to occur in individuals who:

- Do not take their drugs regularly or who do not complete the course of treatment
- Develop TB again after having been treated previously
- Come from a region where drug-resistant TB is common
- Spend time in close proximity with someone infected with drug-resistant TB

Multidrug-resistant TB (MDR TB) is caused by mutated strains that have become resistant to the two most potent TB drugs, isoniazid and rifampin. These drugs are used to treat all persons with TB disease. Estimates show that there are nearly 500,000 cases of MDR TB each year, and only 56 percent of those patients are successfully treated. In 2013, the FDA approved bedaquiline as part of a 24-week treatment regimen for MDR-TB if other agents are unavailable.

Extensively drug-resistant TB (XDR TB) is a rare type of tuberculosis bacteria that is resistant to isoniazid and rifampin, plus fluoroquinolone, and at least one of three injectable second-line drugs (i.e., amikacin, kanamycin, or capreomycin). Patients infected with extensively drug-resistant tuberculosis are left with few options and treatments available are much less likely to be effective. Individuals with HIV/AIDS or other severely immunocompromised conditions are more likely to develop TB disease if exposed and infected. They will have an increased risk of death from drug-resistant TB.

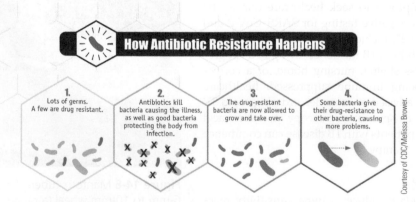

Courtesy of CDC/Melissa Brower.

Figure 14-10 How antibiotic resistance happens.

Patients who must undergo treatment regimens for multidrug and extensively drug-resistant forms of TB may experience potentially life-threatening side effects of the powerful medications used to fight the infection. Serious side effects of drug therapy include depression and psychosis, hearing loss, hepatitis, and kidney failure. In addition, the drug treatment is extremely expensive and the duration of treatment may be years.

Mycobacterium leprae

Mycobacterium leprae is closely related to *M. tuberculosis*; both have the unique waxy cell wall that can only be stained through the acid-fast staining method and both grow slowly. *M. leprae* grows best at temperatures that are slightly below body temperature, which explains the tendency for the bacterial cells to infect the cooler areas of the body, such as the fingers, toes, ears, and nose.

Leprosy

Mycobacterium leprae is the bacterium that causes the disease called leprosy. The more formal term for leprosy is Hansen's disease, named for the Norwegian scientist Gerhard Hansen who identified *M. leprae* as the causative agent. Leprosy is an ancient disease that is described in detail in the Bible and other literature. It was a feared disease, and individuals with leprosy were often shunned and isolated from society.

M. leprae infects both the skin and the peripheral nervous system. The resulting effects are a severe and disfiguring skin rash with the loss of cutaneous sensation. The disease is most likely transmitted from person to person by direct contact or nasal secretions in droplets, similar to route of transmission for TB. There are two forms of the disease, tuberculoid form and lepromatous form.

Approximately 3 to 5 years after becoming infected, a person develops indeterminate leprosy. A few indiscriminate skin lesions form with no effect on the nerves, however, a skin biopsy reveals early evidence of nerve damage that confirms the infection. The infection progresses to either the tuberculoid or the lepromatous form if untreated. Scientists do not know why some people develop tuberculoid leprosy while others develop the lepromatous form. One theory is that the infected individual's genetic structure determines the type of leprosy that will develop.

The immune system of patients with tuberculoid leprosy reacts with an aggressive cell-mediated immune response to control the infection. Usually only a few skin lesions form, but complete loss of nerve sensation is experienced (see Figure 14-11).

Patients whose immune system is not able to contain the infection experience progression into the lepromatous form of the disease. Infected individuals will have a high number of *M. leprae* cells, representing a highly contagious stage of the disease. Skin damage by lesions is extensive and occurs throughout the body, grossly disfiguring the person (see Figure 14-12). The skin lesions are flat or

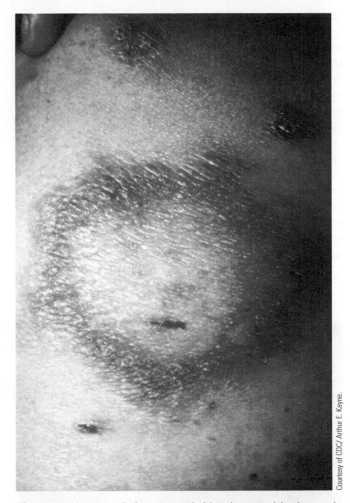

Courtesy of CDC/ Arthur E. Kayne.

Figure 14-11 A well-demarcated skin plaque with elevated border and a loss of sensitivity in its central region due to the tubercular form of leprosy, or Hansen's disease (HD), caused by the bacterium, *Mycobacterium leprae* and characterized by the presence of asymmetrically distributed solitary skin lesions.

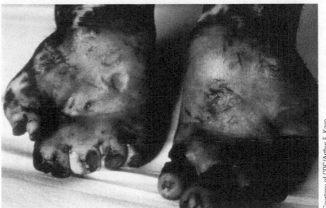

Courtesy of CDC/Arthur E. Kaye.

Figure 14-12 Hands of an individual with leprosy, also known as Hansen's disease, which affects peripheral nerves; note the severe degeneration and mutilation of all of the fingers.

raised lesions, and the bones and cartilage are often damaged. Facial features become thickened and are referred to as leonine (lion-like), a classic characteristic of lepromatous leprosy. The nose may flatten and collapse due to the destruction of the cartilage, there may be a loss of eyebrows, and digits (toes and fingers) may have to be amputated due to extensive bone and cartilage damage (see Figure 14-13).

In 2020, 159 people in the United States and 250,000 around the world contracted Hansen's disease or leprosy. In the United States, leprosy is rare and occurs most often in California, Hawaii, Texas, Florida, Louisiana, New York, and Puerto Rico. Infection cannot be transmitted by casual contact and after a few doses of antibiotic therapy, individuals are no longer contagious and need not be isolated from others. Armadillos, found in southern states, are naturally infected with the bacteria that cause Hansen's disease and could be a potential source of infection, although the risk is considered very low. Avoidance of any contact with armadillos is advised. The US Public Health Service organized and manages the National Hansen's Disease Center in Louisiana. Leprosy patients are given free treatment at that center or six other satellite sites.

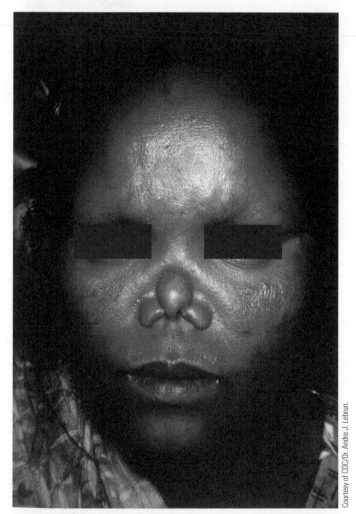

Figure 14-13 Lepromatous leprosy and under who standards, classified as multibacillary (MB) leprosy, caused by *Mycobacterium leprae*; note the saddle-nose deformity due to disintegration of nasal cartilage and lack of eyebrows.

Courtesy of CDC/Dr. Andre J. Lebrun.

Nocardia

Species in the genus *Nocardia* are aerobic *Actinomycetes* that are saprophytes found around the world in soil, decaying organic matter, and in fresh or saltwater bodies. More than 50 species of the genus *Nocardia* have been identified. The taxonomy has been challenging in the scientific community due to its fungal-like characteristics. More than 50 percent of *Nocardia* infections in humans are due to members of the *Nocardia asteroides* complex. The *N. asteroides* complex comprises *N. abscessus*, *N. cyriacigeorgica*, *N. farcinica*, and *N. nova*. Other known pathogenic species of *Nocardia* include *N. transvalensis* complex, *N. brasiliensis*, and *N. pseudobrasiliensis*.

Nocardiosis

Nocardiosis is a relatively uncommon Gram-positive bacterial infection caused by aerobic *Actinomycetes* in the genus *Nocardia*. There are 500 to 1,000 cases reported annually in the United States. Bacteria in this genus have the ability to cause localized or systemic suppurative (pus-forming) disease in both humans and animals. The disease can be transmitted by inhaling contaminated dust or if the soil containing *Nocardia* bacteria get into an open wound. Nocardiosis is regarded as an opportunistic infection; however, approximately one-third of infected patients have no immune deficiency.

Two characteristics of nocardiosis are its ability to spread to almost any organ, particularly the central nervous system (brain and spinal cord), and its tendency to relapse or progress despite appropriate therapy. Eighty percent of nocardiosis cases present as invasive pulmonary infection, disseminated infection, or brain abscess. Twenty percent present as cellulitis. It may also involve the kidneys, joints, heart, eyes, and bones. Pulmonary infection commonly presents with fever, cough, or chest pain. Central nervous system (CNS) symptoms include headache, **lethargy**, confusion, seizures, or sudden onset of neurologic deficit.

In rare cases, *N. asteroids* can cause formation of cutaneous or skeletal mycetoma (a granulomatous inflammatory lesion). Immunocompromised persons are at greatest risk. These include individuals with chronic lung disease, connective tissue disorders, malignancy, organ transplant, HIV/AIDS, or alcoholism, or those using high-dose corticosteroid therapy (see Figure 14-14).

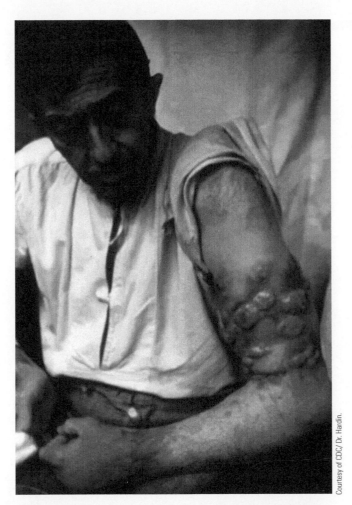

Figure 14-14 Nocardiosis infection of the left upper arm, due to Gram-positive, *Nocardia madurae* bacteria, which had manifested into a cellulitic inflammation known as an actinomycotic mycetoma.

Streptomyces

Streptomyces species, members of the class *Actinobacteria*, are non-motile, filamentous, Gram-positive bacteria that produce spores from aerial filaments called sporophores. These rise above the base colony and form spores called conidia by cross-wall divisions of the filament (see Figure 14-15). The *Streptomyces* were long thought to be fungi due to their method of reproduction and growth, unique among bacteria. *Streptomyces* are found in soil around the world and are important in soil ecology. The characteristic smell of wet dirt comes from chemicals called **geosmins** that are given off by *Streptomyces*. The bacteria can consume almost anything (sugars, alcohols, amino acids, organic acids) by producing extracellular hydrolytic enzymes. Ecologists have shown great interest in these organisms as agents for bioremediation.

Streptomyces spp. are widespread environmental bacteria that rarely cause severe invasive infections and are aerobic

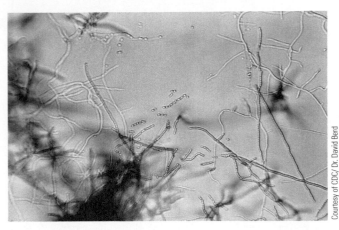

Figure 14-15 Branching filamentous hyphae, abundant aerial mycelia, and long chains of small spores are visible, which is characteristic of all *Streptomyces* species bacteria.

Actinomycetes best known for their use in the production of antimicrobial substances.

The most common clinical sign of *Streptomyces* infection is mycetoma, a chronic, localized, suppurative cutaneous infection that is characterized by inflammatory granuloma formation. The cutaneous *Streptomyces* infection typically results from transmission of the microorganism through a thorn puncture and involves the legs or feet.

Invasive *Streptomyces* infections are extremely rare. Only 10 cases of invasive *Streptomyces* infection (those other than mycetoma or superficial skin infections) were reported in the literature between 1966 and 2000. Invasive infections involved pneumonia, pericarditis, brain abscess, and peritonitis. Most of the patients were HIV/AIDS patients. A pathologic feature of pulmonary infections with *Streptomyces* is the presence of granulomas sometimes associated with focal necrosis.

Streptomyces are also of medical and industrial importance because they synthesize antibiotics. More than 50 different antibiotics, antifungals, and antiparasitics have been isolated from *Streptomyces* species, including streptomycin, neomycin, chloramphenicol and tetracyclines, and ivermectin.

MICRO NOTES

"Killer Armadillo"

It seems that armadillos, those football-shaped, funky-looking animals found in southern states of the United States, have more under those armored plates than you know. Armadillos are natural carriers of Hansen's disease, otherwise known as leprosy. According to the CDC, it is not common; however, you can get leprosy from contact with armadillos. If you have contact with one, you might want to check with your healthcare provider just to be safe and certain.

Under the Microscope

Kim went for the required annual TB screening with the hospital employee health nurse. The PPD injection was 24 hours ago and the area around it is raised and tender with a 3-cm ring of redness around the injection site. Kim is worried how this may impact her job as a CST in L&D.

1. What are the available tests performed for TB testing?

2. What are the steps in reading of a Mantoux test, the results, and implications for a positive test?

3. What are common features and characteristics of the types of *Actinobacteria discussed in this chapter*?

4. Which additional diagnostic studies will Kim have to undergo if the skin test result is positive?

5. How do the *Actinobacteria* infections manifest their signs and symptoms?

6. Will Kim be allowed to continue working if the test is positive for TB infection?

CHAPTER 15

Gram-Negative Cocci and Spirochetes

Learning Objectives

After completing the study of this chapter, you will be able to:

1. Define key terms.
2. Discuss the unique morphological characteristics of spirochetes.
3. Describe methods of disease transmission for *Neisseria* and *Treponema*.
4. Compare and contrast the virulence of *N. gonorrhoeae* and *N. meningitidis*.
5. Describe the prevalence, clinical stages, and long-term effects of syphilis.
6. Apply critical thinking skills in relating chapter material to the surgical environment of care or broader global community.

Key Terms

Asymptomatic	Fibromyalgia	Louse	Ruminants
Cervical os	Gummas	Myalgia	Syphilomas
Chancre	Hyperendemic	Petechiae	Urethral meatus

The Big Picture

Many of the pathogenic organisms discussed in this chapter have caused human suffering for millennia. Despite the clinical effectiveness of antibiotic therapy for treatment of the diseases these microbes cause, many infections progress to debilitating conditions or even fatal outcomes. During your examination of the topics in this chapter, consider the following:

1. Which bacterial infections present the most concern and challenge for public health agencies?

2. What barriers to prevention and/or treatment of infections transmitted by sexual contact continue to exist?

3. The clinical signs and symptoms of which disease progresses the fastest, possibly resulting in fatality in a matter of hours?

4. What long-term complications can result from unrecognized or untreated infections discussed in this chapter?

Clinical Significance Topic

One of the more difficult aspects of the surgical technology profession is witnessing the devastating effects of disease processes on patients coming into the surgical environment of care. Knowing that some of these infections are sexually transmitted diseases, which are preventable with the use of protection such as condoms, it would be easy to be judgmental and critical instead of keeping focus on the problem at hand and not how the patient became infected. Pregnant females may have irreversible damage from pelvic inflammatory disease or infect their fetuses, resulting in permanent damage in utero or during delivery. Understanding the complexity of these diseases, that nobody intentionally becomes infected, and realizing that many may not even recognize that they have been infected, removes that unfair bias or perception and should refocus one's attention on taking care of that patient with the same dedication by all members of the surgical team, as any other patient would deserve and should expect.

Neisseriaceae Family

To briefly review, bacterial microbes that do not retain the crystal violet dye used in the Gram-staining process appear pink or red due to the safranin added as a counter-stain and are therefore categorized as Gram-negative. The family *Neisseriaceae* is a member of the phylum Proteobacteria and class Beta-Proteobacteria and contains the pathogenic Gram-negative aerobic bacteria. Important genera within this family are *Neisseria*, *Kingella*, and *Chromobacterium*. The members of the *Neisseriaceae* family are classified as spherical-shaped cocci; however, some are short, slightly rod-shaped coccobacilli. Specific virulence factors associated with the various types of Gram-negative bacteria are the endotoxins contained within the lipopolysaccharide (LPS) layer of the outer cell membrane and structural characteristics that allow bacteria to adhere to tissues.

Neisseria

The genus *Neisseria* consists of 10 species, 2 of which are human pathogens of significance: *N. meningitidis*, that causes bacterial meningitis, and *N. gonorrhoeae*, that causes gonorrhea. Both of these pathogens have two important virulence factors: they have pili that allow the cells to attach to the tissues of the host more readily, making them more difficult to remove and they have the ability to encapsulate.

Neisseria gonorrhoeae

Neisseria gonorrhoeae is a fastidious, Gram-negative diplococcus that is microaerophilic, capnophilic, and always considered a pathogenic organism. It is identified by culture, Gram stain, and immunodiagnostic techniques. Many strains are antibiotic-resistant, which is discussed in more detail later in the chapter (see Figure 15-1).

Gonorrhea, referred to by some as "the clap," is the disease caused by *N. gonorrhoeae*. It is a common and significant sexually transmitted disease (STD) that affects both males and females and is the second most commonly reported bacterial sexually transmitted infection in the United States in all U.S. regions and among all racial or ethnicity groups.

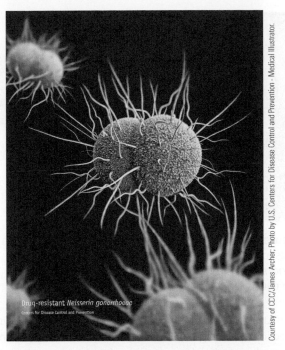

Figure 15-1 3-D computer-generated illustration of drug-resistant *Neisseria gonorrhoeae* diplococcal bacteria with hair-like pili that promote motility and improve surface adherence.

According to the CDC, in 2019, a total of 616,392 cases of gonorrhea were reported, increased by 92.0 percent since the historic low in 2009. During 2018–2019, the overall rate of gonorrhea infections reported increased 5.7 percent. The significantly higher case rate among males could signify increased transmission, increased diagnosis through screening, or both. The highest rates of disease transmission are in those between the ages of 15 and 24 years; however, disease can be transmitted during all types of unprotected sexual contact at any age. Sexually active males who are gay or bisexual, or males who have sex with males (MSM), should be tested for gonorrhea every year. Sexually active females younger than age 25 years and older females with risk factors such as new or multiple sex partners or a sex partner who has a sexually transmitted infection should also be tested for gonorrhea every year.

Clinical Presentation

In the early phase of infection, bacteria attach to the mucous cells of the epithelium in the genitourinary (GU) tract, rectum, or oropharynx. The bacteria then pass through the cells into the sub-epithelial space, where the infection becomes established. The bacteria can also cause secondary infections if spread through the circulatory system. Lesions may appear on skin surfaces or cause debilitating joint inflammation (see Figure 15-2).

Many months may pass after the initial phase, allowing the bacteria to damage and scar reproductive organs. At this stage of the disease, symptoms may or may not appear. In females, the vague symptoms are often mistaken for other types of infection.

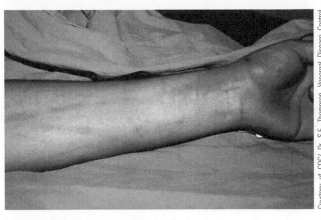

Figure 15-2 Systemically-disseminated *Neisseria gonorrhoeae* seen as the cutaneous lesion on the lateral left wrist, surrounded by an erythematous halo which runs the length of the forearm along the lines of venous drainage.

Symptoms in females include:

- Pain or burning sensation during urination
- Increased vaginal discharge
- Vaginal bleeding between periods

The primary site of infection in females is the cervix because it contains endocervical columnar epithelial cells. The bacteria cannot penetrate the squamous epithelial cells of the vagina in post-pubescent females.

A serious complication of undiagnosed or untreated gonorrhea is pelvic inflammatory disease (PID), which is an acute infection of the abdomen. Females with PID present with a tender abdomen upon palpation or severe chronic pain with vaginal discharge. Females of child-bearing age may become unable to conceive due to formation of adhesions that may require surgery. PID can also cause salpingitis, an inflammation of the fallopian tube or oophoritis, inflammation of an ovary that leaves the structures scarred and results in infertility (see Figure 15-3). Once the infection is

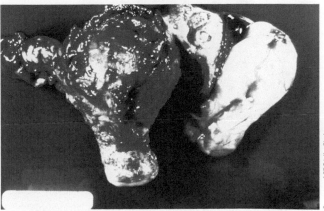

Figure 15-3 Uterus and ovary that had been excised, due to the presence of an ovarian abscess in a case of pelvic inflammatory disease (PID).

fully resolved, surgery for removal of the affected ovary or attempted re-establishment of patency of the fallopian tubes may be performed but may not be successful.

Another complication of fallopian tube adhesions from PID is ectopic pregnancy, which is the implantation of a fertilized egg in the fallopian tube or other areas within the abdominal cavity instead of the uterus. As the embryo grows, it ruptures the tube, causing pain and bleeding and requiring emergency surgery to remove the embryonic tissue and stop hemorrhage (see Figure 15-4).

Pregnant females who are infected can transmit gonorrhea to their newborn during normal vaginal delivery. If a diagnosis is obtained prior to onset of labor, then a Cesarean delivery is performed prophylactically to prevent infection of the neonate.

Infection in males occurs primarily in the urethra. After an incubation period of approximately 2 to 5 days, a urethral discharge with dysuria (painful or difficult urination) may be experienced (see Figure 15-5). Most males will have acute symptoms, including:

- Burning sensation during urination
- A white, yellow, or greenish discharge from the penis
- Painful or swollen testicles (less common)

In some cases, males with testicular infections may develop adhesions of the scrotal structures that produce and transmit sperm, resulting in infertility.

Gonococcal infections of the rectum in both males and females may also not produce symptoms. If there are symptoms present, they may include:

- Anal itching or soreness
- Discharge or bleeding
- Painful bowel movements

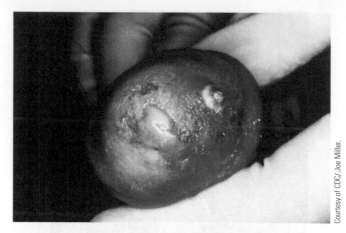

Courtesy of CDC/ Joe Miller.

Figure 15-5 Purulent penile discharge due to gonorrhea caused by the Gram-negative bacterium, *Neisseria gonorrhoeae*, and overlying penile pyodermal lesions, the cause of which was unidentified.

Another type of infection seen is gonococcal pharyngeal infection (pharyngitis). Any individual who engages in oral sex can be infected. The infectious state may be asymptomatic or there may be only a mild sore throat of short duration. Rarely, gonococcal bacteria can disseminate throughout the blood and attack joints. These infections may cause life-threatening sequelae.

Individuals with sexually transmitted diseases, including gonorrhea, have a higher risk of becoming infected with human immunodeficiency virus (HIV). One reason for the increase in risk is the behavior of the individuals that predisposed them to the initial STD. These types of behaviors or circumstances that elevate disease risk include:

- Having unprotected (no condom) vaginal, anal, or oral sex
- Having multiple or anonymous sexual partners
- Risky behavior due to consumption of drugs or alcohol
- Failure to disclose infection status or previous encounters with infected individuals

Diagnosis

Anyone who is sexually active, who has had encounters similar to those described in the previous section, or is experiencing symptoms should seek medical care without delay to prevent potential long-term damage. Physicians usually order a urinalysis for detection of gonococcal infection; however, it may also be necessary to take swab samples of the **urethral meatus** of males or the **cervical os** of females. Additionally, a swab test may be performed in the throat or rectum if the patient has had oral or rectal sexual relations.

The CDC created the Gonococcal Isolate Surveillance Project (GISP) in 1986 as a way to gather statistical data about the prevalence of gonorrhea throughout the United States. Gonococcal infections remain the second most commonly reported sexually transmitted disease (see Figure 15-6). Data are submitted to four to five regional laboratories for analysis

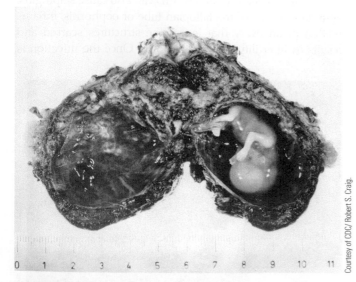

Courtesy of CDC/ Robert S. Craig.

Figure 15-4 An excised ectopic pregnancy showing the trophoblastic capsule surrounding the developing fetus, as well as the placenta that had been implanted outside the uterus, but within the abdominal cavity.

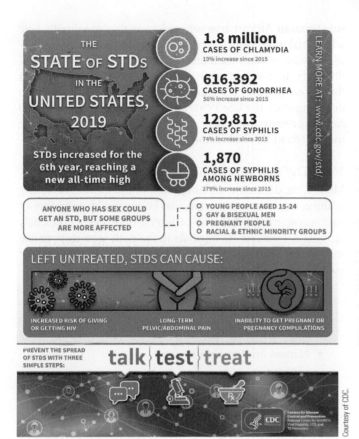

Figure 15-6 Public information graphic, "The State of STDs in the United States, 2019"

and from which the CDC's STD Treatment Guidelines are developed, monitored, and revised as necessary. Clinicians are advised to submit specimens to the GISP labs when standard treatment protocols fail, thus allowing them to assess emergence of new resistant strains.

To facilitate clinical testing for reporting and development of treatment protocols, various diagnostic tests were evaluated and many of those were found to be suboptimal. The Nucleic Acid Amplification Test (NAAT) was developed and approved by the FDA as the most reliable screening test for gonococcal and chlamydial infections. In cases of possible sexual assault and for periodic assessment of antibiotic resistance, standard laboratory culture techniques are still required. The NAAT tests are considered non-culture tests because the specimens collected are not maintained in proper laboratory conditions to allow for culture and sensitivity studies.

Treatment

Antibiotic therapy is the treatment modality for gonorrhea. Over the decades since penicillin was first discovered and used to treat gonococcal infections, *Neisseria gonorrhoeae* has developed increasing resistance to multiple drug treatments, including sulfanilamides, penicillin, tetracycline, and fluoroquinolones, such as ciprofloxacin. More than half of all infections in 2019 were estimated to be resistant to at least one

antibiotic, making continuous monitoring, research, and development of new therapies critical in the fight against these preventable diseases. The CDC released updated gonorrhea treatment guidelines in December 2020, recommending a single 500 mg intramuscular dose of ceftriaxone for cases of uncomplicated gonorrhea.

Ophthalmia neonatorum is a gonococcal eye infection in neonates transmitted through exposure to infected tissues during vaginal delivery. It affects the corneal epithelium and causes microbial keratitis, ulceration, and perforation (see Figure 15-7). Ophthalmia neonatorum is prevented by instillation of erythromycin (0.5 percent) ophthalmic ointment in each eye in a single application. All newborn infants, whether delivered vaginally or by C-section, should be given prophylactic treatment for potential sight-threatening disease, and it is required by law in most states. The United States Preventative Services Task Force (USPSTF) recommends ocular prophylaxis with erythromycin ointment for all neonates within the first 24 hours after birth. Previous treatments with silver nitrate, tetracycline, bacitracin, and povidone iodine are no longer used. Erythromycin is the only antibiotic ointment recommended for use in neonates.

Neisseria meningitidis

Neisseria meningitidis is an encapsulated Gram-negative diplococcus (see Figure 15-8). The bacterium is nearly identical to *N. gonorrhoeae* except for the presence of a polysaccharide capsule that has antiphagocytic properties. There have been 12 different serotypes identified that are based on these capsules. *N. meningitidis* is only found in humans and colonizes the nasopharynx. Experiments have shown that meningococcal cells selectively attach to specific receptors for pili on nonciliated epithelial columnar cells that line the nasopharynx. Non-pili meningococci are not virulent because of their inability to bind with the columnar cells.

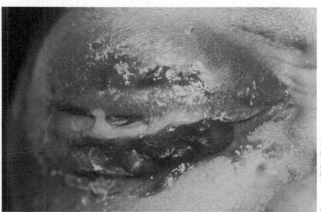

Figure 15-7 Infant's right eye with extensive inflammation due to an ophthalmic infection caused by the bacterium, *Neisseria gonorrhoeae*, referred to as ophthalmia neonatorum or neonatal conjunctivitis.

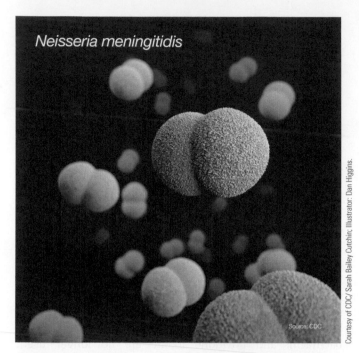

Neisseria meningitidis

Source: CDC

Courtesy of CDC/ Sarah Bailey Cutchin; Illustrator: Dan Higgins.

Figure 15-8 3-D, computer-generated image of a number of diplococcal, Gram-negative, *Neisseria meningitidis* bacteria.

Infections from *N. meningitidis* are often severe or fatal and include infections of the meningeal lining of the brain and spinal cord (meningitis) and bloodstream infections (bacteremia or septicemia). Approximately 10 percent of individuals have *N. meningitidis* present in nasopharyngeal tissues; however, they may not show any signs or symptoms of disease. These asymptomatic carriers may transmit infection through intimate contact such as kissing or through exposure to salivary and respiratory secretions. It is not transmitted through the air or by casual contact with infected persons. There are recognized risk factors associated with *N. meningitidis* infections, including:

- Age: infants, adolescents, and young adults are at increased risk for infection. Highest incidence rates are seen in children younger than age 1 year and in adolescents or young adults between ages 16 and 23 years.

- Community setting: first-year college students (especially those living in dormitories) and military service training facilities where close contact living conditions are routine.

- Certain diseases (HIV), medications, and surgical procedures (splenectomy) may weaken the immune system and increase the risk of meningococcal disease.

Foreign travel: vaccination is recommended (though not required) for persons traveling to countries where *N. meningitidis* is **hyperendemic** or epidemic Meningococcal disease occurs globally, however, the highest rates of disease occur in the

sub-Saharan African area referred to as the "meningitis belt" where major epidemics occur every 5 to 12 years with statistical population rates estimated at 1,000 cases per 100,000 individuals. In the United States, there are three serogroups that cause disease: B, C, and Y. Rates of disease have been declining since the late 1990s and, currently, fewer than 1,000 cases are reported annually. Infections are seasonal, occurring most often in December and January.

Meningococcal Meningitis

Meningitis, defined as inflammation of the meningeal lining of the central nervous system, can be caused by a number of pathogenic microbes, some of which have been previously discussed. *Neisseria meningitidis* is the pathogen responsible for meningococcal meningitis. Classic signs and symptoms of meningococcal meningitis are sudden onset of:

- Fever
- Headache
- Stiff neck (meningismus)
- Nausea and/or vomiting
- Photophobia (severe sensitivity to light)
- Changes in mental state, confusion, or unresponsiveness

As the disease progresses, neurological signs develop due to the irritation and inflammation of the meninges and increased intracranial pressure, including cervical spine rigidity (Brudzinski sign), thoracolumbar rigidity, hamstring spasms (Kernig's sign), convulsions, and exaggerated reflexes.

The classic signs and symptoms listed above may not be observed in new-borns and infants. An infected infant may be slow, inactive, irritable, vomiting, or feeding poorly. There may be bulging of the cranial fontanelles (soft spots) or arching backwards of the head and neck (opisthotonos). In young children, reflexes may be lessened or delayed, which can also be a sign of meningitis.

Any cases of suspected meningitis should be treated immediately. Fatalities can occur within a few hours of onset of symptoms. Non-fatal cases can still result in permanent brain damage or loss of hearing.

Meningococcal Septicemia

Meningococcal septicemia, also known as meningococcemia, is an extremely serious generalized bloodstream infection caused by *N. meningitidis*, which causes damage to blood vessels and bleeding into organs, the skin, and other soft tissues. The bacteria invade the bloodstream by going through the nasopharyngeal epithelium by the process of endocytosis. An endotoxin present in the outer cellular membrane of *N. meningitidis* is responsible for vascular damage, including inflammation of the blood vessel walls, thrombosis, endothelial cell damage, and disseminated intravascular coagulation (DIC). DIC is the widespread formation of thromboses in the microcirculation that inhibit intrinsic coagulation and can cause massive hemorrhaging.

Death can occur in a matter of hours because of meningococcal meningitis. Non-fatal cases may require amputation of fingers, toes, or extremities, or extensive debridement of necrotic tissues with skin grafting (see Figure 15-9). Signs and symptoms of meningococcal septicemia include:

- Fatigue
- Vomiting and/or diarrhea
- Chills
- Cold hands or feet
- Severe body aches and pain
- Rapid breathing and heartrate
- Red, pinpoint rash (**petechiae**)
- Dark purple skin rash (in later stages)

Acute fulminating meningococcal septicemia, also known as Waterhouse-Friderichsen syndrome, is a serious disease that involves multiple organ systems of the body and has a high mortality rate, near 100 percent. It begins abruptly, characterized by a high fever, chills, weakness, nausea, vomiting, generalized **myalgia**, and headache. In just a few hours, the patient becomes restless, apprehensive, and delirious. Petechial skin patches suddenly appear over the entire body. The disease progresses, resulting in devastating DIC with shock, destruction of the two adrenal glands, and pulmonary insufficiency. The majority of patients die within 24 hours of contracting the illness despite antibiotic treatment and intensive treatment of associated complications.

A milder form of meningococcal septicemia can also develop. The patient experiences low-grade fever, arthritis, and small petechial skin lesions for a few days or weeks. The majority of patients are treated with antibiotic therapy with an excellent prognosis.

Other less common infections caused by *N. meningitidis* include pneumonia, urethritis, and arthritis. Meningococcal pneumonia is usually secondary to a respiratory tract infection. The signs and symptoms include chest pain, rales, fever, chills, and chronic cough. Again, the prognosis is excellent with these patients.

Diagnosis

Patients with meningococcal infections can present in three ways: meningococcal meningitis alone (30–50 percent of cases); meningococcal meningitis with septicemia (40 percent of cases); or meningococcal septicemia alone (7–10 percent of cases). Meningococcal septicemia can kill faster than any other infectious disease process, so recognition of the signs and symptoms is crucial for immediate initiation of medical treatment.

A significant challenge for healthcare providers who first encounter patients with meningococcal infections is that laboratory findings in the early stages are often non-specific and unremarkable. Definitive diagnosis is achieved through positive growth of *N. meningitidis* on culture studies of blood, cerebrospinal fluid, synovial fluid, or skin lesions. Other laboratory studies performed in conjunction with these types of cultures include the following:

- Complete blood count (CBC) and differential (white blood cell totals)
- Electrolytes
- Blood urea nitrogen (BUN) and creatinine
- Fibrinogen and C-reactive protein
- Coagulation studies
- Imaging studies

In cases of meningococcal septicemia, antibiotic treatment should be started as soon as possible to prevent systemic shock and death. This disease process progresses more quickly than meningococcal meningitis.

The best specimens for the diagnosis of meningococcal pathogens are blood and cerebrospinal fluid (CSF). Laboratories should be advised in advance that a culture specimen is presumed to be *N. meningitidis* because special handling techniques are required to maintain viability of the microbes. The organisms are highly susceptible to temperature differences below or above 37°C (98.6°F). Cultures should be obtained prior to the start of intravenous antibiotics to allow for accurate culture results.

A lumbar puncture, also known as a spinal tap, must be performed to acquire a sample of CSF. A test indicating the possible presence of *Neisseria meningitidis* yields high levels of white blood cells, high levels of protein, and low levels of glucose. Additionally, staining of spinal fluid with methylene blue indicates the presence of the *N. meningitidis*.

The United Kingdom launched a public health awareness campaign about meningococcal diseases that focused

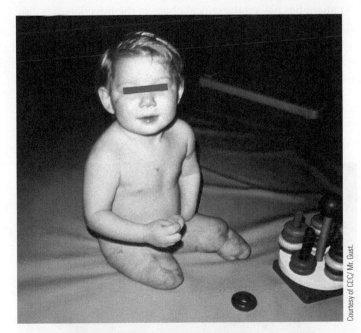

Courtesy of CDC/ Mr. Gust.

Figure 15-9 A 20-month-old infant following amputations of both feet, and left hand due to meningococcal septicemia or meningococcemia, caused by *Neisseria meningitidis* that caused multiple arterial occlusions leading to gangrene.

on the recognition of classic symptoms. A simple, low-tech way to determine if the appearance of a new rash requires immediate attention is called the tumbler test. Parents of small children who cannot communicate symptoms are encouraged to use a clear drinking glass (tumbler) and press it up against the rash area. If the spots remain visible through the glass and do not blanch (fade or pale), then they should seek immediate medical attention. The rate of fatality decreased as a result of the public education efforts.

Meningococcal polymerase chain reaction (PCR) assay is a rapid method for diagnosing CSF infection that is used extensively in the United Kingdom. Spinal fluid PCR provides sensitivity and specificity greater than 90 percent in the diagnosis of meningococcal meningitis. This alternative study is useful when antibiotics have been administered and can be used to rapidly determine serotypes (see Figure 15-10).

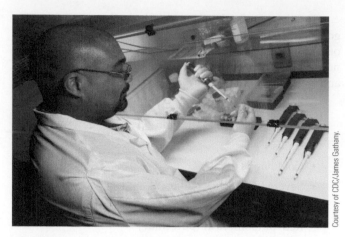

Figure 15-10 CDC biologist preparing a master mix, for use in a multiplex real time polymerase chain reaction (PCR) assay that produces large amounts of replicated DNA, or RNA molecular sequences from very small samples.

Treatment

Penicillin G has traditionally been the treatment of choice for susceptible serotypes of *N. meningitidis*. An alternative is third-generation cephalosporins (cefotaxime or ceftriaxone) for initial therapy until definitive culture results are available or in countries where penicillin-resistant strains of *N. meningitidis* have been identified. During 2019–2020, isolates from 11 cases of penicillin-resistant and ciprofloxacin-resistant *N. meningitidis* serogroup Y (NmY) were shown to contain a mutation that harbored a ciprofloxacin resistance–associated mutation in a chromosomal gene. Thirty-three cases of infection were reported between 2013 and 2020 from 12 separate geographic areas of the United States and represent a concerning increase in penicillin-resistant and ciprofloxacin-resistant meningococcal strain isolates in the United States. The recommended first-line antibiotics, ceftriaxone and cefotaxime, can continue to be used for treatment of bacterial meningitis, but healthcare providers should determine susceptibility of the bacteria to penicillin before switching to traditional treatments with penicillin or ampicillin. In general, antibiotic selection is dependent on patient age, health status, and exposure risk. The medical community has concentrated efforts on the prophylactic treatment of individuals who have been exposed to diseased patients or carriers and are building immunity to the disease-causing serogroups.

Infected patients may require extensive and intensive hospital care. Those with meningococcal septicemia resulting in poor tissue perfusion may require surgical debridement of necrotic or gangrenous tissues (see Figure 15-11). Artificial skin grafts may be used to temporarily cover large areas of skin loss. Autologous grafting can be performed after the patient has passed the critical phase of the infection. It is also recommended that physicians delay surgical amputation of extremities until patients are stable and there is a clear line of demarcation between viable and non-viable tissues. In some cases, fasciotomy may help preserve function of extremities or digits when compartmental pressures rise and threaten circulation. Poor dental tissue perfusion may also require extensive extraction of affected teeth.

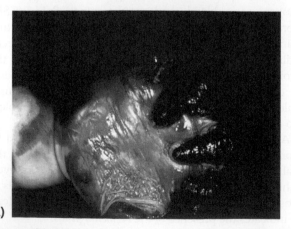

(A)

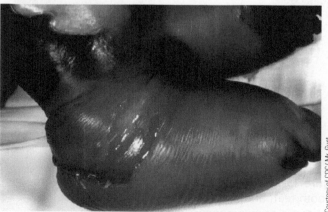

(B)

Figure 15-11 A. 4-Month old infant's right hand with gangrene due to the bacterial infection, meningococcemia from *Neisseria meningitidis*. **B.** Same infant's gangrenous feet.

Prevention

Vaccines have been developed to protect against meningococcal infections. Children who are 11 or 12 years of age old should be given the meningococcal conjugate vaccine and then have a booster dose at age 16 years. Students entering college may be required to have either an initial vaccine or a booster vaccination. Adults aged 56 or older are recommended to have the meningococcal polysaccharide vaccine if they have the risk factors discussed in previous sections. Additional discussion of meningococcal vaccinations is included in Chapter 21.

Moraxella

Moraxella belongs to the phylum Proteobacteria, class Gamma Proteobacteria, order Pseudomonadales, and it is a genus of the *Moraxellaceae* family, representing Gram-negative, non-motile cocci. Members of the genus are strictly aerobic and are coccobacilli, meaning they have a shape between cocci and rods. In the past, the genus has often been reorganized based on nucleic acid analysis. It was formerly placed in the genus *Neisseria*, but scientific information has established that it should be its own genus. Even the species within the genus continue to be reclassified. However, the three most well-known species are *M. nonliquefaciens*, *M. lacunata*, and *M. catarrhalis*.

Moraxella nonliquefaciens colonizes the upper respiratory tract, particularly the nose, and is often indicated as a possible secondary invader in respiratory infections. *Moraxella lacunata* can be isolated from the eyes and is thought to be a cause of conjunctivitis in humans. However, *M. catarrhalis* is the pathogen that is most studied in the genus.

Moraxella catarrhalis

As mentioned, the scientific community has debated for many years about the appropriate classification of *Moraxella* bacteria. *M. catarrhalis* has been previously named *Micrococcus catarrhalis*, *Neisseria catarrhalis*, and *Branhamella catarrhalis*. Studies have shown that *M. catarrhalis* colonize 30 to 100 percent of infants between birth and 1 year of age. By adulthood, these numbers decrease to 1 to 10 percent.

Moraxella catarrhalis is the third most common cause of otitis media in children, after *Streptococcus pneumoniae* and *Haemophilus influenzae*, accounting for an estimated 3 to 4 million cases of otitis media annually in the United States alone. It also has been identified in cases of adult sinusitis, bronchitis, and bronchopneumonia, especially in older adults already compromised by chronic obstructive pulmonary disease (COPD). Patients with COPD experience emphysema and chronic bronchitis. The signs and symptoms are shortness of breath and chronic cough that are exacerbated (made worse) by the presence of *M. catarrhalis*. Often, the infection leads to pneumonia, which can be life-threatening in the older adult. As a pathogenic source of pneumonia, the clinical signs and symptoms are indistinguishable from gonococcal pneumonia, so it is important to perform the appropriate laboratory tests to differentiate between the two organisms. *M. catarrhalis* has been identified as the cause of systemic infections such as meningitis and endocarditis in rare cases.

Treatment

Laboratory cultures of *M. catarrhalis* strains isolated in the United States demonstrate that up to 95 percent produce beta-lactamase. Antibiotics such as penicillin, amoxicillin, and ampicillin are ineffective with bacteria that produce beta-lactamase. In certain geographic regions, more than 90 percent of *M. catarrhalis* is resistant to amoxicillin. Amoxicillin-clavulanate, second-generation and third-generation oral cephalosporins, and trimethoprim-sulfamethoxazole (TMP-SMZ) are the most recommended antibiotic treatment regimens. Azithromycin or clarithromycin can be used as alternative treatments.

Research is ongoing to produce a vaccine to prevent millions of cases of painful otitis media and other potentially serious respiratory and systemic infections in the United States.

Spirochetes

Spirochetes are organisms in the order Spirochaetales, derived from the Greek spira, meaning "spiral," and chaite, meaning "mane." The order has two families: *Spirochaetaceae*, which includes the genera *Spirochaetu*, *Cristispira*, *Treponema*, and *Borrelia*, and *Leptospiraceae*, which includes the genera *Leptospira* and *Leptonema*. Spirochetes are either facultative anaerobes or aerobes. The species that cause human disease are in the genera *Treponema*, *Borrelia*, and *Leptospira*.

Spirochetes are long, snake-like microorganisms that appear as tight coils under the microscope, somewhat resembling the cord of an old telephone or a corkscrew. They are propelled through fluids by axial filaments attached to each pole of the cell that are encased within a Gram-negative outer sheath that surrounds the bacterium. These internal flagella, similar to the flagella of other bacteria, are a unique characteristic of spirochetes. Rotation of these axial filaments allows the organism to rotate along its longitudinal cell axis in a corkscrew-like fashion. The action of the axial filaments, similar to the contraction of a large muscle, allows the spirochete to swim faster in high-viscosity liquids and more easily penetrate tissues. The number and shape of flagella vary among the species. Spirochetes are distinguished by the number of axial filaments and morphology. For example, *Leptospira* cells have a hook at the end, and *Treponema* organisms are thin yet coiled tightly (see Figure 15-12). *Borrelia* species are more loosely coiled and are somewhat thicker than *Treponema*. Laboratory examination of these microbes may require use of dark-field or electron microscopy due to their extreme thinness.

Spirochaeta are free-living, non-pathogenic inhabitants of mud and water and are responsible for a disease referred to

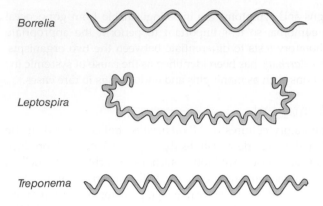

Figure 15-12 Morphology of spirochetes: *Borrelia*, *leptospira*, and *Treponema*.

as endemic syphilis. *Leptospira* affects animals primarily and humans secondarily (see Figure 15-13). The genus *Borrelia* includes several species that are transmitted by lice and ticks and cause Lyme disease and relapsing fever. Many species of spirochetes are saprophytes and can be found in soil, sewage, and decaying matter. They can also be found in standing water. Other species are found within the gastrointestinal tract, oral cavity, and genitals of animals and humans as either normal microflora or pathogens.

The first discovery of pathogenic spirochetes is credited to Otto Obermeier, a German physician who, in 1868, detected highly motile corkscrew-like organisms in the blood of patients with relapsing fever. Obermeier noticed that they were similar to the water spirochete, *Spirochaeta plicatilis*.

Spirochetes are not a particularly large group of bacteria (only six genera); however, they are an important group of organisms that may have a major impact on the lives of humans. Spirochetes are responsible for four diseases that are discussed in this chapter: syphilis, Lyme disease, relapsing fever, and yaws. They are also important symbionts that live in the stomachs of cows and other **ruminants**.

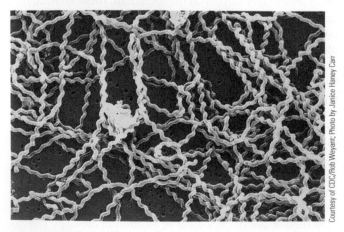

Courtesy of CDC/Rob Weyant; Photo by Janice Haney Carr

Figure 15-13 Digitally-colored scanning electron micrograph (SEM) image depicts a number of corkscrew-shaped, *Leptospira* sp.

Treponema

Treponema species belong to the phylum Spirochaetes, class Spirochaetes, order Spirochaetales, and family *Spirochaetaceae*. They are normal microflora of the oral cavity and include the agents *Treponema pallidum*, which causes syphilis, *Treponema pertenue*, which causes yaws (endemic syphilis), and *Treponema endemicum*, which causes non-venereal endemic syphilis. These diseases are referred to as "treponematoses" and are characterized by distinct primary, secondary, latency, and tertiary clinical stages.

Treponema organisms are delicate, requiring pH in the range of 7.2 to 7.4, temperatures in the range of 30°C to 37°C, and a microaerophilic environment. The cells have high lipid content, which is an unusual characteristic for bacteria. They possess a complex antigenic makeup that is difficult to determine because they cannot be grown in vitro.

Treponema pallidum

The name of the organism comes from the Latin pallidus, meaning "pale." There are four subspecies of *T. pallidum*, although some believe that *T. pallidum* subspecies *pallidum* and *T. pallidum* subspecies *pertenue* are variants that cause different degrees of infection, rather than true subspecies. The four species, which are identical to *T. pallidum* in their morphology, can be distinguished from one other by infectious patterns in humans, by geographical location, and by nucleic acid sequencing. The four subspecies of *T. pallidum* and the diseases they cause are:

- *T. pallidum pallidum*: causes syphilis
- *T. pallidum pertenue*: causes yaws
- *T. pallidum endemicum*: causes bejel (endemic syphilis)
- *T. pallidum carateum*: causes pinta (non-venereal syphilis)

Treponema pallidum was one of the few major bacterial pathogens that microbiologists had been unsuccessful at culturing in vitro (in a test tube) since Robert Koch first identified the spirochete as the causative agent for syphilis more than 100 years ago. This was a barrier to better understanding the organism and its disease expression. In 2018, researchers reported their successful long-term cultivation of *T. pallidum* in a tissue culture system, paving the way for expanding analysis of new information applicable to the diagnosis, treatment, and prevention of syphilis.

Treponema pallidum pallidum

Treponema pallidum pallidum is the most virulent of the spirochetes. It is the causative agent of the sexually transmitted disease venereal syphilis. Syphilis is a slow-evolving disease with short, symptomatic periods related to the rapid multiplication of the bacteria, followed by prolonged **asymptomatic** periods during which the immune system attempts to heal tissues. The incubation period for the disease is from 10 to 90 days and precedes the clinical presentation of signs and symptoms.

Syphilis is transmitted in a manner similar to that of HIV. Because the spirochete requires moist, dark environments to thrive, it is ideally suited to transmission through sexual contact. It can, however, be transmitted to a host through blood transfusions, infected hypodermic needles, breast milk, and saliva. The bacteria can only live on surfaces outside of the human body for approximately 2 hours.

Beginning in around the mid-1400s, practitioners of the medical arts in the more developed nations used mercury to treat syphilis, which did little to treat the disease and more than likely poisoned the patient. Practitioners also used bleeding techniques, most likely infecting themselves with the bacteria in the process.

Historians believe that Columbus and his crew brought the bacteria back from the New World, triggering the "Great Pox" in Europe in the sixteenth century. The Great Pox most likely developed from a milder clinical disease from the Native Americans, mutating into the deadlier strain. Without knowing the origin of the disease, each European country blamed the disease on its geographical neighbor. The French referred to the disease as the "Italian pox," and the English called it the "French pox." A few famous figures in history suspected of having had syphilis include George Washington, Adolph Hitler, and Napoleon Bonaparte. Napoleon had arsenic (a treatment regimen at that time) in his system when he died in exile.

Sir William Osler, considered to be the founder of modern medicine, referred to syphilis as the "great imitator" because of the variable clinical manifestations of the disease. He told his students that if they knew the disease, then they understood medicine.

In the United States, Ehrlich developed Salvarsan (arsphenamine), a treatment that was toxic and difficult to administer. Injections of neoarsphenamine replaced this in 1909, and the progression of the disease was monitored monthly with spinal taps. The U.S. Public Health Service launched an anti-syphilis campaign in 1937, and physicians treated the disease with repeated doses of heavy arsenic chemicals.

Today, syphilis is generally treated with an injection of penicillin or by a 2-week regimen of tetracycline. The first stages of syphilis are curable with these injections, so early detection is important. Early detection in pregnant women can prevent the disease from being transmitted to the unborn fetus.

Clinical Stages of Syphilis

Treponema pallidum is introduced into the body through cuts in the skin or small abrasions of the mucous membranes. It is most commonly transmitted through sexual contact. As with other blood-borne pathogens, transmission through shared contaminated needles is not uncommon as well as transplacental transmission of the infection to the fetus from the mother (see Figure 15-14). Young adults aged 20 to 24 years are most often affected and, because the route of transmission is the same for both diseases, 10 percent of gonorrhea patients are also infected with syphilis. Proper use of a condom can prevent STD infection.

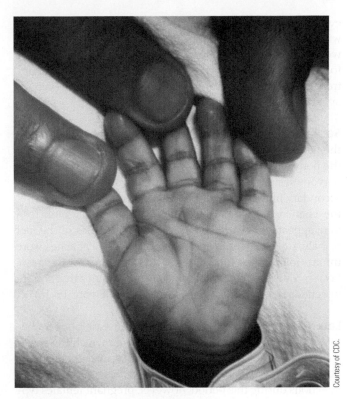

Figure 15-14 A newborn infant's left palm with copper colored rash, characteristic of congenital syphilis caused by the spirochete bacterium, *Treponema pallidum*, and transferred by way of the placenta.

Primary Stage The primary stage of syphilis involves multiplication of the bacteria at the site of entry (typically the genitalia) to produce a localized infection. Ten to 60 days after bacterial exposure, a small, hard, ulcerous lesion appears at the infection site. This lesion, referred to as a **chancre**, may appear on the sexual organs, the anorectal area, or the mouth of the infected individual, depending on the area of sexual exposure. It typically appears as a single primary lesion, but in persons with HIV-AIDS multiple lesions may occur (see Figure 15-15). It initially appears as a slightly red area but

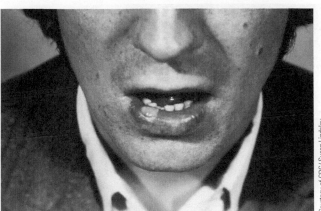

Figure 15-15 Presence of a primary extragenital syphilitic chancre lesion on the lower lip caused by *Treponema pallidum*.

eventually ulcerates, forming a slightly elevated oval lesion with a red rim. The lesion heals without treatment in 3 to 6 weeks. Initial infection during the primary stage is typically followed by swollen and painless lymph nodes and, if left untreated, progresses throughout the body and into the secondary stage of the disease.

Secondary Stage The secondary stage of syphilis is typically the period in which the bacteria are spread to other tissues of the body and may involve any organ of the body. The central nervous system (CNS) is most frequently infected during the secondary phase of the disease. One week to 6 months after the chancre heals, a widespread maculopapular pink rash may appear, concentrated especially on the soles of the feet or palms of the hands and genitals. Fever, headaches, sore throat, joint pains, and weight loss accompany the rash. Lesions often appear within mucous membranes that secrete infectious fluids and last 3 to 6 months (see Figure 15-16).

Latent Stage A latency period for the disease appears between the primary and secondary stages in which the spirochetes continue to invade the host's tissues although no obvious symptoms are visible. The host may or may not be infectious during this period, however, pregnant females typically pass the disease to their unborn children as congenital syphilis infection. The infected host may experience vague discomfort during this period as the spirochetes burrow into the tissues. Approximately 50 to 70 percent of latency-period carriers do not move into the final stage of the disease.

Late (Tertiary) Stage The final stage of syphilis is referred to as the late or tertiary stage and occurs 10 to 30 years after the initial infection. During this stage, the spirochetes inflict serious damage to the invaded tissues. The spirochetes concentrate in specific areas of the tissues and form **gummas** or **syphilomas** (see Figure 15-17).

Spirochetes may invade any tissue of the body, and the disease is labeled according to the system or organs that are

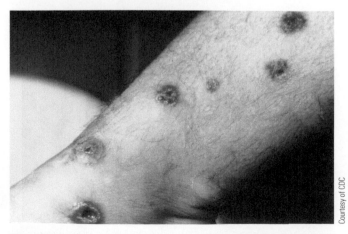

Figure 15-16 A patient's right ankle with of a number of inflamed and draining coin-shaped, scaly lesions due to secondary syphilis, caused by *Treponema pallidum*.

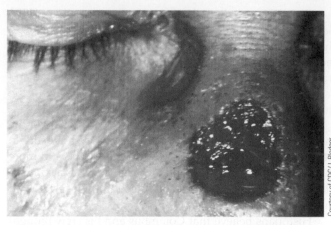

Figure 15-17 Gumma of nose due to a long-standing tertiary syphilitic *Treponema pallidum* infection.

affected. For example, neurosyphilis manifests in the CNS of the host. Spirochetes within nervous tissue of the brain can cause chronic syphilitic encephalitis, resulting in dementia, hemiparesis, or specific neurologic deficits, depending on the area of the brain that is involved. Pleocytosis, elevated protein levels, and lowered glucose levels may be found in the CSF. A positive Venereal Disease Research Laboratories (VDRL) assay from the CSF indicates a definitive diagnosis.

The posterior sensory tracts of the spinal cord are frequently involved in neurosyphilis, resulting in numbness of the extremities. The name for this syphilis-induced malady is tabes dorsalis, which results in a characteristic gait and deformed knees (see Figure 15-18). Without proper feedback to the brain, the joints become malformed from misuse.

Cardiovascular syphilis occurs in the tertiary stage of the disease and affects the cardiovascular system, creating symptoms that resemble cardiovascular disease and often resulting in misdiagnosis. Heart valves may become damaged, and the small vessels that feed the aorta may become inflamed. This inflammation can cause syphilitic aortitis, resulting in aneurysms or dilatations of the ascending aorta. Aneurysm rupture is often fatal, and aortic ring dilatation can lead to aortic valve insufficiency and regurgitation. The coronary arteries may become occluded, resulting in myocardial infarction.

Spirochetes may also invade the skeletal system, destroying bony tissue and resulting in frequent fractures. Damage to nasal and palate bones may result in serious disfigurement requiring extensive facial reconstruction.

Laboratory Analysis of Syphilis

In 1906, the Wasserman test was developed for the diagnosis of syphilis. The test detects the presence of *T. pallidum* through its reaction to substances in the blood. Today, the VDRL test and the rapid plasma regain (RPR) test for the detection of antibodies are used for diagnosis. At least 18 treponemal-specific tests are available in the United States. Use of only one type of serologic test (nontreponemal or treponemal) is insufficient for diagnosis and can result in false-negative

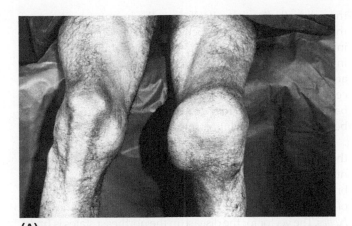

(A)

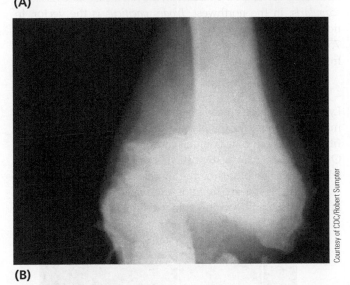

(B)

Figure 15-18 A. Neuropathic arthropathy, known as charcot's joint, seen as the external view of the knee in an individual with tertiary syphilis. **B.** X-ray of the same patient's left knee showing bony and soft tissue destruction of the knee joint.

results among persons tested during primary syphilis and false-positive results among persons without syphilis or previously treated syphilis. The gold standard for diagnosis of syphilis is culture, performed in vivo, by intratesticular inoculation of rabbits with infected exudates, but this remains an expensive and time-consuming method for diagnosis.

Before the appearance of antibodies, detecting spirochetes within the chancres of patients by direct fluorescent antibody test for *T. pallidum* (DFA-TP) or dark-field microscopy is a traditional way of diagnosing the disease in the primary stage. Dark-field microscopy allows bacteria to be viewed by lighting them up against a dark background. Light from the microscope is directed toward the bacteria at an angle so that the light that reaches the objective is reflected directly from the bacteria. DFA-TP is performed with tissue taken directly from a lesion and is more useful than dark-field microscopy because it can differentiate between pathogenic and non-pathogenic treponemes. Persons with a reactive nontreponemal test result should also have a treponemal test to confirm the diagnosis of syphilis infection.

Treponema pallidum pertenue

Yaws is a disease process similar to syphilis but is not sexually transmitted. It is caused by *T. pallidum pertenue*. Yaws occurs in tropical regions and begins as an inflammatory lesion. In highly endemic areas, up to 75 percent of the population may become infected by age 20. It typically affects children and begins as a painless red papule called a "mother yaw" through which the bacteria enter the body. Raspberry-like papules then appear and are scratched by the child, spreading the infection. After a latency period similar to the one involving syphilis, internal and external lesions appear, destroying skin, bones, and other tissues (see Figure 15-19).

Treponema pallidum endemicum

Subspecies *T. pallidum endemicum* is the cause of endemic non-venereal syphilis also called bejel. The disease affects children younger than age 15 years from poorer regions of Asia, Africa, and India. It may be transmitted through contaminated water or through direct contact with mucosal lesions. Proper hygiene habits may prevent the spread of the disease, which is similar in most ways to venereal syphilis. Unlike yaws and pinta, bejel is found in dry arid climates. Previously found in Eastern Europe, it is now rare in that region and seen mainly in nomadic tribes in Saudi Arabia and sub-Saharan Africa.

Treponema pallidum carateum

Subspecies *T. pallidum carateum* causes the disease known as pinta or carate and is the oldest of the human treponemes. It occurs primarily in tropical Central and South America and Mexico. It is characterized by painless primary papules, followed by secondary papules on the hands, feet, and scalp. Pinta, in Spanish, means spot or dot and characterizes the human skin depigmentation that its ulcerative lesions can cause during the secondary and tertiary stages of the disease. The spirochetes for pinta can only be transmitted during the primary stage by

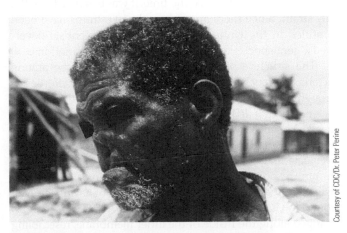

Figure 15-19 78-Year-old man with degenerative changes to the mid-face known technically as rhinopharyngitis mutilans, and commonly as yaws or gangosa, a 50-year history of the nonvenereal endemic syphilis infection caused by the *Treponema pallidum pertenue* spirochete.

direct contact with the lesions, and the only long-term systemic health detriments associated with the disease are related to disfigurement and discoloration of skin. Infected individuals in Nicaragua and Guatemala are referred to as "los morados," which means the purple (or bluish-purple) ones.

Borrelia

Borrelia is part of the family *Spirochaetaceae*. Bacteria in the genus *Borrelia* are helical and have from 3 to 10 loose coils and 15 to 20 axial filaments. They are thicker and less curved than the treponemes. The species include *B. recurrentis*, *B. hermsii*, and *B. burgdorferi*.

Borrelia is transmitted to hosts by lice or ticks. A lice vector transmits *B. recurrentis*, the cause of epidemic relapsing fever. A tick vector transmits *B. hermsii*, the cause of endemic relapsing fever. *Borrelia burgdorferi* causes Lyme disease, and it is transmitted by a tick vector. Collectively, these diseases are called borrelioses.

In 1878, Gregor Münch wrote that recurrent or relapsing fever was transmitted by arthropods such as lice, fleas, or bugs. The French microbiologists Sergent and Foley confirmed this in 1910. The British physicians Dutton and Todd, through their work in the Congo in 1905, discovered that "human tick disease" was caused by a spirochete transmitted by the African soft-shelled tick, *Ornithodoros moubata*. At the same time, the German microbiologist, Robert Koch, investigating East Coast fever in cattle in East Africa, noticed that Europeans traveling to that region were suffering from a recurrent fever that was thought to be malaria. Koch proved that the fever was indeed caused by *O. moubata*, and at the same time demonstrated that spirochetes could be transmitted via eggs to the progeny of infected female ticks.

Borrelia burgdorferi

Borrelia burgdorferi was first isolated from the deer tick by Willy Burgdorfer in 1982. At the time, it was believed to be the only strain. Since then, approximately 100 strains have been identified in the United States alone, and scientists developed a genospecies to subcategorize the many variations.

The structure of *B. burgdorferi* is highly unique among bacteria. It is very large and highly motile, swimming effortlessly through bodily fluids and tissues. It is similar to other *Borrelia* bacteria in that it has a three-layer cell wall with internal flagella. However, what sets it apart from other *Borrelia* is a gel-like coating of glycoproteins, called the slime layer. The slime layer acts like a suit of armor, protecting it from the host's immune response. The arrangement of DNA in *B. burgdorferi* is distinctive and unlike other bacteria. Instead of having DNA all around the inside of its cytoplasm, the DNA of *B. burgdorferi* is arranged along the inside of the inner membrane, resembling a net just below the surface of its outer layer.

The bacterium literally invades a healthy human cell and causes the cell's own digestive enzymes to dissolve the cell. As the bacterium leaves the cell, it drapes itself in a portion of the cell wall, disguising itself from the immune response of the host. Unlike other spirochetes, *B. burgdorferi* can remain in the human body for years in a dormant state. While in this inanimate state, the bacteria are not performing metabolic activities, meaning that antibiotics would have no effect on cell wall synthesis. When conditions become favorable, the bacteria can trigger a relapse in victims who were thought to be disease-free after antibiotic therapy.

B. burgdorferi causes Lyme disease, the most common of the tick-borne diseases in the United States. Transmission to humans is through a deer tick vector that usually occupies brushy areas or tall grass. In the United States, the distribution of the disease matches the distribution of ticks of the genus *Ixodes*. The vector for the disease in the northeast states is *Ixodes scapularis*. In the northwest, *Ixodes pacificus* is the vector. In ticks that have been caught in some areas and examined, up to 75 percent were infected with the spirochete. Transmission from human to human has not been documented.

Lyme Disease

Lyme disease affects many systems of the body at once. Victims may test negative for the disease, leading to a misdiagnosis of **fibromyalgia**, chronic fatigue syndrome, or multiple sclerosis. Other victims may test positive but exhibit no symptoms whatsoever. Symptoms of the disease consist of a bulls-eye skin lesion, erythema migrans, muscle pain, headache, stiff neck, fatigue, and lymph node swelling (see Figure 15-20).

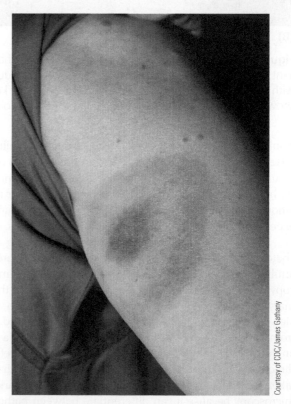

Figure 15-20 An erythematous rash on a woman's upper arm in a "bulls-eye" pattern at the site of a tick bite is shown. Lyme disease was subsequently diagnosed.

Mild symptoms can be easily ignored, leading to more severe complications such as meningitis, encephalitis, Bell's palsy, myocarditis, or arthritis.

Diagnosis Small numbers of the spirochetes in the bloodstream usually prevent diagnosis by direct examination of the blood; however, unlike the treponemes, in vitro culture is possible with the right combination of nutrients. The spirochetes are microaerophilic and grow best in Barbour Stoenner-Kelly (BSK) broth.

Immunologic and molecular diagnostic techniques can detect the spirochetes in tissues. The presence of erythema migrans indicates Lyme disease and may be used for diagnosis. Serologic tests used for diagnosis include the enzyme-linked immunosorbent assay (ELISA) Lyme test, Western blot, borreliacidal antibody assay, Lyme urine antigen test (LUAT), and T-cell activation test. The ELISA and Western blot are the most commonly used diagnostic tests.

Treatment Doxycycline, amoxicillin, or cefuroxime axetil are antibiotics used to treat Lyme disease in the early stages of the infection. Patients with certain neurological or cardiac forms of illness may require IV treatment with ceftriaxone or penicillin. During the later stages, treatment with these antibiotics may be effective for elimination of the spirochetes from the body, but damage done to joints and the nervous system might require further treatment.

Between 10 and 20 percent of individuals who completed antibiotic therapy may suffer with persistent or recurrent symptoms. This condition is called post-treatment Lyme disease syndrome (PTLDS) or chronic Lyme disease.

Borrelia recurrentis and B. hermsii

Borrelia recurrentis, also known as relapsing fever, is transmitted primarily via the human body **louse** (singular of lice), although it can also be transmitted through ticks. Relapsing fever occurs when humans are crowded together under poor sanitary conditions, particularly in areas of North and South Africa, Asia, and Peru. The body louse is called *Pediculus humanus*, and the disease that it causes is often epidemic because of the conditions in which the louse thrives. Typhus fever, another louse-borne infection, often occurs in the same populations.

Tick-borne relapsing fever is typically endemic but can become epidemic under the right circumstances. The largest outbreak of tick-borne relapsing fever in the Western Hemisphere occurred in Washington State in 1968, affecting a group of Boy Scouts on a camping trip.

Relapsing fever derives its name from the fact that the victim experiences 3 to 10 subsequent episodes of fever, chills, and muscle pains that recur in intervals of 5 to 15 days, each less severe than the previous one. During these relapses, *B. recurrentis* circulates throughout the blood of the victim and can readily be observed in stains through a dark-field microscope (see Figure 15-21).

Relapsing fever manifests with similar symptoms. The onset of the disease is abrupt, with a fever that can reach

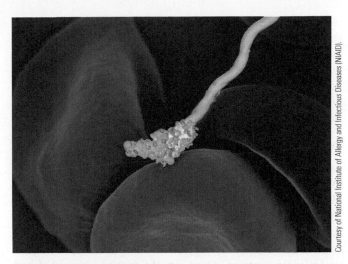

Figure 15-21 SEM image depicts a green-colored, spiral shaped, *Borrelia hermsii* the causative bacterium of tick-borne relapsing fever (TBRF) on top of red blood cells (RBCS).

Courtesy of National Institute of Allergy and Infectious Diseases (NIAID).

104°F. Following transmission and an incubation period of 7 days, the spirochetes begin a massive bodily invasion. Respiratory symptoms, CNS involvement, hepatomegaly, and splenomegaly may occur, and the patient may be jaundiced.

Penicillin is usually effective in treating relapsing fever. Tetracycline and chloramphenicol may also be prescribed. Control of tick and lice infestations is the best preventative measure.

Leptospira

The genus *Leptospira* belongs to the order Spirochaetales and family *Leptospiraceae*. Bacteria in this genus are referred to as leptospires and are thin, flexible, tightly coiled obligate Gram-negative aerobes. They are highly motile and are the smallest and most delicate of the spirochetes. Their structure is similar to other spirochetes, that is, they have a multi-layered outer membrane and flagella located in the periplasmic space, but hooked ends are indicative of *Leptospira*.

Leptospirosis

The disease the spirochete *Leptospira interrogans* causes is called leptospirosis. Disease transmission is through infected animal urine, especially dog, domestic livestock (cattle, swine, horses), or rodent urine. The organism is often lodged in the renal tubules of the host animals and is washed out with their urine. Drinking urine-contaminated water from streams is a common method of transmission, but the spirochetes can also enter the body through cuts or broken skin.

The three subspecies that are most often implicated in leptospirosis are *L. interrogans canicola*, *L. interrogans pomona*, and *L. interrogans icterohaemorrhagiae*. Classic leptospirosis consists of an initial septicemic stage followed by an immune stage. The septicemic stage arises abruptly and is characterized by a high fever and severe headache. Eye pain and photophobia may also be present, and some victims are inflicted with hemorrhagic rash. An asymptomatic stage of 1 to 3 days is followed by an immune stage during which the *Leptospira* are cleared of the blood and an inflammatory reaction develops.

Weil's Disease

Leptospira interrogans icterohaemorrhagiae is the causative agent of Weil's disease, also known as infectious hemorrhagic jaundice. Weil's disease is named for A. Weil, a German physician who, in 1886, documented the intense jaundice and "black vomit" of his patients and noticed that the symptoms were similar to those of hepatitis. Weil noticed that patients spent a good deal of time barefoot in wet, poorly drained places that had been contaminated by animal urine, especially the urine of rats, or the urine of infected humans. Weil's disease can be fatal if left untreated, primarily due to liver or renal damage. Even nonfatal cases are often quite severe, although mild cases do occur.

Diagnosis and Treatment

Dark-field microscopic examination of blood, CSF, or urine often reveals the leptospires. Urine is most often used because the leptospires are harbored there for longer periods of time. Diagnosis by culture of blood or urine is reliable, but serologic analysis, specifically microagglutination or macroscopic slide agglutination, is used by most laboratories for definitive diagnosis. Antibodies appear in the blood 1 to 2 weeks after infection.

Infection by *Leptospira* is most successfully treated with doxycycline or penicillin. Antibiotic therapy works best if treated early in the infectious stage. Sanitary measures can reduce the incidence of the disease. People should avoid areas where animal urine may be present, especially areas of standing water. Vaccines are available for animals but offer only partial immunity. No vaccines are currently available for humans.

MICRO NOTES

"The Cure Is Not Heavy Metal"

No, this is not about the British rock band being classified under punk instead of heavy metal. Heavy metals such as mercury and silver nitrate, along with poisons including arsenic, were long-used, historic treatments given to individuals suffering distressing signs and debilitating symptoms of gonorrhea or syphilis. The sexually-transmitted diseases that have existed for centuries have been blamed on one country or the other as the source, and carried from region to region, continent to continent by conquerors and soldiers until they became common, though feared and ridiculed. These pathogenic diseases remain in modern times, throughout the globe. Before the discovery of antibiotics, mercury had been widely prescribed by early practitioners of the medical arts. The treatments that included ingestion, inhalation, injection, baths, and ointments of mercury created terrible side effects causing neuropathies, kidney failure, severe mouth ulcers, and loss of teeth. Commonly, patients died of mercurial poisoning rather than from the gonorrheal or syphilitic disease. Treatment would typically go on for years and gave rise to the saying from the fifteenth century, "A night with Venus, and a lifetime with mercury". If heavy metal music, however, "cures" what ails you, go ahead and listen to your heart's content.

 ## Under the Microscope

Danielle, a CST at an inner city hospital, is advised of an add-on case of diagnostic laparoscopy for lower abdominal pain in a 28-year-old female with a past history of a sexually-transmitted disease (STD) infection. As the surgeon inspected the peritoneal cavity, the appendix was normal in appearance; however, there were numerous abnormalities involving the adnexal structures (fallopian tubes and ovaries) and requested that cultures be sent to the lab.

1. What conditions based on her history could be the cause for what the surgeon found?

2. What type of bacterial pathogens could be the cause of her previous STD?

3. What impact might this disease process or the clinical history have on this patient's future?

4. How are the types of infections covered in this chapter typically transmitted?

5. Which morphological features of the bacterial species that could possibly cause the patient's signs and symptoms would the pathologist see on microscopic examination?

CHAPTER 16

Gram-Negative Bacilli and Coccobacilli

Learning Objectives

After completing the study of this chapter, you will be able to:

1. Define key terms.
2. Discuss the mechanisms of disease transmission of opportunistic microorganisms.
3. Identify the body systems involved in infections by pathogenic species of Proteobacteria.
4. Compare and contrast pathogenicity and disease expression in the various taxonomic families within class Gamma Proteobacteria.
5. Identify the Gram-negative bacilli frequently responsible for healthcare-associated infections (HAIs).
6. Apply critical thinking skills in relating chapter material to the surgical environment of care or broader global community.

Key Terms

Atherosclerotic plaques

Cytotoxins

Degranulation

Entomopathogenic

Endoscopic retrograde cholangiopan-creatography (ERCP)

Guillain-Barré syndrome

Halophilic

Inflammatory bowel disease

Osteomyelitis

Peyer's patches

Plague

Polymicrobial

Reticuloendothelial system (RES)

Serovars/serotypes

Tracheostomy

Typhoid fever

Vagotomy

Ventriculitis

Zoonotic

The Big Picture

Many of the pathogenic microorganisms responsible for serious infections in humans are Gram-negative bacilli or coccobacilli. Normally found in or on animals and humans, or free-living in nature, these ubiquitous microbes become pathogenic when given access to areas where they do not belong. During your examination of the topics in this chapter, consider the following:

1. Which characteristics of the various microbes discussed enhance the virulence of these types of bacteria?

2. Which groups or special populations are at increased risk for life-threatening infections?

3. Why does modern medical care continue to contribute to serious morbidity and mortality from these types of bacterial infections?

4. Have the types of bacteria responsible for causing massive deadly outbreaks throughout history been eradicated or could they cause new pandemics?

Clinical **S**ignificance **T**opic

Many of the bacterial species discussed in this chapter are part of the normal gastrointestinal microbiome; however, are opportunistic pathogens capable of causing devastating infections. Surgical technologists are taught the importance of strict "bowel technique" in cases involving the gastrointestinal tract to prevent potential contamination of internal cavities, organs, or tissues. The specifics of bowel technique are outlined in the Association of Surgical Technologists (AST) Guidelines for Best Practices in Bowel Technique (available at www.ast.org) in the section on Aseptic Technique. An understanding of the bacteria involved in these surgical interventions and their potential for surgical site infections, combined with skills taught in laboratory and clinical practice, will strengthen the foundational principles of quality patient care the surgical technologist provides as part of a high-functioning, integrated, professional team in the OR.

classes and their families within phylum Proteobacteria include:

- Alpha Proteobacteria: *Brucellaceae* and *Rickettsiaceae* (see Chapter 10)

- Beta Proteobacteria: *Neisseriaceae* (see Chapter 15 for cocci genera), which includes the genera *Kingella* and *Chromobacterium*, and *Alcaligenaceae*, which includes the genus *Bordetella*

- Gamma Proteobacteria:

  1. *Enterobacteriaceae* includes the genera *Escherichia, Enterobacter, Klebsiella, Citrobacter, Morganella, Proteus, Providencia, Serratia, Salmonella, Shigella, Yersinia*, and others.

  2. *Moraxellaceae* (see Chapter 15 for cocci genera), which includes the genus *Acinetobacter*

  3. *Pasteurellaceae* includes the genera *Pasteurella, Haemophilus, Actinobacillus*, and others.

  4. *Vibrionaceae* includes the genus *Vibrio*

  5. *Aeromonadaceae* includes the genus *Aeromonas*

  6. *Pseudomonadaceae* includes the genus *Pseudomonas*

  7. Epsilon Proteobacteria: *Campylobacteraceae* and *Helicobacteraceae*

Phylum: Proteobacteria

The phylum Proteobacteria is broken down into classes: alpha (α), beta (β), gamma (γ), delta (δ), epsilon (ε), and zeta (ζ). Some of the most pathogenic species of bacteria belong to members of Proteobacteria. Members of the delta and zeta classes are not identified as human pathogens. All of the members of this group are Gram-negative bacilli or coccobacilli. Some of the taxonomic

Brucellaceae

Brucella bacteria are small, aerobic, Gram-negative, non-motile, non-encapsulated, intracellular coccobacilli that belong to the family *Brucellaceae* and class Alpha Proteobacteria. *Brucella* are referred to as intracellular parasites of the **reticuloendothelial system (RES)** after they gain entry into the body via breaks in the skin, mucous membranes, conjunctiva, ingestion of unpasteurized milk or undercooked meat, and respiratory inhalation of aerosols. Once in the body, the bacterial cells are phagocytized by monocytes and macrophages, which carry the microbes to the liver, kidneys, spleen, lymph nodes, joints, breast tissue, and bone marrow. Granulomas form in these body structures and, if not treated, the microbes will destroy the organ tissue.

The genus *Brucella* consists of six species, four of which are human pathogens that cause the **zoonotic** infection called brucellosis and are named for the animal in which they are most commonly found: *B. abortus* (cattle), *B. canis* (dogs), *B. melitensis* (sheep and goats), and *B. suis* (swine). The species vary in their ability to survive destruction because they can inhibit leukocyte **degranulation** and are resistant to phagocytosis. *B. melitensis* has the highest degree of pathogenicity followed by *B. suis*, *B. abortus*, and *B. canis*. Brucellosis is discussed further in Chapter 17.

Kingella

The genus *Kingella* is a member of the class Beta Proteobacteria, family *Neisseriaceae*, and includes the species: *Kingella kingae*, *K. denitrificans*, and *K. oralis*. Species in the *Kingella* genus are Gram-negative, short, non-motile coccobacilli that may initially appear as cocci.

Kingella kingae

The species *Kingella kingae* comprises Gram-negative, fastidious, pathogenic coccobacilli that have been identified mainly in children and that colonize the respiratory and oropharyngeal tracts. Cases of invasive disease caused by *K. kingae* include bacteremia in infants, **osteomyelitis** in young children, and endocarditis in school-aged children and adults. Definitive diagnosis of *K. kingae* is frequently missed because invasive disease is uncommon.

Kingella denitrificans and K. oralis

Kingella denitrificans and *K. oralis* are coccobacilli; however, some isolates may appear to be diplococci and are very similar in appearance to *N. gonorrhoeae*. The bacteria in this genus are commensals in the oropharynx and on gums and teeth but are only occasionally pathogenic. Minor oral trauma such as aggressive dental cleaning and brushing may allow transmission of the bacteria into deep tissues and blood vessels. Endocarditis infections may be attributable to *Kingella* bacteria.

Chromobacterium

Chromobacterium is a genus also in the class Beta Proteobacteria and family *Neisseriaceae*. *Chromobacterium* is a large, curved or rod-shaped Gram-negative microorganism that is a facultative anaerobe. It is motile with a single polar and one or two lateral peritrichous flagella. The principal species within the genus is *C. violaceum*. The name indicates that *C. violaceum*

produces a violet-colored pigment known as violacein. The organism is found in water, soil, and animals but is not a part of the normal flora of humans. *C. violaceum* is well-known for inhabiting the south-eastern region of the United States and tropical areas of Southeast Asia and South America. It is the only microorganism that produces a violet-colored pigment that can cause an infection in humans (see Figure 16-1).

Infections with *C. violaceum* are relatively rare in humans and usually occur in persons who have an open traumatic wound contaminated by soil and/or water. Individuals can develop serious complications due to the infection, including cellulitis, wound ulceration, lymphadenitis, septicemia, osteomyelitis, solid organ abscesses, UTIs, and eye infections. Infections have a high mortality rate even with treatment. The virulence of *C. violaceum* is due to the production of an endotoxin that helps the bacterial cells evade phagocytosis.

Recently, researchers have discovered a microbe in the *Chromobacterium* genus, designated *Chromobacterium* sp. Panama or *Csp_P*, in the mid-gut of *Aedes aegypti* mosquitoes. These mosquitoes, along with the *Anopheles gambiae* species, are carriers of and vectors for transmission of malaria (*Plasmodium falciparum*) and dengue fever viruses. The *Csp_P* bacteria do not produce violaceum but instead have shown the ability to reduce both the infectivity of the mosquitoes and the lifespans of larvae and adults. The bacteria were shown to also be antipathogenic and **entomopathogenic** in laboratory cultures. The research provides new strategies of producing a mosquito biopesticide from *Csp_P*, derived from an air-dried, non-living bacterial powder preparation in the fight against these menacing global health threats. Researchers reporting in the May 2020 American Society for Microbiology journal *Applied and Environmental Microbiology*, stated "We demonstrate that the preparation has broad spectrum activity against the larval form of the mosquitoes responsible for the transmission of malaria and the dengue, chikungunya, yellow

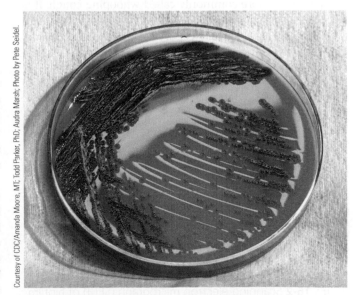

Courtesy of CDC/Amanda Moore, MT; Todd Parker, PhD; Audra Marsh; Photo by Pete Seidel.

Figure 16-1 Dark violet-colored *Chromobacterium violaceum* bacteria grown on sheep's blood agar demonstrating production of violacein.

fever, West Nile, and Zika viruses, as well as mosquito larvae that are already resistant to commonly used mosquitocidal chemicals. Our preparation possesses many favorable traits: it kills at a low dosage, and it does not lose activity when exposed to high temperatures, all of which suggest that this preparation could eventually become an effective new tool for controlling mosquitoes and the diseases they spread." An exciting prospect of using a microbial species of bacteria to control dangerous bacterial and viral pathogens.

Alcaligenaceae

The family *Alcaligenaceae* is a member of the class Beta Proteobacteria and consists of several human pathogenic genera, including *Achromobacter, Alcaligenes,* and *Bordetella.* A number of other species are mammalian and avian pathogens. Related species within the family are Gram-negative bacilli to coccobacilli found in the environment that become opportunistic pathogens in humans.

Achromobacter xylosoxidans, formerly called *Alcaligenes xylosoxidans,* is a water-borne bacterium that can live in saline environments and has been isolated from patients with cystic fibrosis and from the lumens of indwelling central venous catheters after removal. It has been included in publications regarding emerging diseases and healthcare-associated infections (HAIs) in oncology clinics (see Figure 16-2).

Bordetella

Bordetella is the most recognized member of the *Alcaligenaceae* family. *Bordetella* species are Gram-negative, strictly aerobic coccobacilli that occur singly or in small groups (see Figure 16-3). Three species cause disease in humans: *B. pertussis, B. parapertussis,* and *B. bronchiseptica. Bordetella pertussis* is the most virulent of the three organisms and causes the disease pertussis, more commonly called whooping cough. It is still primarily a disease of infants and children, although adults are susceptible. It is especially dangerous in infants younger than 6 months of age. The morbidity rate is not

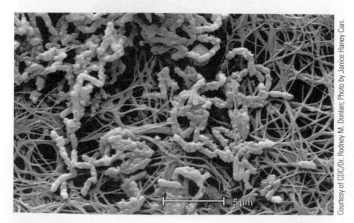

Figure 16-2 Scanning electron micrograph (SEM) of biofilm from lumen of a central venous catheter containing *Alcaligenes xylosoxidans* in association with fibrin-like material on the catheter's surface.

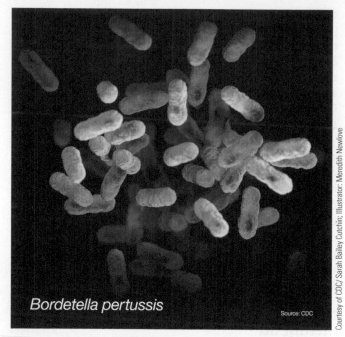

Bordetella pertussis

Source: CDC

Courtesy of CDC/ Sarah Bailey Cutchin; Illustrator: Meredith Newlove

Figure 16-3 A 3D computer image of a group of aerobic, Gram-negative, *Bordetella pertussis* bacteria as seen with SEM.

affected by climate or season. Pertussis is discussed in detail in Chapter 20. Virulence factors of *B. pertussis* include:

- A surface protein located on the cell wall called filamentous hemagglutinin, which aids the ability of the organism to adhere to the cilia of the respiratory tract
- Secretion of pertussis toxin, an exotoxin that increases the release of histamine
- Secretion of adenylate cyclase, a compound that inhibits phagocytosis
- Tracheal cytotoxin, an exotoxin that destroys the tissue of the respiratory tract

Enterobacteriaceae

The microorganisms within the family *Enterobacteriaceae* and its genera have long been referred to as enteric bacteria or "enterics" because most of them are commensals in the gastrointestinal tracts of humans and other mammals. Some of the species are found in plants, water, and soil, so they do not reflect the enteric classification.

In 2020, a change in taxonomy placed the family *Enterobacteriaceae* under the Order Enterobacterales. Researchers stated in a 2021 article in Clinical Microbiology Reviews that "The results of molecular taxonomic and phylogenetics studies suggest that the current family *Enterobacteriaceae* should possibly be divided into seven or more separate families." All of the species within this family are Gram-negative and non-spore-forming. They are either non-motile or motile with the help of peritrichous flagella. They grow best at 37°C (98.6–99°F) and are oxidase-negative and catalase-positive. They ferment glucose and reduce nitrates to nitrites.

Escherichia coli

Probably the most commonly known bacterial species in the class Gamma Proteobacteria, family *Enterobacteriaceae*, and genus *Escherichia* is *Escherichia coli*, frequently identified as the cause of clinical gastrointestinal diseases. *Escherichia coli* are a Gram-negative rod that grows singly. It is part of the normal microbiome of the intestinal tract of humans, and most strains are harmless commensals. Normally, by residing in the intestine and using the nutritive sources available in the intestine, it helps prevent the growth of non-native pathogenic bacteria and synthesizes vitamins necessary for optimal human health. Conversely, *E. coli* is often the cause of endogenous infections (see Figure 16-4).

E. coli Diseases

Escherichia coli bacteria are often identified as the agent of urinary tract infections, sepsis, diarrheal disease, and neonatal meningitis. *E. coli* meningitis is discussed in Chapter 17. Immunocompromised individuals or those who already have a debilitating condition are at higher risk for infection as compared to healthy persons. There are five types of pathogenic strains: enteropathogenic, enterotoxigenic, enterohemorrhagic, enteroaggregative, and enteroinvasive. The types of *E. coli* that cause diarrhea are classified according to their virulence factors that are responsible for the different methods of causing disease. Urinary tract infections caused by *E. coli* as well as the five classes of *E. coli* diarrheal infections are discussed in more detail in Chapter 19.

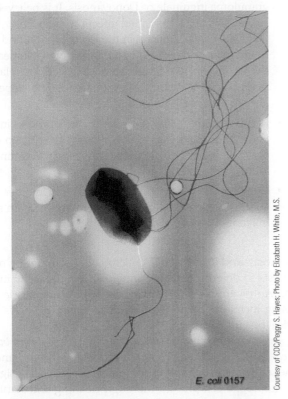

E. coli 0157

Courtesy of CDC/Peggy S. Hayes; Photo by Elizabeth H. White, M.S.

Figure 16-4 Colorized transmission electron micrograph (TEM) of *Escherichia coli* O157:H7.

Enterobacter

Enterobacter is a genus in the class Gamma Proteobacteria, family *Enterobacteriaceae*. The bacteria are Gram-negative, motile, rod-shaped, facultative anaerobes with peritrichous flagella. *Enterobacter cloacae* and *Enterobacter aerogenes* are the species that are highly pathogenic to humans and major contributors to healthcare-associated infections. These bacteria, as with other *Enterobacteriaceae*, have outer membranes that contain lipid-A, an endotoxin which is the major stimulus for the release of cytokines, the mediators of systemic inflammation.

Enterobacter Infections

Known as "ICU bugs," these bacteria are causative pathogenic agents for bacteremia, endocarditis, septic arthritis, osteomyelitis, and infections of the central nervous system, lower respiratory tract, peritoneal cavity, skin and soft-tissues, urinary tract, surgical sites, and eyes. The highest risk factors for *Enterobacter* infections include:

- Admission to the intensive care unit (ICU)
- Hospitalization of more than 2 weeks
- Invasive procedures in the previous 72 hours
- The presence of an indwelling central venous catheter
- History of treatment with antibiotics in the past 30 days or recent use of broad-spectrum antibiotics (cephalosporins or aminoglycosides)
- Age: older adults and neonates.

As with many of the *Endobacteriaceae*, healthy individuals are rarely affected by these opportunistic pathogenic bacteria. Although community-acquired infections have been reported, the majority are HAIs.

Cronobacter sakazakii, formerly called *Enterobacter sakazakii*, has been reported as a cause of sepsis and meningitis, **ventriculitis**, brain abscess, cerebral infarction, and cyst formation in neonates and children younger than age 2 years. *C. sakazakii* is able to survive in very dry environments and has been associated with outbreaks due to contaminated dry powdered formula for infants as well as in other powdered foods (see Figure 16-5).

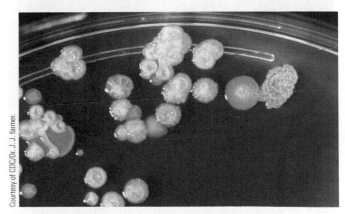

Courtesy of CDC/Dr. J. J. farmer.

Figure 16-5 Soy agar plate culture of *Cronobacter sakazakii* formerly called *Enterobacter sakazakii*.

Diagnosis and Treatment Laboratory cultures are the most important diagnostic studies for *Enterobacter* infections. Two sets of culture specimens, one aerobic and one anaerobic, should be obtained 20 to 30 minutes apart and from two different sites if possible. Gram-staining techniques are important to determine initial bacterial categorization. Other types of diagnostic tests include the following: blood and urine studies; imaging studies such as x-ray, CT scan, or MRI; **endoscopic retrograde cholangiopancreatography (ERCP)** for possible biliary obstruction; soft tissue or bone needle biopsy; surgical drainage and cultures; and lumbar punctures for collection of cerebrospinal fluid samples.

All *Enterobacter* infections require antibiotic therapy; however, the choice of appropriate and effective antimicrobial treatment is extremely complicated. Most species have demonstrated the ability to quickly develop antibiotic resistance, so selection must be carefully considered and clinicians should avoid unnecessary administration or prolonged use of antimicrobial agents.

In cases of ICU outbreaks of *Enterobacter* infections, isolation precautions should be followed. Proper hand washing and use of sanitizing agents must be strictly practiced by all healthcare providers to prevent cross-contamination.

Klebsiella

Klebsiella organisms are named after Edwin Klebs, a nineteenth century German microbiologist. They are non-motile, rod-shaped, Gram-negative, facultative anaerobes that have a prominent polysaccharide capsule. The polysaccharide capsule encases the whole cell, giving it a larger appearance, providing resistance against many host defense mechanisms, and contributing to antibiotic resistance (see Figure 16-6).

Klebsiella bacteria are a part of the normal microflora of the colon, but once outside that enclosed environment, they are pathogenic. The pathogenic species for humans are *Klebsiella pneumoniae, K. oxytoca,* and *K. granulomatis* (formerly *Calymmatobacterium granulomatis*). *Klebsiella pneumoniae* is isolated from the respiratory tract and stool of a small percentage of healthy individuals. It is a Gram-negative, non-motile, aerobic bacterium that is rod-shaped. *Klebsiella* are common pathogens in HAIs. Pneumonia caused by *K. pneumoniae* is discussed in Chapter 20.

Klebsiella Infections

Common sites of healthcare-associated infections from *Klebsiella* include the biliary tract, respiratory tract, urinary tract, and surgical wounds. Clinically, in addition to those mentioned, *Klebsiella* is frequently the causative agent in cases of pneumonia, bacterial septicemia, cholecystitis, diarrhea, osteomyelitis, and meningitis. HAIs from species of *Klebsiella* are linked to invasive devices, ventilator equipment, indwelling urinary catheters, and secondary to inappropriate use of antibiotics. Bloodstream sepsis and septic shock may result from contamination during invasive procedures. Premature infants in neonatal intensive care units (NICUs) have been infected with *K. oxytoca,* resulting in neonatal septicemia.

Less common infections from *Klebsiella* species include:

- Chronic genital ulcerative disease also known as granuloma inguinale or Donovanosis. It is believed to be a sexually transmitted infection caused by *K. granulomatis*. It is rare in the United States and found mainly in parts of India, Papua New Guinea, the Caribbean, and South America. Ulcers are relatively painless, although they are dramatic in appearance in advanced stages (see Figure 16-7).

- Rhinoscleroma, a chronic inflammatory process involving the nasopharynx. Respiratory obstruction can occur secondary to purulent drainage, crusting, and nodule formation.

- Ozena, a chronic atrophic rhinitis mainly in older adults, characterized by necrosis of nasal mucosa and mucopurulent nasal discharge.

Diagnosis and Treatment A microbiology laboratory must run tests to determine which antibiotics will treat the infection. Antibiotic-resistant strains of *Enterobacteriaceae* are causing increasing concerns for public health agencies and clinical practitioners.

Infections involving Carbapenem-resistant *Enterobacteriaceae* (CRE) have been reported in patients having undergone upper endoscopy procedures. The mechanical design of the endoscope can prevent thorough cleaning and sterilization and have been identified as the cause in previous outbreaks. Infections caused by CRE are serious, potentially

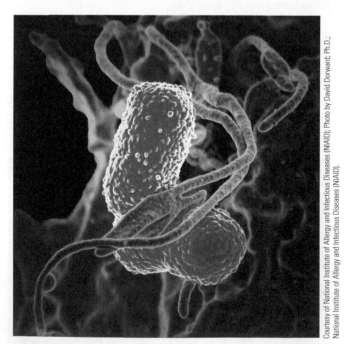

Courtesy of National Institute of Allergy and Infectious Diseases (NIAID); Photo by David Dorward; Ph.D.; National Institute of Allergy and Infectious Diseases (NIAID).

Figure 16-6 Digitally colorized micrograph depicts two pink multi-drug-resistant *Klebsiella pneumoniae* bacteria interacting with a human neutrophil (colored blue).

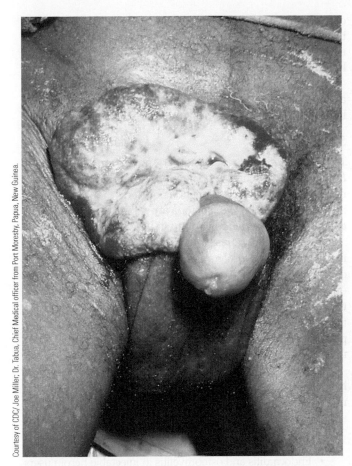

Figure 16-7 An ulcerative cutaneous lesion of the suprapubic skin, penis, and scrotum called granuloma inguinale (Donovanosis), an STD caused by *Klebsiella granulomatis*.

life-threatening, difficult to treat, and may be associated with mortality rates as high as 50 percent for hospitalized patients (see Figure 16-8). CRE infections are discussed further in Chapter 21.

Citrobacter

The species of the genera *Citrobacter* are Gram-negative, opportunistic bacteria that use citrate as their sole source of carbon. They are known to cause severe UTIs, neonatal meningitis, respiratory tract infections, endocarditis, and bacteremia in immunocompromised patients. The two most common *Citrobacter* species are *C. koseri* (previously *C. diversus*) and *C. freundii*.

The mortality rate for individuals with bacteremia is high. *C. koseri* can cause brain abscesses and meningitis in neonates. Some strains have been shown to have a unique protein on the outer cellular membrane, which is thought to be associated with their virulence.

Morganella, Proteus, and Providencia

Within the family *Enterobacteriaceae* are taxonomic "tribes." A tribe is a level above genus, but below family. The three genera grouped as the tribe, *Proteeae*, under *Enterobacteriaceae* are *Morganella*, *Proteus*, and *Providencia*.

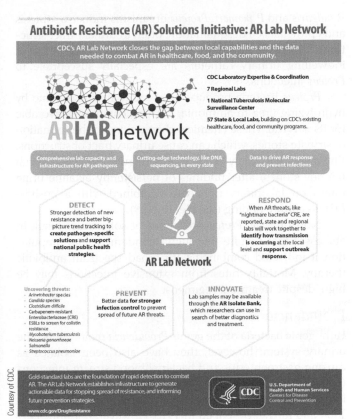

Figure 16-8 CDC graphic of Antibiotic Resistance (AR) Solutions Initiative: AR Lab Network.

Morganella

Morganella has only one species, *M. morganii*, and two subspecies. It is a Gram-negative, rod-shaped, non-encapsulated, motile bacterium that is commensal in the GI tracts of humans, mammals, and reptiles (snakes). *Morganella* bacteria are opportunistic pathogens that are relatively uncommon; however, they have been isolated in cases of UTI, SSI, CNS infections, pericarditis, sepsis, endophthalmitis, empyema, and peritonitis.

Risk factors for *M. morganii* infection include the following:

- History of exposure to ampicillin and other beta-lactam antibiotics
- Diabetes mellitus
- Advanced age
- Recent surgery
- Perinatal exposure
- Soft tissue snakebite infections

Proteus

Proteus bacteria are part of the normal microbiome of the human intestinal tract along with *Escherichia* and *Klebsiella*. Ninety percent of *Proteus* infections are from *Proteus mirabilis*, considered a community-acquired pathogen. Two other species responsible for healthcare-associated infections are

P. vulgaris and *P. penneri*. *Proteus* organisms induce apoptosis and epithelial cell desquamation, often in urinary tract structures. Patients in long-term care facilities with chronic use of indwelling urinary catheters are especially susceptible to *Proteus* infections.

Proteus bacteria produce urease and alkalinize urine by hydrolyzing urea to ammonia, creating conditions favorable for its survival. These chemical changes create the formation of struvite stones, which can cause urinary tract obstructions. Physicians will likely order exams to rule-out renal calculi (kidney stones) after findings of persistently alkaline urine found on laboratory urinalysis combined with a positive *Proteus* culture finding (see Figure 16-9).

Non-urologic *Proteus* infections of soft tissues result in abscesses that require thorough debridement and amputation if indicated combined with broad-spectrum antibiotic therapy. Mortality rates from extensive infections may be high, despite treatment regimens.

Providencia

Pathogenic bacteria of the genus *Providencia* mainly affect the urinary system; however, they have also been isolated as causing gastroenteritis and bacterial blood stream infections (bacteremia). The types of bacteria that would eventually be included in the current taxonomic groups were first noted in 1904 and further described in 1918. However, not until 1951 did the species become grouped into the genus under the family *Bacteriaceae*. It was named for Providence, Rhode Island, where the scientists of Brown University studied them. There are five species currently in the genus *Providencia*, the most common of which is *P. stuartii*.

The typical reservoirs for *Providencia* bacteria are animals such as cats, dogs, birds, sheep, cattle, guinea pigs, penguins, and snakes (boas, pythons, and vipers). As mentioned previously, they are normally found in the urinary tract but have

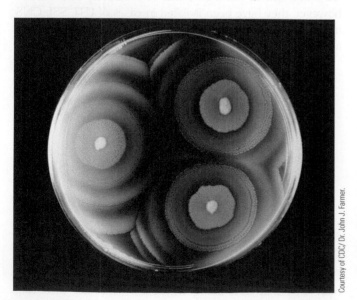

Figure 16-9 Petri dish culture plate with trypticase soy agar, inoculated with *Proteus mirabilis* bacteria, showing a colonial growth pattern referred to the dienes reaction.

occasionally been responsible for food-borne disease outbreaks. Older adults, those with long-term indwelling urinary catheters, and travelers to foreign countries are at highest risk for *Providencia* infections.

Treatment of *Providencia* infections includes appropriate antibiotic therapy as well as surgical intervention if indicated for removal of urinary stones or debridement of abscesses.

Serratia

The genus *Serratia* is another member of the large *Enterobacteriaceae* family. They are small, motile, Gram-negative, rod-shaped, peritrichous bacteria that are opportunistic pathogens. *Serratia* bacteria are widely distributed in the environment but are rarely found in the GI tract of humans.

The most common species, *S. marcescens*, produces a pigment prodigiosin, which ranges from dark red to pale pink, depending on the age of the colonies. Chemical components of the prodigiosin pigment have immunosuppressive and antitumor properties. Postpartum mastitis from *S. marcescens* turns breast milk pink due to the presence of the prodigiosin pigment. Prodigiosin is also being studied as a possible treatment for Chagas disease.

As with most of the other genera in this family, *Serratia* has been discovered in a variety of healthcare-associated illnesses including:

- Infective arthritis following intraarticular injections and in neonatal intensive care units (NICU)
- Endocarditis and osteomyelitis in injectable heroin users
- Meningitis following epidural anesthesia for Cesarean section deliveries or chronic pain therapy
- Bacteremia following central venous access
- Urinary tract infection following surgery or catheter placement
- Respiratory infections following endoscopy procedures or airway intubation for mechanical ventilation
- Ocular and soft tissue infections.

The main risk factor for *Serratia* infections is having undergone some type of healthcare procedure. Rare cases of community-acquired infections have been reported. Diagnosis is made through laboratory culture and treatment is appropriate antibiotic therapy.

Shigella

The genus *Shigella* is a group of Gram-negative facultative anaerobes that are intracellular pathogens discovered more than a century ago by a Japanese microbiologist named Shiga. These bacteria are part of the family *Enterobacteriaceae* and tribe *Escherichieae*. The species are also known as groups and include *Shigella dysenteriae* (Group A), *Shigella flexneri* (Group B), *Shigella boydii* (Group C), and *Shigella sonnei* (Group D). They are non-motile, non-spore-forming, rod-shaped, and non-encapsulated. The species are further divided into serotypes: group A has 13 serotypes; group B has 6 serotypes; group C has 18 serotypes; and group D has 1 serotype.

S. dysenteriae type I, or group A, is the causative agent of deadly outbreaks of dysentery in various developing parts of the world where sanitation may be less than optimal. Groups A and C are rarely encountered in the United States. *S. sonnei*, or group D, is responsible for two-thirds of infections and *S. flexneri*, or group B, causes most other cases in the United States. Shigellosis, the general name given to infections by these pathogens, is discussed in Chapter 19.

Salmonella

Salmonella is a rod-shaped, Gram-negative bacterium that is non-spore-forming. Most species are motile via flagella (see Figure 16-10). There are more than 2,500 serovars (serotypes) of *Salmonella*, the majority of which are human pathogens. The scientific community has debated and struggled for decades over the classification and taxonomy of *Salmonella* species. *Salmonella enterica* finally gained official approval in 2005 as the type species of the genus *Salmonella*. The genus *Salmonella* also contains the species *Salmonella bongori* and *Salmonella subterranean*.

The three major **serovars/serotypes** of *S. enterica* are: Typhi, Typhimurium, and Enteritidis. In an attempt to prevent confusion, the serovar/serotype name is included. For example, what had previously been *Salmonella typhi* is now designated as *Salmonella enterica* ser. Typhi. The serovar/serotype name is not italicized in these cases. Despite the attempts to prevent confusion and due to the use of both new and old taxonomic rules being used in current literature, confusion about the correct naming of various *Salmonella* species may continue. Readers will likely encounter the abbreviated designation of *Salmonella* Typhi (or *S.* Typhi) with the genus name (*Salmonella*) in italics and the serovar name (Typhi) capitalized but not in italics.

Most species are part of the normal intestinal flora of cattle, birds, and rodents; however, some are limited to cold-blooded reptilian and amphibian animals such as turtles and frogs. Members of the genus *Salmonella* are the most

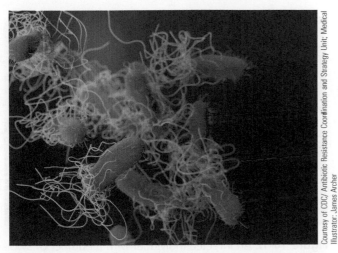

Figure 16-10 Medical illustration for CDC of drug-resistant, nontyphoidal, *Salmonella* sp. bacteria.

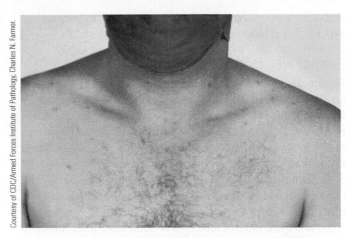

Figure 16-11 Rose spots on the chest of a patient with typhoid fever due to the bacterium *Salmonella* Typhi.

common cause of enterocolitis (diarrhea) due to the ingestion of contaminated foods.

Salmonella Typhi

Salmonella enterica serovar Typhi is the causative agent for **typhoid fever**, the most serious of *Salmonella* infections. Although rarely seen in the United States today, typhoid fever is still seen frequently in developing countries. Symptoms of typhoid fever include, as the name suggests, fever, nausea, vomiting, and diarrhea, and may lead to death. Humans are the only species affected by *Salmonella* Typhi. As with most other intestinal infections, *S.* Typhi is transmitted by the fecal-oral route through ingestion of food or water contaminated with *S.* Typhi bacteria.

This organism, as well as other species of the genus *Salmonella*, can invade non-phagocytic cells, effectively evading the human immune defenses. *S.* Typhi is not destroyed by macrophages and will multiply within them. The microbes that survive the acid environment of the stomach invade the **Peyer's patches** of the small intestine and enter the lymphatic system. From the lymph system the bacterial cells are transported throughout the body via the circulatory system. An inflammatory response is initiated in the lungs, periosteum, and gallbladder. In some cases, patients have a rash consisting of flat, rose-colored spots (see Figure 16-11). Hepatosplenomegaly, an enlargement of the liver and spleen, occurs in many patients. Soon the symptoms of constipation followed by bloody diarrhea appear. *Salmonella* Paratyphi causes a similar infection, but it is much milder.

After recovery from typhoid fever, an individual may carry and excrete *S.* Typhi bacteria for a long period of time (months to years). The cells tend to persist in the gallbladder (especially in the presence of gallstones), common bile duct, hepatic ducts, and cystic duct where bile provides an excellent medium for growth. A very small percentage of persons will become permanent carriers. The first documented carrier of *S.* Typhi, Mary Mallon, nicknamed "Typhoid Mary," was a permanent carrier and was responsible for several outbreaks and deaths before health officials caught up with her and she was forcibly quarantined for the remainder of her life.

Salmonella Typhimurium

Salmonella enterica serovar Typhimurium bacteria are frequently identified in food-borne disease outbreaks, especially in large meat processing plant products. Additionally, infections have been traced back to handling of live poultry, often raised in backyard settings. Pet reptiles have also been found to be carriers of *S.* Typhimurium. Symptoms caused by *S.* Typhimurium are typically less severe than those of *S.* Typhi; however, the at-risk populations (very young, older, and immunocompromised individuals) may suffer exaggerated signs and symptoms of all forms of *Salmonella* infections.

Salmonella Enteritidis

Salmonella enterica serovar Enteritidis has been linked in the past to eggs contaminated with fecal waste during the collection and packing processes. A disease outbreak in the 1970s led to implementation of stringent decontamination and inspection protocols to prevent transmission of *S.* Enteritidis on the surface of eggshells. More recently, transmission has been linked to healthy-appearing hens whose ovaries may be colonized with *S.* Enteritidis, which infects the eggs prior to shell development, thereby remaining unaffected by cleaning and screening practices. Eggs that are eaten raw or are undercooked transmit bacteria even though they are rated Grade A.

Yersinia

The final member of the *Enterobacteriaceae* family discussed here is the genus *Yersinia*. *Yersinia* has three species that are important to the medical community: *Y. pestis*, the agent responsible for bubonic and pneumonic plague, as well as *Y. enterocolitica* and *Y. pseudotuberculosis*, both causing severe gastroenteritis with abscess formation and possible death due to peritonitis. The latter two species are discussed further in Chapter 19.

Yersinia pestis

Yersinia pestis is a Gram-negative, facultative anaerobe that is an obligate intracellular parasitic pathogen. On laboratory study, it is a bipolar-staining (the ends take up more stain than the center of the bacterium) coccobacillus that exhibits slime production due to the presence of a capsular antigen. The microorganism is the cause of three forms of plague: pneumonic, septicemic, and, the most infamous, bubonic **plague**, which is a deadly disease commonly known as the Black Death. It was responsible for some of the greatest epidemics in history. Between the sixth and eighth centuries, what was later called the Justinian plague killed an estimated 25 percent of the population south of the Alps from Asia and India to the Middle East and then over to the Mediterranean region. From the eighth through twelfth centuries, the plague was again responsible for killing an estimated one-third of the world's population between the years 1348 and 1530. The third major endemic plague affected provinces in China from

1855 to 1910 and killed an estimated 10 million. Major pandemics seemed to discontinue, with only occasional outbreaks over the past century. The change is most likely due to improved rodent control and use of insecticides.

Humans can become infected with *Y. pestis* in the following ways:

- Bitten by an infected rat flea carried by infested rodents
- Exposure to and inhalation of droplets expelled during coughing or sneezing by a person with pneumonic plague
- Exposure to blood, body fluids, or tissues of an infected animal, for example, a hunter skinning an infected animal without use of proper PPE or protective apparel

In infected individuals, the bacterial cells lose their capsular layer and most are phagocytized and destroyed by leukocytes. However, a few of the cells enter tissue that provides protection, and this allows the cells to resynthesize their capsules and other virulence antigens. After the capsule has been re-formed, the bacterial cell kills the macrophage and is released with the ability to resist phagocytosis.

The infection quickly spreads to the lymph nodes closest to the site of inoculation. These lymph nodes become swollen, tender, and warm to the touch, and they become hemorrhagic, giving rise to the most notable characteristic of bubonic plague, the bulbous or black-colored buboes responsible for the name bubonic plague (see Figure 16-12). The infection invades the circulatory system, involving the spleen, liver, and lungs. The result is a bacterial pneumonia with violent coughs that expel viable infectious cells into the environment. If left untreated, then the mortality rate is very high because the pneumonic form is extremely difficult to treat and control.

Y. pestis must be quickly diagnosed due to the virulence of the microorganism and the rapid progression of the disease (see Figure 16-13). Death can occur within 24 hours after

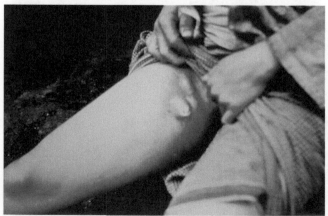

Figure 16-12 An infected individual with a number of swollen inguinal lymph nodes or buboes, caused by a *Yersinia pestis* bacterial infection also known as the plague.

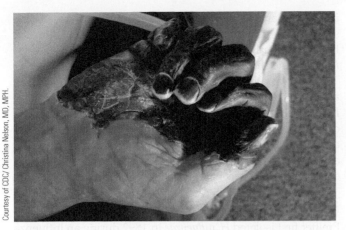

Courtesy of CDC/ Christina Nelson, MD, MPH.

Figure 16-13 Gangrenous condition of the fingers and palm of the right hand of a male infected by the plague bacterium, *Yersinia pestis*.

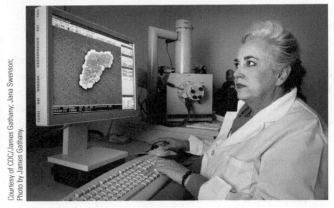

Courtesy of CDC/James Gathany, Jana Swenson; Photo by James Gathany.

Figure 16-14 CDC microbiologist and electron microscopist scanning a specimen of *Acinetobacter baumannii* bacteria.

the patient has exhibited the initial signs of infection. Diagnosis is confirmed by obtaining sputum specimens, blood culture, and lymph node aspiration biopsy.

Y. pestis is susceptible to gentamicin, streptomycin, and tetracycline. Few drug-resistant strains are present. Control measures have centered on the elimination of the rat flea, which is credited with preventing outbreaks during World War II in Europe and during the Vietnam War in Southeast Asia. Attempts at eliminating the rodent reservoir population have been unsuccessful, and it is highly unlikely that the rat flea can be eliminated worldwide. The World Health Organization (WHO) states that 1,000 to 2,000 cases of plague are reported annually, mainly in small rural areas; however, it is believed that actual rates are greatly under-reported.

In the United States, the plague was first documented in 1900, most likely as a result of rodents carrying infected fleas on ships from countries with endemic disease. The CDC reports that between 2000 and 2019, on average there between 1 and 17 cases of plague annually in the United States with only one case reported in 2018 and 2019. Geographically, sporadic infections continue to occur in two major areas: in the northern New Mexico/northern Arizona/southern Colorado area, also known as the 4-corners area, and in the California/southern Oregon/far western Nevada area.

Moraxellaceae

The family *Moraxellaceae* is included in the class Gamma Proteobacteria and includes organisms that are cocci as well as those that are bacilli. The genus *Moraxella* is discussed in Chapter 15. The genus *Acinetobacter* includes numerous species of bacteria that are bacilli to coccobacilli in morphology. They are Gram-negative, non-motile aerobes found in soil and water that rarely affect healthy individuals; however, they may become dangerous opportunistic pathogens in those who are immunocompromised or who have chronic lung disease or diabetes. *Acinetobacter baumannii* is the most

commonly identified member of the *Moraxellaceae* family and genus *Acinetobacter*, which is responsible for healthcare-associated infections (see Figure 16-14).

Acinetobacter baumannii

Acinetobacter baumannii is estimated to cause 80 percent of HAIs within the genus *Acinetobacter*. It grows best in fluid environments but may survive on human skin and inanimate dry surfaces for moderate periods. Typically isolated in critical care areas such as ICUs, infections due to *A. baumannii* are rarely found outside of healthcare settings. Infections may involve various body systems and have been cultured from invasive devices such as central venous catheters, **tracheostomy** tubes, and urinary catheters, and also from open wounds. Bacteria have been found to colonize hospital irrigation and intravenous solutions.

The spread of *A. baumannii* can cause infections of the lungs, bloodstream, urinary tract, and central nervous system. *A. baumannii* is known to have strong antibiotic resistance and clinicians must carefully consider choices of antibiotic therapy to treat infections. Proper hand washing and antimicrobial skin preparation by all healthcare workers are the most effective methods of prevention of cross-contamination between acutely ill patients or contaminated surfaces and vulnerable individuals.

Pasteurellaceae

The family *Pasteurellaceae* belongs to the class Gamma Proteobacteria and includes the genera *Actinobacillus*, *Haemophilus*, and *Pasteurella*. The genera are Gram-negative, non-motile, non-spore-forming, and either aerobic or facultative anaerobes. In the laboratory, they are fastidious organisms that require enriched media.

Pasteurella

Pasteurella (named after Louis Pasteur) are pleomorphic (ranging from bacilli to cocci) and facultative anaerobes. The genus is a commensal in the oropharynx of many animals but it is also the cause of disease. *Pasteurella multocida* is easily grown on blood or chocolate agar in the laboratory. The colonies produce a characteristic foul odor.

Human infections are the result of animal contact, and the microbe is transferred through a scratch, cut, skin abrasion, or animal bite. The species *Pasteurella multocida* is the most commonly known human pathogen, whereas the other species are opportunistic pathogens and rarely cause infections in humans. The four forms of *P. multocida* infections are:

- Localized: areas of cellulitis, lymphadenitis, and pain after an animal bite
- Respiratory: increased pulmonary complications in patients already experiencing chronic respiratory disease
- Septicemia: systemic bloodstream and lymphatic infection in immunocompromised patients (especially in those with hepatic disease)
- Endocarditis: infection of the inner lining of the heart muscle

P. multocida colonizes the upper respiratory tract of most domesticated animals. Animal bites, most of which are caused by domestic animals, are responsible for approximately 1 percent of emergency department admissions. Unless thoroughly cleansed and treated, animal bites can result in serious infections. Because *P. multocida* bacteria are facultative anaerobes, they are able to proliferate in bite wounds that have been irrigated thoroughly and sutured closed.

Pasteurella multocida can also rapidly multiply at the site of injury even in the presence of leukocytes. In the absence of immune antibodies, phagocytosis is also absent, allowing the microbes to multiply in the tissue fluids. Acquired resistance to *P. multocida* is humorally mediated. Infections can be treated with a variety of antibiotics and are highly sensitive to penicillin.

Haemophilus

The genus *Haemophilus* is a member of the *Pasteurellaceae* family. The bacteria are non-motile Gram-negative rods that grow in pairs or short chains. They are typically found in the mucous membranes of the respiratory and genital tracts in humans. They are facultative anaerobes that grow in the presence or absence of oxygen, but optimal growth is obtained in an aerobic environment. *Haemophilus* means "blood-loving," referring to the fact that the majority of the species require one or two factors that are present in blood for metabolism, specifically X factor (hemin) and V factor (nicotinamide adenine dinucleotide or NAD). Transmission of the human pathogen species occurs by inhalation of aerosolized droplets from an infected person or through direct sexual contact.

The most recognized species is *Haemophilus influenzae*, which produces a type b polysaccharide capsule, giving it the name *H. influenzae* type b or Hib. It is the primary cause of bacterial meningitis in infants and children, with peak infection rates occurring between the ages of 5 months and 5 years. It is also a major cause of respiratory tract infections

in children and adults. Older adults are prone to developing severe bacterial pneumonia, especially those who already have an underlying pulmonary disease. Diseases caused by *H. influenzae* are further discussed in Chapter 20.

The two other species that are of significance to humans are *H. influenzae* biotype *aegyptius* and *Haemophilus ducreyi*. *Haemophilus influenzae* biotype *aegyptius* is associated with causing of an acute, highly contagious form of conjunctivitis, called "pink eye." *Haemophilus ducreyi* is the species that causes the sexually transmitted disease characterized by soft chancres and/or ulcers in the groin or genitalia.

Haemophilus influenzae

Pfeiffer first isolated *H. influenzae* in 1892 during an influenza pandemic. The bacteria, however, do not cause the viral infection referred to as the "flu." *H. influenzae* bacteria are subclassified into six serotypes, a, b, c, d, e, and f, based on the antigenic characteristics of their polysaccharide capsules. The capsule is antiphagocytic, a major virulence factor. Strains that produce other capsular types can cause infection, but with less severity than those of type b, and the strains are non-invasive. Other virulence factors include:

- Peptidoglycan: present in the cell wall, damaging the blood–brain barrier
- Exotoxin: inhibits the movement of cilia in the respiratory tract
- Fimbriae: aid cell adherence to tissue
- Adhesins: aid cell adherence to tissue

Haemophilus ducreyi

First discovered by Ducrey in 1889, *Haemophilus ducreyi* is only found in humans. Gram stains of fluid from an ulcer or aspirates from enlarged inguinal lymph nodes reveal small Gram-negative coccobacilli that are arranged in groups or chains. Virulence factors have been difficult to identify. It has been proven that the organism has attachment molecules for epithelial cells and may be able to invade them. It may also produce **cytotoxins** that are responsible for the development of the genital ulcerations. The organism is sexually transmitted. It is thought to be underreported in the United States due to its similarity with other ulcerative sexually transmitted diseases and lack of easy laboratory identification.

The organism is endemic in some developing parts of the world, with high infection rates associated with poor socioeconomic and sanitary conditions. In the United States, infection with the organism is most common among those who abuse injection drugs , sex workers, and those with alcohol addiction. The organism is the cause of the disease called chancroid. The ulcerations are soft chancres, as opposed to the hard chancres seen in cases of primary syphilis. The initial sign of chancroid infection is typically the appearance of one or more raised skin bumps or sores with reddened borders in the groin or on the genitalia. These lesions, referred to as buboes, fill with pus and subsequently rupture, leaving painful open sores (see Figure 16-15).

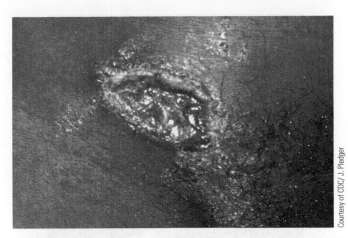

Courtesy of CDC/ J. Pledger

Figure 16-15 Necrotic swollen right inguinal lymph node, referred to as a bubo, as a result of a disease known as chancroid caused by *Haemophilus ducreyi.*

Aggregatibacter

The genus *Aggregatibacter* is another member of the *Pasteurellaceae* family. Most of the species are responsible for disease in animals. The species identified most commonly with humans and responsible for periodontal disease is *Aggregatibacter actinomycetemcomitans*. The taxonomic nomenclature classification of *A. actinomycetemcomitans* was changed in the past few years from the previous *Actinobacillus actinomycetemcomitans* to the new genus name.

The small, fastidious, non-motile, non-encapsulated, capnophilic, Gram-negative bacilli to coccobacilli bacteria are commensals of the human mouth and found on culture of oral secretions in up to 20 percent of healthy people as well as in the great majority of those with localized juvenile periodontitis. *A. actinomycetemcomitans* bacteria have been isolated with other microbial species in dental plaques and biofilms. These co-pathogens may play a role in systemic disease including defective heart valves and atherosclerotic plaques lining blood vessels.

Vibrionaceae

Members of the family *Vibrionaceae* and class Gamma Proteobacteria are Gram-negative, straight or curved, rod-shaped bacteria with flagella at one or both ends. Species of the genus *Vibrio* produce multiple extracellular cytotoxins and enzymes that are responsible for the extensive tissue damage seen in soft tissue infections and cases of septicemia.

Vibrio

There are approximately 12 species of *Vibrio* known to cause disease in humans. The diseases they cause are categorized as either cholera or non-cholera forms. Non-cholera diseases are sub-classified as **halophilic** or non-halophilic, depending on their need for sodium chloride. The non-cholera *Vibrio* infections are often considered food-borne due to the most common route of transmission being ingestion of infected seafood. Other infections, however, such as wound infections are caused by species of non-cholera *Vibrio*.

The following sections examine two species that cause vibriosis, *Vibrio parahaemolyticus* and *Vibrio vulnificus*, as well as *Vibrio cholerae*, which is responsible for the potentially deadly, acute diarrheal disease cholera.

Vibrio parahaemolyticus

Vibrio parahaemolyticus is a natural inhabitant of the coastal salt waters of the United States and Canada and is more abundant in summer months. The bacteria are responsible for infections seen following ingestion of raw seafood, most notably oysters, or wound infections after exposure to sea water. The CDC reports a yearly average of 80,000 cases of vibriosis and 100 deaths occurring mainly between the months of May to October when ocean temperatures are warmer than other months.

Vibrio vulnificus

Vibrio vulnificus is very similar to *V. parahaemolyticus* in its routes of transmission and signs and symptoms of infection; however, it is responsible for more serious infections and higher fatality rates. Immunocompromised individuals who ingest contaminated seafood are at greater risk for complications of septic shock and bacterial septicemia, leading to a 50 percent fatality rate. Additionally, in persons who are immunocompromised, cases of wound contamination by exposure to coastal sea water may lead to ulceration, necrosis, and potentially fatal bloodstream sepsis. Those with liver disease are 80 percent more likely to suffer septicemia than healthy individuals who become infected.

Aggressive and immediate antibiotic treatment should be initiated when *V. vulnificus* is suspected or confirmed. Surgical debridement of infected wounds is indicated and fasciotomy or even limb amputation may be required to stop the spread of tissue damage.

Vibrio cholerae

Vibrio cholerae is the bacterial pathogen responsible for the acute gastrointestinal disease, cholera. It is believed that cholera outbreaks may have been described in ancient literature dating back to Hippocrates during approximately 400 BCE. The two reservoirs of *V. cholerae* are water and humans. Cholera is considered extremely rare in animals.

The normal acid environment of the stomach is usually effective in rendering *V. cholerae* non-infectious. In individuals with hypochlorhydria (reduced gastric acid) secondary to gastric surgery, **vagotomy**, *Helicobacter pylori* infection, or pharmaceutical H2 blocker therapy for gastric ulcer, the risk of *Vibrio* infection is elevated. Malnutrition also elevates the risk for infection.

For unknown reasons, individuals with O blood type have double the risk of becoming infected with *V. cholerae* than those with other blood types. Cholera and non-cholera vibriosis are discussed further in Chapter 19.

Aeromonadaceae

The genus *Aeromonas* is a member of the family *Aeromonadaceae* and the class Gamma Proteobacteria. Bacteria are Gram-negative, non-spore-forming, rod-shaped bacilli to coccobacilli, facultative anaerobes. They are found in both fresh water and salt water as well as in soil, sewage, and some foods. The genus was moved from its previous placement in the family *Vibrionaceae* after researchers were able to perform molecular studies demonstrating its related phylogenetic properties.

Aeromonas consists of two groups. One group has polar flagella that provide motility and six species are known to cause disease in humans similar to other members of the Gamma Proteobacteria phylum. The second group is non-motile and mainly infects fish and other marine species.

Researchers debate the role of *A. hydrophila* in human gastroenteritis infections. In cases of septicemia in those who are immunocompromised, *A. caviae* and *A. sobria* have been isolated as potential causative agents.

Pseudomonadaceae

The family *Pseudomonadaceae* is a member of the class Gamma Proteobacteria and includes the genus *Pseudomonas*, which comprises non-fermentative, Gram-negative bacteria that are short, straight, or slightly curved rods. They are non-spore-forming and motile, with species exhibiting one or more polar flagella and pili that aid in the attachment of the microbial cells to host tissues. Some strains are surrounded by an outer slime layer that consists primarily of polysaccharides. The slime layer may surround individual cells or several cells forming a microcolony. The pili and slime layer add to the virulence of the strains (see Figure 16-16).

Pseudomonas is found worldwide. It can withstand harsh environmental conditions that would destroy most other bacteria. Its ability to survive is related to a highly impermeable cell wall and the production of enzymes that destroy toxic substances. The most commonly known species within the genus, and an excellent example of an opportunistic pathogen, is *Pseudomonas aeruginosa*. It rarely infects healthy individuals or undamaged tissue; however, it can easily invade the tissues when compromised by trauma or disease.

Pseudomonas aeruginosa

Pseudomonas aeruginosa bacteria are easily identified in the laboratory. The colonies produce a fruity odor and an extracellular pigment. The microorganisms are motile and oxidase-positive. Non-pigmented strains that are polymyxin-resistant are difficult to identify, requiring further laboratory tests.

Due to their durability in adverse environmental conditions and their low nutritional requirements, the microorganisms can live in many areas of a hospital, including sinks, drinking fountains, cleansing soaps used by the hospital staff, and patient humidifiers. The pathogen has become highly antibiotic-resistant.

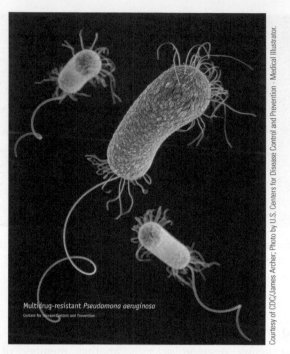

Multidrug-resistant *Pseudomona aeruginosa*
Centers for Disease Control and Prevention

Courtesy of CDC/James Archer; Photo by U.S. Centers for Disease Control and Prevention - Medical Illustrator.

Figure 16-16 3D computer-generated image of multi-drug resistant *Pseudomonas aeruginosa* bacteria.

Individuals who are otherwise healthy can suffer ear and skin infections from exposure to inadequately chlorinated water in hot tubs and swimming pools. Cases of conjunctivitis have occurred following use of extended-wear contact lenses. Patients with weakened immune systems from conditions such as cystic fibrosis, burns, and leukemia are at high risk for development of *P. aeruginosa* infections, as are patients on ventilator assistance or who have a temporary or permanent tracheostomy in place. The wide variety of infections in multiple body systems caused by *P. aeruginosa* is discussed in subsequent chapters.

Campylobacteraceae

The family *Campylobacteraceae* is part of the phylum Epsilon Proteobacteria and order Campylobacterales. Members of this group are Gram-negative, microaerophilic, non-fermentative, spiral-shaped, motile rods with unipolar or bipolar flagella (see Figure 16-17). Two genera, *Campylobacter jejuni* and *C. coli*, are implicated in food-borne infections, whereas *C. fetus* is responsible for spontaneous abortions in sheep and cattle and it is also an opportunistic pathogen in humans.

Campylobacter jejuni

The most commonly isolated *Campylobacter* species is *C. jejuni*, an organism that is highly sensitive to the environment and cannot survive in 21 percent oxygen, heated, dry, or acidic conditions. The bacteria grow best in atmospheric conditions of 3 to 5 percent oxygen and 2 to 10 percent carbon dioxide. *C. jejuni* is often found in birds, including chickens, with no signs of infection. Contaminated chicken and manure-contaminated

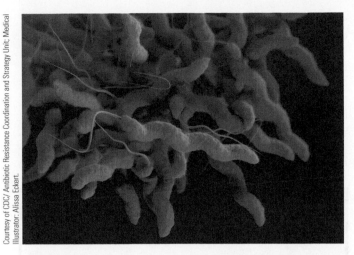

Courtesy of CDC/ Antibiotic Resistance Coordination and Strategy Unit; Medical Illustrator: Alissa Eckert.

Figure 16-17 3D CDC computer-generated medical illustration of a cluster of drug-resistant *Campylobacter* sp. bacteria.

unpasteurized milk from cows can cause the food-borne human infection campylobacteriosis, which is discussed in Chapter 19.

Studies have shown that *C. jejuni* is the leading cause of diarrheal illness in the United States, causing more disease than *Salmonella* spp. and *Shigella* spp. However, the bacteria are not carried by healthy individuals. Most campylobacteriosis diarrheal infections are self-limiting and cause no lasting sequelae. In some cases, however, a patient's immune system is triggered to attack the body's own nervous system, causing a severe disease called **Guillain-Barré syndrome** and resulting in paralysis that can last for weeks. Studies tracking incidence of Guillain-Barré syndrome cases following gastrointestinal infections, including campylobacteriosis, in industrial nations showed a major decline following strict regulation of food (poultry and cattle) processing and preparation practices.

Helicobacteraceae

The family *Helicobacteraceae* is part of the phylum Epsilon Proteobacteria and order Campylobacterales. The genus *Helicobacter* comprises Gram-negative, microaerophilic bacteria that are similar to the *Campylobacter* genus. Both genera are motile, catalase-positive, and exhibit curved cell bodies. *Helicobacter* is thought to be the causative agent of chronic gastritis and stomach and peptic (pyloric) ulcers. *Helicobacter pylori* is the species that clinical evidence points to as the most likely causative agent of peptic ulcers, but the mechanism for pathogenesis is not well-understood. *H. pylori* infection is discussed further in Chapter 19.

Other Gram-Negative Pathogens

It is apparent that there are many species of microbial pathogens that are classified as Gram-negative organisms. Whether they have the morphological features of cocci, bacilli,

spirochete, or a variation such as coccobacilli, they exist all around, on, and inside us. Often, they do no harm until circumstances allow them to seize the opportunity to wreak havoc in susceptible animals and humans.

It may also have become apparent that the scientific community of microbiologists, epidemiologists, virologists, and others face the challenge of trying to identify and appropriately classify these tiny beings into logical groups. Unfortunately, this is a moving target and microbes thought to belong to one taxonomic phylum, class, order, genus, or species may be moved or renamed if improved laboratory analytics demonstrate new or previously undetected properties and characteristics.

The following organisms that are discussed were not included in previously discussed taxonomic groups but are important microbes for study.

Bacteroides

The genus *Bacteroides* is part of phylum and class Bacteroidetes, order Bacteroidales, and family *Bacteroidaceae*. *Bacteroides* contains obligate anaerobic bacteria that comprise the majority of organisms that are part of the normal microbiome of the human digestive tract and are opportunistic pathogens. *Bacteroides* bacteria in humans are found in great numbers in the area of the junction of the terminal ileum and colon. The danger to humans involves the escape of *Bacteroides* from the intestinal tract and colonization of the peritoneal cavity, internal organs, or other tissues. Infections can occur anywhere in the body and are commonly associated with abscess formation. Harmful effects of infection by *Bacteroides* may include: peritoneal cavity and pelvic abscesses; bacteremia; and diarrhea in young children or adults who have **inflammatory bowel disease**.

As a normal inhabitant of the human digestive tract, *Bacteroides* provides a beneficial component for us by:

- Aiding in the biotransformation of bile acid
- Competing with and depleting the food supply needed by pathogens such as *Salmonella*
- Providing a large portion of the energy supply needed by other enterobacteria through anaerobic metabolism
- Breaking down carbohydrates for use that the body otherwise could not.

Bacteroides fragilis

Bacteroides fragilis bacteria are small, pleomorphic, anaerobic, Gram-negative bacilli. They are easily grown on blood agar. Under the microscope, large vacuoles will be seen that look like spores; however, the species are non-spore-forming, non-motile, and have an unusually large polysaccharide capsule. Their pathogenicity is weak because they do not secrete an endotoxin and their primary virulence factor is the capsule. The capsule renders them resistant to phagocytosis and promotes abscess formation. *B. fragilis* infections are discussed further in Chapter 19.

Porphyromonas gingivalis

Porphyromonas gingivalis is a species belonging to the phylum and class Bacteroidetes, order Bacteroidales, family *Porphyromonadaceae*, and genus *Porphyromonas*. The species was previously classified in the *Bacteroides* genus. *P. gingivalis* are Gram-negative, anaerobic, non-motile, rod-shaped, often encapsulated bacteria found in the oral mucosa of humans. In laboratory cultures, they appear black when grown on blood agar plates.

Porphyromonas gingivalis is an opportunistic pathogen that contributes to periodontal disease and the destruction of the supporting tissues of teeth, including the periodontal ligaments, cementum, and alveolar bone. Typically, periodontal infections are caused by biofilms consisting of **polymicrobial** combinations of Gram-positive and Gram-negative bacteria, of which *Porphyromonas gingivalis* is considered a key factor. In addition to the damage to dental structures, *P. gingivalis* has been implicated as a cause of inflammation leading to **atherosclerotic plaques** seen in cardiovascular disease. It may also play a role in rheumatoid arthritis and potentially in dementia.

Fusobacterium

The genus *Fusobacterium* belongs to the phylum Fusobacteria, class Fusobacteriales, and family *Fusobacteriaceae*. These bacteria are similar to *Bacteroides*; however, they are highly virulent Gram-negative, rod-shaped, obligate anaerobes. They are typically long bacilli with pointed or tapered ends. A primary component of the cell wall is a lipopolysaccharide (LPS). The difference between *Fusobacterium* and *Bacteroides* is that the *Fusobacterium* LPS molecules secrete an endotoxin and the *Bacteroides* molecules do not. The most medically important species are *F. nucleatum*, *F. mortiferum*, *F. necrophorum*, and *F. varium*. The species can cause a variety of infections in the body, including head and neck infections, chronic sinusitis, liver abscess, periodontitis, brain abscesses, and abdominal cavity infections.

Most of the infections in which *Fusobacterium* is involved are polymicrobial, causing infections in conjunction with other anaerobes. *Fusobacterium nucleatum* is the most common species that is associated with polymicrobial respiratory system infections. *Fusobacterium periodonticum* is another common species and a common cause of dental abscesses. Brain abscesses are polymicrobial infections in which *Fusobacterium*, *Prevotella*, and *Porphyromonas* species are isolated.

MICRO NOTES

"An Old Pearl of Wisdom"

Wise sayings, or "old wives' tales" as they are also called, often have a basis in fact and advise prudent behavior. One of these involves eating raw oysters only in months that have the letter "r" in them: September, October, November, December, January, February, March, and April. The reason for the warning is the increased chance that oysters will contain pathogenic amounts of *Vibrio vulnificus* or *Vibrio parahaemolyticus*, which are found in greater amounts in warm water areas such as the Gulf of Mexico, especially in the summer months (May, June, July, and August). Oysters filter surrounding water through their shells as part of their normal feeding and the *Vibrio* bacteria that live freely in the oceanic ecosystem concentrate in the oyster tissues during the summer spawning months. When eaten raw, seafood containing these opportunistic pathogens may cause gastrointestinal infections that range from mild discomfort in healthy individuals to being fatal in those with weakened immune systems. And, just to dispel another myth, hot sauce on raw oysters does not kill pathogenic microbes.

 ## Under the Microscope

Mel, a surgical technology student, was assigned to a procedure scheduled as an incision and drainage of multiple traumatic wounds. The patient was transported to the OR from the ICU since being admitted following a hiking fall resulting in multiple deep lacerations to the torso and extremities, including a penetrating injury of the upper abdomen and an open femoral fracture. Prior to the I&D procedure, the surgeon took cultures from the two open wounds. Mel noticed that there were darkened areas in the wounds and a very slight fruity odor.

1. Which type of Gram-negative microorganism has the characteristic signs of darkening and fruity odor?

2. Which other Gram-negative microbes might be associated with an infection in an abdominal wound as a result of penetrating trauma in a mountainous terrain and potential internal organ involvement?

3. Why might the surgeon choose to leave the wounds partially open with sterile antimicrobial packing instead of closing them?

4. What other routes of transmission would be involved in the types of infections attributable to the Gram-negative types of bacilli and coccobacilli bacteria discussed in this chapter?

5. Which of the bacteria covered in this chapter are commonly identified as causing or contributing to healthcare-associated infections (HAIs)?

CHAPTER 17

Diseases of the Circulatory and Central Nervous Systems

Learning Objectives

After completing the study of this chapter, you will be able to:

1. Define key terms.
2. Discuss the mechanisms of contamination of blood products.
3. Identify the pathogens associated with infections of the cardiovascular system.
4. Identify the pathogens associated with infections of the central nervous system (CNS).
5. Describe the various infections caused by pathogenic invasion of the structures within the cardiovascular and CNS.
6. Apply critical thinking skills in relating chapter material to the surgical environment of care or broader global community.

Key Terms

Aneurysm

Anomalies

Auscultation

Bioprosthetic valves

Cardiac arrhythmia

Cardiac tamponade

Cardiomyopathy

Cardioverter-
  defibrillator

Cerebral infarct

Choroid plexus

Congestive heart
  failure

Electrophoresis

Emboli

Empyema

Extrapulmonary

Gallops

Heart murmur

Hemodialysis

Hepatosplenomegaly

Hypotension

Hypothermia

Intractable

Ischemia

Lysis of adhesions

Mastoiditis

Morbidity

Neti pots

Paraphernalia

Parenchyma

Pericardiocentesis

Rales

Sarcoidosis

Stenosis

Subungual

Tachycardia

Transfusions

The Big Picture

Two of the most important body systems for human survival are the cardiovascular and CNS. Pathogenic compromise of either one can have severe or fatal consequences. During your examination of the topics in this chapter, consider the following:

1. As important as blood donation is, what methods are used to ensure that the donated blood products are free from contaminating pathogens and recipients are safe?

2. What types of challenges face healthcare providers in accurately and quickly diagnosing serious infections involving the cardiovascular or neurological systems?

3. Why are pathogenic infections able to readily access and move from the cardiovascular system to the CNS?

4. Are there specific measures individuals can take to reduce their likelihood of becoming infected with diseases of the blood vessels, heart, or nervous system?

Clinical Significance Topic

Blood-borne pathogens are very familiar to surgical technologists and other members of the surgical team. The extensive training in prevention of "sharps injuries" and use of personal protective equipment (PPE) should focus not only on the technical actions but also on the actual risks from unknown or unrecognized microbial pathogens. As vigilant as the surgical team is to protect the patient from potential infection, the team members should apply the same vigilance to their own health and protection. Most patients undergoing surgical care are probably unaware if they are carriers of infectious microbes hiding in their blood. For that reason, Standard Precautions are designed to presume that every individual is potentially infectious. Hands-free, neutral-zone, and no-touch techniques for passing of sharp instruments and devices should be practiced by anyone in the sterile field. Use of blunt suture needles for closure of large or deep wounds should be embraced by surgeons in training as well as into their surgical practice. Wearing proper eye protection to prevent blood transfer to conjunctival membranes should be done for every case, not just the "big" cases. These are just a few examples of the tools we have to be proactive in order to not become unfortunate statistics in the fight against disease transmission.

Hematology and Serology

As a review from anatomy and physiology, hematology is the study of blood and the tissues that form blood; however, it primarily focuses on the cells of the circulatory system:

- White blood cells (leukocytes)—WBCs are involved in the body's defense system against foreign invaders such as bacteria or viruses.

- Red blood cells (erythrocytes)—RBCs transport oxygen and carbon dioxide.

- Platelets (thrombocytes)—thrombocytes help prevent blood loss during injury.

Each of these types of cells is suspended in a solution called plasma. When blood is spun in a centrifuge, the cells conglomerate and separate from the plasma, allowing the plasma to be isolated from the constituent cells.

The total blood volume is the amount of blood within the body's circulatory system. The average adult has 4 to 8 liters (1 liter equals 1.06 quarts). An individual weighing 150 pounds would have an estimated blood volume of 5.5 liters. Blood cells comprise 45 percent of the blood volume, and plasma makes up the other 55 percent. Plasma comprises 90 percent water and 10 percent solids. The solids in plasma consist of proteins, carbohydrates, enzymes, vitamins, lipids, and salts. Whole blood, then, refers to the cellular components of blood and the plasma (see Figure 17-1).

Sera (plural of serum) are the clear liquid portions of any plant or animal fluid that are left after the solid elements within that fluid have been separated. In the context

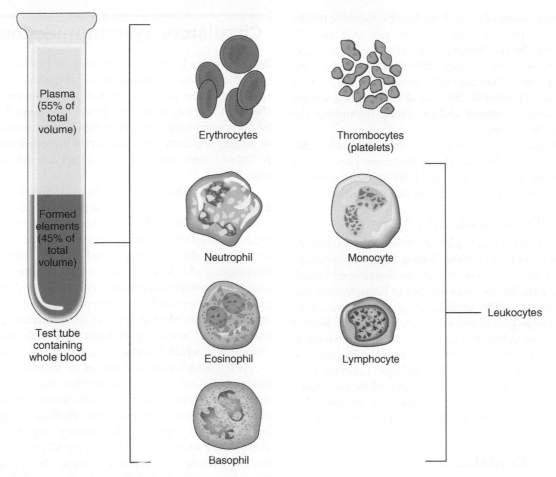

Figure 17-1 The major components of blood.

of this discussion, serum refers to the liquid that remains after plasma has been separated from fibrinogen and blood cells within blood which is the straw-colored portion of plasma that remains in fluid form after blood has clotted.

Serology involves the study of blood serum and the immune responses within it as discussed in Chapters 3 and 21. Previously, serology referred to the in vitro reactions of immune sera: precipitin, agglutination, and complement fixation reactions. Currently, these reactions determine if a blood sample contains antibodies or antigens to infectious diseases by calculating serum titers. Two commonly used laboratory serology tests are the slide agglutination and ELISA tests.

The Western blot test is another serologic test that can identify bacteria within serum. This serologic test is used to identify the bacterium *Borrelia burgdorferi*, which causes Lyme disease. It may also be used to identify HIV. Following separation of proteins from serum by **electrophoresis**, the proteins are transferred to a filter using a blotting technique. Dye-tagged antibodies are then washed over the filter. A positive test is indicated by a colored band left on the filter as a result of the bonding of the antibody with the antigen.

Transmission of Infections from Donated Blood Products

Generally, blood **transfusions** with donated blood products are safe and often life-saving procedures. Very rarely, despite strict donor screening protocols, blood samples can be contaminated with blood-borne pathogenic bacteria, viruses, parasites, or prions. There have been documented cases of individuals receiving blood transfusions suffering serious inadvertent infections as a result of the blood collection process, storage conditions and handling of blood products, or from the presence of undetected microbial contaminants. The infective agents transmitted through subsequent transfusion may proceed to affect the recipient's body systems or tissues in a similar manner as if acquired through other common routes of transmission or may contribute to serious systemic sepsis.

Bacterial Blood Contamination

The Gram-positive bacteria *Staphylococcus aureus* and *S. epidermidis* are two of the most common causes of bacterial contamination of donated blood. It is believed that the percutaneous passage of the hollow-bore hypodermic needle through the skin provides entry of the bacteria that normally reside on and in the skin layers into the blood vessel accessed. Due to the pressure of the donor's blood in drawing the sample out and putting them into collections tubes, the bacteria most likely are transferred into the donated blood sample rather than already present and circulating throughout the donor's vascular system.

Gram-negative bacteria such as *Acinetobacter, Klebsiella,* and *Escherichia* may be underlying infections present in a blood donor and go undetected until the transfusion recipient displays signs and symptoms of systemic infection.

Parasitic Blood Contamination

Donor questionnaires aim to identify individuals who may be undiagnosed carriers of parasitic disease, often due to foreign travel or recreational activities such as camping or hiking. Some of the parasitic diseases capable of being transmitted through blood donation include anaplasmosis caused by *Anaplasma phagocytophilium* and babesiosis from *Babesia microti,* which are tick-borne bacteria capable of surviving in stored blood products. Chagas disease caused by *Trypanosoma cruzi* is spread by triatomine or "kissing bugs." Leishmaniasis, which is transmitted by sand flies, is caused by *Leishmania* protozoa. Malaria, one of the most common parasitic diseases worldwide, is caused by *Plasmodium falciparum,* which is a mosquito-borne disease.

Viral Blood Contamination

Blood donors are asked about their general health, personal habits, and social behaviors to assess whether they may be potential carriers of certain types of viruses. Blood screening methods routinely check for the presence of hepatitis B virus (HBV), hepatitis C virus (HCV), human immunodeficiency virus (HIV), human T-lymphotropic virus (HTLV), West Nile virus (WNV), and potentially others.

The possibility of viral blood contamination and transmission through transfusion also exists with dengue fever, which is spread by mosquitoes, and although no cases of infection have yet been reported through this route, chikungunya or Zika viruses could be spread in the same way. Hepatitis A virus (HAV), spread through the fecal-oral route and contaminated foods, has been reportedly transmitted through blood transfusion.

Prion Blood Contamination

Transmissible spongiform encephalopathies, discussed previously in Chapter 8, are caused by the abnormal folding of normal, non-living, cellular prion proteins in brain or spinal cord tissues, which leads to brain damage and eventually death. In humans, Creutzfeldt-Jakob disease (CJD) and the more rapidly progressing variant CJD (vCJD) can be transmitted through blood transfusion and certain human tissue transplantation such as meningeal dura mater. Individuals with a history of travel to certain countries, including the United Kingdom, may be excluded from donation of blood or tissue.

Circulatory System Infections

Bacteremia is a bacterial infection of the bloodstream. Other microbial pathogens can gain access to the vascular system as discussed in the preceding section; however, bacteria cause the great majority of serious blood infections. The mechanisms of entry vary from minor skin injuries to major trauma or surgery and from dissemination of bacteria from minor infections of other body systems to direct access through blood transfusions.

Healthcare-associated infections (HAIs) of the blood are becoming more common and are often related to surgical procedures or indwelling catheters where microorganisms are introduced either directly into the patient's bloodstream or indirectly through an infected surgical wound. Surgical implantation of a device that is foreign to the body can be the cause of a postoperative wound infection. Surgical technologists must be aware of this when participating in a total joint arthroplasty, ventriculoperitoneal shunt insertion, hernia repair with graft, vascular graft, heart valve replacement, or any procedure in which a device is permanently implanted.

If the body's natural defenses or antibiotic therapy are unable to control and clear an infection, then septicemia may result. Septicemia is an expansion of bacteremia and a serious medical emergency because it can escalate to septic shock, also known as systemic inflammatory response syndrome (SIRS). Data show that approximately 40 percent of patients with septicemia will progress to septic shock and, of those patients, approximately half will die from the infection.

Signs and symptoms of septicemia and septic shock include:

- Hyperthermia or **hypothermia**
- Altered mental status (confusion, dizziness, delirium, coma)
- Skin rash
- **Tachycardia** and **hypotension**

The highest risk populations are the patients who are immunosuppressed or immunocompromised. Individuals in this group include the following: those with HIV/AIDS; those on long-term corticosteroid use for lung disease or following organ transplantation; patients with cancer who are undergoing radiation treatments or chemotherapy; premature neonates in NICU settings; older adults with multiple indwelling catheters or invasive vascular access devices; and those who have been on long-term antibiotic therapy for other conditions.

Gram-positive and Gram-negative bacteria are nearly equally responsible for most cases of septicemia and can be either community-acquired or healthcare-associated infections. The common causative pathogenic agents from other body system infections include:

- Respiratory system infections: *Streptococcus pneumoniae, Chlamydia pneumoniae, Haemophilus influenzae, Legionella* spp.

- Gastrointestinal tract infections: *Escherichia coli*, *Bacteroides fragilis*, Group B *Streptococcus* (in neonates), *Yersinia enterocolitica* (in rare cases)

- Skin and soft tissue infections: *Staphylococcus aureus*, *Streptococcus pyogenes*, *Clostridium* spp., *Pseudomonas aeruginosa*

- Urinary tract infections: *E. coli*, *Klebsiella* spp., *Enterobacter* spp., *Proteus* spp., *Enterococcus* spp.

- CNS infections: *Streptococcus pneumoniae*, *Neisseria meningitidis*, *Listeria monocytogenes*, *E. coli*, *H influenzae*, *P. aeruginosa*, *Staphylococcus* spp.

Infective Endocarditis

Infective endocarditis (IE) is a serious infection of the inner lining (endocardium) of the heart and covers the heart valves. The heart valves suffer valvular incompetence or insufficiency, which may lead to **intractable congestive heart failure** (CHF) and abscesses involving the myocardium.

Infective endocarditis generally occurs in patients with damaged or abnormal heart architecture (physical structure), combined with exposure to opportunistic bacteria that gain access to the vascular system through trauma, dissemination of infection from other body systems, or high-risk activities such as IV drug use and unprotected sex. In cases of IE, **morbidity** is high and, if left untreated, generally fatal (see Figure 17-2).

There are two types of infective endocarditis: subacute native valve endocarditis, a type that is slow to develop, and acute IE, a type that has a sudden onset. Subacute IE is usually caused by α-hemolytic *Streptococcus*, typically found in the oral cavity. *Enterococcus* and *Staphylococcus* bacteria are also common causes of infective endocarditis. Periodontal, pharyngeal, and, less frequently, infections from other parts of the body may cause subacute endocarditis. Dentists will usually prescribe prophylactic antibiotics before tooth extractions to prevent the bacteria from entering the bloodstream

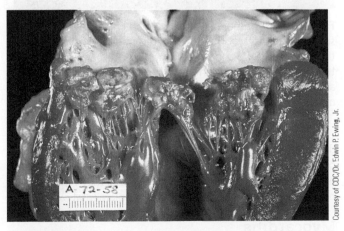

Figure 17-2 Gross pathology of subacute bacterial endocarditis involving mitral valve from the bacteria, *Haemophilus parainfluenzae*.

during the procedure. Without this antimicrobial prophylaxis, bacteria may travel to the heart, colonizing pre-existing lesions on heart valves. These lesions may be left from diseases such as rheumatic fever, mitral valve **stenosis**, or other congenital heart **anomalies**. The colony is protected from phagocytosis by blood clots which, in turn, can eventually break loose and travel to the lungs or brain, resulting in pulmonary thrombosis or **cerebral infarct**.

Acute IE involves normal heart valves and is typically caused by *Staphylococcus aureus* or Group B *Streptococcus*; however, the same bacteria listed in the previous section, which spread through the vascular system, are also potential sources for infective endocarditis. The sudden onset can damage heart valves rapidly, resulting in death if left untreated. As with subacute IE, the bacteria typically arise from an existing infection somewhere in the body and are dislodged, allowing entry into the bloodstream (see Figure 17-3).

Prosthetic valve endocarditis (PVE) is found in patients with implanted prosthetic mechanical or **bioprosthetic valves**, accounting for 5 to 10 percent of all endocarditis infections. Mechanical valves tend to become infected within the first 3 months (early onset) following implantation. The bioprosthetic valves are more likely to become infected after 1 year (late onset). Mitral valves are more likely to be involved in PVE than aortic valves. *S. aureus* is believed to be the most common cause of both early- and late-onset infections, although multiple other bacteria may also cause infection. Individuals with implanted pacemakers and **cardioverter-defibrillators** have similar risk factors for infection and outcomes similar to those with PVE.

Intravenous drug abuse infective endocarditis (IVDA IE) statistics show that up to 75 percent of infections involve normal native heart valves and that 50 percent of those infections involve the tricuspid valve. Fungal IE is found in intravenous drug users and in ICU patients who receive broad-spectrum antibiotics. Blood cultures are often negative, with diagnosis being made only after microscopic examination of large **emboli**.

Bacteria implicated in documented endocarditis infections, although uncommon, include *Bacteroides fragilis*, *Bartonella henselae*, *Escherichia coli*, *Haemophilus influenzae*, *Neisseria meningitidis*, and *Salmonella enteritidis*. Fungal infections of heart tissues may result from colonization of *Candida albicans* or other species of fungi (see Figure 17-4).

Clinical Signs of Infective Endocarditis

Approximately 85 percent of individuals with infective endocarditis will have detectable **heart murmur** on **auscultation**. Classic signs are detected singly or in combination in half the patients with IE. These signs include:

- **Subungual** hemorrhages
- Petechiae of the skin
- Janeway lesions—non-tender maculae on palms of hands and soles of feet

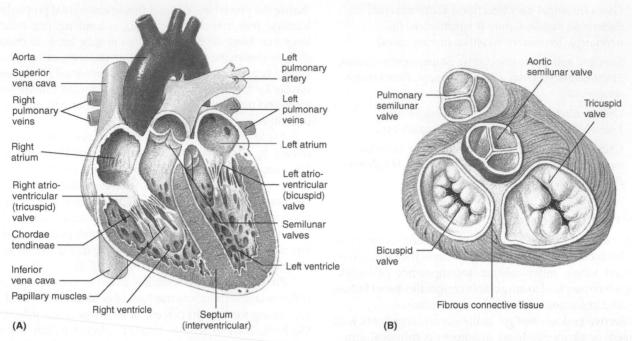

Figure 17-3 (A) The interior structures of the heart and (B) cross-sectioned anterior view of the valves of the heart.

- Osler nodes—tender subcutaneous nodules usually of the distal pads of the digits
- Roth spots—retinal hemorrhages with clear centers, relatively rare (5 percent) in cases (see Figure 17-5).

Other signs of disease that may be observed include:

- Neurological signs of embolic stroke, paralysis, hemiparesis, stiff neck, or delirium
- Distended neck veins and chest x-ray signs of congestive heart failure (see Figure 17-6)
- **Hepatosplenomegaly**
- Pericardial or pleural friction rub
- **Gallops** or **rales**
- **Cardiac arrhythmia**

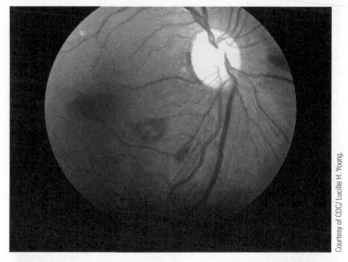

Figure 17-5 A pathologic phenomenon known as a Roth spot (near center of image), located near the point where the retinal arterioles and optic nerve entered the rear of the eyeball and appearing as a hemorrhagic ring with a pale center, a condition caused by immune complex-mediated vasculitis, often following bacterial endocarditis.

Antibiotic therapy is the primary treatment for infective endocarditis; however, surgery for lysis of adhesions or repair/replacement of valves may be required. Patients who suffer renal damage may require **hemodialysis**. Patients may require treatment for congestive heart failure and supplemental oxygen.

Myocarditis

Myocarditis is a condition caused by a number of pathogenic microbes. Common bacterial causes of myocarditis include *Chlamydia, Mycoplasma, Streptococcus, Staphylococcus, Borrelia,*

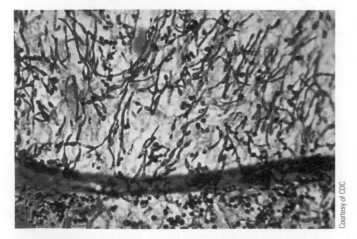

Figure 17-4 Histopathologic changes indicative of endocarditis caused by the fungal organism, *Candida albicans*.

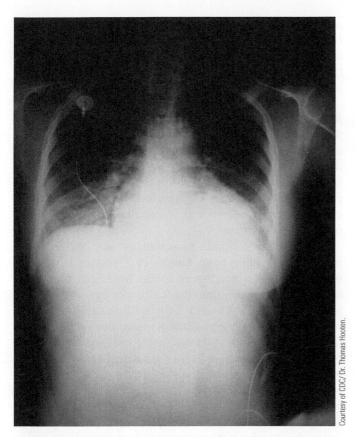

Figure 17-6 An A-P x-ray of the chest of a female with congestive heart failure, with presence of an enlarged cardiac silhouette and fluid accumulation in both lungs, known as pulmonary congestion.

and *Treponema*. Viral causes include Coxsackie B virus, Cytomegalovirus, Epstein-Barr virus, Hepatitis C virus, Herpes simplex, HIV, and Parvovirus. Fungal causes include *Aspergillus*, *Candida*, *Coccidioides*, *Cryptococcus*, and *Histoplasma*.

Often, symptoms are mild or absent, so the infection goes undetected and may lead to **cardiomyopathy**, which is a type of heart failure (see Figure 17-7). Symptoms of myocarditis and possible impending heart failure include the following:

- Abnormal heartbeat and possible fainting episodes
- Chest pain when starting exercise or at rest in bed
- Light-headedness or fatigue
- Stabbing pain in chest radiating to neck or shoulders, similar to classic heart attack signs
- Flu-like symptoms of fever, sore throat, headache, muscle aches, diarrhea
- Swelling of joints, legs, or neck veins
- Decreased urine output

Myocarditis and cardiomyopathy are the leading causes for heart transplantation in the United States.

Pericarditis and Pericardial Fluid

Pericarditis, an inflammation of the pericardium, has several forms. It is typically secondary to other bacterial infections of

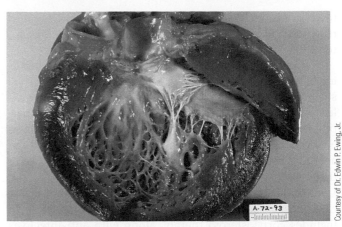

Figure 17-7 Human heart revealing pathologic changes caused by cardiomyopathy, showing a thickened, dilated left ventricle with sub-endocardial fibrosis manifested as increased whiteness of the endocardium.

the body, such as lung abscesses or pneumonia, and is most often caused by *Streptococcus*. Occasionally, pericarditis can be caused by a virus and is referred to as acute non-specific pericarditis. Another form, chronic pericarditis, causes the pericardium to bind to the heart by formation of adhesions. This form may result from acute pericarditis, but usually the origin is unknown. Surgical **lysis of adhesions** may be required. Tuberculosis may cause chronic pericarditis, resulting in deposits of calcium and fibrin that constrict the free movement of the heart, requiring surgical excision.

Tuberculous Pericarditis

Tuberculosis, the highly contagious respiratory disease caused by *Mycobacterium tuberculosis*, is also the causative agent in some pericardial infections. The **extrapulmonary** tuberculosis infection called tuberculous pericarditis causes a thickening of the pericardial sac that may allow serous pericardial fluid to leak from the pericardium and become entrapped in the space between the myocardium and pericardium, leading to a life-threatening condition called **cardiac tamponade**. **Pericardiocentesis** may be required to drain the serous fluid and relieve the pressure off of the heart muscle, allowing it to pump freely. Pericardial fluid may recollect and the procedure may have to be repeated. In the case of a severely damaged pericardium, surgery may be required to remove a portion of the pericardial sac, called a pericardial window.

Tuberculous pericarditis is relatively uncommon in the United States due to the infrequency of TB infections but is seen more commonly in immigrant populations and in foreign countries with a high incidence of tuberculosis. Those living with HIV have increased risk for development of tuberculous pericarditis.

Vasculitis

Inflammation of blood vessels is called vasculitis or angiitis. If arteries are inflamed, then it is called arteritis and inflammation of veins is called venulitis. There are several causes of vasculitis, including bacterial infection, drug or chemical reactions, allergic response, cancer, or rheumatic disease reactions.

Vascular inflammation can lead to the following: narrowing of the internal lumen, reducing blood flow; complete constriction, causing **ischemia** and possible necrosis; or dilatation, leading to **aneurysm** formation. The severity of the disease process is dependent on the size of the vessels and numbers involved, the body systems affected, the amount of oxygen able to reach tissues or organs, and the resulting amount of tissue loss or compromise due to the reduced blood supply. Definitive diagnosis is achieved through biopsy and, in the case of suspected infection, culture results. Treatment often includes corticosteroid therapy along with anti-infectives (antibiotics, antifungals, or antivirals) if indicated.

Pseudomonas aeruginosa Infections

Pseudomonas aeruginosa is a common infectious agent of patients with burns and puncture wounds. The moist surface of the burn and lack of neutrophil response to invasion by *P. aeruginosa* place the patient at risk. It produces a characteristic blue pus due to the pigment pyocyanin produced by the bacteria. Pyocyanin can mediate tissue damage. As the infection progresses, colonization can occur in the intestine, followed closely by bacteremia.

For reasons unknown, the bacterial cells show an affinity for invading blood vessels. This invasion is a syndrome called ecthyma gangrenosum. It begins as superficial skin lesions, usually on the buttocks, perineum, axillary region, or extremities. The lesion invariably grows larger, and the center of each lesion eventually becomes black in color, a result of necrosis caused by the destruction of capillaries, arterioles, and venules. The mortality rate is high among patients who have neutropenia (a diminished number of neutrophils in the blood) in combination with bacteremia. Patients with deep wounds, open bone fractures, and severe burns are also subject to developing osteomyelitis caused by *P. aeruginosa*.

Patients with prosthetic heart valves and IV drug users are prone to endocarditis caused by *P. aeruginosa*. Injection drug users tend to be younger males who usually have no outstanding health problems other than their substance use disorder and acquire the infection from using drug **paraphernalia** contaminated with water-borne bacterial cells. The tricuspid valve between the right atrium and ventricle is more often involved than the other heart valves. A severe form of the infection also may affect the left heart (left-sided endocarditis) and presents the patient with a poor prognosis.

Blood–Brain Barrier

A physiological barrier exists between systemic blood and the brain **parenchyma** (the functional elements of the brain). It is designed to prevent the entrance of antibodies and certain large molecules. The blood–brain barrier remains permeable to water, oxygen, carbon dioxide, and non-ionic solutes such as alcohol, glucose, and anesthetic drugs. Tight junctions between the epithelial cells of the **choroid plexus**, arachnoid cells, and capillary endothelial cells help to establish this barrier but it also makes it difficult to clear potentially harmful invasive substances once the barrier is penetrated.

No barrier exists between the brain and cerebrospinal fluid (CSF). Extracellular fluid in the brain and CSF is in direct contact with brain matter, primarily because the ependymal cells that comprise the walls of the ventricles do not have tight junctions. Free movement between inflammatory cells or pathogenic organisms within extracellular fluid of the brain is restricted however, because the cellular space between neurons is smaller than the diameter of the smallest viruses.

Researchers continue to search for safe and effective methods of treating brain tumors or abscesses by finding ways to bypass the blood–brain barrier. In Oregon, physicians have tried temporarily opening the barrier by using concentrated sugar solutions to shrink the epithelial cells. In France, patients with glioblastoma tumors have been treated with fine ultrasound probes that vibrate the cells and allow for up to 6 hours of dilated opening of the barrier to enhance delivery of chemotherapeutic drugs to the tumor bed and surrounding brain tissue. Researchers in the United States are experimenting with nanoparticle-containing agents and other formulations that combine proteins with chemotherapeutic drugs to facilitate movement of relatively large molecules through the physiological blood–brain barrier to reach cancerous target tissues.

Infections of the Central Nervous System

Nearly 20 percent of a person's total blood volume passes through their brain at any given time, so it would stand to reason that the CNS could be affected by most of the pathogens that are able to invade the vascular system and travel upstream.

Although the tissues of the CNS are remarkably resistant to infection by various pathogens, they are not fully impervious to them. When infection does occur, the resulting damage can be severe. Damage to the brain and spinal cord as a result of invasion by bacteria, viruses, or fungi can result in a wide range of neurological deficits. Expedient diagnosis and treatment for infections of the CNS are critical to prevent death or permanent neurologic damage.

CNS infections are relatively uncommon, considering that the system does not have an intrinsic immune system. However, infections can easily become life-threatening because the brain and spinal cord are protected by bone and meningeal coverings that, when penetrated, compartmentalize the invasive microorganisms. Physiologic mechanisms such as the blood–brain barrier that filters systemic circulation create a challenge for effective delivery of antibiotic therapy where needed.

Prion diseases including Creutzfeldt-Jakob disease (CJD), vCJD and other transmissible spongiform encephalopathies are discussed in Chapter 8.

Meningitis

Bacteria and other pathogens can reach the meninges and other areas of the brain through the bloodstream, or they can enter through a penetrating wound or as a result of a surgical procedure. Abscesses can spread from adjoining structures such as the nasal sinuses or periodontal infections. The following sections discuss meningitis and encephalitis infections based on the classification of pathogen responsible (see Figure 17-8).

Non-infectious diseases such as **sarcoidosis** and some cancers, as well as drugs used to treat cancer and prevent organ rejection, can inflame the meninges and cause symptoms similar to those of infectious meningitis.

Bacterial Meningitis

Acute bacterial meningitis is defined as an infection of the meningeal pia mater and arachnoid layers. It is a life-threatening disease that requires immediate medical treatment. Some of the most common pathogens responsible for bacterial infection are *Haemophilus influenzae* type B, *Streptococcus pneumoniae*, *Neisseria meningitidis*, and *Escherichia coli*. These bacteria are normal residents of the nose, upper respiratory system, or gastrointestinal tract and often infect the CNS when a person's immune system is depressed. Meningitis may also occur as a complication of other diseases such as endocarditis, pneumonia, or otitis media (middle ear infection). Any penetrating injury (including surgery) of the skull can also allow the entrance of bacteria into the CNS. Patients with advanced kidney disease are more susceptible to infections from *Listeria* bacteria.

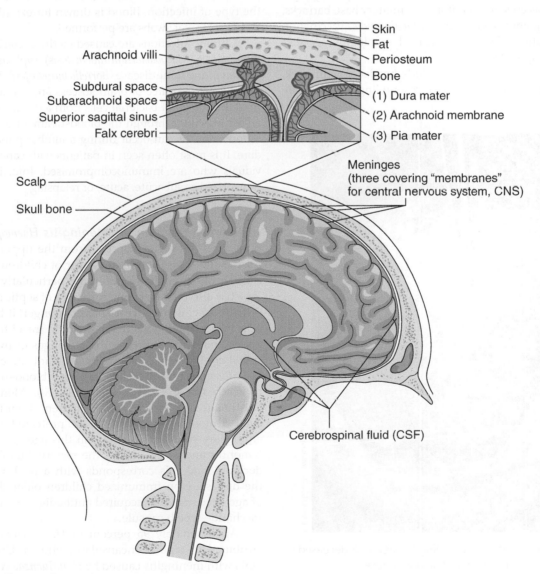

Figure 17-8 The meninges.

Meningitis occurs frequently in small children because of their immature immune systems and susceptibility to infections in general. In the immediate neonatal period, infections from group B *Streptococcus*, *E. coli*, or *Listeria monocytogenes* are most common. In infants older than age 1 month, the infections are usually from *Streptococcus pneumoniae*, *Haemophilus influenzae* type B (Hib), and *Neisseria meningitidis*.

The mortality rate for infant *E. coli* meningitis is high, in the range of approximately 40 to 80 percent, with the majority of survivors suffering neurologic deficits and/or developmental abnormalities. Neonates can be exposed to the microorganism during childbirth. Studies have indicated that the maternal intestinal tract is colonized by an increased number of *E. coli* cells during pregnancy. However, it is not understood how the increase in number of bacterial cells predisposes the infant to developing meningitis.

Except for a surgical infection or head injury, bacterial meningitis in adults is usually caused by *N. meningitidis*, *S. pneumoniae*, and *L. monocytogenes* (see Figure 17-9).

Outbreaks may occur in areas where groups of people reside, such as college dormitories or military base barracks, and are frequently caused by *N. meningitidis*. Vaccination recommendations for meningococcal meningitis are discussed in Chapter 15.

Symptoms of meningitis include headache, stiff neck, sore throat (usually following or resembling a respiratory illness), and vomiting. A physician examining a patient will try to lower the patient's chin to the chest and may find it too painful for the patient to achieve. Older children and adults may become irritable and confused, with eventual progression from drowsiness to stupor, followed by coma and death. Waterhouse-Friderichsen syndrome is caused by *N. meningitidis* and results in severe diarrhea, seizures, vomiting, internal bleeding, hypothermia, and shock. Death often results without immediate treatment.

Children younger than age 2 years present with a high fever, lethargy, vomiting, and seizures. A red or purple spotted skin rash and overall blue skin color resulting from cyanosis may be present. The physician may note that the child's legs pull up when the head is brought down to the chest. The physician must quickly determine if the origin of the infection is bacterial, fungal, or viral to properly determine treatment. A spinal tap (lumbar puncture) is performed and CSF is examined under a microscope and cultured. Glucose level, protein elevation, and white blood count also help determine the type of infection. Blood is drawn for examination, and nasal and throat swabs are performed.

Chronic infections are caused by the bacteria that cause tuberculosis (*Mycobacterium tuberculosis*), syphilis (*Treponema pallidum*), and Lyme disease (*Borrelia burgdorferi*). *Pseudomonas aeruginosa* is a source of brain abscess and meningitis either from the spread of bacterial cells from a distant site (such as an ear infection) through the bloodstream, or through direct introduction, as can occur during a lumbar puncture procedure. It is most often seen in patients with cancer and individuals who are immunocompromised. Infections can be categorized as subacute, acute, or relapsing.

***Haemophilis influenzae* Meningitis** *Haemophilus influenzae* type b (Hib) can spread from the upper respiratory tract to the sinuses and middle ear of children and adults, causing otitis media. Children are particularly vulnerable. Type b is also the most common cause of septic arthritis and cellulitis in children 2 years old or younger. If the bacterial cells invade the bloodstream, they can travel to the lymph nodes and possibly invade the meninges of the brain and spinal cord, causing meningitis. It is not understood how *H. influenzae* type b cells cross the blood–brain barrier to reach the CNS (see Figure 17-10). Meningitis is a life-threatening infection in children. Infants who are aged 3 months and younger are protected by maternal antibodies, so infection is rare in this age group. Between 6 months and 1 year of age, the maternal antibodies have declined, and this corresponds with a peak incidence in the disease. Non-immunized children older than 3 years of age have naturally acquired antibodies against the polysaccharide type b capsule.

Approximately 95 percent of *H. influenzae* cases are attributed to type b encapsulated strains. Untreated infants with meningitis caused by *H. influenzae* type b have a

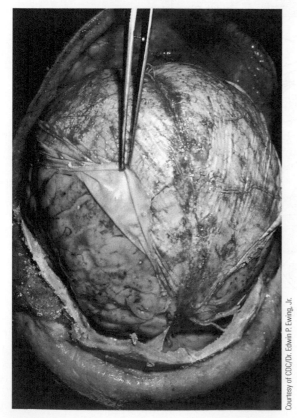

Figure 17-9 Pneumococcal meningitis seen in a deceased patient's brain with a history of alcohol abuse.

Courtesy of CDC/Dr. Edwin P. Ewing, Jr.

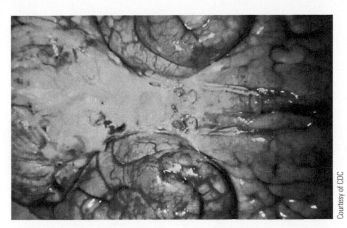

Courtesy of CDC

Figure 17-10 An inferior view of a post-mortem human brain infected with Gram-negative, *Haemophilus influenzae* bacteria, causing meningitis showing an overall inflammatory response and purulent exudate of the midbrain, cerebellum, and spinal cord.

very high fatality rate, with past rates reported as high as 90 percent. Mortality in treated cases declines to approximately 3 to 6 percent. Neurologic sequelae or enduring deficits after recovery from meningitis can include hearing loss, blindness, chronic seizures, hydrocephalus, and developmental disabilities.

Diagnosis, Treatment, and Prevention Cerebrospinal fluid obtained through a spinal tap to collect CSF, samples of blood, sputum, nasopharyngeal swabs, and exudates from infected conjunctivae are types of specimens obtained from a patient suspected to have a *Haemophilus* species infection. Blood cultures are highly effective in isolating the bacteria involved. Identification of the specific bacterial agent is critical to prescribing the optimal antibiotic therapy because other types of bacteria can cause ear infections and meningitis.

The Hib vaccine is a routine childhood immunization in the United States. Currently, three monovalent conjugate Hib vaccines and three combination vaccines that contain Hib conjugate are available. Depending on the type of vaccine used, infants are given a series of injections at ages 2, 4, and 6 months or at ages 2 and 4 months. Booster doses are recommended at 12 to 15 months. Since the vaccine protocols have been in place, the incidence of Hib infections in children younger than age 5 years has decreased 99 percent in the United States.

Fungal Meningitis

Certain fungal infections, especially *Cryptococcus*, develop slowly in comparison with acute bacterial infections and can result in chronic meningitis. Other fungi known to cause meningitis are *Histoplasma*, *Blastomyces*, and *Coccidioides*, which are found in the soil, and *Candida*, which is nearly always an HAI.

Immunosuppression from pre-existing disease such as HIV/AIDS or rheumatoid arthritis, corticosteroid therapy for cancer or lung disease, transplant anti-rejection therapy, or surgery are all risk factors for fungal infection that could spread through the blood to cause meningitis.

Parasitic Meningitis

A rare form of meningitis caused by the microscopic amoeba, *Naegleria fowleri*, is called primary amoebic meningoencephalitis (PAM). The parasite gains access into the body through the nose when diving or swimming in bodies of warm freshwater such as lakes, ponds, rivers, underchlorinated pools, or warm springs. Additionally, water from contaminated water heaters used to irrigate sinuses with devices such as **Neti pots** has been reported as a mechanism of infection. The parasite travels to the brain through the sinuses. Drinking contaminated water is not a route of transmission. *Naegleria fowleri* is not found in saltwater bodies such as coastal waters.

There have been 148 reported PAM infections in the United States from 1962 through 2019 with only four survivors. Between 2003 and 2012 there were only 31 cases, however, each of them was fatal. Initial symptoms mimic those of bacterial meningitis; however, once symptoms begin, the disease progresses quickly, destroying brain tissue and resulting in death in approximately 5 days. Preventative measures for keeping water from these areas from entering the nose are the most effective against possible parasitic infection.

Other parasitic infections of the CNS include acute and chronic encephalopathies. As with PAM, acute infections are typically caused by free-swimming amoebas and trichinosis, resulting in meningitis or encephalitis. African trypanosomiasis (also known as chronic sleeping sickness), chronic cerebral granulomas caused by *Schistosoma japonicum*, or brain abscesses caused by *Toxoplasma gondii* are chronic parasitic encephalopathies.

Cysticercosis, as discussed in Chapter 10, is the most common of the parasitic CNS infections and is caused by the larvae form of *Taenia solium*. These larval infections cause much of the episodes of basilar arachnoiditis and parasitic cysts of cases in South America and Asia, resulting in seizures and hydrocephalus.

Viral Meningitis

Viral meningitis is the most common form of meningitis infections. The non-polio enteroviruses, coxsackievirus, enterovirus, echovirus, and parechovirus, are often the cause, although many who become infected with non-polio enteroviruses never suffer meningitis.

Other frequent causes include mumps (paramyxovirus of the genus Rubulavirus), herpesviruses (including herpes simplex virus and varicella-zoster virus), measles virus, influenza virus, West Nile virus, and lymphocytic choriomeningitis virus. Cytomegalovirus and HIV/AIDS may also result in a chronic infection.

Encephalitis

Encephalitis is defined as an inflammation of the brain parenchyma and is considered to be clinically more dangerous than viral meningitis. The condition may be caused by the viruses listed here as well as arboviruses and rabies.

Herpes simplex encephalitis is the most common type that occurs in the United States. If left untreated, fatality rates reach 70 percent. This virus can cause severe destruction in the anterior temporal lobe and orbital frontal region. Approximately one-third are due to primary herpes simplex infections, and two-thirds are due to reactivation of a latent herpes simplex virus (HSV) agent. CSF may contain red blood cells and white blood cells. Acyclovir, an antiviral agent used to treat HSV, is effective, especially if administered early in the infection.

Mosquito-borne arboviruses cause specific types of encephalitis such as eastern equine encephalitis, western equine encephalitis, Venezuelan equine encephalitis, Japanese B encephalitis, La Crosse encephalitis, and St. Louis encephalitis. This type of virus causes epidemic encephalitis throughout the world.

Paralytic poliomyelitis is a virus that targets select motor neurons of the CNS. Initial symptoms include sore throat, gastrointestinal upset, low-grade fever, and mild headache. As discussed in Chapter 8, the virus spreads and the patient suffers from an increased fever, severe headache, vomiting, and stiff neck. The polio virus enters the bloodstream, gaining access to the CNS and infecting the motor neurons of the anterior horn of the spinal cord and within the brain. Hemiplegia and reflex losses ensue (see Figure 8-13 in Chapter 8); 10 to 15 percent of victims experience difficulty in swallowing or speaking, and CSF exhibits an increased white blood count and elevated protein.

Rabies is a type of encephalitis that causes problems in developing countries where the lyssavirus responsible for the disease known as rabies is often endemic in local canine populations. In the United States, it is endemic in wild animals, especially skunks, foxes, raccoons, and bats. Transmission to humans is through a bite from an infected animal. Clinical manifestations include fever, headache, seizures, hydrophobia, and aerophobia. If the rabies vaccine is not administered before clinical symptoms manifest, then death is imminent. The virus has a characteristic bullet shape when viewed under a scanning electron microscope (see Figure 17-11).

Brucellosis

Brucellosis affects both the cardiovascular system and the CNS. The disease has been given a number of names based

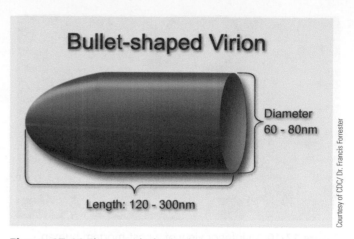

Figure 17-11 The morphologic characteristics observed in a single rabies virion, which is referred to as being bullet shaped.

on the areas where outbreaks occurred, such as Malta fever, fever of Crete, or Mediterranean fever, or based on the clinical presentation (undulant fever or gastric remittent fever). It was first isolated by David Bruce during an epidemic among British soldiers on Malta Island in 1887. He isolated the bacteria from the liver and spleen of patients.

Brucellosis continues to be a reportable disease; however, in the United States it has become rare. Globally, more than 500,000 cases occur and are mainly in developing countries with predominantly agrarian societies. In countries where there is routine and stringent screening of domesticated animals by veterinarians, human disease transmission is infrequent. The World Health Organization continues to monitor brucellosis as a serious public health concern.

Acute brucellosis infections present with symptoms similar to the flu, such as fever, chills, sweating, fatigue, headache, weakness, headache, weight loss, and abdominal, joint, and back pain. Most cases of acute brucellosis resolve with appropriate antibiotic treatment; however, chronic disease is possible in some individuals, with or without treatment. Chronic cases, similar to tuberculosis, can cause recurrent symptoms for years. The most serious complications of brucellosis are infective endocarditis, meningitis, and encephalitis.

Brain Abscess

A brain abscess is a collection of pus, usually found within the frontal or temporal lobe of the cerebrum. Pus may be free or encapsulated and may occur in multiple areas of the brain. It is typically secondary to another infection somewhere in the body. Cases of otitis media, sinusitis, or **mastoiditis** are typical primary infections. Bacteria may also travel to the brain from an infected tooth or from infections within the heart or lungs.

Symptoms are those that are typically associated with abnormally increased intracranial pressure (ICP) and include headache, nausea, vomiting, visual disturbances, and hemiplegia (weakness on one side of the body). Computed tomography (CT) or magnetic resonance imaging (MRI) scans help to diagnose the location. Surgery is required to eliminate the mass, and intravenous antibiotics are necessary to clear the infection from primary and secondary sites.

A subdural **empyema** is a collection of pus just beneath the dura of the brain. It is frequently a complication of sinusitis or otitis media, but it can also result from bacteria entering through a penetrating head injury. Surgery may be required to drain the pus and relieve intracranial pressure. Intravenous antibiotics are used to clear the remaining infection.

MICRO NOTES

"I Have a Hot Tip for You!"

Did you know that Dr. Harvey Cushing, considered to be the father of modern neurosurgery, and Dr. William Bovie, a biophysicist and inventor, collaborated in 1926 to create the first "Bovie" electrosurgical unit? After Dr. Cushing was unable to complete the resection of a very vascular brain tumor, Dr. Cushing provided him with the tool that would cut through tissue and cauterize bleeding vessels with high-frequency electrical current. The electrosurgical unit has become one of the most widely used surgical devices across every surgical specialty, but it was exceedingly valuable in surgical procedures to treat various diseases and infections of the CNS, during which the use of strands of suture material as ligatures was tedious and often impractical. One can hardly imagine how modern complex surgeries could be done now without it.

 ## Under the Microscope

A craniotomy was scheduled for excision of left-sided intracranial lesion. Dr. Nelson reached the lesion and an encapsulated mass filled with purulent material was noted. Two sets of cultures were taken and they proceeded to remove the capsule and purulent collection. The circulating nurse was asked to look back at the referring physician's history and found that the patient had recently been treated for anemia which required a blood transfusion in the hospital.

1. Based on your review of the chapter materials, what type of lesion did Dr. Nelson most likely find and remove?

2. What is the relevance of the patient's past history to the findings at surgery?

3. In general, what other types of infections could cause intracranial findings?

4. Which other types of infections can be spread through the circulatory system or contaminated blood products?

5. What are examples of ways to prevent infections affecting the circulatory and central nervous systems?

CHAPTER 18

Diseases of the Skin and Internal Tissues

Learning Objectives

After completing the study of this chapter, you will be able to:

1. Define key terms.
2. Describe the general classifications of skin infections.
3. Identify the pathogens associated with infections of the integumentary system.
4. Identify the pathogens associated with infections of internal tissues.
5. Describe the routes of transmission for pathogens of the skin and internal tissues.
6. Apply critical thinking skills in relating chapter material to the surgical environment of care or broader global community.

Key Terms

Arthritis	Edematous	Interstitial fluid	Sheath
Autoimmune disease	Emphysema	Leprosy	Tenosynovitis
Bifurcated	Erysipelas	Mastectomy	Vesicles
Crepitus	Erythematous	Papillomas	
Debridement	Folliculitis	Pseudomonad	
Ecthyma	Ganglion	Schwann cells	

The Big Picture

The first line of defense that humans have against the environment is our skin. As effective as it normally is, there are numerous ways in which the protective mechanisms can be disrupted, exposing our internal tissues to external microbes that become opportunistic pathogens. During your examination of the topics in this chapter, consider the following:

1. How do microbes that normally reside in our epidermal tissues protect us from other transient microbes?

2. What could be potentially negative implications to frequent and constant use of antimicrobial cleansers and skin preparations?

3. Which diseases of the skin and internal tissues have been affecting humans for centuries?

4. Which types of infections discussed in this chapter have the potential for requiring surgical intervention?

Clinical Significance Topic

Suture closure of a laparotomy incision is performed in multiple layers. Typically, following resolution of the pathology that was the reason for surgery, the peritoneum is closed first, followed by the fascia and muscle as a unit, the subcutaneous layer, and then the skin. The subcutaneous layer comprises fatty tissue that resembles chicken fat and small blood vessels. Even though the fatty tissue provides no strength to the wound closure, it is an ideal place for bacteria to multiply if the tissues are not approximated (brought together) and dead space (open gap) is not eliminated. The serosanguinous fluid that seeps from incised tissue postoperatively accumulates in the dead space and acts as the perfect culture medium for bacteria that spread to the other tissue layers and surrounding area, causing a surgical site infection (SSI). If the patient is very thin and has almost no fatty tissue, then the "sub-q" layer might not need to be closed. Suture materials such as the Ethicon absorbable Plus sutures available in Vicryl®, Monocryl®, PDS®, and the barbed Stratafix™, PDS™ and Monocryl options are manufactured with an anti-microbial (Triclosan) coating that reduces potential wound layer infections from contamination of the suture material by indigenous or transient normal and opportunistic bacteria including *S. aureus*, *S. epidermidis*, MRSA, MRSE, *E. coli*, and *K. pneumoniae*. These anti-microbial sutures have been recommended by both the World Health Organization and the Centers for Disease Control and Prevention as effective surgical practices that reduce the potential for SSI.

The Integumentary System

The human integumentary system comprises the skin, hair, nails, sweat glands, sebaceous glands, and sensory receptors, and is the largest organ of the body. The skin functions as the first line of defense against the outside world, including infection by foreign microorganisms, environmental irritants, and harmful radiation from the sun. It weighs approximately 6 pounds in an average adult and receives approximately one-third of all the blood circulating through the body. Skin is waterproof but helps regulate the internal temperature of the body by releasing water.

It consists of two layers: the epidermis, a layer of stratified epithelial tissue that is further divided into sublayers, and the dermis, found just underneath the layers of the epidermis. The dermis is dense connective tissue that connects the skin to the tissues below it (adipose and muscle tissue) and contains nerves and nourishing blood vessels. The hair follicles, oil gland ducts, and sweat gland ducts of the dermis provide passageways for potential pathogens to make their way past the protective skin and infect deeper body tissues. The epidermis and dermis combine to comprise the cutaneous tissues of the body, and the layer beneath this cutaneous layer is called the subcutaneous layer (see Figure 18-1).

The skin is home to many resident bacterial species that penetrate the protective barrier as a result of a traumatic injury or planned surgical incision. Surgical technologists and other sterile team members are educated in how to prevent surgical site infections and the bacterial species involved in them. This chapter examines diseases and infections of the skin and soft tissues beneath it.

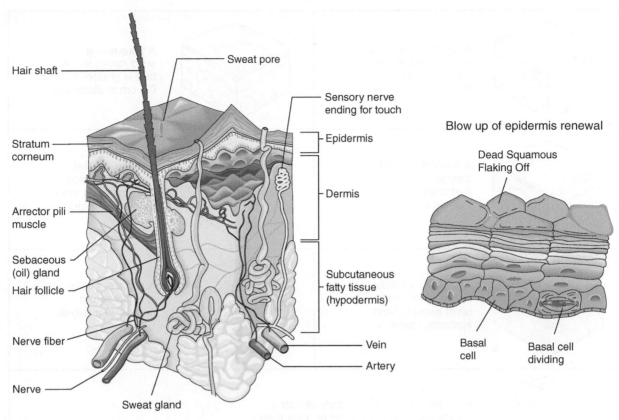

Figure 18-1 The layers of the skin with separate cross-section of the epidermis.

Indigenous Microbiota of the Skin

The skin is covered with microorganisms considered the indigenous microbiota of the skin or resident microbes, more commonly called the normal microflora or just normal flora. Growth of the microbial population is influenced by the amount of moisture on the skin, pH, and temperature. Successful commensals tend to be those that thrive in high-salt environments and are resistant to drying. The species *Staphylococcus epidermidis* and *Propionibacterium acnes* can be found anywhere on the skin. *Staphylococcus aureus* and mycobacteria are also common residents but in fewer numbers. Corynebacteria are found primarily in moist areas, such as armpits, the groin, or perineum. Other resident skin microbes include Gram-positive organisms such as bacillus, diphtheroids, micrococci, streptococci, and yeast. Gram-negative bacilli can also be found on the skin.

Researchers have studied resident skin microbes and found that they provide a mechanism of protection by crowding out more pathogenic species, taking up space in pores and on surfaces. Additionally, several species produce substances toxic to other bacteria, preventing colonization by competitors.

Transient microbes are those acquired through interaction with the surrounding environment and can include almost any type of microbe that remains on the skin surface until washed and wiped off or sloughed off with normal epidermal skin cell shedding.

Bacterial Skin Infections

The microbiota of the skin is so abundant that skin infections are relatively common even though the skin has its own defense mechanisms. Wound infection occurs when the skin is broken and the opportunistic microbes make their way into the deeper layers. Once past the barrier, they can get into lymph or blood and cause septicemia.

Skin lesions do not necessarily indicate skin infection, but they may be a manifestation of a more serious systemic infection. Vesicles are small fluid-filled lesions. Vesicles larger than 1.0 cm are called bullae. Flat, reddened lesions are called macules. Raised, pus-filled lesions are called pustules, and they vary in size, shape, and color. An ulcer is a skin depression in which the epidermis and a portion of the dermis have been destroyed. These are common in pressure areas on patients who are bedridden or otherwise immobile for long periods (see Figure 18-2).

Staphylococcal Skin Infections

Staphylococci are the most common skin pathogens. They are responsible for boils, abscesses, and superficial **folliculitis**. *Staphylococcus aureus* is the most pathogenic of the staphylococci and is a serious problem for hospitals because it is carried and easily transmitted by patients, employees, and visitors. Untreated infections can lead to tissue

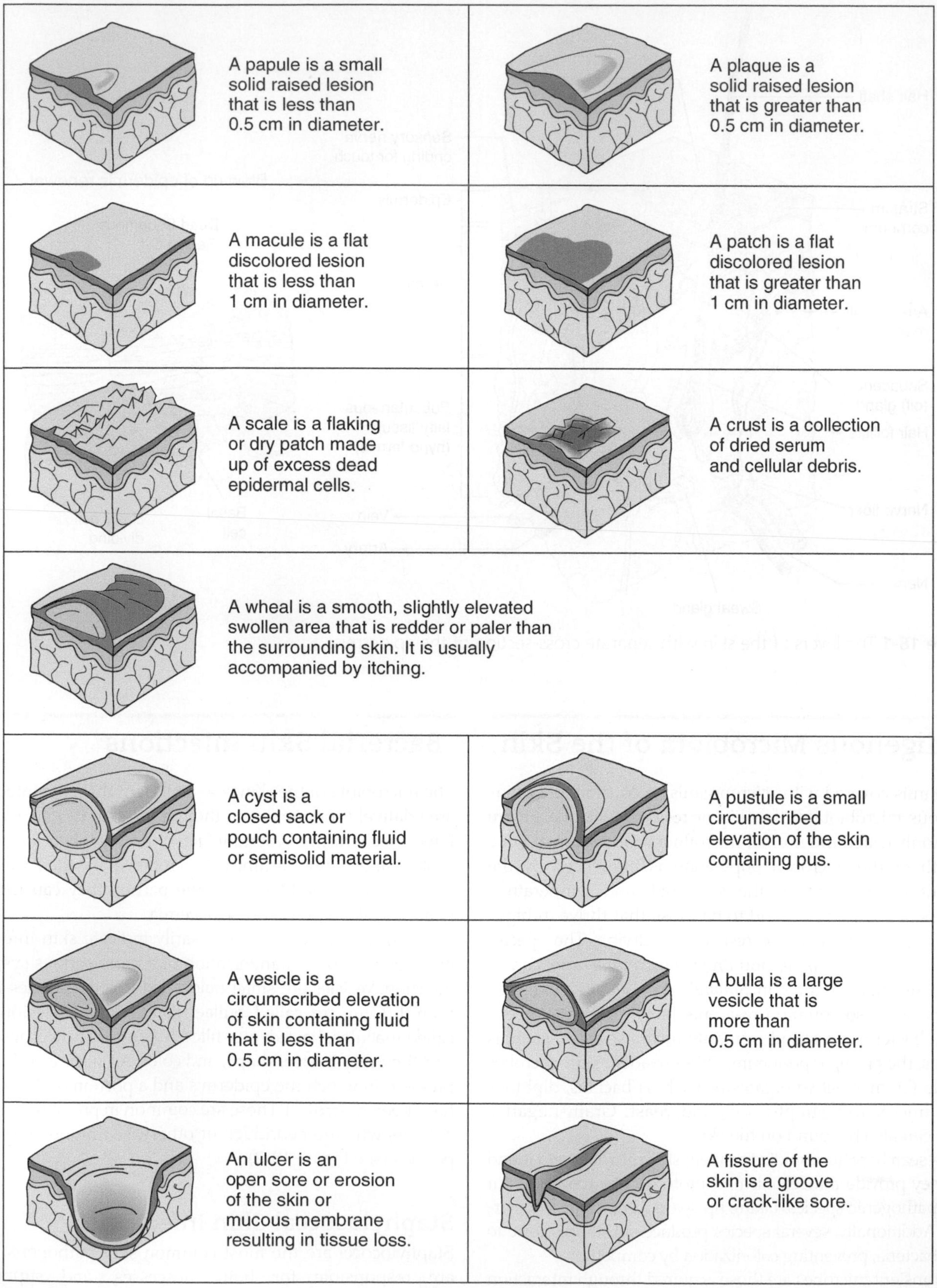

A papule is a small solid raised lesion that is less than 0.5 cm in diameter.

A plaque is a solid raised lesion that is greater than 0.5 cm in diameter.

A macule is a flat discolored lesion that is less than 1 cm in diameter.

A patch is a flat discolored lesion that is greater than 1 cm in diameter.

A scale is a flaking or dry patch made up of excess dead epidermal cells.

A crust is a collection of dried serum and cellular debris.

A wheal is a smooth, slightly elevated swollen area that is redder or paler than the surrounding skin. It is usually accompanied by itching.

A cyst is a closed sack or pouch containing fluid or semisolid material.

A pustule is a small circumscribed elevation of the skin containing pus.

A vesicle is a circumscribed elevation of skin containing fluid that is less than 0.5 cm in diameter.

A bulla is a large vesicle that is more than 0.5 cm in diameter.

An ulcer is an open sore or erosion of the skin or mucous membrane resulting in tissue loss.

A fissure of the skin is a groove or crack-like sore.

Figure 18-2 Examples of various skin lesions.

necrosis or cellulitis. Antibiotic-resistant strains are common because the microorganism is exposed to so many different antibiotics. Staphylococcal enterotoxin B can even cause infection on intact skin.

Staphylococcus aureus is present in large numbers in the nasal passages. The bacteria are aerosolized after a sneeze or spread to the hands of the host after touching the nose. *S. aureus* can attach to hair follicles, causing folliculitis, which often appears as a pimple. If it gets into the follicle of an eyelash, it causes a sty (sometimes spelled stye). A badly infected follicle can form into a furuncle, also known as a boil (see Figure 18-3). A furuncle is a large, raised lesion full of pus and surrounded by inflamed tissue. It is often treated by incision and drainage (I&D) of the pus and possibly additional debridement of the inflamed tissue. Furuncles, carbuncles, and boils can be severe and also be seen with other types of dermatologic infections such as cutaneous anthrax infection.

Staphylococcus aureus and *Streptococcus pyogenes* are the causative agents for impetigo, characterized by thin-walled vesicles on the skin that rupture and crust over. The bacteria can penetrate deep into the dermis, creating a crater-like ulcer called an **ecthyma**. The disease typically affects toddlers and school-aged children and is spread through skin-to-skin contact (see Figure 18-4).

Streptococcal Skin Infections

Streptococcus pyogenes (also known as group A β-hemolytic streptococci) is the causative agent for many diseases, including toxic shock syndrome, necrotizing fasciitis, and streptococcal pharyngitis. As mentioned previously, the microbe is one of the causative agents for the condition called impetigo. It also causes a serious dermal disease called **erysipelas** that manifests as red patches, typically on the skin of the face, but may appear on other skin surfaces. The disease is usually preceded by streptococcal pharyngitis (see Figure 18-5).

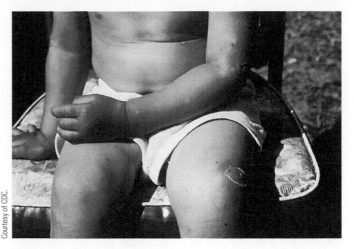

Figure 18-4 A child with macro-papular impetigo lesions.

As the streptococci colonies grow, they secrete toxins called hemolysins; species are characterized by the hemolysin that they produce (α hemolytic and β hemolytic). The β-hemolytic streptococci are virulent pathogens, producing toxins that lyse red blood cells (erythrocytes).

Streptococci that simply affect the skin are usually localized and easily treated, but those that make it into deeper tissues can cause serious destruction through the production of streptokinases, which are enzymes that dissolve blood clots. These bacteria also produce hyaluronidase, an enzyme that dissolves hyaluronic acid, the substance that cements connective tissue, and deoxyribonucleases, which degrade DNA.

Necrotizing fasciitis is a disease that results from invasion by group A streptococci (called flesh-eating bacteria). The enzymes produced by the bacteria destroy muscle and its fascial covering. One of the bacterium's toxins, called exotoxin A, triggers the immune system to attack the area by acting as an antigen, contributing to the localized damage.

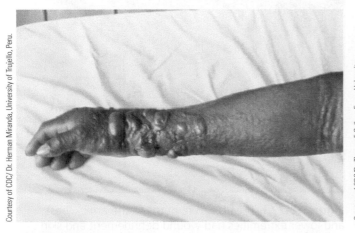

Figure 18-3 Right forearm and hand with a cluster of boils, or carbuncles from, in this case, a cutaneous anthrax infection, caused by *Bacillus anthracis*.

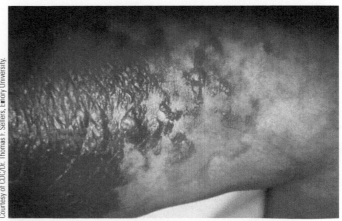

Figure 18-5 Lateral view of a right thigh with erythematous dermatologic condition (erysipelas) of the skin and subcutaneous tissue from a ß-hemolytic streptococci bacteria.

The disease is relatively rare; however, any case becomes highly publicized if picked up by the media. Refer to Chapter 12 for additional images and information regarding *Streptococcus* infections.

A rare skin condition often mistaken for necrotizing fasciitis is called pyoderma gangrenosum. The non-infectious and non-contagious, ulcerative cutaneous condition is an immunologic disorder commonly associated with systemic disease and frequently precipitated by trauma. The ulcerations of the skin may be mistaken for surgical site infection when they occur post-operatively. Subsequent debridement of the area may actually exacerbate the skin destruction if a definitive diagnosis is not made and appropriate non-surgical, immunosuppressive therapy is not initiated. To complicate the condition, the initially non-infected ulcerated areas may become colonized with opportunistic bacteria such as *Pseudomonas aeruginosa* (see Figure 18-6).

Pseudomonas Infections of the Skin

Pseudomonas aeruginosa is found in great numbers in hot tubs that have low chlorine levels. The Environmental Protection Agency (EPA) has set strict standards regarding public hot tubs/whirlpools. Prior to the standards, outbreaks of folliculitis were frequently reported. Folliculitis is an infection of the hair follicles resulting in a rash. The rash can be localized or widespread and can develop into severe ecthyma gangrenosum within 24 hours in individuals who are immunocompromised.

Dermatitis from *P. aeruginosa* has also been linked to vigorous scrubbing of skin, as with use of abrasive pumice stones or loofa sponges. Depilation (hair removal) by waxing, using hot or cold methods, may cause minor skin damage sufficient for bacterial entry into deeper skin layers.

Pseudomonas aeruginosa is an opportunistic species that causes infection in patients with severe burns, and it is nearly impossible to prevent patients with burns from being infected with *P. aeruginosa*. The goal is to keep the bacterial cell count as low as possible to prevent the patient from developing septicemia; however, *P. aeruginosa* is often the contributing factor to the mortality rate of severe burn victims. Topical creams have limited success in controlling the colonization of *P. aeruginosa*. Burn patients undergo frequent surgical **debridement** of necrotic skin in an effort to control the infection (see Figure 18-7).

The species grows easily in dilute disinfectants, and hospital personnel must take special precautions to prevent infections. More **pseudomonad** species are becoming antibiotic-resistant.

Acne Infections

Acne is a bacterial skin disease that is characterized by inflammatory pustules, cysts, and papules. The pathogens responsible for acne are *Propionibacterium acnes*, *Staphylococcus aureus*, and *Corynebacterium*. Most teenagers have some form of the disease, an indication that the disease can be triggered by fluctuating hormones during stages of puberty. Teens and young adults may suffer a severe form called cystic acne, which leaves scars on the face and upper body.

The disease is caused by blocked channels in the skin that are designed for the passage of sebum to the outside of the body. Sebum accumulates and forms whiteheads. As the top portion of the whitehead is exposed to air, it becomes a blackhead. *Propionibacterium acnes* metabolizes the sebum and forms free fatty acids that lead to inflammation. White blood cells and **interstitial fluid** accumulate and create cysts that rupture and cause scarring. Acne vulgaris is a severe form of acne caused by *P. acnes* (see Figure 18-8). Topical creams of varying strength and oral antibiotics are used to treat more serious acne infections.

Hansen's Disease

Hansen's disease, more commonly known as **leprosy**, was once a highly feared disease that dates back centuries, is mentioned in ancient literature, and discussed in Chapter 14.

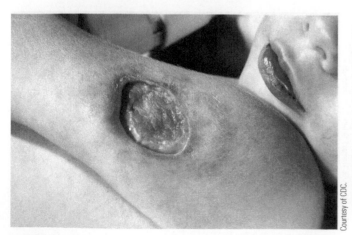

Courtesy of CDC.

Figure 18-6 Pyoderma gangrenosum ulceration of the left lateral upper arm with a positive finding of a *Pseudomonas* infection.

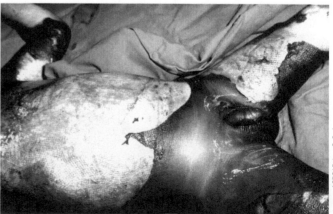

Courtesy of CDC/ Robert S. Craig.

Figure 18-7 Child with severe burns to the arms, chest, and lower extremities had wound debridement and skin grafts over some of the burned areas, however much more was required to remove remaining necrotic skin to reduce bacterial contamination.

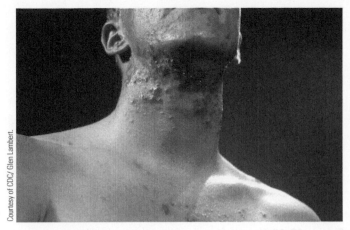

Figure 18-8 Dermatopathological condition known as acne vulgaris, or acne, with a cutaneous papular outbreak of inflamed papules over the neck, lower jaw, and upper chest.

Leprosy is caused by *Mycobacterium leprae*, an acid-fast, obligate intracellular bacillus. The pathogen may be found in macrophages, **Schwann cells**, muscle cells, and endothelial cells. There are two forms of the disease: the neural, tuberculoid form that results in **erythematous** skin macules and peripheral nerve lesions and the cutaneous, lepromatous form that results in progressive, disfiguring skin nodules, papules, and macules and occurs throughout the body (see Figure 18-9).

Cutaneous Anthrax

Bacillus anthracis, the bacterium that causes anthrax, takes four forms based on the route of transmission: cutaneous, inhalation, gastrointestinal, and injection. These are discussed in Chapter 13.

Cutaneous anthrax is the least dangerous and most common form of anthrax, although all forms are capable of becoming life-threatening systemic infections. It is transmitted by cuts or scrapes in the skin during contact with the hides, hair, or wool of infected animals. Small bumps or blisters in the skin appear anywhere from 1 day to 2 months

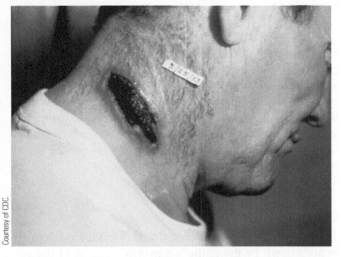

Figure 18-10 Cutaneous anthrax lesion on the neck.

after exposure. After the blisters fade, a lesion with a necrotic black center will remain and eventually slough and heal if proper treatment is given (see Figure 18-10). Without treatment, approximately 20 percent of cutaneous anthrax cases may be fatal.

Gas Gangrene

Also discussed in Chapter 13, gas gangrene (myonecrosis) is a serious infection of skin or surgical wounds. *Clostridium perfringens* is the most common cause; however, group A *Streptococcus, Staphylococcus aureus*, and *Vibrio vulnificus* are also possible pathogens. Persons with atherosclerosis, diabetes, or colon cancer are at greater risk for gas gangrene infections. The toxins released by *C. perfringens* produce painful swelling and subcutaneous **emphysema** (air under the skin), which creates **crepitus** when pressed (see Figure 18-11). The progression of the tissue necrosis is extremely rapid, so immediate IV antibiotics and surgical debridement or amputation of the extremity is crucial for survival. Subsequent hyperbaric oxygen therapy may be used to support wound healing.

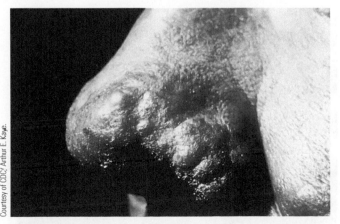

Figure 18-9 A patient's nose with reddish-brown nodular cutaneous changes, from lepromatous leprosy caused by bacterium *Mycobacterium leprae*.

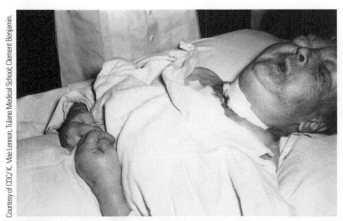

Figure 18-11 A patient after a traumatic fall down a flight of stairs resulting in a fractured rib and subsequent leakage of air into the subcutaneous tissues of the head and neck, known as crepitation, or subcutaneous emphysema.

Fungal Skin Infections

Many fungi are responsible for various skin infections. The cutaneous mycoses may invade skin, hair, and nails and grow as filaments (hyphae). Fungi are typical aerobes that affect only the outer, dead layer of skin and cannot grow into the deeper regions. They can, however, secrete toxic substances that diffuse into the dermal regions, which results in a reddened area. Additional information can be found regarding fungal microbes in Chapter 11.

Cutaneous Mycoses

The superficial fungal infection tinea is a cutaneous mycosis better known by the name "ringworm" because of the appearance of a red ring around a healing white scaly region. Scalp and hair infections are called tinea capitis. When hair is infected, the hyphae may invade the internal hair shaft and cause the hair to break off, causing the infected area to appear bald.

Superficial fungal infections in other parts of the body are given specific names as well: tinea pedis (athlete's foot) is a fungal infection of the foot; tinea cruris (jock itch) affects the groin; tinea corporis affects the body; and tinea barbae affects the beard area (see Figure 18-12). Tinea unguium affects the nails, which become yellow and start to deteriorate soon after infection. Nail fungal infections are almost always secondary to a primary fungal infection elsewhere in the body (see Figure 18-13).

Collectively, these superficial fungal infections are called dermatomycoses and are easily spread. Each scale of an infected area contains hyphae and spores, and these can grow readily if passed from one individual to another. Indirect transmission can occur in shower stalls or through personal toiletries. The pathogens responsible for the dermatomycoses are various species of *Microsporum*, *Epidermophyton*, and *Trichophyton*. Treatment is usually topical anti-fungal agents.

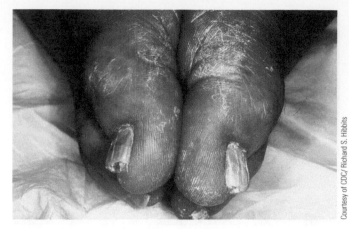

Courtesy of CDC/ Richard S. Hibbits

Figure 18-13 The great toes of a patient with dry, crusty tinea pedis lesions of the toes diagnosed specifically as tinea unguium.

Subcutaneous Mycoses

Subcutaneous fungal infections are more serious than the superficial cutaneous infections. Some fungi, usually soil-dwelling fungi, are able to penetrate the skin and enter deeper areas of the dermis. The most common form of subcutaneous fungal infection is called sporotrichosis, which is caused by *Sporothrix schenckii*. This disease often infects gardeners who do not wear gloves. The fungus enters an opening in the hand and gets into the lymphatic and circulatory system, where it can travel to different areas and cause lesions (see Figure 18-14).

Candidiasis is caused by *Candida albicans*, yeast-like organisms that are resident microflora in the mouth and gastrointestinal tract. Certain conditions, such as a patient who is immunocompromised, has diabetes, or is on steroid or antibiotic therapy, can cause the microorganism to proliferate and even change its growth form. Pregnant females and those who are immunocompromised are prone to *Candida* vaginitis. Images of *Candida* can be found in Chapter 11.

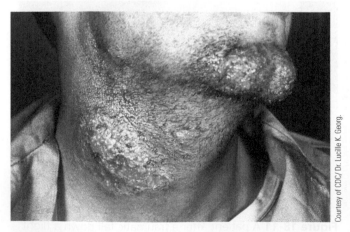

Courtesy of CDC/Dr. Lucille K. Georg.

Figure 18-12 Patient with a dermatophytic fungal infection in the bearded diagnosed as a case of tinea barbae, caused by the fungus, *Trichophyton mentagrophytes*.

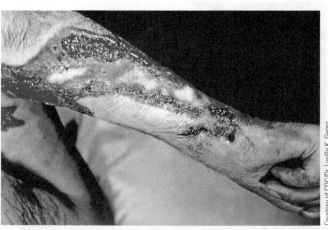

Courtesy of CDC/Dr. Lucille K. Georg.

Figure 18-14 Sporotrichosis of arm caused by the fungus *Sporothrix schenckii*.

Systemic Mycoses

Systemic fungal infections are the most serious forms of the mycoses. Those infected most commonly inhaled the spores that live as saprophytes in the soil. The spores can lodge in the lung and begin to grow. If the host's immune system does not destroy these invaders, then lesions can form that interfere with breathing. From the lung, the fungi can enter lymph and blood and spread to other areas of the body.

Viral Skin Infections

Viral diseases of the skin may be minor (warts) or major (smallpox), as outlined in Chapter 8. Warts are called **papillomas** and are caused by more than 50 types of papillomavirus. Often, warts are removed with liquid nitrogen or acids in a doctor's office. The term "pox" is Latin for "spotted" and a term used for any type of skin infection manifested by serious rash or pustule formation.

Chickenpox

Chickenpox is a respiratory infection caused by the varicella zoster virus (VZV), characterized by local vesicular lesions on the skin of the face, thorax, and neck. The **vesicles** fill with pus, rupture, and form scabs. Vesicles may form in the mucous membranes. The disease is usually mild and self-limiting, but encephalitis or pneumonia can occur in a few susceptible individuals (see Figure 18-15).

Shingles

Varicella zoster virus remains latent in the body for a lifetime after initial infection. It moves to the peripheral nerves and ends up in the dorsal root **ganglion** near the spine. It may be reactivated by stress or aging and move into superficial sensory nerves, resulting in a painful condition known as shingles (herpes zoster). Shingles is basically a different form of the disease chickenpox but is less severe because of the partial immunity that results from the initial infection. It exhibits lesions similar to chickenpox, but they tend to be more localized and typically occur on only one side of the body. Because the virus exists in the nerve ganglion and manifests in cutaneous nerves, it is a more painful condition than chickenpox. If the nerves are damaged, more serious complications can occur.

It usually begins as a tingling feeling in the torso or extremities of one side of the body and is followed by severe pain and rash of the trunk or extremities. The rash begins as a band or patch of raised dots on one side of the trunk, face, abdomen, arms, or legs. The rash typically occurs on only one side of the body, like a band or belt. The word shingles comes from a Latin word meaning belt or girdle, and zoster is Greek for "belt." The most common sites of shingles are on one side of the chest (front or back, like half of a belt) and on one side of the forehead and scalp. After a few days, the spots become blisters filled with fluid (see Figure 18-16).

Treatment goals for shingles are to reduce pain and discomfort, to hasten healing of blisters, and to prevent the

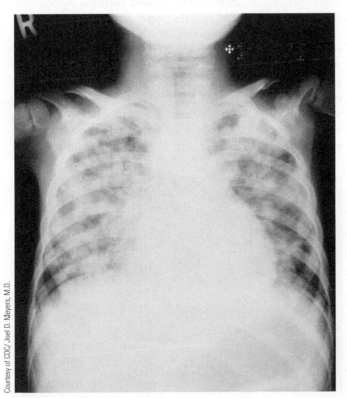

Courtesy of CDC/ Joel D. Meyers, M.D.

Figure 18-15 AP x-ray showing bilateral pulmonary infiltrates throughout the entirety of each lung field in a child with leukemia who contracted chickenpox pneumonia.

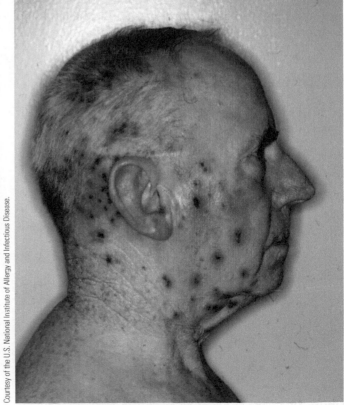

Courtesy of the U.S. National Institute of Allergy and Infectious Disease.

Figure 18-16 Varicella zoster virus rash of head and neck.

disease from spreading. Because a virus causes shingles, the main treatment is antiviral medication. Other drugs such as corticosteroids may be given to relieve the inflammation. Prescription pain relievers and low doses of antidepressant medication should be given to ease the pain. If the pain, also called post-herpetic neuralgia, is debilitating, then a nerve block may be performed.

Shingles can be prevented with a vaccine given prior to an outbreak. The CDC recommends that adults 50 years of age or older get the shingles vaccine called Shingrix, a recombinant zoster vaccine, in two injections separated by 2 to 6 months even if you have previously had a shingles outbreak, are not sure if you had chicken pox as a child, or if you had the previous Zostavax vaccine previously. The Shingrix vaccine provides greater than 90 percent protection initially and maintains approximately 85 percent protection for at least four years after vaccination according to the CDC.

Smallpox

Smallpox is a disease caused by the variola virus. There are two forms: variola major, with a 30 percent or higher mortality rate, and variola minor, with a mortality rate of less than 1 percent. Variola major has four types: ordinary, which is the most common form and accounts for 90 percent of smallpox infections; modified, which is a mild form seen in previously vaccinated individuals; flat; and hemorrhagic. Flat and hemorrhagic variola major are both very rare but are usually fatal.

Transmission is through respiratory aerosol and from the lungs. Variola virus can infect many internal organs before blood carries it to the skin. The lesions that form on the skin are the recognizable sign of the disease and are highly disfiguring (see Figure 18-17).

Smallpox is a serious disease that was eradicated from the world's population by an effective vaccine and the fact that the disease has no animal reservoir. The last case in the United States was in 1949. The last naturally occurring case of smallpox was in Somalia in 1977. The last known death from smallpox which occurred in 1978, was an English woman who worked as a photographer for Birmingham University Medical School. She worked above the university's Medical Microbiology research lab where smallpox was being studied by staff and students. It took 9 days for clinicians to diagnose her with smallpox and she died within a month of showing symptoms, starting with a rash.

The CDC in the United States maintains laboratory samples of the virus for clinical study and it is believed that there may also be samples maintained in other countries such as Russia. Smallpox has the potential for use as a biological weapon and research stockpiles are closely guarded and protected. The CDC states that, currently, there are adequate supplies of the smallpox vaccine for every person in the United States in case of a bioterrorism incident.

Smallpox Vaccination

Routine smallpox vaccinations of the public were discontinued due to the determination of eradication of the disease and cases of severe side effect reactions from the vaccine. The live vaccinia virus is used instead of smallpox for the vaccine and produces a vigorous immune response; however, there is no possibility of actual smallpox infection. Unlike other vaccines, a hypodermic needle is not used. Instead, a **bifurcated** needle is dipped into the live vaccinia vaccine and the upper arm of the recipient is then pricked multiple times (see Figure 18-18). A powered special vaccine injector apparatus that has multiple circular rows of small needles has also been used in extensive smallpox eradication campaigns (see Figure 18-19). The normal reaction is development of a pustule that fills, drains, scabs over, and then sloughs off over a 3-week period. Care must be taken during the period when the lesion contains or drains pus, because the live virus can be spread to other parts of the body or to others.

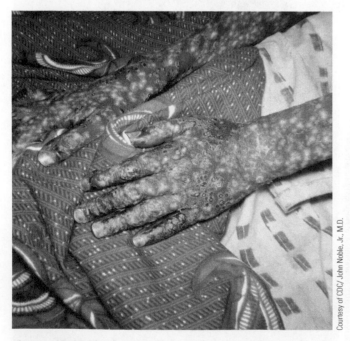

Courtesy of CDC/ John Noble, Jr., M.D.

Figure 18-17 The hands of an adult with smallpox showing the characteristic maculopapular rash due to the smallpox variola virus.

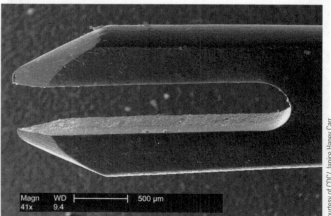

Magn	WD		500 µm
41x	9.4		

Courtesy of CDC/ Janice Haney Carr.

Figure 18-18 SEM image of the roughened tip of a bifurcated smallpox vaccination needle used to abrade the skin at the vaccination site to introduce the vaccinia virus into the tissues.

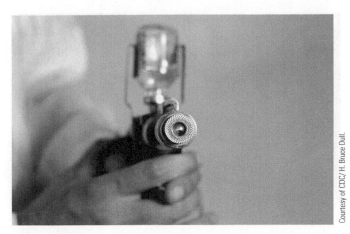

Courtesy of CDC/ H. Bruce Dull.

Figure 18-19 A hand-held vaccine jet-injector invented by Aaron Ismach in 1960 and used throughout the world during mass smallpox eradication campaigns.

Progressive vaccinia, also called vaccinia necrosum, is an ongoing infection of skin with tissue destruction caused by vaccination in persons with inadequate immune responses. The statistically rare post-vaccination infection progresses rapidly and is frequently fatal. A small number (14–52) out of 1 million persons vaccinated in the past suffered devastating reactions (see Figure 18-20).

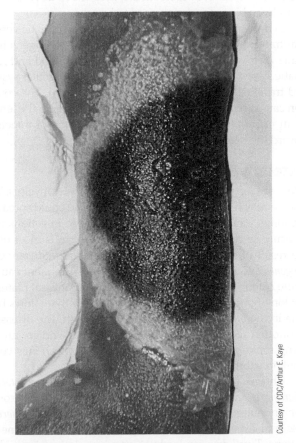

Courtesy of CDC/Arthur E. Kaye

Figure 18-20 Vaccinia necrosum reaction following smallpox vaccination in a 70-year-old woman from Wales who had pre-existing chronic lymphocytic leukemia is shown. The reaction was progressive and eventually fatal.

Vector-Borne Skin Infections

Parasitic and viral infections of the integumentary system are commonly caused by bites of insect vectors. Ticks, mosquitoes, lice, mites, fleas, spiders, and flies are usually unaffected by the parasitic pathogens they carry and transmit to humans. The skin at the site of the bite may shows signs of tissue damage and inflammatory reaction or may appear normal, depending on the extent of the infectious process. Some infections will enter the bloodstream and become systemic, whereas others may stay localized in the immediate area of the bite. Species belonging to the family *Rickettsiaceae* are responsible for diseases such as typhus, scrub typhus, Q-fever, and Rocky Mountain spotted fever. These microbes and diseases are discussed in Chapter 10.

Infections of Internal Tissues

Internal tissues, such as the breast, fascia, tendon **sheaths**, bone, joints, and lymph nodes, are susceptible to infection by many of the same pathogens as the various body systems. Infections involving the skin may extend beyond the localized area and penetrate into the internal tissues, normally free from bacteria.

Breast Tissue Infections

Infections of the breast, referred to as mastitis, may be either generalized or localized and are typically associated with breastfeeding or pregnancy. Although breast infections are relatively uncommon, they occur more frequently in females who are lactating. In fact, breast infections can be classified as those that occur in females who are either lactating or not. Infections in pregnant or lactating females produce a generalized pain that affects the entire breast.

Localized breast infection of a female who is not lactating is associated with cellulitis (a diffuse inflammation of the solid tissues, usually the loose tissues beneath the skin), folliculitis, or other skin infections.

Lactational Mastitis

Lactational mastitis occurs when a female is breastfeeding and her nipples become cracked. Bacteria from the nursing infant's mouth enter through the cracks in the nipple and make way into the milk ducts. The milk supplies nutrients that allow the bacteria to multiply rapidly and can eventually block the duct. The breast becomes firm, reddened, swollen, and painful. Warm compresses, massage, and antibiotics are suggested to unblock the duct and relieve the infection. If the infection becomes severe, then it may form an abscess that requires surgical incision and drainage.

Staphylococcus aureus from the infant's mouth and nasal passages is the most common pathogen. Other bacteria from the mouth and nares of the infant may also cause infection. The newborn may become inoculated by nursery personnel who transfer the bacteria to the infant from their hands. After handling an infant that is colonized with bacteria, the healthcare worker may handle other infants, cross-contaminating them. If healthcare workers are carriers of antibiotic-resistant bacteria such as methicillin-resistant *Staphylococcus aureus* (MRSA) and transfer the bacteria to the newborn, infection could affect both the mother who is nursing and her infant.

Chronic subareolar abscess occurs when sebaceous glands around the nipple become infected. Pus and tissue fluids accumulate during the inflammatory response and the area becomes painful, red, and **edematous**.

Non-Lactational Mastitis

Non-lactational mastitis is similar to lactational mastitis; however, it is usually localized and may occur subsequent to a primary infection from the skin or cellulitis. Females who have had lumpectomy (surgical removal of a lump in the breast) or partial **mastectomy**, followed by radiation therapy, may develop this form of mastitis. Females with diabetes or whose immune systems are compromised may also be at risk for mastitis infection.

Fasciitis and Tendonitis

An infection of the fascia, the sheet of fibrous connective tissue that lines muscles, is called fasciitis. Infections may occur because of penetration of the epidermis that extends into the dermis and allows opportunistic pathogens to infiltrate the deeper fascial layers. Necrotizing fasciitis, discussed in Chapter 12, is a fulminating group A streptococcal infection that begins as extensive cellulitis and spreads to the superficial and deep fascial layers.

Bacterial tendonitis is uncommon and involves the tendon sheath. It should not be confused with tendonitis that is an inflammatory process following repetitive movement and strain. Tendon sheaths consist of a visceral layer that encloses tendons. These tube-shaped structures are lined with a synovial membrane that secretes lubricating synovial fluid. Infection of the tendon sheath, or **tenosynovitis**, is usually the result of direct inoculation of bacteria from a traumatic wound that breaks the skin. Infection usually spreads along the course of the sheath. Increased pressure within the sheath may impair oxygen and nutrient flow, resulting in necrosis. Symptoms are pain on extension, tenderness along the course of the tendon, and edema of the affected area. Lymphadenopathy (lymph node swelling) and fever may be present in some individuals.

Lymphadenitis

Lymphadenitis is the inflammation and possible visible and palpable enlargement of a lymph node and is the result of benign, localized, or generalized infections. Enlargement may affect a single node or a localized group of nodes. Generalized lymph node enlargement is common in infectious mononucleosis, cytomegalovirus infection, brucellosis, secondary syphilis, and disseminated histoplasmosis. Regional lymph node enlargement is prominent in streptococcal infection, tuberculosis, primary syphilis, plague, chancroid, and genital herpes simplex (see Figure 18-21).

Lymphadenitis may be acute, subacute, or chronic. Node enlargement is due to a proliferation of cells intrinsic to the node, such as lymphocytes, plasma cells, monocytes, or histiocytes. It can also result from infiltration of cells external to

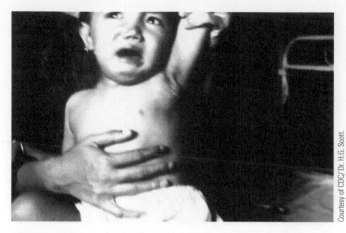

Figure 18-21 A child infected with the plague bacterium, *Yersinia pestis* from an infected flea vector and showing the left axilla with swelling from an inflamed lymph node, also known as an axillary bubo.

Courtesy of CDC/ Dr. H.G. Scott.

the node such as malignant cells or neutrophils. Viruses, bacteria, protozoa, rickettsiae, or fungi can cause lymphadenitis. In some infections, the overlying skin becomes inflamed, as seen in cellulitis. Abscess formation may lead to draining sinuses from the nodes.

Treatment depends on the underlying condition, with resolution of the disease leading to reduced lymph node size. If the inflammation does not abate, then the nodes may need to undergo biopsy and may need to be removed.

Lymphangitis, an inflammation of the lymphatic vessels that transport lymph fluid, is a sign that the pathogens have made their way through the defenses of the blood and lymphatic systems and are circulating within the vascular system and traveling throughout the body (septicemia). The condition causes red streaks just under the skin, running the length of an extremity away from the original source of infection, toward the heart.

Osteomyelitis

Infections of the bone are referred to as osteomyelitis. The disease may result in destruction of bone and could spread to the joints, causing stiffening and pain. These infections may be acute or chronic in nature. The acute form is most often the result of invasion by *Staphylococcus aureus*. *Streptococcus pyogenes* and *Haemophilus influenzae* are less frequent causes. Acute osteomyelitis primarily affects the epiphyseal plates of the long bones due to decreased blood flow that allows bacteria in the bloodstream to settle and flourish. The disease is most often seen in children and adolescents who are undergoing rapid growth. Osteomyelitis in growing bones could result in shortening of the extremity.

Chronic osteomyelitis is usually caused by *Mycobacterium tuberculosis* and is often a secondary infection arising from a primary pulmonary infection. *Salmonella, Pseudomonas aeruginosa*, and *Treponema pallidum* may also cause chronic bone infections. *T. pallidum* can lead to severe bone lesions in children with congenital syphilis (see Figure 18-22). Chronic osteomyelitis is most likely to affect the vertebrae, although bones of the hands, feet, hips, and knees may also be affected.

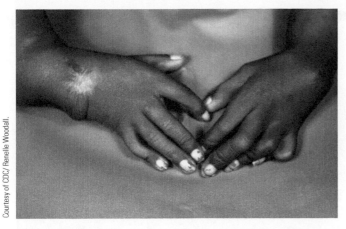

Courtesy of CDC/ Renelle Woodall.

Figure 18-22 Congenital syphilitic bone disease of the hands including osteoperiostitis, ulnar deviation of the middle fingers, and shortening of the little finger (Du Bois sign) from placental transfer of the spirochete *Treponema pallidum*.

Arthritis

Arthritis is an inflammatory disease of the joints, causing pain, edema, and restricted motion. The two main forms are osteoarthritis and rheumatoid arthritis. Rheumatoid arthritis is a chronic systemic disease with inflammatory changes occurring throughout the body's connective tissues. It is regarded as an **autoimmune disease** in which the body produces antibodies against its own cells and tissues (see Figure 18-23).

Septic arthritis is a result of bacterial invasion of the joint from the bloodstream (bacteremia) or from direct inoculation of the joint from penetrating trauma (see Figure 18-24). Once again, *S. aureus* is the most common pathogen, although *H. influenzae* and *Salmonella* may cause septic arthritis in children. These pathogens usually only affect a single joint, but rare infections caused by *N. gonorrhoeae* can affect many joints in a condition known as polyarthritis. Hip or knee joints may be infected by *M. tuberculosis*.

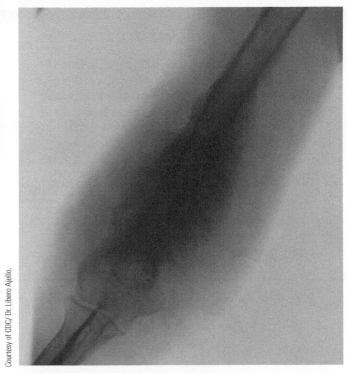

Courtesy of CDC/ Dr. Libero Ajello.

Figure 18-24 A-P x-ray of a right distal humerus showing the markedly swollen soft tissue silhouette around the bony infection of actinomycotic mycetoma caused by the Gram-positive *Nocardia asteroides*.

MICRO NOTES

"You're Such a Flake"

Humans shed 500 million skin cells each day at the rate of 0.001 to 0.003 ounces of skin flakes every hour. Every 2 to 4 weeks, our entire superficial epidermal layer is replaced with new cells. These cells sloughed off by normal movement and friction are a substantial component in "house dust." They also contribute to contamination of the operating room environment and are the reason for the recommendation that non-scrubbed team members wear long-sleeved cover jackets while in the OR.

A study published in the American Chemical Society's journal, *Environmental Science & Technology*, explained that human skin flakes contain oils partly comprising cholesterol and squalene, a compound produced by the liver. Previous research by the researchers suggested that squalene from airline passengers' skin had a role in reducing levels of ozone, a component of indoor, or in this case in-cabin air pollution. They wrote, "More than half of the ozone removal measured in a simulated aircraft cabin was found to be a consequence of ozone reacting with exposed, skin, hair, and clothing of passengers." Next time you are scrubbing the oil off of your face, consider that maybe it is there for a reason and may not be such a bad thing to "shine" a little after all.

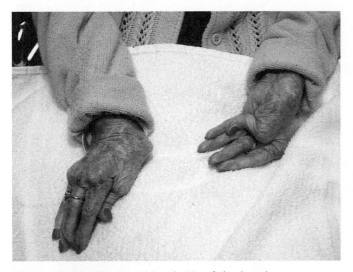

Figure 18-23 Rheumatoid arthritis of the hands.

Under the Microscope

Patients coming to surgery may present with a wide range of skin conditions including diseases, infections, or traumatic burns or penetrating injuries that may prevent them from having non-emergent procedures until these conditions have been addressed or be at risk of having serious post-operative complications, including surgical site or systemic infections.

1. How does loss or violation of intact skin contribute to risk of systemic infection?

2. Which types of skin and soft tissue diseases, infections, or burns require surgical debridement to remove devitalized tissue?

3. Which pathogens are most often associated with serious skin and internal soft tissue infections?

4. How do infections in the skin and internal soft tissues become systemic infections?

5. What benefits do the normal or indigenous microbes present in the layers of the skin provide?

CHAPTER 19

Diseases of the Gastrointestinal and Genitourinary Systems

Learning Objectives

After completing the study of this chapter, you will be able to:

1. Define key terms.
2. Describe the general classifications of gastrointestinal and genitourinary tract diseases.
3. Identify the pathogens associated with infections of the gastrointestinal system.
4. Identify the pathogens associated with infections of the genitourinary system.
5. Discuss the consequences of untreated sexually transmitted diseases.
6. Apply critical thinking skills in relating chapter material to the surgical environment of care or broader global community.

Key Terms

Adenocarcinoma	Ectopic pregnancy	Hematuria	Periodontium
Amines	Endometriosis	Hemodialysis	Polymorphonuclear
Atrophic	Enteroaggregative	Hemolytic anemia	Postpartum
Crohn's disease	Enterohemorrhagic	Infectivity dose	Pyelonephritis
Cystogram	Enteroinvasive	Intubation	Synergism
Dental caries	Enteropathogenic	Metaplasia	Vaginosis
Diverticulitis	Enterotoxigenic	Nephropathogenic	Verotoxin
Dysplasia	Erythema nodosum	Neutralizes	
Dysuria	Flaccid paralysis	Periodontitis	

The Big Picture

One of the ways educators tackle the daunting task of teaching about the human body and diseases that may affect it is to divide it into separate and distinct systems. This is appropriate for exploration of similar functions performed by these systems. However, the complex physiological interactions and anatomical structural design of our human bodies combine to create one organism in which every system is affected by changes, diseases, or infections in another system. During your examination of the topics in this chapter, consider the following:

1. How do microbes that normally reside in our gastrointestinal or genitourinary systems protect us from other transient microbes?

2. In what ways are humans often ultimately responsible for many GI and GU diseases or infections due to the choices they make in everyday life?

3. Which diseases or infections tend to run their course without the need for medical treatment?

4. Why do some types of infections often go undiagnosed or untreated for extended periods with potentially devastating results?

Clinical Significance Topic

An open total abdominal hysterectomy (TAH) is performed through an incision in the lower abdomen and pelvis to remove the entire uterus. To remove the uterus, the gynecologist dissects the cervix, which creates an opening of the pelvic floor into the vagina. The peritoneal cavity is considered sterile as a closed space with no natural connection to the external environment. The vagina, a natural body orifice open to the outside, is considered relatively contaminated in comparison. After the surgeon has removed the uterus with the cervix attached to it, the surgical technologist should recognize that the instruments used for traction during closure of the pelvic floor structures are contaminated and should be isolated appropriately. Despite the fact that the vagina was prepped with an antimicrobial agent preoperatively, the resident microbiota remains. The instruments exposed to the vaginal vault can cause cross-contamination of the tissues of the abdominal cavity by manipulation of tissues and instrument placement. The principle of isolating contaminated instruments to reduce the potential for surgical site infection (SSI) is similar to bowel technique discussed in Chapter 16.

The Gastrointestinal System

The body system probably most commonly associated with bacteria is the gastrointestinal system, also known as the GI tract or alimentary canal. The GI system is a continuous pathway beginning with the mouth and ending with the rectum and anus. Most structures within it are teeming with resident bacteria as part of the normal microbiome and many transient microbes that pass through the system in ingested food and fluids. These transient microbes are potential pathogens but are kept in check by the resident microflora of the intestinal tract. Microbial populations are also controlled by enzymes secreted in the mouth and subsequently by strong acids and the low pH level of the stomach and duodenum (see Figure 19-1).

The population of resident bacteria is mediated as many of them are flushed out along with the transient microbes. Various ingested substances, such as alcohol and simple sugars, affect the normal microbiota. Alcohol can kill resident microbes and sugars feed even unfavorable bacteria, upsetting the natural balance. Antibiotics designed to kill the pathogenic bacteria may also destroy the resident microbial inhabitants of the GI tract.

Most of the intestinal flora are obligate anaerobes, chiefly *Bacteroides* and *Fusobacterium* species. Facultative anaerobes are less abundant but are easier to isolate and cultivate. These include *Escherichia*, *Enterobacter*, *Proteus*, and *Klebsiella* species.

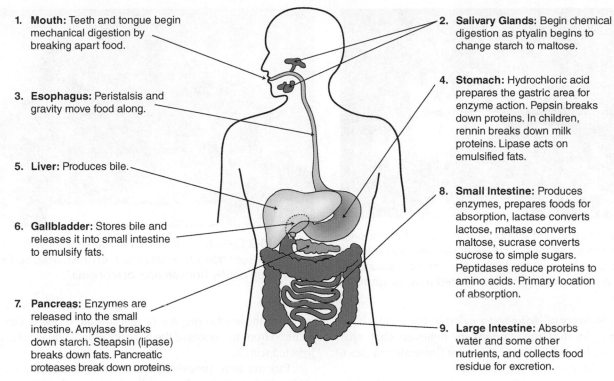

1. **Mouth:** Teeth and tongue begin mechanical digestion by breaking apart food.

2. **Salivary Glands:** Begin chemical digestion as ptyalin begins to change starch to maltose.

3. **Esophagus:** Peristalsis and gravity move food along.

4. **Stomach:** Hydrochloric acid prepares the gastric area for enzyme action. Pepsin breaks down proteins. In children, rennin breaks down milk proteins. Lipase acts on emulsified fats.

5. **Liver:** Produces bile.

6. **Gallbladder:** Stores bile and releases it into small intestine to emulsify fats.

7. **Pancreas:** Enzymes are released into the small intestine. Amylase breaks down starch. Steapsin (lipase) breaks down fats. Pancreatic proteases break down proteins.

8. **Small Intestine:** Produces enzymes, prepares foods for absorption, lactase converts lactose, maltase converts maltose, sucrase converts sucrose to simple sugars. Peptidases reduce proteins to amino acids. Primary location of absorption.

9. **Large Intestine:** Absorbs water and some other nutrients, and collects food residue for excretion.

Figure 19-1 An overview of the process of digestion.

Diseases of the Gastrointestinal System

All of the bacteria in the GI tract have the potential to become pathogenic if they escape their normal environment or if they over-multiply within it. Microorganisms survive by attaching to the many folds of the intestinal epithelium where they multiply. The large intestine contains the majority of the bacterial population, due in part to the slower rate of peristalsis than that of the small intestine. Chapter 16 examines Gram-negative bacilli and coccobacilli bacteria, including the *Enterobacteriaceae* family, which contains many of the microbes associated with gastrointestinal infections. The following sections discuss a few of the more common diseases, infections, and pathogens of the GI system.

Oral Disease

Teeth encounter large amounts of bacteria that proliferate on their surface (dental plaque) and cause decay (**dental caries**). Oral bacteria convert sugars into lactic acid, which erodes tooth enamel. Although there are hundreds of bacterial species in the mouth, the bacterium that causes the most damage to teeth is *Streptococcus mutans*, a Gram-positive coccus capable of creating stubborn polymicrobial biofilms that adhere to crevices in the enamel surfaces of teeth and are protected from the shearing action of chewing.

Infection of the gums (gingivitis) is characterized by bleeding and soreness of the gums. An assortment of streptococci, actinomycetes, and anaerobic Gram-negative bacteria causes these infections. Untreated gingivitis progresses to a chronic condition called **periodontitis** (see Figure 19-2). Pus pockets form around the teeth, destroying bone and tissues that anchor the teeth. This condition is caused primarily by *Porphyromonas gingivalis*.

Fusobacterium Infections

Fusobacterium and spirochetes such as *Treponema* work synergistically to cause acute necrotizing ulcerative gingivitis (ANUG), commonly called "trench mouth," a serious infection of the mouth that causes bleeding, pain, and difficulty with chewing. Other names include Vincent's angina or Vincent's infection. It is a non-contagious periodontal disease that affects the **periodontium**, causing ulceration and necrosis of the gum tissue and resulting in crater-like defects. Those individuals who are infected usually have fever, bone destruction, tissue destruction, and a foul odor due to tissue necrosis. The tissue necrosis results from the production of lactic acid and endotoxin production secondary to poor oral hygiene and influenced by overcrowded living conditions where there is frequently malnutrition of the population.

Gastric Ulcer Disease

The inside of the stomach was believed to be a sterile environment due to the gastric acid and low pH level until

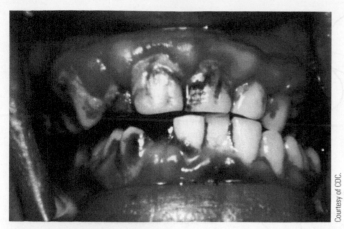

Courtesy of CDC.

Figure 19-2 Incisors and surrounding gingivae show the presence of advanced periodontal disease manifested as calcified plaque build-up between the teeth, affecting the surrounding gums in an inflammatory process referred to as gingivitis.

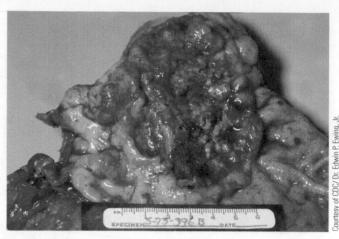

Courtesy of CDC/Dr. Edwin P. Ewing, Jr.

Figure 19-3 Gross section of interior mucosal lining of the stomach tissue showing an ulcerated, erythematous surface and a rolled border from an adenocarcinoma.

the 1982 discovery of *Helicobacter pylori* in the stomach and duodenum. At that time, scientists believed that spicy foods, hectic lifestyles, and stress were the major causes of gastric and duodenal or peptic ulcers.

It is now understood that urease produced by *H. pylori* bacteria **neutralizes** gastric acidity, converting the gastric urea to ammonium ions. The flagella that provide motility help the bacterium pass from the acidic gastric lumen into the mucus of the stomach. The other important defense of *H. pylori* is that the body's immune system cannot attack or destroy the bacterium within the mucous lining. In fact, the body's defenses contribute to the development of a peptic ulcer. Leukocytes, killer T-cells, and other immune system components respond to the infection. These cells are unable to penetrate the internal lining of the stomach; however, they do not disappear. The body continues to provide nutrients to the leukocytes, which the *H. pylori* cells also use to survive. In many cases, persons infected with *H. pylori* are asymptomatic; however, the infected individual can develop gastritis that can lead to development of a peptic ulcer. So, it may not be the *H. pylori* that are directly responsible for a peptic ulcer, but rather the inflammation (gastritis) of the stomach lining in response to the invasion by *H. pylori*.

Steps in the slow progression of *H. pylori* infection include:

- Chronic gastritis
- **Atrophic** gastritis
- Intestinal **metaplasia** that may evolve into **dysplasia**
- Gastric **adenocarcinoma**

Infection with *H. pylori* does not guarantee development of gastric cancers. Multiple factors must align to produce adenocarcinoma, only one of which may be *H. pylori* (see Figure 19-3).

Helicobacter pylori is transmitted by the oral–oral or fecal–oral routes. Fecal matter can be ingested from contaminated water or food or transmitted from the surfaces of unwashed

hands of those who prepare or ingest food. *H. pylori* can be cultured from the stools of the majority of individuals who are infected with it.

Patients were previously treated with H2 blockers and acid-reducing agents. The medications would relieve ulcer symptoms, heal gastritis, or even heal the ulcer itself, but they did not treat the bacterial infection. After acid-suppressing drug therapy was discontinued, the majority of patients would experience a recurrence of the ulcer. Currently, treatment with antibiotics effective against *H. pylori* aids in the removal of the infection and significantly reduces the recurrence rate.

Campylobacter Diseases

Campylobacteriosis is the GI disease caused by *Campylobacter* bacteria. *Campylobacter jejuni* is the primary cause of diarrheal disease in humans and a leading cause of gastroenteritis worldwide. Campylobacteriosis is a zoonotic disease transmitted to humans by animals or animal products. The main route of transmission is the ingestion of raw or undercooked meats, unpasteurized milk, or contaminated water. Rarely is the disease fatal, except in infants, older adults, or persons who are immunocompromised. The disease occurs more frequently in the summer months than in the winter. In an outbreak investigation by the CDC, between January 2019 and March 2021, 56 people infected with a strain of *Campylobacter jejuni* were reported from 17 states, 9 of whom were hospitalized, but with no reported deaths. The laboratory and epidemiologic evidence gathered showed that the most likely source was the handling of mainly pet-store puppies.

The unique shapes of the bacterial cells and flagella are useful in laboratory Gram stain identification and diagnosis. Treatment of campylobacteriosis is usually not indicated and the infection is self-limiting; however, those infected are at risk for dehydration. The only effective method of eliminating *Campylobacter* from contaminated foods is through proper cooking or pasteurization.

Clostridioides difficile

The Centers for Disease Control and Prevention (CDC) placed *Clostridioides difficile* (formerly called *Clostridium difficile*) at the top of their Antibiotic/Antimicrobial Resistance Urgent Threat list in 2019. The other five bacteria listed under the heading of "urgent" are Carbapenem-resistant *Enterobacteriaceae* (CRE), Carbapenem-resistant *Acinetobacter, Candida auris,* and drug-resistant *Neisseria gonorrhoeae.* Unlike the other pathogenic bacteria discussed in this chapter, *C. difficile* is considered one of the most common healthcare-associated infections (HAI) seen mainly in individuals who have had antibiotic therapy for other infections or those who have been treated in healthcare settings. Community-acquired *C. difficile* infections have developed as well. There were an estimated 224,000 infections in 2017, resulting in 12,800 deaths and $1 billion in excess medical costs from *C. difficile* infections in the United States. *C. difficile* is discussed further in Chapter 13.

Escherichia coli Infections

Escherichia coli bacteria are often identified as the agent of urinary tract infections, sepsis, diarrheal disease, and neonatal meningitis. Individuals who are immunocompromised or those who already have a debilitating condition are at a higher risk for infection as compared to healthy persons. There are five types of pathogenic strains: **enteropathogenic, enterotoxigenic, enterohemorrhagic, enteroaggregative,** and **enteroinvasive.** The types of *E. coli* that cause diarrhea are classified according to their virulence factors that are responsible for the different methods of causing disease.

E. coli Diarrheal Disease

Infants may become infected with enteropathogenic *E. coli* (EPEC). It is the least understood strain of the five. It is often the pathogen responsible for diarrheal disease outbreaks in nurseries. During the course of the infection, the microvilli that line the intestinal tract are destroyed. The disease usually resolves in 5 to 15 days, but the infant can have a relapse. Chromosomal genes code for adherence factors that allow the *E. coli* cells to adhere to the mucosal cells of the small bowel. Infants can quickly become dehydrated, so fluids must be constantly administered, typically intravenously.

The commonly known diarrhea caused by enterotoxigenic *E. coli* (ETEC) is referred to as "traveler's diarrhea." The bacterial cells adhere to the epithelial cells of the small bowel. Many of the organisms produce one or two exotoxins whose expression is under the control of genes found in the plasmids. The exotoxins are responsible for producing the diarrheal symptoms. In severe cases, antibiotic therapy may be initiated as well as administering fluids to maintain hydration and electrolyte balance. Individuals who live in countries where ETEC is prevalent will often have protective antibodies against the toxins.

A severe form of bloody diarrhea known as hemorrhagic colitis is caused by enterohemorrhagic *E. coli* (EHEC),

listed in biological reference manuals as *E. coli* O157:H7. The combination of numbers and letters refers to the markers that are found on the cell surface and distinguish it from other types of *E. coli.* The "O" antigen is located on the outer cell membrane, and the "H" is part of the flagellum.

Enterohemorrhagic *E. coli* cause disease by making a toxin called Shiga toxin and are also called Shiga toxin–producing *E. coli,* or STEC. These EHEC/STEC bacteria are also sometimes called verocytotoxic *E. coli* or VTEC. The Shiga toxin is divided into two forms, Shiga toxin 1 and Shiga toxin 2, which tends to be more virulent due to the ability of the bacteria to adhere to tissues. Some *E. coli* strains can have both toxins present simultaneously. These toxins are responsible for hemorrhagic colitis. **Verotoxin** destroys the endothelial cells that line the inner layer of blood vessels. The genitourinary tract is invaded when the verotoxin is absorbed systemically. Both toxins are identical to the toxin produced by *Shigella dysenteriae.* The CDC currently uses the designation of STEC for the strains of *E. coli* that produce Shiga toxins with the individual letter and numeric identifiers as in STEC O157 rather than EHEC. They estimate from public health network reporting that tracks outbreaks that 265,000 STEC infections occur annually in the United States with 3,600 cases requiring hospitalization, 30 fatalities, and that STEC O157 is responsible for approximately one-third of them.

The strain of Shiga toxin–producing *E. coli* O104:H4 that caused a large outbreak in Europe in 2011 was frequently referred to as EHEC. The most commonly identified STEC in North America is *E. coli* O157:H7.

Serogroups of *E. coli* that are classified as non-O157 STEC include STEC O145, O26, O111, and O103; however, most clinical laboratories have limited ability to definitively identify these variations that frequently cause severe manifestations of STEC disease, including bloody diarrhea and hemolytic uremic syndrome (HUS).

HUS involves thrombocytopenia (low blood platelet count), acute renal failure, and **hemolytic anemia.** Those infected will most likely require **hemodialysis** and blood transfusions. Once HUS symptoms appear, antibiotic therapy is ineffective and the disease must be allowed to run its course while supportive therapy is provided until the patient recovers. Five to 10 percent of individuals infected with STEC O157 develop HUS, and most of the patients are children 5 years of age or younger or adults over age 65. Survivors of HUS often have chronic genitourinary complications due to kidney and urinary tract damage.

Various *E. coli* strains, including STEC, are found in the intestines of healthy cattle. During the slaughter and processing of meat, the microbes can be mixed into the beef where the pathogen is acquired by ingesting raw or undercooked ground beef, unpasteurized raw milk or apple cider, soft cheeses made from raw milk, and other raw foods. Meat contaminated with *E. coli* looks and smells normal. It is thought that only a small number of cells needs be ingested to cause infection.

Other methods of becoming infected with STEC include:

- Swimming in or drinking sewage-contaminated water (see Figure 19-4)

- Person-to-person contact among families and in child daycare centers. The bacteria in stools can be passed if proper hygiene habits are not practiced.

In 2014, there were two major food recalls due to STEC contamination. One involved ground beef and the other included raw clover sprouts. A number of infected individuals were hospitalized, but there were no deaths reported.

Enteroaggregative *E. coli* (EAEC) has become a recognized cause of diarrhea in children in developing and industrialized countries. EAEC has been particularly associated with persistent diarrhea (more than 14 days duration), which is a major cause of illness and death. Both sporadic diarrhea and outbreaks (possibly food-borne) have been described. Not all strains of EAEC are equally pathogenic and the mechanisms of pathogenesis and virulence are being studied.

The last type of diarrheal *E. coli* discussed is enteroinvasive *E. coli* (EIEC). This strain causes a type of dysentery similar to shigellosis, but the strain is not as virulent. EIEC invades the epithelial cells that line the intestinal mucosa and produces a mild infection. Children are most susceptible to developing these infections, although it is also common among travelers.

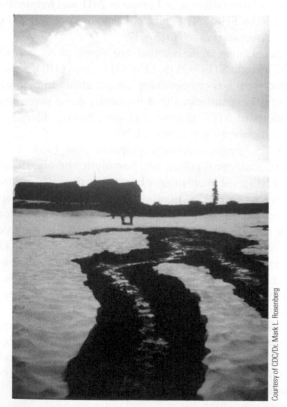

Figure 19-4 Contamination of the drinking water supply by *E. coli* after an outbreak in Oregon was demonstrated by fluorescent dye placed in a toilet flowing out of a sewer manhole.

Courtesy of CDC/Dr. Mark L. Rosenberg

Diagnosis and Treatment

The most common method of identifying *E. coli* as the causative agent of disease is detecting the bacterial cells in the stool of the patient. Laboratories do not routinely test for *E. coli*; the test must be specifically ordered. Most individuals with diarrhea usually do not seek medical assistance unless complications occur such as dehydration because the course of the infection is typically short in duration. As a result, *E. coli* is not identified in many cases. However, individuals who suddenly have diarrhea with bloody stools should immediately be tested for *E. coli* O157:H7. Treatment of *E. coli* diseases includes replacement fluids in cases of dehydration and appropriate antibiotic therapy if indicated (see Figure 19-5).

Shigella Infections

Shigellosis, also known as bacillary dysentery, is an acute bacterial infection that affects the lining of the small and large intestines. It is characterized by bloody diarrhea with mucus and pus, nausea and vomiting, fever, and convulsions. It is caused by serotypes of *Shigella dysenteriae*, *Shigella flexneri*, *Shigella boydii*, and *Shigella soneii*. As part of the same tribe as *Escherichia*, *Shigella* bacteria have very similar characteristics and are often mistaken for *E. coli* infections.

The Shiga toxins produced by *E. coli* are also produced by *Shigella* and add to their virulence profile (see Figure 19-6). Another virulence factor is the number of individual organisms required for causing detectable signs and symptoms of infection. *S. dysenteriae* require only 10 bacteria to cause disease. This **infectivity dose** (ID) is extremely low in comparison to the 100 to 200 organisms of *S. flexneri* or *S. sonnei* required to cause disease.

Humans are the natural reservoir for *Shigella*, but primates may also become colonized. Food may become contaminated with *Shigella* by poor hygiene practices of those in the food production and preparation industries. Field crops may become contaminated by human fecal waste if sanitation facilities are unavailable for workers or if raw sewage is released in flooding events. *Shigella* bacteria may also be transmitted through ingestion of contaminated water from untreated public recreational water attractions.

At-risk populations for serious illness from *Shigella* infections include:

- Children younger than age 5 years and their caregivers, especially in daycare settings

- Men who have sex with men (MSM)

- Individuals with HIV/AIDS

- Individuals in custodial care (prisons, nursing homes, etc.)

- Refugees in crowded living conditions with poor or suboptimal sanitation facilities

- Travelers to international destinations, especially developing countries

The CDC reported in 2020 that there are an estimated 450,000 cases of shigellosis annually. The analysis of the

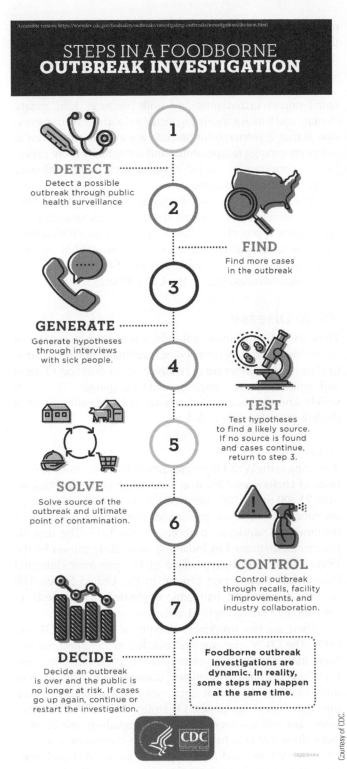

Figure 19-5 Steps in a foodborne outbreak investigation.

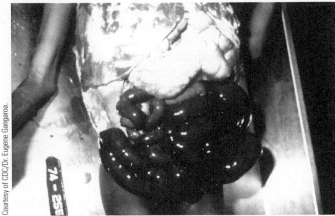

Figure 19-6 Fatal necrosis of the intestines due to a shigellosis infection.

The *Salmonella* bacterium is a Gram-negative facultative anaerobe that lives in the intestines of humans and other animals. CDC published statistics from 2021 show that *Salmonella* bacteria are the cause of 1.35 million infections annually and 26,500 hospitalizations with 420 deaths in the United States. In the majority of these infections, the source is food-borne. *Salmonella* has several serotypes within the genus and is discussed in more detail in Chapter 16.

Botulism

Botulism is a serious disease caused by *Clostridium botulinum*. There are four categories of botulism infection: infant, wound, iatrogenic, and food-borne. The *C. botulinum* bacterium is found primarily in soils and improperly canned foods. Spores have even been isolated from animals. The toxin may be released in the GI system after ingestion of the food-borne bacteria. The toxin is a deadly bacterial toxin and only miniscule amounts are needed to cause disease. Once ingested, the toxins are absorbed into the bloodstream, where they act to block neurotransmission of peripheral nerve synapses. **Flaccid paralysis** results and leads to muscle weakness and respiratory failure. Timely **intubation** and respiratory support have reduced mortality significantly. More information on *C. botulinum* and botulism is discussed in Chapter 13.

Yersinia Infections

Yersiniosis is a gastrointestinal infection in humans manifested by severe diarrhea with necrosis of the Peyer's patches, liver and splenic abscesses, and chronic lymphadenopathy. The causative bacterium, *Yersinia enterocolitica*, has been isolated from wounds, feces, mesenteric lymph nodes, and sputum of patients. Yersiniosis is characterized by diarrhea, vomiting, fever, and abdominal pain. The signs of the infection can mimic appendicitis because the patient often reports right lower quadrant pain, leading to incidental appendectomy. Yersiniosis infection may be identified during pathological examination of an inflamed appendix following appendectomy, providing a definitive diagnosis. Other incorrect

microbial species involved demonstrated previous statistical data showing that *S. sonnei* cause 75 percent of infections and up to 95 percent of *Shigella* infections may go unrecognized and unreported.

Salmonella Infections

Members of the genus *Salmonella* are the most common cause of enterocolitis due to the ingestion of contaminated foods.

differential diagnoses based on the signs and symptoms that yersiniosis mimics include mesenteric lymphadenitis and **Crohn's disease**.

Post-infection complications include reactive arthritis and bacteremia. Arthritis may occur in the absence of symptoms. The frequency of post-enteritis arthritis is approximately 2 to 3 percent. Bacteremia is rare. Diagnosis is made by isolating the organism from the patient's feces, blood, or vomit. The three main symptoms of diarrhea, pain, and fever are the most reliable clinical symptoms.

Yersinia pseudotuberculosis

Yersinia pseudotuberculosis was first reported in the United States in 1938. It is a pathogen of rodents and birds but can also infect humans. It is easily distinguished from other *Yersinia* species because of its motility. It causes fever and acute abdominal pain due to mesenteric lymphadenitis that can also be mistaken for appendicitis. It can cause severe enterocolitis, producing large nodules in the Peyer's patches and intestinal abscesses. If the abscesses cause permanent damage, the patient may have to undergo an intestinal resection. Secondary manifestations of *Y. pseudotuberculosis* infections include **erythema nodosum** and reactive arthritis (see Figure 19-7). The source of the infection has been identified in only rare cases.

Yersinia enterocolitica

Yersinia enterocolitica is a pleomorphic, Gram-negative bacillus in the genus *Yersinia* and family *Enterobacteriaceae*. In some countries, *Y. enterocolitica* has become a more prominent pathogen in cases of bacterial gastroenteritis over *Shigella* and almost as prevalent as *Salmonella* and *Campylobacter*. Infection of the small bowel can cause superficial necrosis of the mucosa with ulceration.

Y. enterocolitica is a known pathogen found mainly in pigs, but also in cattle, sheep, horses, dogs, cats, rabbits, and rodents. Once the infected animal recovers, it becomes a healthy carrier for life. The bacteria isolated in pigs are found mainly in tonsil tissues. The microorganisms are excreted in the feces of animals and can contaminate dairy products and drinking water. Humans are more commonly infected by eating raw or undercooked pork.

Other potential transmission sources include contaminated unpasteurized milk and milk products, tofu, meats, oysters, and fish. A concerning factor in food-borne transmission is that *Y. enterocolitica* bacteria are able to grow even in refrigerator-range temperatures and are actually more prevalent in countries of cooler climates such as Scandinavia, northern Europe, and Japan.

Most infections are self-limiting; however, patients with co-morbidities are at elevated risk for serious sequelae and may require appropriate antibiotic therapy. Cases with definitively identified bacterial species of *Y. enterocolitica* account for an estimated 117,000 infections with 640 hospitalizations and 35 deaths on average in the United States.

Vibrio Disease

Vibriosis is a gastrointestinal infection caused by species of the genus *Vibrio*. Most cases of gastrointestinal vibriosis due to *V. parahaemolyticus* are of relatively short duration (3 days) and typically do not require antibiotic therapy. The more widely known disease and serious public health threat is cholera caused by *Vibrio cholerae*.

Cholera

According to the WHO, there are approximately 1.3 to 4.0 million cases of cholera resulting in a wide range of death estimates from 21,000 to 143,000 worldwide. Cholera outbreaks can be endemic, epidemic, or pandemic. There have been seven documented pandemic outbreaks since 1817. The first six pandemics originated in India and were likely caused by the *Vibrio cholerae* O1 biotype. Five of the pandemics affected Europe and four caused disease in the United States. The seventh documented pandemic originated in Indonesia in 1961 and by 1992 had spread to five continents.

There are two toxigenic serotypes of *V. cholerae*: O1 and O139. The O139 type was first isolated in 1992 and has not been identified in any cases outside of Asian countries. *V. cholerae* O1 has two biotypes: classical and El Tor. Each of those biotypes has two distinct serotypes: Inaba and Ogawa. Infections from the classical O1 strain of *V. cholerae* have become rare and are seen mainly in Bangladesh and parts of India. Strains of non-toxin-producing *V. cholerae* produce less severe symptoms and are designated as non-O1 and non-O139 *V. cholerae*. The route of transmission is the fecal-oral route through ingestion of cholera-contaminated water in areas with insufficient or compromised water sanitation facilities. The bacteria are shed in the feces of infected individuals, and the bacteria are then released back into the environment and spread through the water supply.

Infected individuals often display mild or no symptoms. In those with weakened immune systems, the very young, or in much older adults, symptoms include frequent watery diarrhea, vomiting, abdominal cramping, hypotension, tachycardia,

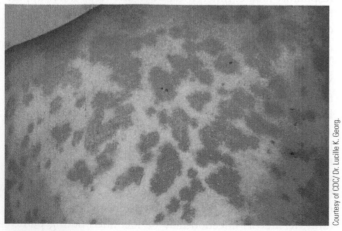

Figure 19-7 Upper back of a patient with a skin sensitivity reaction rash known as erythema nodosum.

Courtesy of CDC/ Dr. Lucille K. Georg.

restlessness, dry mucous membranes, and loss of skin elasticity. The signs are indicative of severe dehydration and the most critical treatment is rehydration with either large amounts of liquids taken orally or intravenous fluids with electrolytes in more severe cases.

A coalition of 50 groups including academic institutions, non-governmental organizations (NGOs), and United Nations agencies created the Global Task Force on Cholera Control (GTFCC) and in 2017 developed a strategic plan for reducing cholera entitled *Ending Cholera: A global roadmap to 2030*. The goal of the task force's partner countries seeks to eliminate cholera in up to 20 different countries with high endemic infection rates and reduce deaths from cholera by 90 percent by 2030. The strategies include widespread use of three oral cholera vaccines (OCVs) that have gained WHO pre-qualification. The three vaccines require two doses for full protection; however, it is stressed that they do not eliminate the critical need for local health education programs that take culture and beliefs into consideration (see Figure 19-8). These public health educators promote community adoption of good hygiene including hand-washing with soap, safe food preparation and storage, and safe disposal of the feces of infants and young children.

Healthcare workers, including surgical team members who volunteer for medical mission or disaster response service in countries where cholera is prevalent, or following natural disasters such as earthquakes or tsunamis that wipe out existing infrastructure for clean water provisions, should carefully research the options for vaccination or other requirements prior to traveling.

Bacteroides Infections

Infection from *Bacteroides* typically occurs when trauma to the gastrointestinal (GI) tract permits the bacteria to escape from the wound and contaminate surrounding tissues. The infection is actually a polymicrobial process that involves **synergism**. Examples of circumstances in which *B. fragilis* causes infection include GI surgery, perforated appendix, perforated intestinal ulcer, blunt and sharp trauma, **diverticulitis**, and inflammatory bowel disease. Synergism has been clearly established in infections involving *B. fragilis* and *E. coli*. After the intestinal wall has been compromised, the normal microflora spill into the peritoneal cavity. During the first stage of infection (within approximately 20 hours), the aerobes such as *E. coli* are active, causing tissue destruction. Once the aerobes have consumed much of the oxygen, the anaerobic *B. fragilis* begin multiplying, and these bacteria predominate during the second stage of the infection.

Bacteroides fragilis contributes to the synergistic infection in three ways:

- Stimulation of abscess formation
- Resistance to phagocytosis by **polymorphonuclear** leukocytes (PMNs)
- Inactivation of antibiotics by producing βeta lactamase.

Abscesses are a major complication of abdominal infections. A fibrous membrane that contains the infectious fluid typically surrounds abscesses. The fluid is composed of dead PMNs, cellular debris, and bacterial cells. Abscess formation is a response by the immune system to the presence of the polysaccharide capsule of *B. fragilis*. The response of the immune system is designed to wall off the infection and protect the host. What actually occurs is that bacterial cells are shielded from exposure to antibiotics and the immune system, therefore allowing the bacteria to remain viable and multiply.

A serious and often fatal gastrointestinal infection in neonates is necrotizing enterocolitis (NEC) in which the intestinal and intraperitoneal organs become ischemic from a drop in blood flow for unknown reasons and bacteria likely exacerbate the tissue damage due to an undeveloped immune system capability in premature and newborn infants.

Treatment

If left untreated, the abscess will continue to grow and eventually rupture, releasing the infectious material and causing peritonitis. Peritonitis can lead to septic shock and death if not aggressively treated (see Figure 19-9). Surgical intervention involves incision and drainage (I&D), sometimes referred to as irrigation and drainage. If the body is able to contain or "wall off" the abscess, then the prognosis is more favorable. If, however, the infectious abscess fluid spills out into the abdominal cavity, there is a higher likelihood that it may enter the bloodstream, causing bacteremia. The surgical technologist should be prepared for a surgical procedure that may turn from a relatively simple I&D into a complex procedure involving the entire peritoneal cavity. A bowel resection may have to be performed and wound drains placed for postoperative drainage.

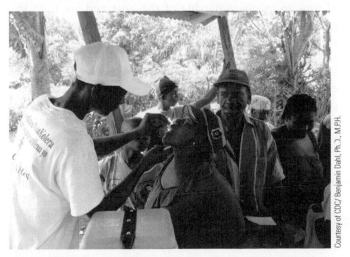

Courtesy of CDC/ Benjamin Dahl, Ph.D., M.P.H.

Figure 19-8 Oral cholera vaccine (OCV) campaign team member administering the oral cholera vaccine to a Haitian woman in live with other recipients of all ages.

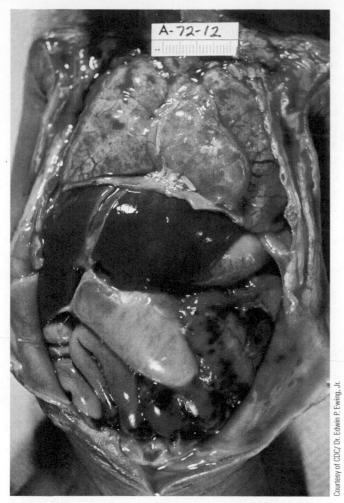

Courtesy of CDC/ Dr. Edwin P. Ewing., Jr.

Figure 19-9 Autopsy of an infant with exposure of the thoracoabdominal organs, showing pathologic changes of abdominal distension, intestinal necrosis and hemorrhage, and peritonitis due to necrotizing enterocolitis.

Staphylococcus Infections

Staphylococcus aureus produces enterotoxins that, when ingested from contaminated foods, causes acute episodes of food poisoning. Many common foods can be contaminated by *S. aureus* and include meats and poultry, prepared deli meats, salads prepared with mayonnaise, milk and other dairy products, and egg products including custard and cream-filled pastries. Additionally, food can be contaminated by the skin of preparers who fail to keep hands clean with proper hand hygeine.

Hepatitis Infections

As an important component of the digestive system, the liver has multiple functions. It produces many of the chemicals required by the body for normal functioning. The liver also breaks down, filters, and detoxifies substances in the body. It is responsible for the production of bile for breaking down ingested lipids for digestion. Finally, it acts as a storage unit for crucial vitamins and other chemicals.

Hepatitis is an infection involving the liver caused by various viruses such as Hepatitis A (HAV), Hepatitis B (HBV), Hepatitis C (HCV), Hepatitis D (HDV), and Hepatitis E (HEV). There are others that have been reported; however, research is ongoing and the viruses are not fully understood. Infections from HAV and HEV are acute and the least serious, similar to many other gastrointestinal infections. HBV and HCV are blood-borne pathogens capable of transmission through sexual intercourse or sharps injuries. The viral pathogens may cause chronic infections that may go undiagnosed for years until signs of serious liver damage such as cirrhosis or liver cancer develop. Treatment for the most severe cases of hepatitis is usually liver transplantation.

Lactobacillus

The genus *Lactobacillus* has a number of species, most of which are part of the normal resident microbiome of the gastrointestinal and female genitourinary systems. Other than *L. delbrueckii*, which has been documented as a cause of some urinary tract infections, most species of *Lactobacillus* are considered "friendly" bacteria. There is evidence that they help break down food, absorb nutrients, and fight off pathogenic "unfriendly" organisms that cause intestinal infections and serious diarrhea. *L. acidophilus* is a common ingredient in milk, yogurt, and other dairy products and is sold as a type of health supplement called "probiotics."

Lactobacillus, a normal part of the vaginal microbiota, may be a crucial component in inoculating neonates during vaginal delivery with their first intestinal bacteria. *Lactobacillus* is needed for the breakdown of breast milk and may reduce digestive difficulties in newborn infants. Chapter 13 evaluates the benefits and properties of *Lactobacillus*.

Gastrointestinal Parasites

The intestinal tract can be home to many species of protozoa and worms. Most of those that cause disease are acquired through the fecal–oral route. Worm larvae require a period of time to incubate outside of the host and are then ingested through contaminated food. Some worm larvae can penetrate directly through the skin and make their way to the intestinal tract through various routes. Animals that are infected with the worms may themselves be slaughtered and eaten, infecting humans who then become hosts. Protozoan pathogens include *Entamoeba histolytica*, *Giardia lamblia*, and *Cryptosporidium parvum*. The diseases they cause are characterized by cysts and trophozoites (the active, motile feeding stage of a sporozoan parasite) in the feces.

Symptoms may be acute or chronic, with severe or mild diarrhea and inflammation. Infections can be life-threatening if the parasites make their way to other parts of the body, such as the brain, lungs, or liver. *Entamoeba histolytica* infection is common in subtropical and tropical countries. The larvae reside within the large intestine, typically as harmless commensals feeding on bacteria. As they reproduce, they exit the host's body in the form of a cyst and can be ingested in contaminated food, continuing the infection cycle in new hosts.

Giardiasis, caused by *G. lamblia*, affects the duodenum and causes severe gas, bloating, abdominal pain, and damage to mucosa. Stools are loose, foul-smelling, and fatty. The disease is usually mild and self-limiting, but chronic forms are not uncommon. Refer to Figure 10-3 in Chapter 10 for an illustration of the life cycle of *G. lamblia*.

Complications include amebic dysentery, which is characterized by blood and pus in the stool. If the parasite perforates the intestine, then peritonitis can result. Trophozoites can enter the bloodstream and spread to the liver or brain, where they form cysts and abscesses.

Diseases of the Genitourinary System

The anatomy of the genitourinary system predisposes it to potential infection from opportunistic resident microbes of the skin or GI tract and through mechanical means such as invasive surgical procedures or during sexual relations. Examples of human genitourinary diseases include:

- Parasites: *Trichomonas vaginalis*
- Fungi: *Candida albicans, Cryptococcus neoformans*
- Bacteria: *Chlamydia trachomatis, Enterococcus* spp., *Escherichia coli, Gardnerella vaginalis, Haemophilus ducreyi, Klebsiella pneumoniae, Mycoplasma hominis, Mycoplasma genitalium, Neisseria gonorrhoeae, Proteus mirabilis, Providencia, Pseudomonas, Serratia, Staphylococcus aureus, Streptococcus* A, *Streptococcus agalactiae, Treponema pallidum*, and *Ureaplasma urealyticum*
- Viruses: herpes simplex 1 and 2 viruses, human papillomavirus, human immunodeficiency virus, hepatitis B and C viruses

Parasitic Infections

Trichomoniasis is a sexually transmitted disease (STD) caused by the protozoan parasite *Trichomonas vaginalis*. In the United States, approximately 3.7 million males and females are infected; however, only one-third has symptoms or is aware of the infection. "Trich" is considered the most curable STD. If symptoms do manifest, they typically include itching, burning, discharge, or redness of genitalia. Pregnant females with this STD are at risk for pre-term labor. Treatment with a single dose of oral anti-infective medication (metronidazole or tinidazole) is prescribed. Individuals can become reinfected if all sexual partners are not treated effectively.

Fungal Infections

Vulvovaginal candidiasis (VVC) is commonly known as a "yeast infection" and is caused by *Candida albicans*, a member of the vaginal microbiome. Nearly 75 percent of adult females have had at least one infection, which occurs when the normal balance of acidity or hormone levels in the vagina is altered (see Figure 19-10). Males can also be infected with candidiasis. Symptoms include itching, burning, odor, and "cottage cheese-like" discharge. Treatment consists of oral or vaginal suppository anti-fungal medications.

Cryptococcus neoformans is a fungal pathogen associated with lung infections or meningitis; however, in patients who are immunocompromised such as those with HIV/AIDS, it can also become a source of genitourinary infection.

Bacterial Infections

It is probably evident by the extensive list of pathogens presented that bacteria, whether resident or transient, can become the source of opportunistic genitourinary infections. Only those most commonly associated with the GU system are discussed in this section.

Chlamydia trachomatis

As with most STDs, *Chlamydia* can be transmitted through vaginal, anal, and oral sex. Often there are no symptoms for either males or females, but when there are they include itching, burning, painful urination, and possible vaginal discharge and minor bleeding. The major risk of undiagnosed *Chlamydia* is the potential for pelvic inflammatory disease (PID) or non-viable **ectopic pregnancy** due to blockage of fallopian tubes (see Figure 19-11). Pregnant females can pass the infection in the form of conjunctivitis or pneumonia to their newborns during vaginal delivery. Antibiotic treatment is effective, but reinfection is possible with unprotected sex with infected partners.

E. coli Urinary Tract Infections

E. coli is a common cause of urinary tract infections (UTIs) in infants who wear diapers, individuals with indwelling urinary catheters, and females in general. It is responsible for causing more than 80 percent of community-acquired UTIs and the majority of healthcare-associated infection (HAI) UTIs. The bacterial cells can invade any portion of the GU tract, including the kidneys, causing a severe infection called **pyelonephritis**.

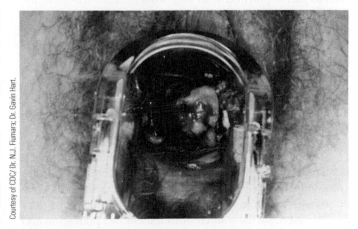

Courtesy of CDC/ Dr. N.J. Fiumara; Dr. Gavin Hart.

Figure 19-10 Purulent discharge surrounding the cervix and cervical os in the vaginal canal due to candidiasis, or moniliasis caused by the fungal organism, *Candida albicans*.

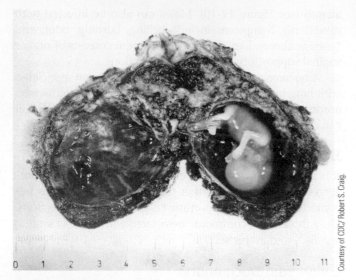

Figure 19-11 A tissue specimen showing early development of a fetus from a female with an ectopic abdominal pregnancy that implanted outside of the uterus and developed the trophoblastic capsule and placenta seen.

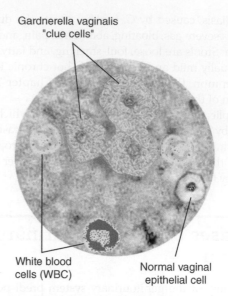

Figure 19-12 Clue cells: vaginal epithelial cells.

Nephropathogenic *E. coli* (NPEC) has a capsule and pilus that add to its virulence. Individuals with UTIs typically experience flank pain that radiates to the back, **dysuria**, frequent urination, and **hematuria**. Indwelling catheters require removal until the infection is resolved by antibiotics.

Gardnerella vaginalis

Gardnerella vaginalis is a pleomorphic, non-motile bacterium that does not possess a capsule and cannot form spores. Its shape resembles a Gram-negative bacillus, but the cell wall structure resembles Gram-positive organisms and adheres to the surfaces of epithelial cells in the vagina and vaginal fluids. The bacteria are facultative anaerobes that grow very slowly in the laboratory.

Gardnerella vaginalis is a part of the normal microbiome of the vagina in 50 to 70 percent of healthy females. It is usually seen as part of polymicrobial **vaginosis** infections. Because inflammation is not present, the term vaginosis is used instead of vaginitis. Other clinical signs of vaginosis include an increase in pH (higher than 4.5) and reduction in lactobacilli. It is not known if the decrease in acid-producing lactobacilli with a corresponding increase in pH is a cause or effect of the general vaginal microbial changes. Diagnosis is supported by the finding of "clue cells." Clue cells are epithelial cells that are covered with Gram-positive or Gram-variable bacilli and curved Gram-negative bacilli (see Figure 19-12).

The condition can be sexually transmitted but has been known to occur in females who are not sexually active. Males are asymptomatic but can contribute to recurring infections in females. Symptoms include a copious grey-white discharge that has a fishy smell from the **amines** putrescine and cadaverine, which are present in rotting fish.

Risk factors for developing vaginosis include invasive procedures (hysterectomy, endometrial biopsy), change in sexual partners, menopause, diabetes mellitus, being immunocompromised, and poor hygiene. *G. vaginalis* may play a role in **postpartum** bacteremia, postpartum **endometriosis**, premature birth, low birth weight, and neonatal septicemia. The standard treatment is the antibiotic metronidazole, which does not affect the normal lactobacilli, returning the vaginal microbiome to its normal pH level.

Haemophilus ducreyi

Discussed previously in Chapter 16, *Haemophilus ducreyi* is the causative agent of chancroid infections that are STDs characterized by painful, open, draining sores on genitalia. On clinical presentation the appearance of genital ulcers and regional lymphadenopathy are typical for chancroid infection (see Figure 19-13).

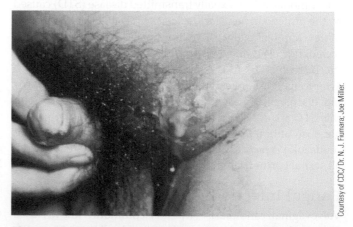

Figure 19-13 A male patient with a chancroid lesion on the glans penis and a left inguinal lymph node, referred to as a bubo, which had ruptured, draining purulent contents and caused by the Gram-negative bacterium, *Haemophilus ducreyi*.

Neisseria gonorrhoeae

Neisseria gonorrhoeae is the bacterium responsible for gonorrhea, a serious STD in both males and females. Similar to chlamydia, risks of undiagnosed gonorrhea include the potential for pelvic inflammatory disease (PID) or ectopic pregnancy due to blockage of fallopian tubes. Pregnant females can suffer miscarriage, pre-term labor, or rupture of membranes, and pass the infection in the form of gonococcal conjunctivitis during vaginal delivery. Males may become sterile from damage to or blockage of the structures of the testicles. Antibiotic treatment is available and patients are counseled to complete the course prescribed and to avoid sexual contact until all parties have been treated. Drug-resistant *Neisseria gonorrhoeae* has been included on the CDC's urgent threat level of the *Antibiotic Resistance Threats in the United States, 2019.*

Treponema pallidum

Treponema pallidum are spirochetes responsible for the STD venereal syphilis. Syphilis is characterized by phases of disease progression and is discussed extensively in Chapter 15. Primary infections involve the genitourinary system; however, as the disease progresses into the subsequent phases, systemic signs and symptoms develop, including cutaneous lesions of areas distant from the genitalia (see Figure 19-14). In 2013, 75 percent of reported primary and secondary cases of syphilis were in men who have sex with men (MSM). Pregnant females can pass the infection to the fetus, potentially resulting in miscarriage or severe birth defects. Antibiotic treatment is successful if used appropriately, but damage already caused will not be reversed by treatment.

Viral Infections

Viruses are discussed in Chapter 8. Those that primarily affect the GU system include herpes simplex virus 2 (HSV-2) and human papillomavirus (HPV). HSV-1 is typically associated with harmless cold sores of the lips and mouth. HSV-2 is associated with lesions of the genitals and anus. Herpetic lesions begin as fluid-filled blisters that rupture and cause pain until resolved in approximately 1 week. Initial "outbreaks" may be more severe and be accompanied by flu-like symptoms. Transmission to a partner during sex is possible even when no visible lesions are present. Pregnant females with active lesions in the perineal region will likely need to undergo C-section to prevent possible transmission to the neonate in a vaginal delivery (see Figure 19-15).

Human papillomavirus (HPV) is the most common sexually transmitted infection. According to the CDC, nearly all sexually active males and females will become infected with HPV at some time during their lives. Currently, it is estimated that 42 million Americans are infected, with 13 million new cases occurring annually.

Often the infection will clear on its own and produce no symptoms or lasting effects. In other cases, signs and symptoms of genital warts may develop. In undiagnosed or untreated infections, cancer of the cervix, vulva, penis, anus, or oropharynx (throat) may occur. Of those infections, annually 36,000 individuals, male and female, will develop cancer as a result of HPV.

A vaccination is available for prevention of the most common types of HPV and should be given to pre-teen males and females prior to their first sexual encounter to prevent infection (see Figure 19-16). Controversy exists, however, due to some parents' sensibilities about addressing the topic of sex with their younger children.

Condyloma

Condyloma, more commonly known as genital warts, is a sexually transmitted infection caused by the human papilloma virus (HPV) and found in the perineal region.

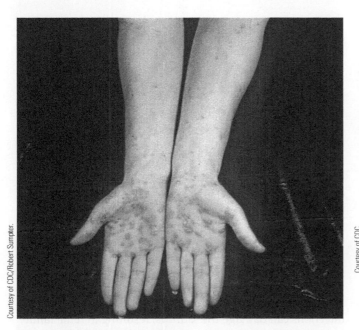

Figure 19-14 Palmar syphilids due to secondary syphilis.

Courtesy of CDC/Robert Sumpter.

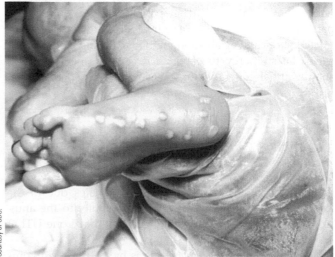

Courtesy of CDC.

Figure 19-15 Left foot of an infant born with a herpes simplex infection known as neonatal herpes or herpes simplex neonatorum manifested by development of maculopapular lesions of the heel and sole of the foot.

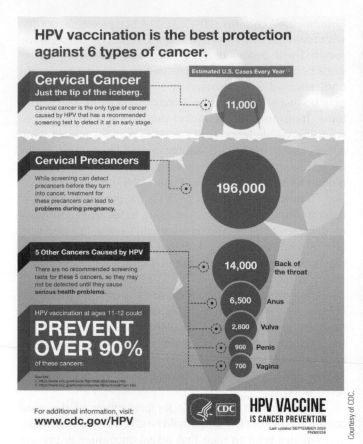

Courtesy of CDC.

Figure 19-16 CDC poster: HPV vaccination is the best protection against 6 types of cancer.

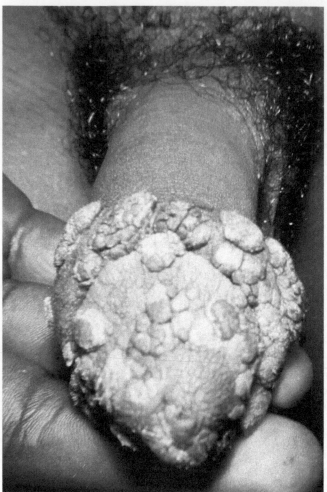

Courtesy of CDC.

Figure 19-17 A male patient's glans penis with numerous rough, nodular, cutaneous lesions diagnosed as condylomata acuminata (CA), or venereal warts caused by human papilloma virus (HPV).

The infection can range from small, flat (condyloma lata) lesions with little or no symptoms to large, dry growths that resemble cauliflower (condylomata acuminata) and spread throughout the genitalia, anus, and up to the suprapubic region (see Figure 19-17). Humans are the carriers and reservoirs for HPV infections. They pass them between intimate partners until both parties are treated. Condyloma may be treated surgically by ablation methods utilizing electrosurgical or laser energy to vaporize infected tissue or excised sharply under general or local anesthesia.

Types of Urinary Tract Infections

Urinary tract infections occur frequently in the human population but affect females far more than males due to the length of the female urethra and its proximity to the anus. Approximately one-half of all females will have one UTI at some point in their lives.

Gram-negative *Escherichia coli* is by far the most common pathogen that causes ascending UTI (ascending from the urethra to the bladder to the kidney). Healthcare-associated UTIs are often caused by *Klebsiella, Enterobacter, Serratia* spp., and *Pseudomonas aeruginosa* because these

microorganisms tend toward antibiotic resistance. Very few viruses or parasites cause UTI.

Upper and Lower Urinary Tract Infections

UTIs are diagnosed as either upper or lower UTIs, depending on the structure or organ affected (see Figure 19-18). Upper UTIs include ureteral infections (ureteritis) or kidney infections (pyelonephritis). Lower UTIs include urethral infections (urethritis) or bladder infections (cystitis). Acute lower UTIs can cause dysuria (pain when passing urine), urgency (an urgent need to pass urine), and increased frequency for urination. The urine is typically cloudy from the presence of pus and bacteria.

Upper UTIs can only be distinguished from lower UTIs by examining urine directly from the ureter through catheterization. Pyelonephritis patients become febrile and also experience lower UTI symptoms. These types of recurrent infections can damage the kidneys, resulting in renal failure or hypertension.

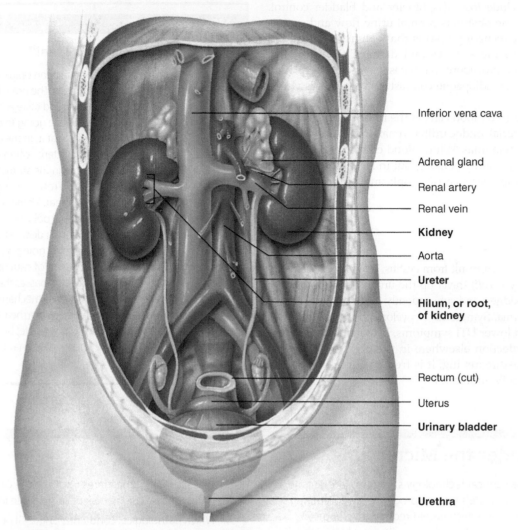

Inferior vena cava

Adrenal gland

Renal artery

Renal vein

Kidney

Aorta

Ureter

Hilum, or root, of kidney

Rectum (cut)

Uterus

Urinary bladder

Urethra

Figure 19-18 Organs of the urinary system.

Complicated and Uncomplicated Urinary Tract Infections

UTIs can be further divided into complicated or uncomplicated infections. A complicated UTI is one in which a patient has trouble with normal urination because of mechanical or neurological problems related to the infection (usually pyelonephritis). These types of infections are often caused by indwelling catheters or other conditions that allow bacteria to ascend and persist over time. These bacteria are often resistant to many antibiotics because of repeated exposure and treatment. Complicated UTIs are difficult to treat.

Uncomplicated UTIs are often seen in sexually active females and do not interfere with urination. Gram-positive *Staphylococcus saprophyticus* is a common pathogen in these infections that responds well to antibiotic treatment.

Cystitis

Most bladder infections (called cystitis) are acquired from bacteria entering from the urethra, and they occur more frequently in females. Cystitis is rare in males, but when it does occur it usually involves the prostate. *Enterococcus* species can leave the urethra and infect the bladder. Most cases of cystitis are caused by *E. coli*. They thrive in urine and can cause a severe form of cystitis.

Mechanical factors can predispose a patient to cystitis. These include any device that facilitates bacterial access to the bladder or conditions that result in the inability of the bladder to empty completely. Urinary catheterization is a major cause of UTI because bacteria from the urethra are transmitted to the bladder on the surface of the catheter. Catheterized patients should periodically have their urine tested for microbes. Urine that has been standing in the catheter drainage bag should not be used as a specimen because microbes may have multiplied since initial drainage from the bladder. Non-catheterized patients should not be catheterized to obtain a urine specimen unless otherwise ordered by a physician.

Residual urine of more than 3 mL can cause a bladder infection and is commonly seen in individuals with neurologic deficits that include loss of sphincter and bladder control. The residual urine obstructs normal urine flow and creates a condition for recurring cystitis that can ascend through the ureters into the kidneys and damage those organs. A **cystogram** is a procedure that measures the residual urine by instillation of a radiopaque contrast solution that is visible on x-ray.

Hematuria (red blood cells in the urine) may be associated with bacterial endocarditis, renal trauma, stones, or urinary tract carcinomas. White blood cells in the urine are often present in healthy persons, but in large numbers they may indicate the presence of neoplasms (tumors), calculi (stones), or a UTI.

Pyelonephritis

Kidney infections can result from cystitis, especially in females. Bacteria (usually *E. coli*) travel up the ureter from the bladder and infect the kidney, and subsequently into the bloodstream, causing septicemia. Symptoms of pyelonephritis include back pain, fever, and lower UTI symptoms. Pyelonephritis is often the result of infection elsewhere in the body. Because it is considered life-threatening, it is treated aggressively with broad-spectrum IV antibiotics.

MICRO NOTES

"I Just Can't Stomach This!"

You may not think that your brain has an opinion about what you eat, but you'd be incorrect. The brain is in control of interpretation of senses of smell and taste and reflexes such as vomiting. If something we are going to eat smells or tastes bad, our brain tells us not to eat it. In the case of food that is infected with pathogenic bacteria, often there are no smell or taste clues; however, once in the stomach, the brain figures out that there is something rotten going on and initiates vomiting to remove the threat. Vomiting after binge drinking is protection against alcohol poisoning. In morning sickness during pregnancy, the brain decides, whether correct or not, that there is something going on that might threaten the fetus and errs on the side of caution, causing vomiting. Once what you've ingested passes the stomach, the digestive system takes over with its mechanisms of increasing peristalsis, better known as diarrhea, to push through infected food as quickly as possible, but it's actually your brain telling it to do so. Those tidbits may be hard to swallow, but it's true.

 ## Under the Microscope

Pat, who is a surgical technology student in the second year of the Associate's Degree program, was preparing for an assignment which would require teaching classmates about pathological conditions of the GI and GU systems and developed the following questions for the group to discuss.

1. Which anatomical areas of the gastrointestinal and genitourinary tracts are most likely to be infected if opportunistic pathogens gain access or disrupt the normal microbial balance?

2. Which types of GI or GU infections might require surgical intervention as a course of treatment?

3. Which surgical procedures involving the GI or GU systems have a higher risk of surgical site infection?

4. Which pathological conditions of the GI or GU system have non-surgical treatment options or are preventable by vaccination?

5. Which types of GI or GU infections pose the greatest risk for the special patient populations (neonates, older adults, patients who are immunocompromised) or on long-term antibiotic therapy, and those living in areas with inadequate sanitation or access to clean water?

CHAPTER 20

Diseases of the Eyes, Ears, and Respiratory System

Learning Objectives

After completing the study of this chapter, you will be able to:

1. Define key terms.
2. Describe the most common types of eye and ear infections.
3. Identify the pathogens responsible for infections of the eyes, ears, and respiratory system.
4. Compare and contrast the range of diseases associated with the respiratory system.
5. Discuss preventative measures available for prevention of respiratory diseases.
6. Apply critical thinking skills in relating chapter material to the surgical environment of care or broader global community.

Key Terms

Alveoli	Convalescent stage	Idiosyncratic	Rheumatic fever
Arthrospores	Cystic fibrosis	Keratitis	Trachoma
Blastomycosis	Dacryocystitis	Microvilli	Vasoconstrictors
Blepharitis	Eustachian tube	Otitis externa	
Catarrhal stage	Histoplasmosis	Otorhinolaryngology	
Coccidioidomycosis	Idiopathic	Paroxysmal stage	

The Big Picture

Prior to the COVID-19 pandemic, infections affecting the respiratory system have been some of the most common among humans and are part of normal life. Parents often stand by helplessly as their children go through the stages of respiratory, eye, and ear infections and look for any way to relieve the pain and suffering they are experiencing. During your examination of the topics in this chapter, consider the following:

1. Why are many respiratory infections such as colds and the flu more common in seasonally colder months?

2. Which preventative measures are effective in blocking transmission of the bacterial, viral, and fungal respiratory system diseases?

3. Which infections involving the eyes, ears, nose, and throat are relatively common in neonates or young children?

4. Which specific patient populations are at elevated risk from various types of pneumonia infections?

Clinical Significance Topic

It may seem that there is a perpetual shortage of employees working in different positions in the OR. To make things worse in the fall and winter months, people start coming down with colds and the flu. Even more than that, now there is the risk of COVID-19 infection present year-around. A standard requirement for most hospital employees has been flu vaccination. Currently, many, if not most health-care facilities and other businesses require employees to be vaccinated against COVID-19 as well as HBV and other communicable diseases that are preventable and easily spread. Staff members may have not felt secure in calling in sick when they have had a cold or the flu for fear of repercussions by administrators. During the heights of the pandemic, healthcare workers already stretched too far, were torn between personal and family safety and the passion they have always had to help those patients with highly-transmissible diseases. If you find yourself in this situation, follow the CDC recommendations on how to use appropriate PPE, social distancing, vaccinations, and hygiene measures to minimize your potential for infection so that you remain healthy for yourself and those you care for.

Diseases Involving the Eyes, Ears, Nose, and Sinuses

The surgical specialties covered in this section are ophthalmology and **otorhinolaryngology**. The infections and diseases involving these body systems are common in humans in particular and maybe most frequently in pediatric populations.

The resident microbial population of the external ear is generally the same as that of other skin. *Streptococcus pneumoniae* and *Pseudomonas aeruginosa* may be recovered from the external auditory canal. The middle and inner ear are sterile, kept free from bacteria by the barrier of the tympanic membrane; however, pathogens gain access to the middle ear from the pharynx into the **eustachian tube**.

Tears contain a natural form of antimicrobial fluid and keep the eye relatively free of microorganisms. When infections do occur, coagulase-negative staphylococci are commonly cultured from the eye (see Figure 20-1).

Sinuses may be populated by the same indigenous microbiota as the nasopharynx, including *S. pneumoniae*, *Haemophilus influenzae* (excluding group B), *Neisseria* species, aerobic streptococci, and occasionally Gram-negative rods or *Staphylococcus aureus*.

Conjunctivitis

Eye infections can come from a variety of microbes, including bacteria, fungi, and viruses. Conjunctivitis, commonly known

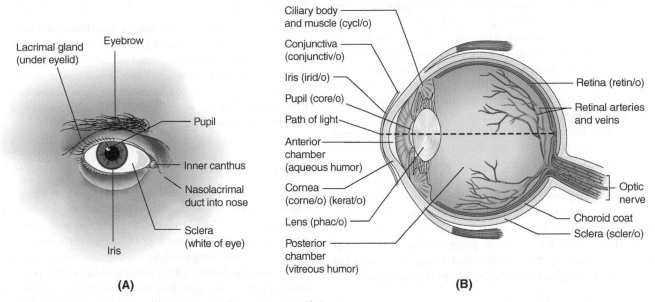

Figure 20-1 (A) External view of the eye and (B) structures of the eye.

as "pink eye," is an inflammation of the conjunctiva that can be caused by bacteria or viruses. Bacteria typically seen in conjunctivitis include *Staphylococcus aureus, Streptococcus pneumoniae, Haemophilus influenzae,* and *Pseudomonas aeruginosa.* Sexually-transmitted diseases that have been disseminated through the vascular system may also produce remote sign of infection of the eyes in adults. Neonatal infections can also occur and are discussed in the next section. Bacterial conjunctivitis produces a thick white discharge or pus and is treated with appropriate antibiotic eye drops or ointments (see Figure 20-2).

Pseudomonas aeruginosa is often the causative agent of conjunctivitis, **keratitis**, and other eye infections that resolve with the patient suffering severe end-effects. The infections are often a result of trauma or postoperative infection after surgery. The lens of the eye can be destroyed

due to a corneal ulcer. As the infection progresses, the tissue of the entire eye can be destroyed unless prompt treatment is provided (see Figure 20-3).

Eye infections can occur in those who use contact lenses and leave the lenses in place for extended periods. Giant papillary conjunctivitis is an infection that produces red bumps on the inner eyelids, itching, tearing, and heavy discharge. Contact wear should be discontinued until the infection is resolved. A change in contact lens formulation may be indicated.

Viral conjunctivitis, also referred to as pink eye, is highly contagious and caused by airborne viruses, possibly in conjunction with viral upper respiratory infections. Discharge is typically watery fluid. Antibiotics are ineffective against viral infections. Medications to reduce inflammation and **vasoconstrictors** may be prescribed.

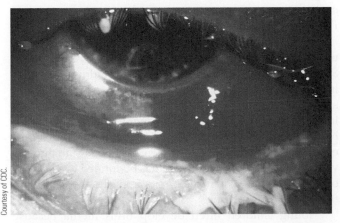

Figure 20-2 Left eye with marked erythematous gonorrheal conjunctivitis due to the systemic dissemination of *Neisseria gonorrhoeae* bacteria causing partial blindness.

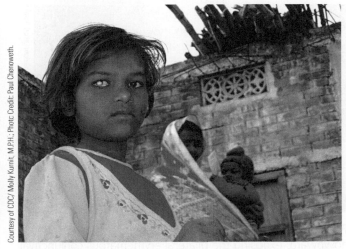

Figure 20-3 Young girl who had sustained a severe corneal ulceration of her right eye due to measles infection.

Non-infectious conjunctivitis causes pink eye–type symptoms of a transient nature and may be caused by numerous environmental irritants such as smoke and chemicals. Allergic conjunctivitis is a non-infective inflammatory response to seasonal or environmental allergens. Over-the-counter (OTC) eye drops and allergy medications may help reduce symptoms until the source of the allergic reaction is eliminated.

Stevens-Johnson syndrome is an **idiosyncratic**, delayed hypersensitivity reaction involving the skin and mucous membranes. Signs and symptoms involving the skin include erythema, edema, sloughing, blistering, ulceration, and necrosis. Signs involving structures of the eye include **blepharitis**, conjunctivitis, and keratitis (see Figure 20-4). Researchers debate the etiology of the syndrome, proposing reactions to drugs, infections, or malignancies; however, approximately half of the documented cases are **idiopathic**. There may be a genetic predisposition to the syndrome.

Neonatal Conjunctivitis

Conjunctivitis can occur in neonates who have eye patches placed while undergoing phototherapy for neonatal jaundice from elevated bilirubin levels. The infection may spread to adjoining structures such as the lacrimal glands (**dacryocystitis**) or the eyelids (blepharitis).

A serious type of conjunctivitis is acquired as the infant passes through the vagina of its mother who has gonorrhea. The infection called neonatal gonorrheal ophthalmia is caused by *Neisseria gonorrhoeae* and if left untreated or if treatment is delayed, ulcerations of the corneas develop and result in blindness. Silver nitrate was once the treatment of choice for this disease but has been replaced with targeted antibiotic therapy.

Chlamydial conjunctivitis caused by *Chlamydia trachomatis* is also acquired by infants as they pass through the birth canal. This type of eye infection can also be acquired from exposure to unchlorinated swimming pool water and is treated with antibiotic eye ointments.

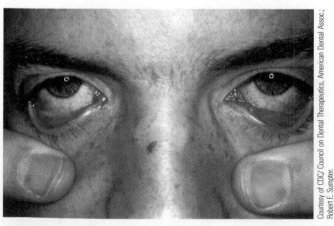

Courtesy of CDC/ Council on Dental Therapeutics, American Dental Assoc.; Robert E. Sumpter.

Figure 20-4 Eyes of a 19-year-old with lower lids pulled downward, exposing the bilateral erythematous conjunctival membranes attributed to Stevens-Johnson syndrome (SJS), also known as erythema multiforme major.

Trachoma

Chlamydia trachomatis also causes **trachoma,** an infectious disease that causes scarring on the surface of the eye, resulting in blindness. Trachoma occurs primarily in the arid portions of Asia and Africa; however, it is also seen occasionally in the southwestern United States, especially in Native American populations. Trachoma is the world's leading cause of preventable blindness.

Ear Infections

Pseudomonas aeruginosa has been identified as the primary cause of **otitis externa**. The bacterial microorganism will inhabit the external auditory canal when it is wet, providing a region for growth. Frequently, children who spend a lot of time in the swimming pool during the summer are diagnosed with "swimmer's ear." Otitis externa is itchy and painful but has a short course and does not present any complications. During the infection the child is treated with topical antibiotics and drying agents to keep the external canal dry (see Figure 20-5).

Malignant external otitis is a more virulent form of ear infection and occurs frequently in older individuals and those with diabetes. It can penetrate the mastoid bone, damage cranial nerve VIII, and is life-threatening. Aggressive antibiotic therapy must be initiated and surgical intervention may be necessary to irrigate and debride the bone surrounding the auditory region.

Fungal organisms are the cause of approximately 10 percent of external ear infections. Otomycosis also known as fungal otitis externa may be caused by *Aspergillus* and *Candida* and in some cases may invade the middle ear as well. Fungal ear infection from *Aspergillus* fungal spores will produce gray, black or yellow colored dots in the ear canal visible on otoscopy and under magnification will show the cotton-like fungal spores (see Figure 20-6). *Candida* fungi will not typically produce visible spots, however, will cause a thick, creamy white pus discharge. Middle ear infections are frequently the result of bacterial invasion by *Staphylococcus aureus, Streptococcus pneumoniae, Streptococcus pyogenes, Pseudomonas aeruginosa,* and *Haemophilus influenzae*.

Otitis media is defined as an infection of the middle ear, usually as a result of infection by viruses or the bacteria *S. pneumoniae*. The tympanic membrane (eardrum) becomes inflamed, pus compresses it resulting in pain and fever. If antibiotics are not a successful treatment or if recurrent infections become frequent, a myringotomy procedure may be performed and tiny, typically plastic or silicone pressure-equalizer (PE) vent tubes are placed into the eardrum through very small incisions. The procedure is performed for the relief of pressure and for drainage of pus from the medial side of the tympanic membrane.

Young children often develop otitis media because their immune systems are not fully developed and because the eustachian tube that connects the middle ear to the throat is smaller and easily obstructed by pus and bacteria.

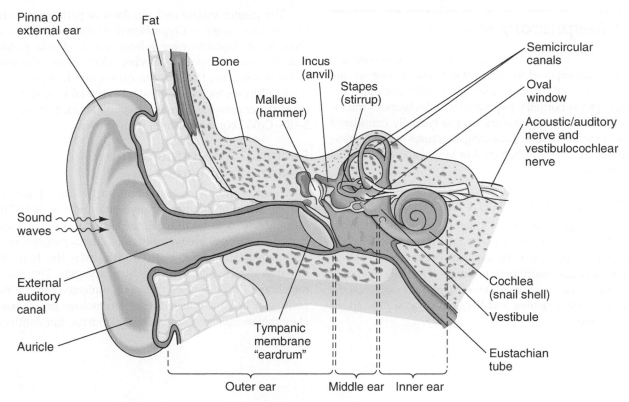

Figure 20-5 Structures of the ear.

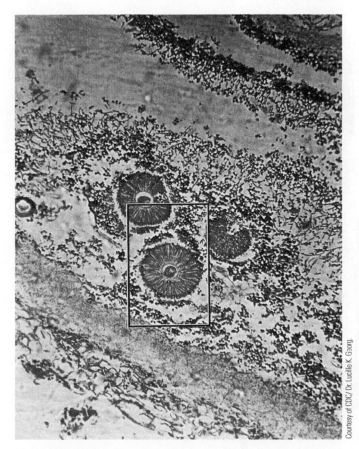

Figure 20-6 Histopathologic changes from ear tissue of a patient with otomycosis caused by *Aspergillus*.

Additionally, the eustachian tube in young children has a very slight (10 degree) slope before connecting to the nasopharynx, making drainage of mucous secretions less efficient than the 35 degree slope seen in adults. This allows pooling and proliferation of bacteria within the middle ear. Clinical signs and symptoms include the following:

- Fever
- Intractable pain due to pressure from fluid build-up
- Flattening of the tympanic membrane
- Scarring of tympanic membrane from repeated infections
- Perforation of tympanic membrane if pressure is untreated
- Potential developmental delay in children with recurrent otitis media

Nasal and Sinus Infections

Nasal sinuses can become infected with *S. pneumoniae* and *S. pyogenes*, a condition known as sinusitis. Mucous membranes that line the sinuses become inflamed and develop a heavy discharge of mucus. The mucous membrane may swell, and flow of mucus becomes blocked. Pressure builds within the cavity and causes pain or headache. Antibiotics are used as treatment; however, in more complicated cases, drainage may be required. Untreated infection can transmit to the brain.

The Respiratory System

The respiratory system is a common site for infection because it is constantly exposed to potential airborne pathogens due to its structure and function (see Figure 20-7). The upper respiratory tract is normally populated with indigenous microflora, but the lower respiratory tract is typically considered cleaner or sterile. Diseases affecting structures of the respiratory system may be viral, bacterial, or fungal and may be mild to life-threatening.

The Respiratory System Microbiome

Similar to the gastrointestinal system, the normal microbiome of the upper respiratory tract contains resident "friendly" microbes that compete with transient opportunistic pathogens for space and nutritional resources. Normal respiratory microflora includes certain species of *Staphylococcus*, *Neisseria*, *Streptococcus*, *Haemophilus*, and *Micrococcus*, as well as spirochetes and yeast.

The greater variety and numbers of pathogens include *Streptococcus pyogenes*, *Corynebacterium diphtheriae*, *Neisseria gonorrhoeae*, *Mycobacterium tuberculosis*, *Bordetella pertussis*, *Brucella* species, *Legionella* species, *Mycoplasma pneumoniae*, *Chlamydia* species, *Pneumocystis carinii*, and *Histoplasma capsulatum*. Viruses include respiratory syncytial virus (RSV), adenovirus, enterovirus, herpesvirus, influenza, parainfluenza, SARS-CoV-2 coronavirus and rhinoviruses.

Bacterial Infections of the Respiratory System

Infections of the upper respiratory tract include pharyngitis (inflammation of the throat), laryngitis, and tonsillitis. These infections tend to be from either bacterial or viral sources. Bacterial infections are typically caused by *S. pyogenes* (group A ß-hemolytic streptococci), which is why the term strep throat is used when referring to pharyngitis. The mucous membrane of the sinuses that communicate with the nasal cavity may become infected with *Streptococcus pneumoniae* or *Haemophilus influenzae*, resulting in sinusitis. Epiglottitis is a

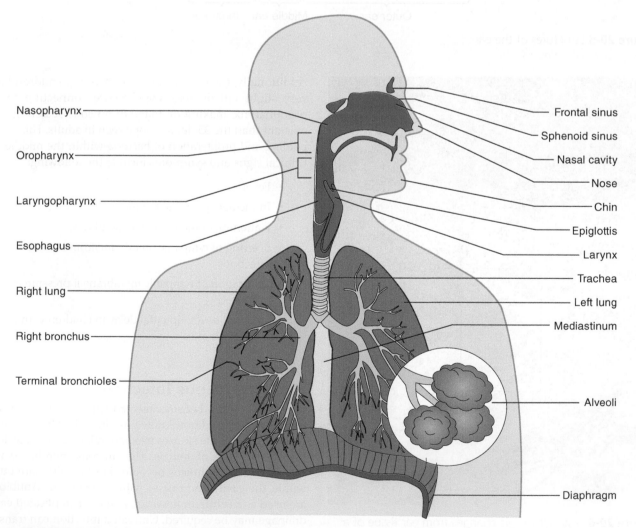

Figure 20-7 Structures of the respiratory system.

severe and dangerous infection of the epiglottis caused by *H. influenzae* that requires immediate treatment and endotracheal tube (ET) intubation due to respiratory obstruction.

Streptococcal Pharyngitis

The primary cause of streptococcal pharyngitis is *S. pyogenes*. The disease is an acute bacterial infection of the pharynx that results in fever and pain. The tonsils are often involved, with white patches on the surface epithelium (see Figure 20-8). The bacteria can travel to the middle ear, resulting in otitis media. If left untreated, the infection could lead to secondary complications of **rheumatic fever** or glomerulonephritis. The disease is transmitted from person to person by direct contact, aerosolized droplets, or in saliva.

Rheumatic fever is a sequela of only pharyngeal infections, but glomerulonephritis can follow pharyngeal or skin infections. Acute rheumatic fever can cause permanent damage to the heart valves, resulting in the need for heart valve replacement surgery (see Figure 20-9). Less than 1 percent of strep throat infections result in rheumatic fever but recurrences of rheumatic fever are common and may require prolonged or even life-long antibiotic therapy.

Acute glomerulonephritis results from the invasion of antigen–antibody–complement complexes on the kidney glomeruli. The occurrence of acute glomerulonephritis has decreased in the United States. Recurrences are rare and antibiotic therapy after the infection has been resolved is unnecessary.

The bacteria that cause pharyngitis are collected by standard throat swab and identified by laboratory culture grown on a blood agar plate, use of fluorescent antibody technique, or by demonstrated susceptibility to bacitracin disks. To expedite diagnosis, a rapid antigen detection test is performed by taking a throat swab and then utilizing an enzyme or acid technique to extract bacterial antigens that can be measured by various laboratory assays. It is relatively common for the rapid antigen detection test to provide a false-negative result for findings of *S. pyogenes*, therefore the recommendation is for standard throat cultures to be performed when a negative rapid antigen detection test result is obtained to definitively rule out infection.

Tuberculosis

Tuberculosis (TB) is an acute or chronic mycobacterial infection of the pulmonary (lung structures) tract. The pathogen is

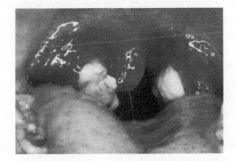

Figure 20-8 Streptococcal pharyngitis.

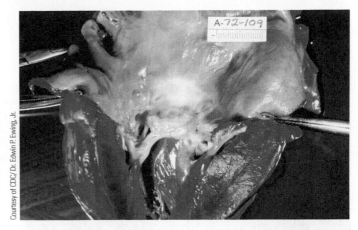

Courtesy of CDC/ Dr. Edwin P. Ewing, Jr.

Figure 20-9 Human heart with severe thickening of the mitral valve and chordae tendineae and left ventricular myocardial hypertrophy due to rheumatic heart disease.

Mycobacterium tuberculosis, a slow-growing Gram-positive bacillus that is highly resistant to environmental stresses. These bacteria can survive for weeks in sputum and are resistant to destruction by many antiseptics and disinfectants. TB is transmitted by inhaling aerosolized tubercle bacilli, although only a few survive to make it to the deeper bronchioles. The few that do are easily phagocytized by alveolar macrophages. If they manage to survive, they are protected from antibodies by the macrophages because they begin to multiply within them. The macrophages accumulate and form a protective wall that results in a lesion called a tubercle. The macrophages release toxins that accumulate and contribute to localized inflammation. The tubercle may become caseous (cheese-like). In this form the tubercle bacilli are dormant. If the tubercle heals, it calcifies (called Ghon complexes) and is clearly visible on chest x-ray.

If the tubercle liquefies instead of becoming caseous, it leads to a proliferation of the bacilli within an enlarged cavity around the tubercle. In this form, the bacilli begin growing outside of the macrophages. The liquid containing the bacilli becomes an aerosol, making the disease highly transmissible, and bacilli begin to spread from the lungs to the circulatory and lymphatic systems. Concerning trends in multidrug resistance of TB are discussed in detail in Chapter 14.

Diphtheria

Diphtheria is an acute respiratory disease that can cause myocardial and neural tissue damage. The disease is caused by *Corynebacterium diphtheriae*, which produces toxins that can lead to systemic infections. The disease is transmitted via aerosol droplets, direct contact, or fomites. It can also be transmitted through ingestion of contaminated food or drink. The bacteria produce a grayish necrotic exudate called a pseudomembrane that covers the larynx, pharynx, and tonsils and may obstruct the airway. The cervical lymph nodes are usually enlarged, giving the victim a "bull-neck" appearance (see Figure 20-10). Conjunctivitis and severe myocarditis may also develop from diphtheria infections. Diphtheria is also discussed in Chapter 14.

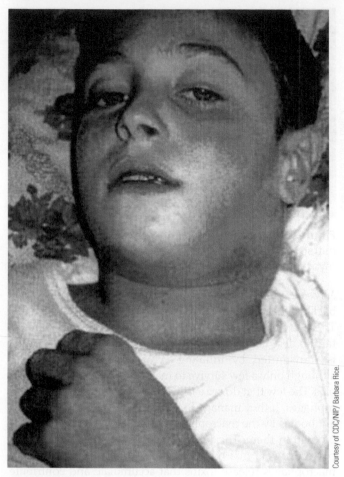

Courtesy of CDC/NIP/ Barbara Rice.

Figure 20-10 A 10-year-old child with a case of severe diphtheria.

Whooping Cough

Bordet and Gengou discovered *Bordetella pertussis* as the bacterial agent responsible for the disease pertussis, commonly called "whooping cough" in 1906. The disease is acquired by inhaling the cough droplets of an infected person and is highly transmissible. Prior to the development of a vaccine, the disease had devastating worldwide effects. In the United States the disease peaked in 1934, when 265,000 cases were reported and 5 out of every 1,000 children died. In China, pertussis is known as the "100-day cough" because it sometimes can last in excess of 10 to 12 weeks. The disease progresses through three stages:

- **Catarrhal stage:** Begins with non-specific cold-like symptoms that progress to a cough
- **Paroxysmal stage:** Frequent, violent coughing attacks that cause the patient to gasp for breath, resulting in the characteristic sound for which the disease received its name, whooping cough
- **Convalescent stage:** Resolution of symptoms and disease

As previously mentioned, the bacterial cells attach to the cilia of the respiratory tract, preventing movement and progressively destroying them, although the cells do not invade the tissues of the respiratory tract. This ciliary destruction prevents mucus that collects from being effectively expelled by the patient, adding to respiratory distress. As the patient attempts to cough up and expel the mucus build-up, the coughing spells become more violent. Infants younger than 1 year of age may not present with the characteristic cough but will experience respiratory distress requiring hospitalization and may die from the disease.

Complications that can occur during the second (paroxysmal) stage include broken ribs (especially in children) due to the violent nature of the coughs, inguinal hernia (primarily in males), rectal prolapse, and severe difficulties in breathing that require the patient to be placed on a ventilator. Otitis media can also occur in children as a secondary infection.

Bordetella parapertussis causes a milder form of whooping cough. It lacks the toxins of *B. pertussis*, reducing its virulence. *Bordetella bronchiseptica* is a pathogen of animals, causing what is commonly known as "kennel cough" in both dogs and cats. It rarely causes disease in humans; however, there have been documented cases of pneumonia infections in patients with HIV/AIDS or other immune disorders. The infection may be mistaken in these patients for *Pneumocystis* species. *Bordetella bronchiseptica* has also been occasionally reported in cases of respiratory and wound infections. It is easily recognized in the laboratory due to its motility, whereas the other two species are non-motile.

Diagnosis, Treatment, and Prevention A specimen for culture is obtained by inserting a polyester, nylon, or rayon swab on the end of a wire through the nose into the nasopharyngeal tract that is left in place while the patient coughs. Cotton swabs are not used because the fatty acids in the cotton fibers inhibit the growth of *Bordetella* species. A more recent method that has shown success is nasopharyngeal aspiration.

Time is a critical factor in treatment of those infected with pertussis. Clinical treatment recommendations are to initiate antibiotic therapy even prior to definitive confirmation of test results for infants and those whose clinical history is strongly suggestive of exposure to pertussis. Individuals who are infected are contagious from the onset of symptoms (catarrhal stage) through the end of the third week after onset of paroxysms (severe coughs). After that time, with or without antibiotic treatment, the patient ceases to be contagious, even if coughing continues. Antibiotic therapy given immediately will reduce the contagiousness status to 5 days after the start of treatment.

The CDC recommends that pregnant females should be vaccinated with the Tdap (tetanus, diphtheria, and pertussis) vaccine during each and every pregnancy (regardless of past vaccination frequency) at 27 to 36 weeks of gestation to maximize the maternal antibody production and transfer of passive immunity to the fetus. Post-partum vaccination is not recommended because it takes up to 2 weeks for antibodies to develop, and that leaves the neonate at risk for exposure to maternal infection. Only in cases of the mother having never been vaccinated previously is post-partum vaccination recommended.

In other age groups, it is theorized that immunity gained from vaccination lasts 4 to 20 years and declines over time.

Current recommendations by the CDC for vaccination are as follows:

- Infants and children: DTaP (diphtheria, tetanus toxoids, and acellular pertussis vaccine) for children at 2, 4, and 6 months, between 15 and 18 months, and between 4 and 6 years of age for a total of 5 doses
- Children 7 to 10 years: dose of Tdap only required if incompletely vaccinated with DTaP, per recommendations
- Ages 11 to 18: Tdap dose recommended preferably between 11 and 12 years of age; however, if not between those ages, then a booster dose should be given prior to age 18
- Adults older than age 19: Tdap if a recommended schedule has not been followed, then a booster dose is recommended as soon as possible, as is re-boosting every 10 years thereafter
- Healthcare workers (HCWs): blood titers may be drawn to assess immunity status or booster doses given, with priority placed on HCWs who work with infants younger than 12 months of age

There were 15,609 cases of whooping cough reported to the CDC in 2018, including cases reported in every state.

Outside of the United States, pertussis remains one of the leading causes of vaccine-preventable deaths. The 2018 WHO estimates showed that there were 151,074 cases reported globally. Other current reports show much higher estimates of 48.5 million cases with nearly 295,000 deaths annually, mainly in infants who are unvaccinated or not fully vaccinated.

Viral Infections of the Respiratory System

Viruses are responsible for many respiratory tract infections. One of the most common infections is what is called the common cold. Viruses of the upper respiratory tract trigger a flow of fluid from the nasopharynx that is full of viruses that are discharged into the air after a sneeze. These viruses are seldom life-threatening but can cause the infected person to feel quite ill for some time.

The Common Cold

Approximately half of all colds are caused by the rhinovirus, with the other half of colds caused by various other common viruses including non-COVID-19 coronaviruses. The rhinovirus alone has more than 100 serotypes, rendering a vaccine an impractical solution. Colds become fewer in number per year with age because the immune system is better able to prevent them. Children tend to have several colds every year. A cold is spread through aerosol droplets that contain large quantities of the virus that are expelled during sneezing. Viruses are also present on the hands of infected persons and are spread to others during physical contact.

The virus implants in the nasopharynx by attaching surface molecules firmly to host cells or their cilia or **microvilli**. This prevents them from being washed away by the same nasopharyngeal secretions they trigger. Cells infected with the viruses then spread to neighboring cells, and distant cells are reached by the secretions. If the viruses reach the middle ear, then otitis media may be the result. If the viruses invade the sinuses from the pharynx, then it may cause sinusitis.

Influenza

Commonly known as the "flu," influenza is a dangerous and common disease. It is characterized by fever, chills, cough, headache, and muscular pains. Many are killed every year by influenza, usually those who are immunosuppressed due to age or underlying diseases, such as pneumonia. The virus thrives during the coldest months of the year, primarily because people are inside more and transmission is easier in enclosed spaces.

The 1918 influenza pandemic was the most severe pandemic in the twentieth century. It was caused by an H1N1 virus with genes of an unidentified avian origin (see Figure 20-11). It is estimated that 500 million people were infected, representing about one-third of the world's population at that time. The global fatality rate was estimated at 50 million, with approximately 675,000 deaths in the United States. The influenza virus and other respiratory viruses are discussed in Chapter 8.

COVID-19

The 1918 flu pandemic was an almost unfathomable event for almost exactly a century, that is until the discovery of a

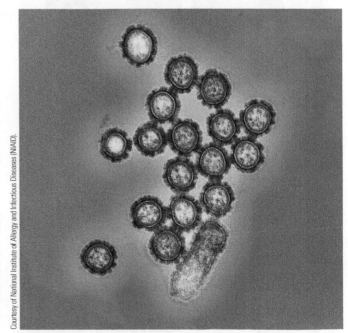

Figure 20-11 Digitally colorized TEM image of H1N1 influenza virus particles showing the surface proteins of the outer layers of the virus particles in black.

novel coronavirus designated as SARS-CoV-2 which is responsible for the respiratory disease COVID-19 so named because CO stands for corona, VI for virus, and D for disease, and first recognized in late 2019. The world was caught off guard by the incredible rate of disease transmission which overwhelmed the healthcare systems of countries around the world. At the start of 2022, there were over 300 million cases of COVID-19 and nearly 5.5 million reported deaths globally, although these numbers may be underreported. In the United States, there were approximately 60 million cases reported and over 800,000 deaths.

The multiple mutations of the original virus into even more transmissible forms such as the delta and omicron variants has contributed to the ongoing progression of the disease, despite availability of effective vaccines. Compounding the basic characteristics of transmissibility and virulence of the new disease have been the public health challenges of widespread misinformation, vaccine hesitancy, pandemic fatigue of the public, and ineffective disaster preparations prior to the need for them. There will be ongoing research studies and refinement of public health protocols in the coming years following the lessons learned from the COVID-19 pandemic and much more information will be available as researchers gather more data and develop strategies for prevention. In the meantime, the known preventative measures of vaccination, wearing masks, proper hand and cough hygiene, and social distancing when possible are simple steps toward protecting everyone at risk (see Figure 20-12).

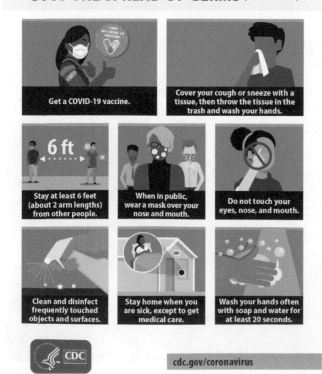

Figure 20-12 Stop the spread of germs—COVID-19

Fungal Infections of the Respiratory System

Because fungi produce airborne spores that can be inhaled, fungal respiratory infections are not uncommon. **Histoplasmosis** is a fungal disease that closely resembles TB, although the initial symptoms resemble a mild respiratory illness. The fungi can spread via lymph and blood to other organs, leaving lesions that can be detected on x-ray (see Figure 20-13). These lesions which may be diffuse and have a "snowstorm" pattern, may be mistaken initially for carcinoma of the lungs. The organism responsible is *Histoplasma capsulatum*, which has a yeast-like morphology in tissue growth and thrives within macrophages. The transmission is through exposure to soil containing bird and bat droppings that provide a nitrogen source for fungal growth. The spores become airborne and are inhaled into the lungs of humans. Bats carry the fungus and spread it to new sites when dropping their feces.

Coccidioidomycosis is a pulmonary fungal disease caused by *Coccidioides immitis*. The disease, also known as Valley Fever, is endemic in the American Southwest and northern Mexico, where the soil is ideal for fungal growth. The organism creates filaments in soil that reproduce through the formation of **arthrospores**, which are carried by the wind to new infection sites. Within tissues, the organism constructs a thick-walled lesion filled with spores that can cause aggressive skin and soft tissue infections, and the identification of these lesions in tissue is the best method for diagnosis (see Figure 20-14). Respiratory symptoms closely resemble TB.

Blastomycosis is caused by the fungus *Blastomyces dermatitidis* and is a disease seen primarily in the Ohio and Mississippi River valleys and the Great Lakes region. Most infections are relatively asymptomatic, but a few deaths occur each year. The disease is characterized by an infection within the lungs that may spread to the bones, joints, central nervous system, or skin, causing cutaneous ulcers that lead to tissue destruction in those with weakened immune systems (see Figure 20-15).

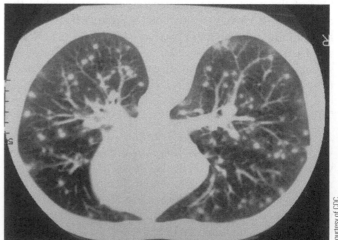

Figure 20-13 CT scan of the thoracic cavity showing the classic "snowstorm" appearance of a fungal histoplasmosis infection in both lungs due to *Histoplasma capsulatum*.

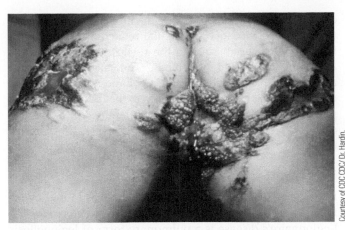

Figure 20-14 Buttocks and posterior upper thighs with large inflammatory cutaneous nodular and papular lesions from coccidioidomycosis, a fungal infection due to *Coccidioides*.

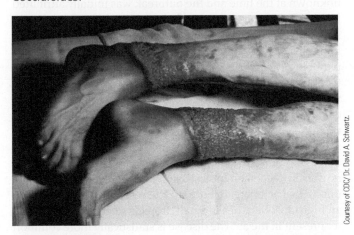

Figure 20-15 Blastomycosis caused by the fungal organism *Blastomyces dermatitidis* in lower extremities of a patient undergoing radiation therapy for unknown reason.

Pneumonia

Pneumonia is an acute infection of lung tissues and alveolar spaces that is caused by a variety of pathogens including bacteria, fungi, protozoa, and viruses. Pneumonias are named for the portion of the respiratory tract that they infect; for example, bronchopneumonia is named for the bronchi and alveoli that are affected. Pneumonia is often a secondary bacterial infection that results from a primary viral infection. Symptoms include fever, cough, acute chest pain, and respiratory distress.

Bacterial pneumonia is most often caused by *Streptococcus pneumoniae*, an organism that forms cell pairs with a thick capsule. This type of pneumonia is referred to as pneumococcal pneumonia and involves both the bronchi and the alveoli. Patients often develop pleurisy (inflammation of the pleurae) and a severe stabbing pain in the chest. The CDC estimates that in the United States 150,000 hospitalizations annually are a result of pneumococcal pneumonia and in 25–30 percent of

those infections, patients develop systemic bacteremia that leads to death in up to 7 percent of those cases. Pneumococcal pneumonia can also lead to empyema, pericarditis, and respiratory failure, more commonly in older adults.

The inflammatory response produces the clinical symptoms of pneumococcal pneumonia. When the chest region is x-rayed or tapped, it looks and sounds like a solid organ. The classic sign of labored breathing is due to this fluid accumulation. The body's natural inflammatory response is not effective in stopping the infection. Because the bacterial cell wall is surrounded by a thick polysaccharide capsule, it is highly resistant to phagocytosis. The pneumococci continue to rapidly multiply and may enter the chest wall lymph nodes or vascular system.

Children, older adults, and patients who are immunocompromised are at greater risk for progression of the disease and worsening symptoms, even when treated, and therefore have the highest mortality rate. Patients who do not have secondary processes usually recover with the administration of antibiotics and persistence of their own immune defenses. Approximately 6 to 10 days into the course of the illness, the fever "breaks," which is an indication of the infection being resolved.

Infection with *S. pneumoniae* does not typically cause permanent damage of the lung. This is another distinguishing feature of the infection; as other types of bacterial pneumonia often damage the lungs.

The spleen also plays an important role in the recovery process. It serves as a filter in removing pneumococci from the bloodstream, which allows the splenic macrophages to process pneumococcal antigens. The next physiologic response is the signal to splenic lymphocytes to produce specific antibodies. Individuals having undergone splenectomy are more susceptible to pneumococcal sepsis. After recovery, patients develop permanent immunity to that particular pneumococcal serotype; however, because there are more than 80 pneumococcal serotypes, subsequent pneumococcal infections can still occur.

Mycoplasmal pneumonia is caused by *Mycoplasma pneumoniae*, an organism that does not have a cell wall and therefore does not grow under the same conditions as other pneumonia-causing bacterial species and is frequently misidentified as viral. This type of pneumonia is commonly seen in young adults and children and is often referred to as "walking pneumonia" because the symptoms are relatively mild.

Klebsiella pneumoniae

Klebsiella pneumoniae is the cause of numerous bacterial pneumonias in the United States whether healthcare-associated or community-acquired. *Klebsiella pneumoniae* tends to affect persons who already have a comorbid disease such as diabetes, alcohol use disorder, or chronic pulmonary disease, and rarely affects healthy individuals. Older adults are prone to developing a serious complication referred to as hemorrhagic necrotizing consolidation of the lungs, also called lobar pneumonia. The bacterial cells are responsible for the necrotic destruction of **alveoli,** abscess formation in the lung, and production of sputum that is thick and red in appearance due to the presence of blood. The sputum is commonly referred to as "currant jelly" sputum because of its dark red appearance.

The bacterial cells are surrounded by a gelatinous capsule that inhibits phagocytosis. If not quickly and aggressively treated, the infection is often fatal. *Klebsiella pneumoniae* can also cause milder respiratory tract infections such as bronchitis or bronchopneumonia. Chest x-rays will reveal lung abscesses in advanced cases. Pus may also surround the lung, a condition called empyema, which irritates lung tissue and causes the formation of scar tissue (see Figure 20-16).

Individuals with an alcohol use disorder are the main population at risk in *K. pneumoniae*, and they constitute approximately 65 percent of people affected by this disease. Mortality rates may be as high as 50 percent and approach 100 percent in persons that also develop bacteremia. *Klebsiella pneumoniae* is highly resistant to antibiotics. The bacterium's drug resistance is attributable to acquisition of plasmids as well as changes to its chromosomal gene structure.

Pseudomonas aeruginosa Pneumonia

Primary pneumonia caused by *P. aeruginosa* most often occurs in patients who already have a debilitating condition such as a pulmonary disease or congestive heart failure. **Cystic fibrosis**, a generalized hereditary disorder that causes an accumulation of thick and tenacious mucus that places individuals at greater risk for infections with *P. aeruginosa*. The microbial

cells colonize the respiratory tract, beginning as an inflammatory response with a consequential reduction in pulmonary function. Once established in the tissues, the bacterial cells are almost impossible to eliminate. The cells form a biofilm around multiple cells creating microcolonies within the bronchi thereby making patients with cystic fibrosis prone to pneumonia and tracheobronchitis (inflammation of the trachea and bronchi), which complicate the disease and contribute to the disease's high mortality rate.

Legionellosis

Legionellosis is an acute bacterial pneumonia caused by infection with *Legionella* species, especially *Legionella pneumophila*. Legionnaire's disease is a pulmonary form of legionellosis that acquired its name when an outbreak occurred during an American Legion convention in Philadelphia in 1976. The aerobic Gram-negative bacillus that caused the outbreak was unknown at the time and the outbreak was initially attributed to a virus. The organism has been isolated in showerheads, sink faucets, hot tubs, hot water tanks and heaters, decorative fountains, central air cooling systems, and complex building plumbing systems. *Legionella* have been found in hospital water lines, prompting hospital facilities engineers to control the water temperature of the hot water lines to prevent bacterial contamination. The bacillus is resistant to low levels of chlorine. Water which is kept or used at cooler temperatures should be routinely tested for bacteria.

Symptoms are similar to other forms of pneumonia, but no person-to-person transmission has been documented. The infectious bacteria gain entry to the respiratory system when an individual breathes in small droplets of contaminated water present in the air. The disease is statistically more common in older males with a past history of or who are currently tobacco users or have an alcohol use disorder. In severe cases of legionellosis, secondary scarring of the lung tissue may remain after the primary infection has resolved.

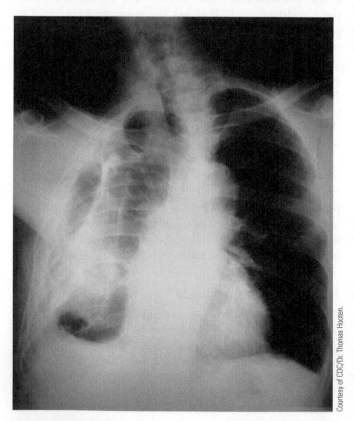

Courtesy of CDC/Dr. Thomas Hooten.

Figure 20-16 This AP chest x-ray revealed the presence of a right fibrothorax due to a previous empyema.

MICRO NOTES

"I've been itching to tell you..."

Have you ever thought about how many expressions we use actually refer to signs and symptoms of disease? "Cough it up." "Spit it out." We use these when we want someone to tell the truth. "That's nothing to sneeze at." This refers to something substantial that should be acknowledged. "Your smile is contagious." That's a good thing. "It gave me the chills." Maybe not a good thing. "They were working at a feverish pace." That would depend on what they're working on. "Don't be a snotty brat." Well, if you're talking to a 2-year-old, they probably can't help it. "I got all choked up." Happy, proud, sad, or surprised? Maybe the next time you say or hear these types of phrases, it'll make you chuckle a little. Just be sure to explain why.

Under the Microscope

Jo, a CST who works in a busy labor and delivery (L&D) department woke up in the middle of the night with a cough, mild difficulty breathing, low-grade fever and redness in the right eye. The schedule for the next day is very busy and they are short-staffed due to illnesses in co-workers. Jo has to make a decision whether to go to work or call the night supervisor and explain the situation.

1. What are possible reasons Jo might be experiencing the signs and symptoms described?

2. Which general groups of pathogens might cause disease in the eyes, ears, or respiratory system?

3. Who might Jo put at risk of transmission of infection by deciding to go into work because of the staffing and scheduling issues?

4. What types of comorbid conditions could complicate Jo's current condition if not appropriately treated?

5. Which types of preventative measures could be taken by anyone in a healthcare facility to mitigate the risk of transmission of infections related to the eyes, ears, or respiratory system?

CHAPTER 21

Control of Microbial Growth

Learning Objectives

After completing the study of this chapter, you will be able to:

1. Define key terms.
2. Discuss the three lines of defense of the human body.
3. Compare and contrast innate, adaptive, and herd immunity.
4. Compare and contrast active and passive immunity.
5. Describe disinfection, decontamination, and sterilization of patient care items.
6. Apply critical thinking skills in relating chapter material to the surgical environment of care or broader global community.

Key Terms

Abstinence

Aeration

Agammaglobulinemia

Anaphylaxis

Antigenic determinants

Aseptic techniques

Attenuated

Bioburden

Biological indicator

Bronchospasm

Chemical indicator/ integrators

Chemotaxis

Complement cascade

Decontamination

Dialysis

Disinfection

Electrosurgical smoke plume

Epinephrine

Erythroblastosis fetalis

Ethylene oxide

Exophthalmos

Free radicals

Glutaraldehyde

Humoral

Hydrogen peroxide

Hyperthyroidism

Hypovolemia

Immunoglobulins

Infrastructure

Interleukins

Invaginates

Irreducible minimum

Kinins

Laryngospasm

Lumen

Lymphokines

Mast cells

Myeloid progenitor stem cells

Peracetic acid

Phagolysosome

Phototherapy

Plasma

Prostaglandins

Pyrogen

Radiofrequency

Sterilization

Sub-pathogenic

The Big Picture

I t is probably obvious to you at this point that escaping contact with microbes is an impossible task. The fact is that humans could not survive without microbes; however, they are also capable of causing great harm and suffering. Controlling the growth and spread of microbes to prevent disease is the ultimate goal. During your examination of the topics in this chapter, consider the following:

1. What are the innate or non-specific defense mechanisms used by the human body to prevent infection by pathogens?

2. What is the impact of immune system malfunction or deficiency on overall human health?

3. How can individuals in a neighborhood or healthcare community contribute to the general health and welfare of their members by following public health protocols and recommendations?

4. How are potentially pathogenic microbes reduced or eliminated in the perioperative and other healthcare settings?

Clinical Significance Topic

Decontamination, disinfection, and sterilization are rarely favorite topics of surgical technology students, or even some instructors. However tedious the material may seem, the truth is that failures of these processes are often implicated in root cause analyses of incidents of surgical site infections (SSIs) or devastating healthcare-associated infections (HAIs) such as carbapenem-resistant *Enterococcus* (CRE), methicillin-resistant *Staphylococcus aureus* (MRSA), vancomycin-resistant *Enterococcus* (VRE), or *Clostridioides difficile* (C. diff). Eliminating HAIs and assuring that surgical instruments are properly disinfected or sterilized prior to use on patients are the responsibilities of everyone working in the surgical environment of care. Without taking the time to understand the mechanisms of infection and transmission, mistakes will be made routinely and remain unrecognized until it is too late. Surgical technologists must be vigilant in following infection control practices and in maintaining the highest levels of performance of aseptic and sterile techniques, even if studying the basics isn't very "flashy."

Control of Microbial Growth

There are numerous ways in which pathogenic microbes can be managed or controlled. As previous chapters have discussed, there are nearly unlimited microorganisms that outnumber humans many times over. The advantage we have is our ability to study them and learn how they impact us and make choices about how to proceed. The majority of microbes are harmless to humans. Many species live nearly everywhere around us. They only become pathogenic in certain situations, and often only if we let down our guard. Our bodies have learned how to coexist with many microbes or realized how to use natural lines of defense against those microscopic invaders able to harm us. Chapter 9 discusses methods of microbial disease transmission and the human body's responses, some of which are briefly reviewed in this chapter.

Surgical technologists learn specific ways to reduce the microbial populations to irreducible numbers for protection of the patients undergoing invasive surgical interventions. This chapter explores the natural methods of controlling or preventing disease and infection as well as the physical, chemical, and thermal methods of disinfection, decontamination, and sterilization.

The Three Lines of Defense

The body is equipped with three basic lines of defense:

- The structural design of the human body itself: the skin and mucous membranes

- Circulatory and chemical responses

- Immunity: active or passive, innate (natural), or adaptive (acquired)

First Line of Defense: The Human Body

The first line of defense of the body includes the external and internal barriers presented by the skin, mucous membranes, and specialized secretions. These barriers are part of the innate (natural, non-specific) immune system, which is a collection of protective mechanisms and responses with which humans are born. The uninjured, intact skin prevents microbes from entering the body. When the skin is damaged, as it is when the surgeon makes the initial skin incision for a procedure, it immediately creates an opening for the invasion of microbes such as *Staphylococcus aureus* that is a part of our normal skin microflora. Burns, lacerations, and abrasions are other examples of non-intact skin that allow microbes to penetrate the body.

The skin further aids the body by secreting lactic acid from the sweat glands and fatty acids from the sebaceous glands that either kill or inhibit the growth of pathogenic bacteria. The low-pH environment of the skin also inhibits the growth of the microbes.

Mucous membranes and cilia line the nose, nasal passages, trachea, and bronchi. The cilia trap inhaled dust, dirt, and pathogens. They move back and forth in a rhythmic movement, sweeping the trapped material forward into the throat, where an individual eliminates the material by sneezing, coughing it up, or swallowing it. In addition, some Gram-positive bacteria are killed by the lysozymes of the nasal secretions, tears, and saliva.

The digestive secretions in the intestine and stomach kill microbes. The secretions of the stomach are highly acidic and those of the intestine are alkaline. The mucous secretions of the intestinal tract help in trapping the pathogens, which then present an easier target for the phagocytes and enzymes. The physiological actions of peristalsis and defecation also remove pathogens from the intestinal tract.

The genitourinary tract is protected from harmful pathogens because of the frequent flushing by urination and vaginal mucosal secretions in females.

Second Line of Defense: Blood and Chemicals

As pathogens penetrate the body's first line of defense, they encounter the second line of defense: the elements found in the circulatory system, including phagocytes, complement and other blood proteins, interferon, fever production, iron balance, and the body's response to injury or infection called the inflammatory response. These protective responses and mechanisms discussed in more detail in Chapter 9 are also part of the innate immune system and briefly reviewed in this section.

Phagocytes

Phagocytosis, the engulfing of bacteria and debris, is necessary in the fight against foreign invaders, but the process also routinely removes dead blood cells and other debris, such as unused cellular secretions. Leukocytes, also called white blood cells, consist of basophils, eosinophils, lymphocytes, monocytes, and neutrophils which are separated into two categories: granulocytes (neutrophils, eosinophils, and basophils) and agranulocytes (monocytes and lymphocytes).

All phagocytes are leukocytes, but not all leukocytes are phagocytes (see Figure 21-1). Phagocytes are the garbage collectors of the human body. The specific phagocytic cells are granulocytes and macrophages. Monocytes (part of agranulocytes) mature into macrophages in body tissues. Granulocytes include neutrophils and eosinophils. Neutrophils are the most abundant and efficient phagocytes. Eosinophils play a more efficient phagocytic role during the allergic response (see Table 21-1).

Phagocytosis is described as a movement in which the phagocyte approaches, surrounds, and engulfs the bacterium for digestion and destruction in the following steps:

1. The phagocyte approaches a bacterium. The process of the phagocyte's attraction to the bacterium is called **chemotaxis**. The chemical attraction is not fully understood; however, it is known to be the result of **lymphokines** that are produced by T-lymphocytes and the activation of complement.
2. The bacterium attaches to the leukocyte.
3. The phagocytic membrane indents or **invaginates**. Two pseudopods extend from the leukocyte to surround the bacterium. The pseudopods entrap the bacterium, forming a vacuole called a phagosome.
4. Within the leukocyte, the organelle called the lysosome that contains digestive enzymes attaches to the phagosome to form a **phagolysosome**.
5. Inside the phagolysosome, the bacterium is quickly destroyed. The digestive process is called degranulation because the granules in the granulocytes are depleted and subsequently decrease in number (see Figure 21-2).

Fixed phagocytes are cells that are attached to the liver, bone marrow, spleen, linings of the blood vessels and intestinal tract, and lymph nodes. The reticuloendothelial system (RES) is composed of these tissues. The function of the lymph nodes is to remove microbes from the lymph before they

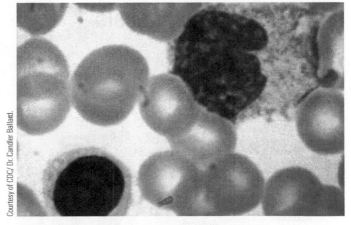

Courtesy of CDC/ Dr. Candler Ballard.

Figure 21-1 Photomicrograph of two different types of WBCs (leukocytes), the larger in the upper right is a monocyte (macrophage) and in the lower left was a lymphocyte.

Table 21-1 Cellular Components of the Blood

Medical Term	Common Term
Erythrocytes	Red blood cells
Thrombocytes	Platelets
Leukocytes	White blood cells
Granulocytes	
Basophils	
Eosinophils	
Neutrophils	
Monocytes that differentiate into macrophages	
Lymphocytes	
B cells	
T cells	
Helper T cells	
Suppressor T cells	
Cytotoxic T cells	
Delayed-hypersensitivity T cells	

reach the major lymph ducts that empty into the bloodstream. If the bacteria are able to escape past the lymph nodes, then the phagocytes of the spleen, liver, and bone marrow assist in filtering out the invaders.

Blood Proteins

Complement is a group of proteins that are found in the plasma and are inactive until needed. Complement is considered a second line of defense and is non-specific because it binds to many variations of antigen–antibody complexes. Complement facilitates the lysis of bacterial cells through the

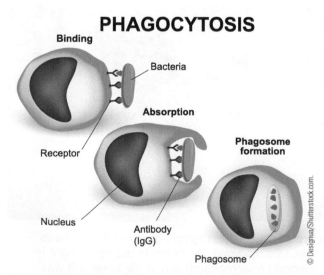

PHAGOCYTOSIS

Figure 21-2 Phagocytosis.

process called the **complement cascade**. The sequence causes an accumulation of fluid that continues until the lysis of the cell membrane occurs and the cell ruptures.

Complement is activated by substances present on the surface of the pathogen that trigger the complement proteins to respond and coat the pathogen to enhance phagocytosis. Antibodies are not required for the initiation of the response. This immediate activation is part of the innate or natural immune response.

Prostaglandins are unsaturated fatty acids that have potent effects in low concentrations. The prostaglandins, including prostacyclin, have a variety of effects to include:

- being potent inhibitors of platelet aggregation.
- controlling the immune response and inflammation.
- increasing capillary permeability.
- being active in the autoimmune response.
- pain production.
- treatment of gastric hyperacidity and asthma.

Interleukins and Interferons

Interleukins are a group of polypeptides produced primarily by T-cells or macrophages. There are several types of interleukins, and each has complex biochemical actions. Most interleukins direct other cells to divide and differentiate. The receptors on cells are specific for the interleukin that attaches to the cell. IL-1 through IL-4 are the interleukins involved in the immune response. Their functions are as follows:

- IL-1: This interleukin has numerous immune functions, including activating resting T-cells, macrophages, and endothelial cells; stimulating the synthesis of lymphokines; and aiding in the inflammatory response. IL-1 is also known as an endogenous **pyrogen.**

- IL-2: Initiates the proliferation of active T-cells. IL-2 is used in the laboratory to grow T-cell clones.

- IL-3: Supports the growth of the bone marrow stem cells and is a growth factor for **mast cells**.

- IL-4: Growth factor for active B-cells, non-activated T-cells, and mast cells.

The last secretion is β-lysin, another polypeptide that is released from platelets during an infection. It destroys Gram-positive bacteria by causing lysis of their plasma membranes. The substance is also located inside phagocytes and aids in their digestion of microbes.

Interferons are proteins produced when leukocytes, T-lymphocytes, and fibroblasts are infected. They inhibit or "interfere" with viral replication within infected cells.

Fever

Fever is a non-specific, systemic host defense initiated by the hypothalamus of the brain to elevate the body's temperature. Many pathogens produce pyrogenic secretions that trigger fever.

The increase in body temperature produces the following reactions:

- Stimulation of the production of IL-1
- Stimulation of leukocytes to migrate to the area of infection and attack pathogens
- Reduction of the availability of iron in the plasma, limiting growth of pathogenic bacteria that require iron for synthesis of toxins

Inflammatory Response

The human body responds to injury, bacterial toxins, and pathogens by initiating an inflammatory response. The inflammatory process is marked by the four classic signs of the battle occurring between the body and pathogens: swelling (edema), redness (blood flow to the area), heat, and pain. The formation of pus is also a sign of the process. A synopsis of the inflammatory process is as follows:

1. There is an injury and the skin is penetrated.

2. Injured cells, mast cells, platelets, and basophils release the chemicals: histamine, bradykinin, heparin, and other **kinins** to increase the permeability of the capillaries and venules and to prevent blood clotting. They also promote vasodilation.

3. The vasodilation and increased permeability allow more blood to enter the area. The blood carries the needed clotting agents and leukocytes for phagocytosis and antibody production.

4. Macrophages are attracted by chemotaxis to the secretions of the damaged cells.

5. Edema results from the collection of fluid, referred to as inflammatory exudate. If the exudate is of a greenish-yellow color, it is called purulent exudate or pus (see Figure 21-3).

6. Erythrocytes collect in the region, producing redness.

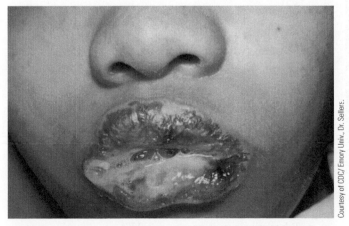

Figure 21-3 Severe erythematous lesions of the mouth and lips from erythema multiforme, which had become pustular in nature.

Courtesy of CDC/ Emory Univ., Dr. Sellers.

7. The cellular activities associated with destruction of microbes, dead cells, and toxins produce heat and fever.

8. The pain is the result of damage to nerve fibers sustained from the initial injury, irritation by toxins, or the edema that places pressure on the nerve endings.

9. When the body wins the battle, the inflammatory response ends.

10. Phagocytes continue to clean the area by engulfing the leftover debris.

11. Cells repair the damaged tissue so it can return to normal functioning.

Third Line of Defense: Immunity

The third line of defense is immunity, defined as the resistance to an infection or disease brought about by production of specific antibodies that protect against pathogens responsible for the initial infection or disease.

Adaptive Immunity

In the adaptive or acquired immune response, antibodies are produced by lymphocytes that bind with microbes to inactivate and destroy them. These **humoral** antibodies are found in the lymph fluid, plasma, and other body secretions. The antibodies are stimulated to form due to the presence of specific pathogens. Two primary types of acquired immunity are adaptive acquired immunity also known as active adaptive immunity and passive adaptive immunity.

Active Adaptive Immunity Individuals who have had a specific infection have partial or total resistance to reinfection by that specific microbial pathogen. The antibodies are produced by the stimulated lymphocytes, and this is referred to as natural active adaptive immunity. Resistance to the disease may be permanent, as is the case with the mumps or measles, or may be temporary, as with influenza. There is no immunity gained against reinfection by some diseases, such as tuberculosis or gonorrhea.

Artificial active adaptive immunity is the second type of actively acquired immunity, and it is gained by vaccination. The vaccine contains a sufficient number of pathogens or their markers to cause the person to form antibodies against that particular pathogen.

Vaccines have traditionally been made from inactivated, **attenuated** living pathogens, or from the toxins they secrete. Vaccines created from living microbes are the most effective but must be prepared from a harmless microbe that is closely related to the pathogen or weakened pathogens that have been genetically modified to render them non-pathogenic. This laboratory process of weakening pathogens is called attenuation. Pasteur developed the attenuated vaccine for rabies, and Sabin developed the attenuated oral vaccine for polio.

Smallpox is a serious disease and deadly disease that may have been present in the human population for over

3,000 years. A vigorous global eradication program declared smallpox eradicated from the world in 1980, therefore vaccination of the general public is not recommended. Due to the potential for use of the variola virus to be used for bioterrorism, there are government stockpiles of the smallpox vaccine in the U.S. to vaccinate anyone who had been exposed if a smallpox outbreak were to occur.

The smallpox vaccine is a weakened live vaccine because it is derived from the cowpox virus (vaccinia) that usually causes a mild infection in humans. In some people, the reaction to the live virus can cause serious to life-threatening reactions. Development of a serious rash caused by widespread skin infection known as eczema vaccinatum can occur mostly in individuals with pre-existing eczema or atopic dermatitis. These at-risk individuals may simply come in contact with the inoculated area of a vaccinated person and contract the vaccinia virus (see Figure 21-4).

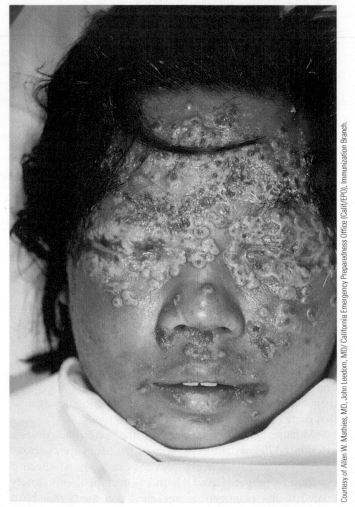

Courtesy of Allen W. Mathies, MD, John Leedom, MD/ California Emergency Preparedness Office (Calif/EPO), Immunization Branch.

Figure 21-4 A 28-year-old female with inactive atopic dermatitis who developed eczema vaccinatum after acquiring the vaccinia virus from her smallpox-vaccinated child. She was given vaccinia immune globulin and other medications resulting in healed lesions without scarring or lasting ocular damage.

Dead pathogens that have been killed by chemicals or heat are more commonly used to make vaccines. They can be manufactured faster and more easily; however, they are less effective when compared to live vaccines and they produce a shorter period of immunity. Vaccines produced in this manner are used to vaccinate against whooping cough, cholera, Rocky Mountain spotted fever, plague, and many types of respiratory diseases.

A third type of vaccine, specifically used to prevent diphtheria and tetanus is the toxoid vaccine. Toxoid vaccine is prepared from exotoxins that are inactivated by chemicals or heat. The vaccine is injected to cause the formation of antibodies that neutralize the exotoxins secreted by some pathogens. A serum that contains specific antibodies is called an antiserum. An antiserum that contains antibodies against toxoids is called an antitoxin.

The newest form of vaccine that was developed and used in response to the COVID-19 pandemic is messenger RNA or mRNA vaccines. This new type of vaccine teaches our cells how to make a protein or a specific portion of a protein that then triggers an immune response from our bodies. The antibodies created as part of that immune response to the protein are what provide protection from infection if the real virus gains entry, unlike the other vaccines discussed that rely on a weakened or inactivated pathogen introduced into the body.

The following is a list of vaccines available in the United States for routine childhood and adult immunizations, for travelers to foreign countries where endemic disease may be present, and for pre-exposure or post-exposure to certain pathogens:

- Chickenpox (Varicella)
- COVID-19
- Diphtheria
- Hepatitis A and Hepatitis B viruses
- Hib (*Haemophilus influenzae* **type B**)
- HPV (Human papillomavirus)
- Influenza (flu)
- Measles
- Meningococcal meningitis
- Mumps
- Pertussis (whooping cough)
- Pneumococcal meningitis
- Polio
- Rabies
- Rotavirus
- Rubella (German measles)
- Shingles (Varicella zoster)
- Smallpox (vaccinia virus, post-exposure only)
- Tetanus (lockjaw)
- Tuberculosis (not common in US)
- Typhoid fever
- Yellow fever

Passive Adaptive Immunity Passive adaptive immunity differs from active immunity in that antibodies formed in one individual are transferred to another. Because the recipient did not produce the antibodies, the immunity is temporary. Passive adaptive immunity has two subcategories: natural passive adaptive immunity and artificial passive adaptive immunity.

In natural passive adaptive immunity, antibodies present in the bloodstream of a pregnant female cross the placenta to reach the fetus. Additionally, colostrum, the precursor to breast milk, contains maternal antibodies that are passed on to the infant. Artificial passive adaptive immunity is created by transferring antibodies from an immune person to a susceptible person. During the Ebola epidemic in 2014, plasma from convalescent (recovering) patients was administered to others in an attempt to expedite the immune response, if not to fully confer artificial passive adaptive immunity. In 2021, the FDA issued new recommendations to healthcare providers and investigators on the use of COVID-19 convalescent plasma from donors who had recovered from infection by the SARS-CoV-2 virus. The process was expedited through an emergency use authorization (EUA) order and investigational new drug (IND) guidance during the public health emergency created by the global pandemic.

Antigens and Antibodies

An antigen is any foreign substance that enters the body and stimulates the production of antibodies. Antigens are also referred to as immunogens and the response they initiate is called immunogenic. Antigens can be formed from many types of biochemical substances, but the best known types are foreign protein antigens. Antigens have one or more sites called **antigenic determinants** to which antibodies or lymphocytes can bind. Antigens are foreign substances that the body does not recognize as being part of itself, stimulating the production of antibodies.

The mechanism used by the body to recognize "self" is a group of proteins in the major histocompatibility complex (MHC), which is produced by the body's own genes. Nearly all human cells have proteins that are called human leukocyte antigens (HLA). When a foreign antigen enters the body, it is perceived as "non-self" and the immune complex initiates an immediate response.

Antibodies are glycoproteins produced by B-lymphocytes (B-cells). Antibodies bind to the receptor site of the specific antigen that stimulated their production. A bacterium has several antigenic determinant sites on its cell membrane, cell wall, capsule, and flagella that stimulate the production of the antibodies.

Antibodies are placed in a class of proteins called **immunoglobulins** (Ig). The term antibody is used to refer to the specific type of immunoglobulin involved in the immune response. Immunoglobulins are also found in lymph fluid, colostrum, tears, and saliva. The type and number of antibodies produced in reaction to the presence of antigens is dependent on the:

- Site of antigen stimulus
- Number of antigens
- Type of antigen and its actions
- Number of times an individual is exposed to the antigen

After the individual has been exposed to the antigen, there is a delayed response in the production of antibodies called the lag phase. During the lag phase, the antigen is involved with macrophages, T-cells, and B-cells. Some antigens require only B-cells (see Figure 21-5).

Eventually B-cells develop into larger plasma cells that can produce antibodies by protein synthesis. This first step of the immune response is called the primary response. When the number of antigens declines, the number of antibodies in the bloodstream also declines as the plasma cells die. Other B-cells become memory cells that can be stimulated to produce antibodies quickly when the body is exposed to the same antigen in future exposures. The production of antibodies following subsequent exposures to the antigen is called the secondary response. This is why blood titer counts are performed to measure the concentration of antibodies present and why booster shots are given to return the antibody concentrations to the level of the secondary response. Protection against the hepatitis B virus (HBV) for surgical personnel is achieved by the three-shot HBV series and have titer counts, with booster shots performed if indicated. Another option is the newer two-shot Heplisav-B® (HepB-CpG) vaccine for incompletely-vaccinated or previously unvaccinated adults 18 years of age and older with a specific risk for infection, or who lack a risk factor but want protection. HBV vaccination is required in most institutions for all healthcare personnel and surgical technology or other allied health students in clinical practice.

Persons may be born with an inherited gene that leaves them without the ability to produce antibodies so have no gammaglobulin in their blood. This condition is called **agammaglobulinemia**. Others with very low levels of antibody production have hypogammaglobulinemia. They are both susceptible to a wide variety of infections, any of which can prove fatal (see Figure 21-6). One surgically successful treatment for these genetic conditions is a bone marrow transplant. The precursor leukocytes transferred to the patient become lymphocytes that eventually implant in the lymph nodes. These become capable of being stimulated by antigens to produce antibodies.

Patients scheduled for an organ transplant procedure receive immunosuppressive drug therapy to reduce the potential for organ rejection. One of the most devastating immunosuppressive diseases is HIV infection, which destroys the helper T-cells that are required for the processing of T-dependent antigens and are also important in the cell-mediated responses. These individuals are at risk for numerous secondary infections, some of which are otherwise uncommon or rare in humans.

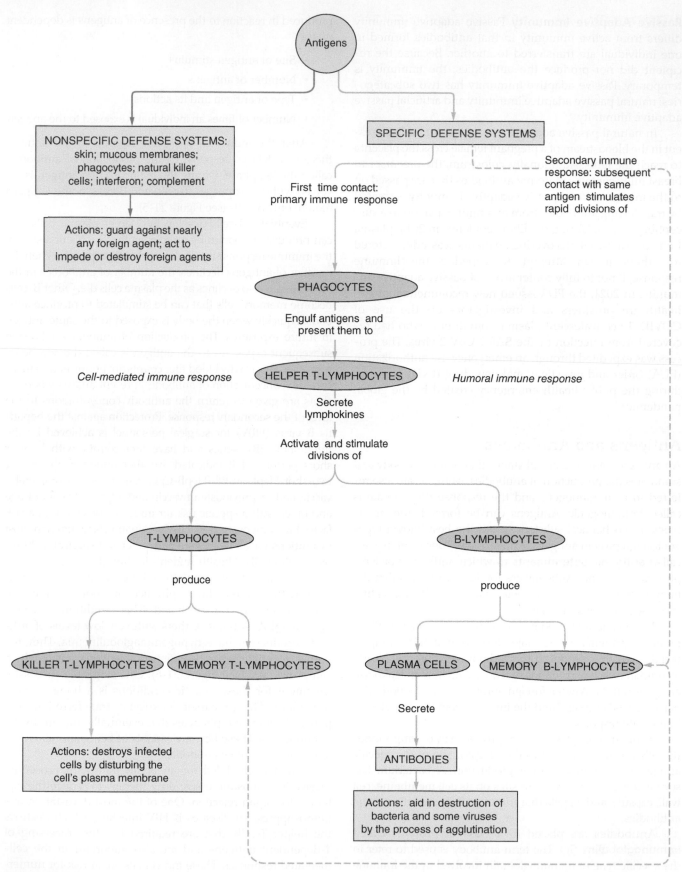

Figure 21-5 Overview of the body's defense mechanisms.

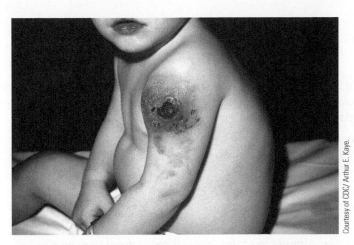

Courtesy of CDC/ Arthur E. Kaye.

Figure 21-6 A 22-month-old with the rare disease Bruton's hypogammaglobulinemia after smallpox vaccination; note the large necrotic area at the vaccination site due to CMI defect (T-cell deficiency).

Components of the Immune System

Immune cells originate in bone marrow as stem cells that develop into a variety of specialized cells. The cells of the body that function as the first-line responders in infectious disease are neutrophils, eosinophils, mast cells, monocytes, macrophages, and dendritic cells, which are products of common **myeloid progenitor stem cells** (CMPs) in the bone marrow and which are the precursors to innate immune cells.

Adaptive (acquired) immune cells develop from common lymphoid progenitor stem cells (CLPs) and include two cell lineages: B-cells (bursa-derived) and T-cells (thymus-derived). Several of the stem cells migrate to the thymus gland to differentiate into one of the four types of T-cells: helper T-cells, suppressor T-cells, cytotoxic T-cells, and delayed-hypersensitivity T-cells. The differentiation, or process of specialization of action, of the T-cells in the thymus gland begins soon before birth. The T-cells are not involved in humoral antibodies but are involved in the cell-mediated immune (CMI) response and control of the production of antibodies.

The other stem cells do not migrate to the thymus. Instead, they differentiate in the lymphoid regions of the intestine, liver, and spleen. The B-cells (bursa-derived) originate from those two regions. B-cells migrate to the lymphoid tissues and produce antibodies that circulate in the lymph system and bloodstream, providing humoral immunity. B-cells only live approximately 1 to 2 weeks. When stimulated by an antigen, the B-cells are capable of immediate mass production of antibodies.

Natural killer (NK) cells also come from myeloid progenitor stem cells, although they display behaviors similar to both the innate and adaptive immune cells. NK cells are also known as cytotoxic cells. As a group, B-cells, T-cells, and natural killer cells are also called lymphocytes.

The B-cell response and T-cell response to specific microbial markers from previous exposures are what is called immunological memory. B-cells are ultimately responsible for humoral immunity and T-cells are responsible for cell-mediated immunity.

Humoral Immunity

The humoral immune system is based on immunoglobulins (antibodies) produced by B-cells, which stick to foreign antigens, marking them for destruction by phagocytes. When the complex is formed, complement is activated to lyse invading bacterial cells, neutralize toxins, and increase phagocytosis. Antibodies are molecules made of four peptide chains arranged in the shape of a "Y." The short ends comprise variable amino acid sequences that result in different shapes capable of binding to antigens. The base portion is called the constant region and determines the isotype classification. There are countless possible antigen–antibody combinations.

Types of Antibodies

Antibodies circulating in the bloodstream are referred to as humoral or circulating antibodies. Five isotypes (classes) of antibodies are designated as IgA, IgD, IgE, IgG, and IgM (see Table 21-2).

Cell-Mediated Immunity

Antibodies cannot enter cells, even those with intracellular pathogens in them. However, cell-mediated immunity (CMI) relies on macrophages and T-cells to control chronic infections. CMI is able to control the cause of the infection but it does not eliminate it.

The herpes virus, for example, travels through the body fluids from a lysed cell seeking to infect the next normal cell. While moving through the body fluids, the virus is exposed to the antibody–complement complex and is destroyed, thereby controlling the viral infection. When the virus is established inside the body cell, the CMI response is able to destroy the infected cells. If the virus escapes the destruction of the cell, it can become latent in the nerve ganglion cells of the body (see Figure 21-7).

CMI is composed of helper T-cells that work with B-cells to initiate the antibody response. Helper T-cells trigger the release of macrophages to seek out "non-self" cells. They also produce interleukins, which leads to rapid creation of new T-cells and B-cells. Suppressor T-cells ensure that the cytotoxic T-cells do not become overly abundant and that the immune response is effective, although not destructive to the body's tissues.

NK cells and cytotoxic T-cells are effective in destroying pathogens inside infected cells. Examples include infected liver cells that are killed during hepatitis infections. The decrease or depletion of helper T-cells impairs the functions of both the humoral and CMI immune systems. An example of this is seen in diseases such as HIV/AIDS.

Table 21-2 **Functions of Antibodies**

Antibody Class	Functions
IgA	Protects mucous membranes and internal body cavities against infection. Known as the secretory antibody since it is found in the saliva, colostrum, tears, bloodstream, and intestine. Prevents pathogens from adhering to mucosal surfaces.
IgD	Function not well understood. Controls antigen stimulation of B cells. May be involved in determining which antibody type a plasma cell produces. Found on surface of B cells and in bloodstream.
IgE	Is the cause of allergies, anaphylaxis, drug sensitivity, and immediate hypersensitivity in skin test reactions. Cause of rash or hives in allergic reactions, runny nose and itchy eyes of hay fever, asthma, and shock in anaphylaxis.
IgG	Most abundant and smallest of the antibodies. Attaches to phagocytes and complement, making it easier for bacteria to be destroyed by phagocytes or lysed by complement. Crosses the placental barrier. Protects against disease. Found in the bloodstream and lymph fluid.
IgM	Largest antibody. First antibodies formed in response to infection. Especially lethal against Gram-negative bacteria. Activates complement. Increases the process of phagocytosis. Found in the bloodstream and lymph fluid.

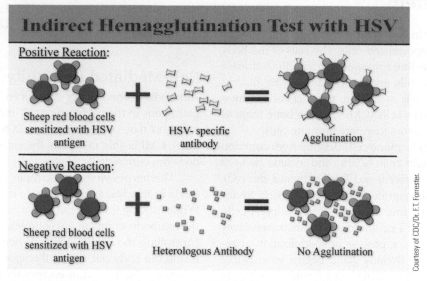

Figure 21-7 Diagram illustrating indirect hemagglutination (IHA) inhibition test, which implements the herpes simplex virus (HSV) antigen to detect the presence of the HSV-specific antibody.

Hypersensitivity Reactions

Hypersensitivity reactions represent an immune response that is abnormal, and the response can be mild to life-threatening. Instead of providing protections, the antibodies damage cells of the body. There are several categories of hypersensitivity reactions and all are represented by the presence of an antigen and T-cells that have been sensitized to that particular antigen.

Hypersensitivity reactions are divided into two primary categories: immediate and delayed. An immediate reaction is one that occurs within a few seconds to 24 hours. There are four subcategories of hypersensitivity reactions described as:

- Type I: also called an immediate reaction. This includes allergic responses to hay fever, animals, grasses, and trees. Other responses under this type include hives due to food allergies, drug allergies, allergic responses to insect bites or stings, and anaphylactic shock. Type I allergic responses can be the most dangerous and life-threatening. The reactions involve the IgE antibodies and release of histamine from basophils and mast cells.

- Type II: also called an antibody-dependent reaction is also immediate. This involves IgG or IgM antibodies and complement. Type II allergic responses are cytotoxic reactions seen when the wrong blood is given to a patient during a blood transfusion and include the Rh incompatibility reactions sometimes seen in pregnant females.

- Type III: also called an immune complex reaction. This involves IgM or IgG antibodies, neutrophils, and complement. Type III reactions are seen in autoimmune diseases such as rheumatoid arthritis.

- Type IV: also called delayed-type (or cell-mediated) hypersensitivity reaction. It does not directly involve antibodies, but it does involve sensitized T-cells that secrete lymphokines due to a subsequent exposure to the antigen.

Immediate Hypersensitivity

Type I is the most common type of hypersensitivity observed, because most humans are allergic to at least one thing. Persons with allergies produce IgE antibodies when exposed to allergens (see Figure 21-8). The type and extent of the allergic reaction depend on the following factors:

- Number of antigens that entered the body
- Route of entry
- Individual's production of IgE
- Length of time between exposures to the antigen

The allergic reaction occurs when IgE antibodies present on mast cells in connective tissue or basophils in the blood are exposed for the first time to the antigen (allergen). During the second exposure, the mast cell or basophil with IgE binds to the allergen. The sensitized cells respond by releasing histamine, prostaglandins, serotonin, bradykinin, and other substances that are responsible for symptoms of sneezing, rhinitis (runny nose), and itchy eyes.

Localized Reaction

Hay fever is an example of localized allergic reactions. The symptoms and reactions depend on how the allergen enters the body and where the IgE attaches. For example, if the allergen is inhaled pollen, it is deposited on the mucous membranes of the respiratory tract. The IgE antibodies will then attach to the mast cells in the respiratory tract. The second exposure causes the mast cells with IgE to bind with the allergen, causing the mast cells to release large amounts of histamine. This produces the hay fever symptoms. Over-the-counter (OTC) or prescribed anti-histamines bind to the histamine sites, thus blocking the histamine and its ability to produce the symptoms.

Anaphylactic Reaction

Anaphylaxis is the most severe and potentially life-threatening type of hypersensitivity reaction. The reaction occurs following exposure to the antigen to which the person has previously been sensitized. Most commonly, the antigens are drugs or insect venom (see Figure 21-9).

The reaction can occur in a few seconds to a few minutes. Initial signs and symptoms include the following:

- Itching
- Flushing of the skin
- Headache
- Ringing in the ears, particularly with drug reactions
- Metallic taste in the mouth, particularly with drug reactions
- Difficulty breathing due to **laryngospasm** and **bronchospasm**
- Hypertension
- Tachycardia
- Restlessness

Late signs and symptoms include:

- Rapid hypotension
- Nausea and vomiting
- Confusion and inability to focus mentally
- Respiratory failure

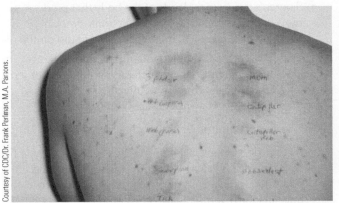

Courtesy of CDC/Dr. Frank Perlman, M.A. Parsons.

Figure 21-8 Patient undergoing allergen sensitivity test.

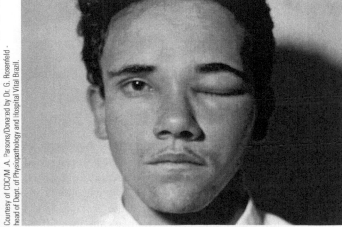

Courtesy of CDC/M .A. Parsons/Dona ed by Dr. G. Rosenfeld - head of Dept. of Physiopathology and Hospital Vital Brazil.

Figure 21-9 This patient presented 31 hours after having been bitten on his face by a *Loxosceles* spp. spider, also known as brown recluse spider.

If not immediately treated, loss of consciousness and death can occur. Treatment involves:

- Administration of 100 percent oxygen
- Injection of **epinephrine**: causes bronchodilation, reduces laryngospasm, elevates blood pressure
- Injection of steroids: stabilizes mast cells to slow the chain reaction
- Administration of IV fluids to maintain fluid volume
- Injection of a vasopressor agent to increase blood pressure

The best course of action in healthcare settings is to identify the patients with known allergies and make this information available to medical personnel. For the surgical team, allergies are clearly marked on the outside of the patient's chart and on their hospital identification bracelet. Outside of healthcare settings, individuals with serious allergies can alert the public by wearing metal ID alert bracelets that indicate allergy status. Auto-injector type devices such as EpiPen® are premeasured doses of epinephrine available for individuals with known history or risk of anaphylactic reaction and should be kept nearby at all times when there is risk of allergy exposure.

Hemolytic Transfusion Reaction

Hemolytic transfusion reactions are an example of a type II immediate hypersensitivity reaction. If blood to be transfused is not properly matched to the patient's blood type, a massive systemic transfusion reaction can occur. Hemolytic reactions are potentially fatal without immediate treatment.

The conscious patient most often verbalizes a lack of energy. Symptoms include shortness of breath, rapid pulse, and skin pallor. In surgery, the patient receiving general anesthesia will not display these signs. The only noticeable signs may be diffuse bleeding at the surgical site and decreased blood oxygen saturation level (SaO_2) due to the inability of the erythrocytes to carry oxygen.

The first step in response is to stop the blood transfusion. A blood sample from the blood bag should be sent to the blood bank to rule out a mismatch. Steroids are given and urine output is closely monitored because **hypovolemia** is common in these patients. In some cases, the patient may have to undergo **dialysis** to aid in the removal of the mismatched blood.

Rh Incompatibility Reaction

Rh incompatibility occurs when a pregnant female's blood type is Rh negative and the fetus is Rh positive. If red blood cells from the fetus mix with the mother's blood through the placenta, the mother's body initiates a hypersensitivity response and produces antibodies against the "foreign" blood of the fetus. If the antibodies cross the placenta, they attack the blood cells of the fetus. Mild reactions may cause jaundice of the fetus, which can be treated by **phototherapy** following delivery. More serious reactions may result in fetal demise,

brain damage, or subsequent developmental delays. First pregnancies typically produce either no reactions or mild reactions, because the body has not built up stocks of available antibodies. Pregnancies subsequent to abortions, miscarriages, or previous births may produce more serious reactions. Rh incompatibility is uncommon in areas where prenatal care is available due to treatment with RhoGAM (Rho D immune globulin human) injections, which prevent the hypersensitivity reaction. Hemolytic disease in newborns (HDN) is also known as **erythroblastosis fetalis** and may require blood transfusion in severe cases.

Autoimmune Disease

Type III hypersensitivity reactions are the result of an autoimmune disorder. Autoimmune diseases develop when the immune system fails to recognize a body tissue as being part of "self." The immune system attempts to destroy the tissue perceived as foreign. These diseases may be directed to single organs or may be systemic. Examples of systemic autoimmune disorders include:

- Rheumatoid arthritis: a crippling and progressive disease in which the immune system has turned against the collagen tissue of the joints.
- Lupus erythematosus: a chronic, inflammatory, connective tissue disease that can affect the joints and many organs, including the skin, heart, lungs, kidneys, and nervous system.
- Multiple sclerosis: disorder of the central nervous system caused by destruction of the myelin sheaths of neurons and results in signs and symptoms of generalized muscle weakness, numbness, loss of coordination or bladder control, and problems with vision and speech.
- Scleroderma: fibroblasts are stimulated to produce excess collagen. The excessive collagen forms thick connective tissue that builds up within the skin and internal organs, causing hardening and malfunctioning. Joints and blood vessels may also be affected.
- Reiter's syndrome: also called reactive arthritis, involves the joints, urethra, and eyes, which become swollen and inflamed in response to infections.
- Sjogren's syndrome: glands of the body that produce moisture (tears, saliva, vaginal secretions, synovial fluid) are disrupted, leading to dryness and discomfort.
- Crohn's disease: also called inflammatory bowel disease (IBD); multiple factors including immune disorder in which chronic formation of intestinal ulcerations causes excessive diarrhea and abdominal pain.

Single-organ autoimmune disorders include:

- Insulin-dependent diabetes mellitus (IDDM) or type I diabetes mellitus: also called juvenile diabetes; the body attacks beta cells in the pancreas, which produce insulin, eventually causing complete loss of insulin production.

- Grave's disease: antibodies that mimic thyroid-stimulating hormone (TSH) cause thyroid to overproduce thyroxine (T4) and triiodothyronine (T3), which control body metabolism and lead to **hyperthyroidism** symptoms including tachycardia and **exophthalmos**.

- Myasthenia gravis: disease characterized by muscle weakness during periods of activity that improves after rest and involves muscles that control eye movement, facial expression, mastication, talking, swallowing, respiration, and possibly neck or extremity movement. The thymus gland may be implicated in production of antibodies that block acetylcholine, a neurotransmitter responsible for muscle movement.

Delayed Hypersensitivity

Delayed, or type IV, hypersensitivity is unique in that sensitized T-cells secrete substances in the absence of antibodies. For example:

1. Antigens invade the body
2. When the antigen is being phagocytized by macrophages, the T-cells that are attached to the macrophage are sensitized by the antigen
3. When the sensitized T-cells are exposed to the antigen a second time, they secrete lymphokines (cytokines produced by lymphocytes)
4. The lymphokines directly destroy the antigen

The tuberculin skin test is a classic example of displaying the action of T-cells, macrophages, and lymphokines. The localized reaction is seen within 48 hours and the patient displays fever with redness and swelling in the inoculated area. Similar reactions occur with poison ivy.

A more serious reaction is one that may be experienced by recipients of transplanted tissues or organs. The reaction can cause rejection of the transplanted tissue or organ. The donor organ must match the recipient's blood and tissue types. The optimal donor is an immediate family member, such as a sibling or parent. The rejection process is similar to that described, with the exception that antibodies and lymphokines are the cause of transplant rejection. The patient is given immunosuppressive drug therapy pre-operatively and post-operatively to lessen the possibility of tissue/organ rejection. Great care must be taken to minimize exposure, because the patient with a suppressed immune system is far more likely to contract a wide range of infectious diseases.

Immunodeficiency Disorders

Any part of the immune system may be affected by immunodeficiency disorders. Typically, these conditions occur when T-lymphocytes or B-lymphocytes (or a combination of both) malfunction and when too few antibodies are produced. The disorders may be primary or acquired. There are more than 180 documented primary immunodeficiency disorders.

Primary genetic or inherited disorders include hypogammaglobulinemia or agammaglobulinemia. Infections from *Streptococcus pneumoniae*, *Haemophilus influenzae*, and *Staphylococcus* spp. are frequent and may be abnormally severe to life-threatening due to the inability of the body to produce enough (or any) lymphocytes (B-cells or T-cells) to fight the infections. Areas infected most commonly are the skin, upper and lower respiratory tract, and gastrointestinal system.

Acquired immunodeficiency disorders are complications of HIV, malnutrition, chemotherapy or anti-rejection regimens, and absence of the spleen. Older adults and individuals with diabetes are also at increased risk for immunodeficiency.

Herd Immunity

Prior to the COVID-19 pandemic, mainly epidemiologists and public health groups were interested in the concept and goal of achieving herd immunity in the general public. Herd immunity, also known as community immunity, is a phenomenon of protection of a large group or community of people from communicable disease when the majority of those in the group have been properly vaccinated. Those few individuals who have not been vaccinated due to allergies to the vaccine, immunocompromised status, or religious/moral objections are unlikely to become infected due to the near total lack of widely circulating pathogens. In certain diseases such as measles, approximately 95 percent of the community must be vaccinated against measles for herd immunity to be effective. Prior to widespread vaccination campaigns, each individual infected with measles in turn infected an average of 11 to 18 others.

In 2020, there were only 13 cases of measles, one third the number reported in 2021, however, this may have been chiefly a factor of measures taken in response to the pandemic that limited contact in public places and transportation. The CDC reports that there were 1,282 cases of measles reported in 31 states in the United States in 2019, the highest annual rate since 1992. Prior to that concerning rise in annual measles cases, an outbreak of measles occurred in 2015 among visitors to California's Disneyland in late December 2014. By midyear, 178 cases of measles in 24 states had been recorded with 66 percent (117) of the cases directly linked to the Disneyland exposure. Statistical models showed higher rates in areas with groups known to have objections to routine vaccination of children. Because the measles virus is capable of remaining viable on inanimate surfaces for hours after inoculation, transmissibility potential was sufficient to disseminate measles to a large group (see Figure 21-10).

Objection to vaccination of children has been mainly linked to erroneous information reported by a discredited British researcher, Andrew Wakefield, who linked autism in young children to vaccines in a study published in a British medical journal in 1998. Wakefield was found to have falsified his data and changed the histories of the study subjects.

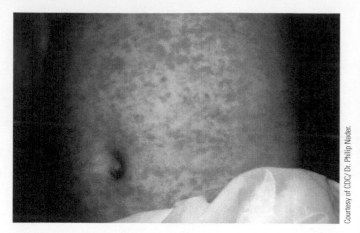

Courtesy of CDC/ Dr. Philip Nader.

Figure 21-10 The torso of a child infected with the morbillivirus known as measles or rubeola, and the characteristic rash associated with the viral infection.

He also failed to disclose that his research had been funded (at least in part) by attorneys seeking to develop a program of class-action law suits against manufacturers of the MMR vaccines. The more recent spread of false and misleading misinformation in certain groups and on social media regarding the COVID-19 vaccinations cannot as easily be attributed to an individual source, however, the end results have been similar. In addition to the damage to the overall scientific research and reliance on medical and public health communities, the ultimate damage done to the larger societal community caused by fear and distrust has now resulted in ever-increasing numbers of outbreaks of vaccine-preventable infections and ever-decreasing attainment of adequate herd immunity thresholds.

Behavioral Factors

Benjamin Franklin said, "An ounce of prevention is worth a pound of cure." This is a perfect rallying cry for the topic of controlling microbial growth and prevention of infection. Human behavior is frequently the main causative factor in the transmission of disease, even though it is nearly always unintentional and unrealized. Prevention of infection is cheap, but treatment is costly. Behavioral factors that impact control or prevention of disease transmission include:

- Sexually transmitted infections (STIs) or STDs from blood-borne pathogens or in bodily fluids can be prevented by routine safe-sex practices including proper use of condoms or even **abstinence** if risk of transmission is likely. Negative screening for STIs and monogamous, long-term relationships may provide sexual partners with a sense of assurance and allows for choice of discontinuation of protection if desired. Risky behaviors elevate risk of infection and disease (see Figure 21-11).

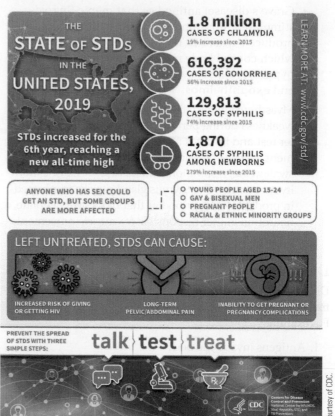

Courtesy of CDC.

Figure 21-11 The state of STDs in the united states 2019.

- Careful food preparation and storage methods can help prevent most cases of food-borne infections. Cross-contamination of kitchen surfaces by raw meats or eggs, failure to reach adequate internal temperatures during cooking of certain foods, selection of unpasteurized dairy items for consumption, failure to maintain sufficiently cold temperatures of prepared foods, unwashed raw fruits and vegetables, and fecal–oral contamination of foods from unwashed hands of food preparers are all examples of easily preventable sources of contamination by and transmission of pathogenic bacteria (see Figure 21-12).

- Adherence by the public to recommendations for routine vaccinations to eliminate preventable diseases and protection of vulnerable pediatric and older adult populations contributes to the phenomenon of herd immunity for the greatest majority of the public.

- Local government **infrastructure** mechanisms must be adequately maintained and monitored to prevent contamination of public water supplies for drinking and irrigation of crops. Additionally, measures to eliminate widespread contamination during flooding events should be developed. Municipal public health departments must offer control of vector-borne diseases by spraying of insecticides in areas of high mosquito presence. Animal control departments should contain animals with potential for disease.

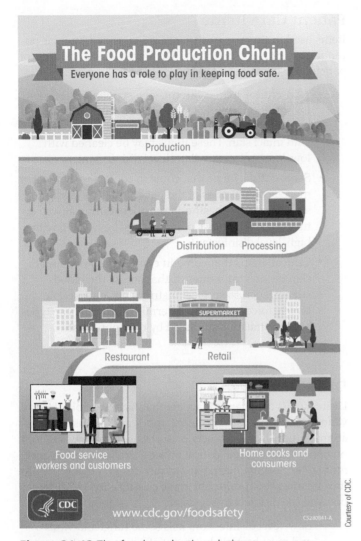

Figure 21-12 The food production chain

- Pet owners should maintain a schedule for routine vaccinations for their house pets and recognize potential for infectious bacteria in cat or dog urine or feces when young children or pregnant females are in the household.
- Healthcare workers, including physicians, must practice appropriate infection control techniques such as proper hand washing or skin antisepsis before and after every interaction with patients and after eating or using the restroom. Use of personal protective equipment (PPE) when indicated also helps reduce potential for cross-contamination between patients or between patients and caregivers. Administration of antibiotic therapy should be carefully evaluated to reduce the increase in antibiotic resistance of pathogenic microbes. Environmental cleaning and decontamination of surfaces in healthcare settings should be adequate to prevent dissemination of unseen pathogenic microbes throughout the facility and reduce potential for deadly and costly healthcare-associated infections.

Prevention of Disease Transmission in the Surgical Environment of Care

Surgical technology students are provided extensive education in the areas of **decontamination** of areas, surfaces, and equipment within the operating room suite; **disinfection** of patient care items; and **sterilization** of surgical instrumentation. The following sections are a brief synopsis of some of those areas of critical importance in controlling microbial growth and transmission for the safety of surgical patients and personnel in the surgical environment of care.

Environmental Controls

Surgical suites are designed to minimize the potential for cross-contamination of clean and contaminated items by creation of traffic patterns and zoning. Architectural and engineering plans are developed to address the following specifications and challenges.

- Air entering individual operating rooms is filtered by high-efficiency particulate air (HEPA) filters. The rooms are maintained with positive pressure, meaning the pressure in the OR room is higher than the air in the adjacent corridors/hallways. This keeps airborne contaminants in the less clean corridors from entering the cleaner operating room when the doors are opened. The entire volume of room air is replaced at a rate of 15 to 20 air exchanges per hour to dilute accumulated airborne bacteria and other fumes such as **electrosurgical smoke plume** or escaped anesthetic gases. The flow of air into the room is unidirectional from ceiling level to floor level. This one-way flow prevents dust and bacteria on the floor from being disturbed and disseminated from air turbulence and potentially resettling on the sterile field.
- Floors must be non-grouted and waterproof for flooding with cleaning solutions and removal with wet-vacuums during terminal cleaning. Walls and other surfaces in the OR must be non-porous to prevent microbes from accumulating in cracks or crevices and must be able to withstand frequent cleaning with strong disinfectants.
- Temperatures are kept cool (68–73°F) to reduce microbial growth. Microbes have an optimum temperature at which they grow best, a minimum temperature below which they cease to grow, and a maximum temperature above which they will be destroyed. The range of temperature varies among microbes. Generally, microbes grow slowly at lower temperatures and faster at higher temperatures. Humidity levels are maintained to prevent growth of mold and mildew as well as reduce static electricity on surfaces.

Attire and Zoning

Personnel entering the surgical suite wear proper surgical attire and components of PPE depending on the zone they enter and the task to be performed. Proper OR attire consists of freshly laundered scrubs, shoes that prevent soaking through with blood or body fluids from the surgical field, and hair covers that contain all hair on the head (or face) to prevent shedding of bacteria from hair, dandruff, or skin cells. Cover jackets are recommended for non-scrubbed personnel to prevent microbial shedding from exposed skin of the arms. Shoe covers are recommended to keep shoes clean but are not required for protection of the environment.

Unrestricted areas or zones include locker rooms, front desks, and pre-operative (holding) or post-anesthesia (recovery) care units and may have no restrictions regarding attire. Semi-restricted areas or zones may be storage areas and peripheral inner corridors (hallways) and require proper surgical attire, including head covers. Restricted areas or zones require the addition of surgical facemasks. Restricted areas include ORs where sterile supplies are open or surgical procedures are in progress, clean-core storage areas, or anywhere otherwise designated by that facility as restricted. Facemasks reduce transmission of airborne or droplet particles from breathing and talking.

Skin Preparation

Surgical technologists learn the process of a surgical scrub to remove transient microbes and reduce the resident microbial population on the skin of their hands and forearms to an **irreducible minimum**. The procedure renders the skin "surgically clean," but not sterile, as many believe. Living skin is incapable of being sterilized. Sterility is defined as the absence of all living microorganisms, including spores. There will always be living microbes in the layers of living skin. The process of the surgical scrub includes use of an antimicrobial soap and brush and water from a scrub sink. The water used is tap water and also not sterile. For these reasons, the surgical scrub procedure is actually an aseptic technique and not a sterile technique. Asepsis is defined as the absence of infection. **Aseptic techniques** are used to prevent transmission or potential for infection, as in reduction of microbes on the skin of the surgical team members. The skin of the patient is similarly prepped by the circulating nurse prior to draping with sterile drapes and commencement of the surgical procedure. The prep reduces the patient's microbial count in an attempt to prevent opportunistic bacteria from being pulled into the wound from surrounding areas of skin.

For clarification, surgical technologists and other scrubbed members of the team perform a surgical scrub or a chemical skin preparation and then don (put on) a sterile gown and gloves to establish and work within the sterile field. Students will learn the areas of the gown that are considered sterile and those that are not when they learn principles of scrubbing, gowning, and gloving. They are then considered part of the sterile team and interact only with sterile items or surfaces.

Patient Care Items

Items used in the care of patients are classified by their potential for causing infection. The three classifications of patient care items developed by Earle Spaulding are:

- Non-critical: items with the lowest potential for causing infection include blood pressure cuffs, pulse-oximeters, or other items that only come in contact with intact skin. These items may be cleaned with low-level or intermediate-level disinfectants.

- Semi-critical: items that come in contact with intact mucous membranes of the patient such as laryngoscopes used by anesthesia providers during airway intubation. These types of items must be cleaned with high-level disinfectants.

- Critical: items that come in contact with non-intact skin or internal tissues or that access the bloodstream, such as surgical instruments, endoscopic biopsy forceps, and hypodermic needles. These types of items must be sterilized by the appropriate method.

Disinfection

Disinfectants are chemical agents that have the ability to kill various classes of pathogenic microbes and are used on inanimate (non-living) objects or surfaces. They may be used on non-critical or semi-critical patient care items or for environmental cleaning of inanimate surfaces and equipment in the operating room suite. The three classifications of disinfection and the disinfectants used are:

- Low-level disinfection: kills some fungi and viruses and most bacteria but is not effective against spores and *M. tuberculosis*. Low-level disinfectants are less commonly used than higher-level disinfectants.

- Intermediate-level disinfection: kills all bacteria, fungi, and non-hydrophilic viruses, but is not capable of killing spores or certain hydrophilic viruses. These disinfectants may be used on countertops, OR furniture, floors, and other surfaces, and instruments that only come into contact with the intact skin of the patient.

- High-level disinfection: kills all microorganisms except microbial spores and prions (CJD).

Disinfectants vary regarding the types of microbes they can kill. Selection of a disinfectant is based on the item to be disinfected and whether it is a critical, semi-critical, or non-critical patient care item. The amount of time the disinfectant must have contact with the item is also based on its classification and manufacturer's recommendations. Disinfectants used for environmental cleaning must make contact with all surfaces to be effective. The chemical composition of most disinfectants may be hazardous to employees and safety data sheets (SDS), previously called material safety data sheets, should always be available in circumstances of spills or personnel exposure.

To be approved for use in hospitals, a disinfectant must be able to destroy *Pseudomonas aeruginosa*, *Salmonella*, and *Staphylococcus aureus*. Disinfectants can be labeled with the term germicide as long as the agent is effective in killing growing and vegetative bacteria. If the agent is effective against *Mycobacterium tuberculosis*, it can be labeled as tuberculocidal. If effective against viruses it is virucidal; if it kills fungi it is fungicidal; if effective against bacteria it is bactericidal; and if it is able to kill spore-forming bacteria it is sporicidal. Two commonly used disinfectants are isopropyl alcohol and sodium hypochlorite.

Isopropyl Alcohol

Isopropyl alcohol in a concentration of 60 to 70 percent destroys microbes by coagulating the cellular proteins. It is most commonly used as a disinfectant for wiping down the surfaces of furniture and shelves in the operating room. Alcohol is tuberculocidal, bactericidal, virucidal, and fungicidal, but it is not sporicidal.

Sodium Hypochlorite

Sodium hypochlorite, also known as household bleach, is an effective disinfectant for surfaces, floors, and equipment. Sodium hypochlorite disrupts cellular metabolism and is effective and fast-acting, bactericidal, virucidal, tuberculocidal, and effective against HIV, HBV, and other viruses. The CDC recommends its use in cleaning blood and body fluid spills.

Decontamination

Contamination is defined as the presence of pathogenic microbes. This can involve human tissues as well as surgical instrumentation used for surgical procedures. Decontamination is the process of reducing the microbial population to **sub-pathogenic** levels. The process of instrument decontamination begins with initial cleaning at the point of use, in other words, in the OR at the time of the procedure. Instruments should be rinsed of blood and tissue to reduce the **bioburden** present on the surfaces.

Following transport to a decontamination area in the OR suite or in a sterile processing department, the instruments are rinsed with cool or lukewarm water before being placed into mesh-bottom trays. Instruments that are delicate or have motors may need to be cleaned manually. The majority of surgical instruments are designed to withstand frequent cleaning and sterilization methods. Those instruments are placed into an automated washer-sterilizer or washer-decontaminator that acts like a large dishwasher (see Figure 21-13). At the end of the washer-sterilizer cycle, the instruments are subjected to high-pressure steam and sterilized. They are not ready for patient use because they require testing, reassembly in trays, packaging, and sterilization in closed, filtered containers before being sent back to the supply room for storage until they are needed again.

Sterilization

Sterilization is the process of destroying all living microorganisms, including spore-forming bacteria, because they are

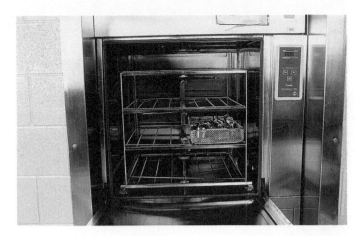

Figure 21-13 Washer-sterilizer.

the most resistant type of microbe due to their ability to withstand harsh environmental conditions. Critical patient care items such as surgical instrumentation must be sterile to prevent surgical site infections (SSIs). Hospital central sterile processing departments utilize various methods to achieve sterility dependent on the properties of the instruments.

Thermal methods include steam under pressure for items that are able to withstand high temperatures and moisture. Dry heat is similar to an oven and used for items that can withstand high heat but not moisture, however, this method is not commonly used in hospital facilities. Chemical sterilization can take the form of liquids, gas, or gas **plasma**. These methods utilize lower temperature modalities and rely on the lethality of the chemical agents to render items sterile. Ionizing radiation is a sterilization method used mainly in large-scale industrial manufacturing where large quantities of supplies may be sterilized without the need for high temperatures or chemicals; however, strict regulation of ionizing radiation exposure makes it inappropriate for hospital use.

Steam Sterilization

Steam under pressure is the most widely used method of sterilization. It is inexpensive, reliable, safe, and appropriate for the majority of surgical instrumentation. The combination of time and temperature that is required to destroy a type of microbe in the laboratory is called the thermal death point or thermal death time. Steam sterilization cycles consist of time, temperature, and pressure settings determined to achieve the destruction of all microbial life. Steam at normal atmospheric pressure is incapable of sterilizing; however, the addition of pressure in a closed space increases the temperature rapidly (see Figure 21-14).

Direct contact of the steam with every surface of the items to be sterilized is the primary principle of steam sterilization. If any portion of the surface and/or **lumen** of an item is not contacted by steam, the item is considered unsterile because there was a failure in the process. The steam must remain in contact with the items for a set period of time to destroy all the microbes, including bacterial spores. That period is referred to as the exposure time. The correlation is that increased pressure increases temperature and reduces time needed to complete the process.

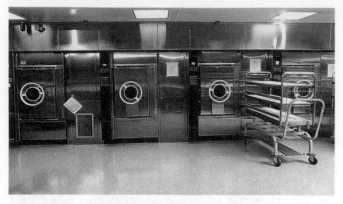

Figure 21-14 Steam sterilization area.

Pressure is important from the point of view that it only aids in increasing the temperature, but it has no direct effect on the destruction of microbes. Several types of steam sterilizers are used and will be covered extensively in the surgical technology student's program curriculum.

Chemical Sterilization Methods

Chemicals that are approved for use as sterilants are available in gas, liquid, or plasma form. The chemicals briefly discussed are **ethylene oxide**, **hydrogen peroxide** gas plasma, **glutaraldehyde**, and **peracetic acid**.

Ethylene Oxide Gas Ethylene gas sterilization is used to process heat-sensitive or moisture-sensitive materials that cannot be processed using steam sterilization. Ethylene oxide (EO) was once the predominant chemical sterilization process used to sterilize plastics, rubber, and other materials that would be damaged by the high temperature and moist steam method. EO is effective against all forms of microbes and is sporicidal. It does not corrode metal. Many hazards exist with use of ethylene oxide. It is flammable, carcinogenic, toxic, and requires long **aeration** times. Although it is used by large manufacturers of surgical products, its use in the hospital setting has dramatically decreased due to the dangers to personnel and the availability of alternative methods of sterilizing heat and moisture sensitive items.

Hydrogen Peroxide Gas Plasma Hydrogen peroxide gas plasma (HPGP) sterilization has replaced ethylene oxide in many facilities and uses gas plasma at low temperatures to sterilize heat-sensitive and moisture-sensitive items. One example of a gas plasma sterilization system, commercially referred to as Sterrad™, uses hydrogen peroxide in plasma form. The process involves diffusion of hydrogen peroxide in a gaseous state with the addition of a strong electrical field created by **radiofrequency**, which passes through the gas, creating a cloud of plasma. Hydrogen peroxide is a highly reactive molecule that creates **free radicals** (hydroxyl and hydroperoxyl), inactivating all microbial life.

Glutaraldehyde Glutaraldehyde, often marketed as Cidex™, is a low-temperature method of liquid chemical disinfection and sterilization used for heat-sensitive devices that can withstand complete immersion in an activated disinfectant solution. The liquid must contact all surface areas of the item, including cannulas, lumens, or tubes. Rigid and flexible endoscopes are two kinds of surgical instruments which may be decontaminated or sterilized using glutaraldehyde. All items disinfected with glutaraldehyde must be thoroughly rinsed with sterile water (do not use tap water because this will re-contaminate the item) before use on the patient to prevent the tissue of the patient from being chemically injured. Ten hours of complete submersion in glutaraldehyde is required to render an item sterile. For high-level disinfection, a minimum exposure time of 20 minutes at room temperature is required.

Peracetic Acid Peracetic acid is another low-temperature liquid chemical sterilization method that has largely replaced glutaraldehyde. Liquid chemical sterilization is an alternative to steam under pressure and EO. It is generally safe for items that are heat-sensitive but moisture-stable, however, peracetic acid is corrosive to some metals. One example of the chemical sterilant, peracetic acid, is the Steris System™. Newer technology of vaporized peracetic acid (VPA) is proving to be another option for use of peracetic acid but has wider application to critical patient care items that cannot tolerate liquid immersion.

Sterilization Process Assurance Monitors

The sterilization processes require several methods of assurance monitors to verify success. Mechanical indicators are the printouts generated by the sterilizer unit that records the cycle times and critical parameters.

Validation of the chemical process is achieved by use of **chemical indicator/integrators** that are designed to turn color when exposed to the type of sterilant for which they are designed to test. This provides a visual assurance that the tray or pack has been through the sterilization process; however, it does not guarantee that the items within the pack or tray are sterile (see Figure 21-15). The indicators/integrators, are strips, dots, or symbols inserted into the middle of instrument trays or packs (internal indicator) and on the outside of the prepared package (external indicator) prior to sterilization.

Biological indicators (BIs) are devices that contain a small, measured dose of a specific type of bacteria that is

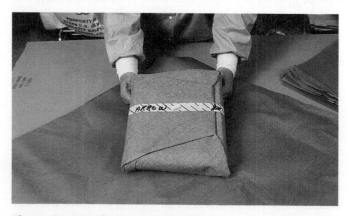

Figure 21-15 Indicator tape showing color change appropriate for exposure to the steam sterilization process.

normally killed when exposed to specific sterilizing conditions. The bacterial sample is in the spore stage and highly resistant to destruction. The BI is the only test that demonstrates that the method of sterilization used is capable of killing microorganism that otherwise could survive them. The logical presumption is that items are sterile and the conditions necessary for sterilization have been met.

A biological indicator is placed in the sterilizer. After the sterilization cycle is complete, it is removed. The BI vial is gently broken, which releases the growth medium and covers the spore-impregnated disk. The growth medium is a red nutrient broth. Following the 24-hour incubation period, if the broth remains red, the test is considered negative and the spores have been killed. If, however, the broth turns yellow, then the test is positive and the spores were not killed, meaning the conditions for sterilization were not met. The items in the load must be considered unsterile. The items in the sterilizer load must be immediately recalled and reprocessed. The sterilizer is taken out of service until the next negative BI result is achieved.

Due to the need for quick turnover of instrument trays, often brought in by industry vendors, newer methods of rapid-read out testing have been developed that provide results in 3 hours and others that may be read in as little as 24 minutes. The rapid and super-rapid read-out tests detect and measure the ultraviolet (UV) fluorescent by-products of the enzymes that living, spore-forming bacteria produce. A test result showing the absence of the enzymes, that would be present if the microbes were living, provides a high level of assurance that the bacteria were killed during the sterilization process and instruments and items sterilized in that load are safe for use in the surgical procedure and for implantation in the body.

The BI for steam sterilization contains the bacterial spore *Geobacillus stearothermophilus*, which is highly resistant to steam sterilization but is harmless to humans. For ethylene oxide, spores of *Bacillus atrophaeus* are used. These spores are the most resistant to EO but also harmless to humans.

Administrative controls involve the record-keeping of all three types of process monitors in case of inspection by agencies such as the Joint Commission or in instances of tracking for sterilizer failure.

MICRO NOTES

"Science (in) Fiction"

You may have seen a version of the movie or read the book *War of the Worlds* by H. G. Wells. The story involved many literary themes; however, from the perspective of the science of microbiology, it was an interesting analogy to the topics of disease transmission, infection, and immunity. Spoiler alert: if you have not read or seen it, the end of the story is discussed here. Ultimately, these very unfriendly alien invaders who attacked humans and consumed them were defeated by the smallest inhabitants of the planet Earth—microbes. The invading extraterrestrials had no experience with these microscopic residents and were defenseless against life forms new to them and their immune systems (presuming they had them). The symbiotic relationship we have developed over our combined evolutionary history saved us from being exterminated by the alien invaders. Maybe common colds aren't such a bad thing after all.

 ## Under the Microscope

Emma was called in for an emergency laparotomy and possible splenectomy for blunt force trauma. During the pre-op surgical time-out, the anesthesia provider mentioned to the team that the patient expressed a desire to receive the COVID-19 vaccine booster dose which they had not had a chance to get prior to this accident and was concerned that being in the hospital might expose them to potential breakthrough infection. The circulating nurse informed the team that the patient wore a medical alert bracelet indicating allergy to penicillin, and that there was compatible blood available in case of excessive intraoperative blood loss. Emma, the surgical technologist, verified the availability and sterility of the surgical instruments for the procedure. The patient was prepped with an antiseptic skin prep agent and draped with sterile drapes to establish the sterile field prior to the start of the procedure. The patient did end up having extensive intraoperative blood loss from the splenic laceration and required infusion of donated blood.

1. What would be the long-term effects of the patient having the splenectomy on their future health?

2. Which safety measures or process monitors are related to the preoperative or intraoperative routines outlined in the scenario that apply to the topics covered in this chapter?

3. What are important risk factors related to the patient's immune system that must be considered regarding the noted allergy status as well as the need for donated blood from the blood bank?

4. What are the routine processes and routines that Emma took to ensure that any risk of SSI was eliminated when preparing for this patient's procedure?

5. What type of protections do the original and booster vaccine doses provide that would protect the patient and others in the community from widespread transmission of infection?

CHAPTER 22

Emerging, Recurring, and Reappearing Diseases

The Big Picture

The expression "too much of a good thing" may apply to the use of antibiotics. The primary risk factor for development of antibiotic resistance is the use of antibiotics. This presents healthcare providers with a difficult challenge in how to be good stewards of antibiotic prescribing and treat infections without causing additional harm. Healthcare providers must also develop treatment strategies for newly emerging, recurring, and reappearing diseases that should have been eliminated. During your examination of the topics in this chapter, consider the following:

1. What are the factors that can lead to the development of antibiotic resistance?

2. Which classifications of diseases would be described as emerging, recurring, or reappearing diseases?

3. How can patients take measures to positively influence and advocate for their own health and wellbeing in healthcare or community settings?

4. What are factors that should be considered within the United States healthcare system that would ensure better preparedness in dealing with emerging diseases previously associated with other countries, as well as domestically recurring and reappearing diseases previously thought to be eradicated?

Clinical Significance Topic

A nurse from Dallas was the first person to contract Ebola in the United States. She became ill after caring for a patient who had traveled to and returned from West Africa and presented to the emergency department at Texas Health Presbyterian Hospital in Dallas in September 2014. Subsequently, another nurse who also cared for the patient contracted Ebola. Both were treated and survived the illness. In 2015, the first nurse announced that she was suing the hospital where she worked and was exposed to Ebola for failing to develop policies to adequately train personnel in how to treat patients with highly contagious infections such as Ebola. One of the important lessons to be learned from this case is the importance of training and practice in how to use personal protective equipment (PPE) correctly to prevent transmission of any pathogenic disease. In the OR, surgical team members may have no idea what a patient's full health status is, and therefore they must presume every patient to be potentially infected with any and every possible type of disease to which they might have been exposed. With that mindset, we must all take personal responsibility for knowing how to use the PPE provided and then choose to use them each and every time we participate in a surgical procedure.

Microbes in the Media

The true story highlighted in the Clinical Significance Topic is very closely related to the weaknesses of the healthcare system when the United States and the entire population of the planet had to suddenly deal with a global disease pandemic. Despite the media attention placed on the exposure of a small handful of healthcare workers to a deadly, but very rarely encountered Ebola pathogen in this country, the COVID-19 pandemic focused attention on the lessons that should have been learned from that experience. The global COVID-19 pandemic placed incredible stress and pressures on the healthcare providers who had to find unique solutions to supply-chain shortages of critical PPE and acute care equipment to deal with massive numbers of critically ill and dying patients not seen since the 1918 influenza pandemic.

In recent years before 2020, hardly a week went by without a story in the news about an outbreak of some type of infectious disease. Some stories involved newer diseases that have been seen primarily in foreign countries, and with the vast expansion of travel, tourism, and trade, have gained entry to the United States. Other emerging diseases are linked to the broad scope of the U.S. healthcare system and include increasing numbers and types of mutated strains of pathogenic and potentially antibiotic-resistant bacteria.

Some media stories focus on recurring diseases and sporadic outbreaks, often in food contamination. Other recurring diseases are due to a wide range of human behavior factors and include ongoing preventable sexually-transmitted infections and other lifestyle choices that predispose individuals to transmissible diseases.

The last group involves diseases previously eradicated or held in check by effective and accepted national vaccination campaigns, public health initiatives, and herd immunity that are currently reappearing due to growing numbers of individuals opting out of established vaccination recommendations.

The year 2014 saw the largest outbreak of the Ebola virus in western Africa since its discovery in the 1970s. New cases continue to arise, with an outbreak in early 2021 in which 16 cases (12 deaths) of Ebola infection were documented in Guinea on the African continent in the same area as the 2014 outbreak. Ebola is only one of several types of **hemorrhagic fever** viruses that have continued to cause outbreaks in other parts of the world.

New viruses have caused concerning infections in children including the deadly delta and highly transmissible omicron variants of the SARS CoV-2 virus which causes COVID-19. Other common viruses such as measles, previously under control by virtue of routine vaccination programs, have reappeared due to parents failing to follow public health vaccine schedule recommendations.

Emerging Viral Diseases

Viruses are naturally equipped to **mutate** and evolve to adapt to changing environments. Viral relationships with infected host cells cause subtle and cumulative changes in the host cells over time. Changing conditions, coupled with transmission of mutated viruses from animals, allow new viruses to infect and affect humans in all regions of the planet. Humans are now more mobile than ever before in history, allowing viruses to quickly move about and infect globally, whereas in the past many infections were localized. *Aedes albopictus,* a mosquito vector for Dengue fever, established itself in several American states after being transported to Houston in used tires from Asia, and it continues to cause disease in endemic regions.

Most emergent viruses are zoonotic (transferred from animal hosts). Conditions that allow interactions between animals and humans increase the chances that an animal virus that has successfully mutated for human infection can be transmitted to a human host. HIV was believed to have originated as a simian virus (SIV) that was transferred to a human through a bite from a primate (type of mammal including apes).

Viruses develop an evolutionary balance between transmissibility and virulence, with an advantage held by those strains that are more readily transmitted and over prolonged periods.

Viral Hemorrhagic Fevers

Dengue, Ebola, Marburg, and Lassa fevers are the most common of the hemorrhagic diseases caused by viruses. Dengue

fever was documented as far back as 1779. Lassa fever was first described in the early 1950s. Marburg was first discovered in 1967. The Ebola virus was first identified in 1976.

Hemorrhagic fevers share common characteristics: high fever, headache, myalgia, diarrhea, vomiting, and internal hemorrhaging. Leakage of plasma through vessel walls causes hypovolemic shock. Because of the horrible nature of these viruses, outbreaks have caused fear throughout the world, and the media are quick to cover and sometimes sensationalize them when they do occur. Globalization has created the opportunity for epidemics to become pandemics and for previously unaffected countries having to learn to deal with these deadly diseases on home soil.

Ebola Hemorrhagic Fever

Ebola hemorrhagic fever (EHF) is a fatal viral disease that affects humans and primates. The Ebola virus is a member of the filovirus (*Filoviridae*) family of RNA viruses characterized by long filaments and threads that emerge from the central body (see Figure 22-1). They are highly variable in length; however, the average length of an infectious virion appears to be 920 nm. **Replication** within the host cell occurs quickly, destroying the host cell and releasing large numbers of infectious **virions** that spread rapidly through the bloodstream and take hold in multiple organs, causing severe and rapid necrosis. The central lesions appear to be those affecting the vascular endothelium and the platelets. As these structures deteriorate, uncontrolled bleeding occurs, especially in the mucosa, abdomen, and pericardium. Intravascular volume depletion results in intractable (difficult to manage) systemic shock, respiratory failure, and death.

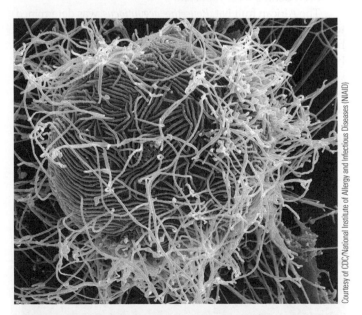

Figure 22-1 NIAID produced 25,000x magnification digitally-colorized scanning electron micrograph showing filamentous ebola virus particles (green) budding from a chronically-infected vero E6 cell (orange). Vero E6 cells are a cell line from the kidneys of African green monkeys.

EHF was first recognized as an emerging viral infection in 1976 and was named after a river in the Democratic Republic of the Congo (formerly Zaire). The virus is zoonotic and the host for the Ebola virus had long been unknown; however, Ebola and Marburg viruses have been isolated in species of fruit bats in the endemic areas. Transmission of filoviruses involves close personal contact between an infected individual's body fluids and another susceptible individual. Limiting or preventing contact between the uninfected and those infected results in a reduction of new filovirus infections. As the disease progresses rapidly, infected individuals are debilitated and unable to care for themselves. Caretakers of those who are infected have a high risk of becoming infected if strict contact precautions and use of adequate PPE are not practiced (see Figure 22-2). Medical aid workers and doctors providing humanitarian care also contracted Ebola along with the patients they were treating in the region. By July 2015, the year-long outbreak had resulted in a cumulative toll of over 11,200 deaths.

Marburg Hemorrhagic Fever

The Marburg virus, another member of the *Filoviridae* family of hemorrhagic fever viruses, was first recognized in 1967. Research laboratory workers in two labs, one in Marburg, Germany and the other in Belgrade, Serbia (formerly Yugoslavia), working with African green monkeys and their tissue samples were infected. In total, 31 individuals became ill. At first, the laboratory workers began showing signs and symptoms of the hemorrhagic fever, and then medical personnel and family members who had cared for them also fell ill. Seven deaths were reported.

The African fruit bat, *Rousettus aegyptiacus*, was determined to be the natural reservoir for the Marburg virus. Infected fruit bats show no obvious signs of illness and infect primates and humans, with resulting high mortality rates. Outbreaks are rare, with two travelers becoming infected in 2008. Four individuals in a family in Uganda were infected in 2017 and one case is still under investigation in Guinea in 2021.

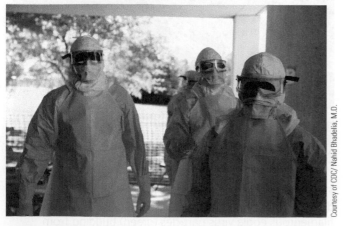

Figure 22-2 CDC 2014 Domestic Ebola ETU training course for healthcare workers.

Dengue Fever

Dengue fever (DF) first appeared in the 1770s in areas of Africa, Asia, and North America. The CDC estimated in 2021 that upwards of 400 million people are affected every year with 100 million becoming ill and of those, 40,000 die. Dengue fever is caused by any of four serotypes: Dengue 1, Dengue 2, Dengue 3, and Dengue 4. Infection with one serotype does not protect against the others. Multiple or sequential infections increase the risk for developing Dengue hemorrhagic fever (DHF) and Dengue shock syndrome (DSS).

The Dengue virus is a member of the genus *Flavivirus* and the family *Flaviviridae*. It has a long viral genome consisting of a single-strand positive-sense RNA. The virus is transmitted by the mosquito *Aedes aegypti*. **Viremia** in humans persists for 2 to 12 days.

The symptoms of Dengue fever begin approximately 5 days after infection with what is known as break-bone fever that manifests by severe myalgia, **arthralgia**, high fever, headache, and rash on extremities. **Leukopenia** and **thrombocytopenia** are also commonly noted. If fibrin aggregation is present, then the severe DHF form of the disease begins. Loss of appetite, abdominal pain, vomiting, headache, and hypotension ensue. Hypovolemic shock occurs when plasma leaks through vessel walls. Death occurs in 50 percent of all cases of DHF.

Lassa Fever

Lassa fever was first described in the 1950s and was isolated in 1969 when two missionary nurses in Nigeria contracted the virus and died. The disease is endemic in large areas of Africa, including Sierra Leone, Liberia, Guinea, and Nigeria; however, surrounding countries are also at risk. In 2015, a traveler returning to New Jersey from Liberia was found to have been infected with Lassa fever.

The virus that causes Lassa fever belongs to the *Arenaviridae* family of viruses, so named because of the sand-like appearance on their surface (arena is Latin for "sand"). In human diseases, members are usually associated with rodent vectors and each virus is associated with a particular rodent host species. The viral particles are spherical and have an average diameter of 110 to 130 nm. The virions are enveloped in a lipid (fat) membrane (see Figure 22-3).

The natural rodent host is the *Mastomys natalensis* rat, which transmits the disease through its urine and feces, which may produce aerosols of viral particles that are inhaled or ingested. The virus is highly contagious and can be transmitted from person to person. Laboratory personnel must take extreme precautions when working with viral hemorrhagic fever specimens to prevent potential infection or cross-contamination (see Figure 22-4).

Signs and symptoms of Lassa infection include fever and fatigue, with gastrointestinal (abdominal pain, nausea, vomiting, diarrhea), respiratory (pharyngitis, coughing), cardiovascular (pericarditis, hypertension), and neurologic systems (encephalitis, meningitis, confusion, seizures) affected. The 2019 CDC estimates show that approximately 100,000 to 300,000 infections occur annually, with 5,000 resulting deaths.

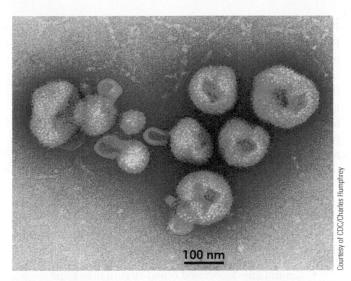

Figure 22-3 Transmission electron micrograph depicts eight virions (viral particles) of Lassa fever, a member of the genus, *Arenavirus*.

Hantavirus

Unlike the previous viral diseases, Hantavirus is not a hemorrhagic fever virus. It belongs to family *Bunyaviridae,* a group of RNA viruses with three segments of negative-sense single-strand RNA. There are dozens of types, but only two

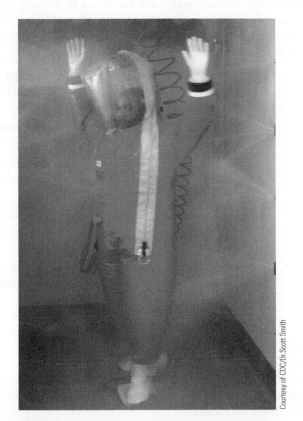

Figure 22-4 A CDC microbiologist showering inside a Biosafety Level 4 (BSL-4) laboratory decontamination booth prior to exiting the sealed confines of the BSL-4 laboratory where viral hemorrhagic fever samples are studied.

members of the family cause serious diseases: Hantavirus pulmonary syndrome (HPS) and hemorrhagic fever with renal syndrome (HFRS).

The virus that causes HFRS is found in East Asia. The HPS-causing strain is endemic to North America and South America. The most prevalent strain of the HPS-causing virus is the Sin Nombre virus (SNV), also known as the Four Corners virus, named for the region in the United States where the first outbreak occurred (the combined geographic border for Utah, Colorado, New Mexico, and Arizona).

The Hantavirus was named for the Hantaan River in Korea where the virus was first isolated from a field mouse in 1976. The Hantaan virus was eventually classified under its own genus, Hantavirus. HFRS was first recognized in the Western hemisphere after a 1951 outbreak among US troops stationed in Korea. It is estimated that in China, 100,000 people contract HFRS annually after exposure to the Asian striped field mouse (*Apodemus agrarius*), the rodent vector for the virus. Characteristics of HFRS include fever and myalgia followed by petechiae. Gastrointestinal hemorrhage, pulmonary edema, and acute renal failure ensue. Death is due to shock and loss of blood volume.

In 1993, several members of the Navajo Nation in New Mexico died from a mysterious respiratory ailment that scientists called unexplained adult respiratory distress syndrome (UARDS). Most of the victims were young and healthy and died soon after reaching the hospital. Researchers eventually found that UARDS created antibodies that were also produced by the Hantavirus. The pattern of reactivity, which was low-titer but cross-reactive with several Hantaviruses, suggested that UARDS was caused by a new strain of Hantavirus. Rodent trappings at the homes of the victims led to the recognition that the HPS-causing virus is primarily carried by deer mice (*Peromyscus maniculatus*). Humans are exposed to the virus in places where rodent infestation is high, and the virus is transmitted when the victim breathes in infected urine or feces aerosols. Most incidences occur in rural areas.

Characteristics of HPS are flu-like symptoms (fever, myalgia, and chills), which are the first clinical signs. Eventually, the lungs begin to fill with fluid from the circulatory system and respiratory distress ensues, resulting in death in two-thirds of all cases. Onset of respiratory distress is much quicker than in other respiratory diseases.

Chikungunya Virus

For the first time in late 2013, the chikungunya virus was found in the Americas on islands in the Caribbean including the territories of Puerto Rico and the US Virgin Islands. It is now considered a nationally notifiable disease by the CDC. Asia and the Americas have been the regions most affected by chikungunya. Pakistan and India have had approximately 70,000 in the last five years. North, Central, and South America and the Caribbean have had 185,000 reported cases with Brazil accounting for greater than 90 percent of those cases. Chikungunya outbreaks were also reported in 2018 in Sudan, in 2019 in Yemen, and in Cambodia and Chad in 2020.

Symptoms are very similar to Dengue fever and the virus is transmitted by *Aedes aegypti* and *Aedes albopictus* mosquitoes. There is no vaccine to prevent or medicine to treat chikungunya virus infection.

Other Viral Infections

Zika virus is a mosquito-borne flavivirus transmitted by *Aedes* species mosquitos. The zoonotic virus was first isolated in monkeys in Uganda in 1947 and later found in human infection in1952 in Uganda and Tanzania. Subsequent outbreaks of Zika virus have been recorded in Africa, the Americas, Asia, and the Pacific Islands. A large outbreak of Zika virus infections occurred in French Polynesia in 2013, later followed by a large outbreak in 2015 in Brazil where researchers recognized the association between Zika virus and microcephaly of infants born to mothers infected during pregnancy. An increased risk of neurologic complications has also been linked to Zika virus infection in adults and children to include neuropathy, myelitis, and Guillain-Barré syndrome. Most people infected with Zika virus are asymptomatic and, for those who do show mild signs of illness, they typically include fever, rash, conjunctivitis, muscle and joint pain, malaise, and headache. These usually last for 2–7 days. According to the WHO in 2018, 86 countries have had evidence of mosquito-transmitted Zika infections. In addition to transmission by mosquitos, the virus can be transmitted through unprotected sexual intercourse through blood or semen of an intimate partner who has been infected.

Sporadic outbreaks of viral infections have been reported over the past decade and include Middle East respiratory syndrome (MERS) a respiratory coronavirus, Enterovirus EV-D68, a severe respiratory virus that affects mainly children with pre-existing asthma, and a respiratory illness that has been named acute **flaccid myelitis** that affected children with sudden onset of weakness in one or more arms or legs. MRI scans showed inflammation of the gray matter of the spinal cord. Although not confirmed, there is a possibility of a link between the cases of EV-D68 and the cases of acute flaccid myelitis. In addition to these viruses, the delta variant of COVID-19 has proved to be a deadly new viral pathogen and the extremely transmissible omicron variant with cases and research about the mutations likely to be ongoing for some time.

Recurring Diseases

As mentioned earlier, some of the diseases that are recurring and ongoing include food-borne infections, viral gastrointestinal infections, and many sexually transmitted diseases, despite years of public education campaigns and media attention. More relevant to surgical technology students are the recurring healthcare-associated infections (HAIs), which have been the focus of attention by government and private agencies for years. A sampling of recurring diseases is discussed in this section.

Healthcare-Associated Infections

Formerly called nosocomial infections, healthcare-associated infections (HAIs) have been a focus of media attention and oversight organizations such as the Joint Commission and the Centers for Medicare and Medicaid Services (CMS). In general, HAIs are preventable, and for that reason, providers are being increasingly held accountable for the incredible expense of managing infections that patients might never have acquired had they not passed through the healthcare system (see Figure 22-5).

Despite the numerous initiatives designed to educate healthcare workers about infection control and prevention, HAIs continue to occur in all areas of the country and are among the leading causes of preventable deaths. Attention has been focused on several areas, including:

- Central line-associated blood stream infections (CLABSIs)
- Catheter-associated urinary tract infections (CAUTIs)
- Surgical site infections (SSIs)
- Ventilator-associated pneumonia (VAP)

The broad issues concerning healthcare-associated infections are multifactorial. No single group is responsible for causing or is able to resolve these complex problems. The issues require and will continue to demand the cooperative efforts of the various healthcare members to identify risks, assess impact, develop strategies, and implement work practice controls to protect the patients who enter the healthcare system. Some of the issues to be considered include:

- Long-established standards of antibiotic administration contributing to growing antibiotic resistance in an increasing variety of microbial pathogens
- Non-compliance of healthcare workers with infection control policies and procedures
- Failure of adequate training and/or insufficient supplies or distribution of effective personal protective equipment (PPE)
- Increasing complexity of instrument and device structural designs preventing adequate decontamination and disinfection
- Increase in unrecognized or undiagnosed community-acquired diseases in individuals entering healthcare settings

Microbes Linked to Healthcare-Associated Infections

The CDC has compiled a list of pathogenic bacteria and viruses most frequently linked to or responsible for the majority of HAIs. These microbes are:

- *Acinetobacter*
- *Burkholderia cepacia*
- *Candida auris*

- *Clostridioides difficile*
- *Clostridium sordellii*
- Carbapenem-resistant *Enterobacterales*
- ESBL-producing *Enterobacterales* (including *E. coli* and *Klebsiella pneumoniae*
- Gram-negative bacteria
- Hepatitis viruses
- Human immunodeficiency virus (HIV/AIDS)
- Influenza virus
- *Klebsiella*

- Methicillin-resistant *Staphylococcus aureus* (MRSA)
- *Non-tuberculous Mycobacterium abscessus* (NTM)
- Norovirus
- *Pseudomonas aeruginosa*
- *Staphylococcus aureus*
- *Mycobacterium tuberculosis* (TB)
- Vancomycin-intermediate *Staphylococcus aureus* (VISA)
- Vancomycin-resistant *Staphylococcus aureus* (VRSA)
- Vancomycin-resistant Enterococci (VRE)

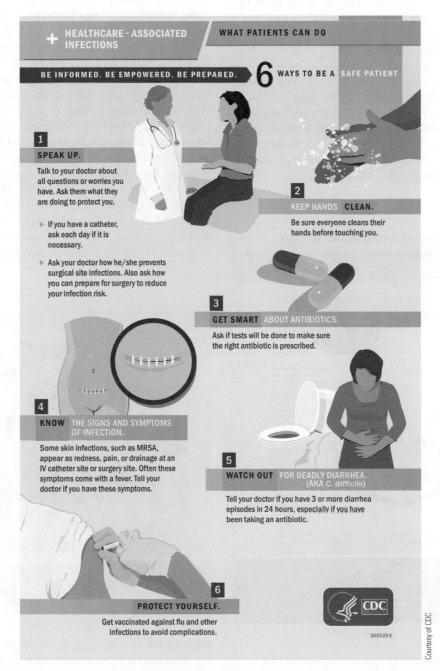

Figure 22-5 CDC-created infographic intended to help patients become more informed about their medical condition.

Antibiotic Resistance

It is estimated that 2.8 million infections from antibiotic resistant bacteria occur annually and result in more than 35,000 deaths. Nearly 223,900 people in the United States in 2017 required hospitalization for *C. difficile* infection and approximately 12,800 of those patients died. Antibiotics are possibly the most common of all medications prescribed. In nearly half of all cases, the antibiotics prescribed are done so inappropriately (wrong type, wrong dose, unnecessary for the encountered infection). Animals raised for food are routinely given low doses of antibiotics to enhance their growth and development. This practice leads to antibiotic resistance in bacterial species, including *Salmonella* and *Campylobacter*. Finally, transmission of antibiotic-resistant pathogens between individuals broadens their reach among members of a population (see Figure 22-6).

Antibiotic-resistant infections are most commonly spread in community settings; however, the healthcare system must then care for those who become infected. Once in the healthcare setting, the antibiotic-resistant pathogens are easily spread to patients who are more vulnerable and immunocompromised. The CDC published a report in 2019 outlining the top 18 drug-resistant threats in the United States. These threats were categorized based on level of concern: urgent, serious, and concerning (see Table 22-1).

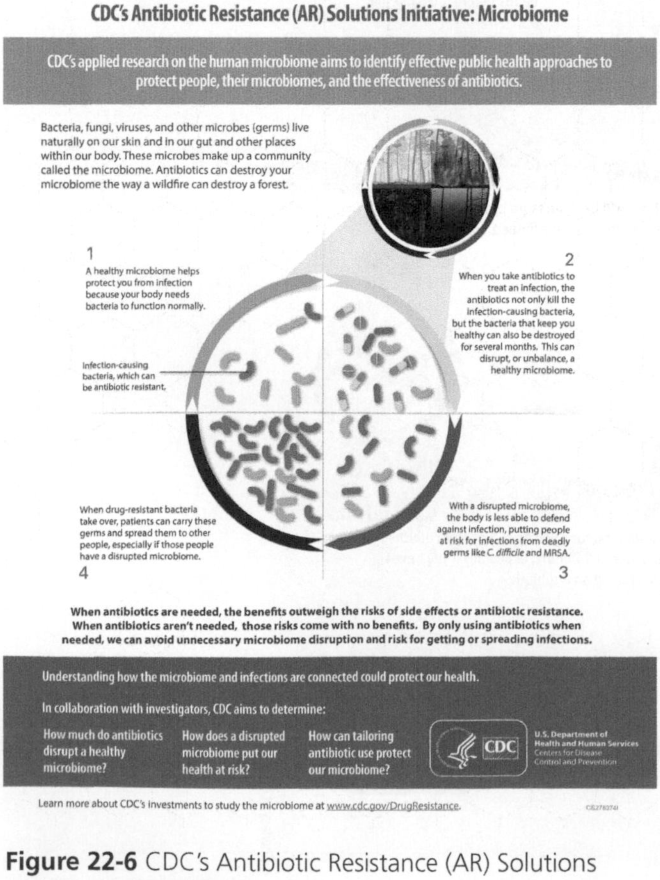

The current emphasis on prevention of antibiotic resistance is addressed in the CDC *Antibiotic Stewardship Implementation Framework for Health Departments*. Antibiotic stewardship is described as coordinated interventions designed to improve the use of antibiotics. The focused programs have demonstrated an increase in optimal prescribing for therapy and prophylaxis, improvements in overall quality of patient care, and reduction of adverse events such as *C. difficile* infections associated with antibiotic over-use and resistance.

Gastrointestinal Viruses

Norovirus and rotavirus are two of the more pathogenic members of the *Caliciviridae* family of enteropathogenic viruses that cause GI infections from food sources, contaminated surfaces, or person-to-person contact (see Figure 22-7). Annually in the United States, there are 2,500 outbreaks resulting in 19 to 21 million cases of vomiting and diarrhea illnesses, 109,000 hospitalizations, and 900 deaths from complications of the infections, mainly in adults age 65 and older. Norovirus outbreaks have been featured in news reports about cruise ships having to cut trips short due to overwhelming sickness in the majority of passengers. Other outbreaks have been seen in schools and nursing homes where groups of individuals spend prolonged periods in close quarters. Food-borne infection sources include restaurants, banquet facilities, private homes, healthcare facilities, schools and daycare centers, and other venues.

The disease is extremely contagious, requiring transmission and inoculation of only 18 viral particles to cause disease in another individual. The viruses may remain in feces for

CDC's Antibiotic Resistance (AR) Solutions Initiative: Microbiome

CDC's applied research on the human microbiome aims to identify effective public health approaches to protect people, their microbiomes, and the effectiveness of antibiotics.

Bacteria, fungi, viruses, and other microbes (germs) live naturally on our skin and in our gut and other places within our body. These microbes make up a community called the microbiome. Antibiotics can destroy your microbiome the way a wildfire can destroy a forest.

1 A healthy microbiome helps protect you from infection because your body needs bacteria to function normally.

Infection-causing bacteria, which can be antibiotic resistant.

2 When you take antibiotics to treat an infection, the antibiotics not only kill the infection-causing bacteria, but the bacteria that keep you healthy can also be destroyed for several months. This can disrupt, or unbalance, a healthy microbiome.

4 When drug-resistant bacteria take over, patients can carry these germs and spread them to other people, especially if those people have a disrupted microbiome.

3 With a disrupted microbiome, the body is less able to defend against infection, putting people at risk for infections from deadly germs like *C. difficile* and MRSA.

When antibiotics are needed, the benefits outweigh the risks of side effects or antibiotic resistance. When antibiotics aren't needed, those risks come with no benefits. By only using antibiotics when needed, we can avoid unnecessary microbiome disruption and risk for getting or spreading infections.

Understanding how the microbiome and infections are connected could protect our health.

In collaboration with investigators, CDC aims to determine:

How much do antibiotics disrupt a healthy microbiome?

How does a disrupted microbiome put our health at risk?

How can tailoring antibiotic use protect our microbiome?

CDC U.S. Department of Health and Human Services Centers for Disease Control and Prevention

Learn more about CDC's investments to study the microbiome at www.cdc.gov/DrugResistance.

Figure 22-6 CDC's Antibiotic Resistance (AR) Solutions Initiative: Microbiome

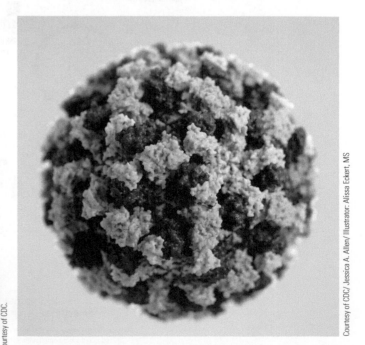

Figure 22-7 3-D illustration of a single norovirus virion and the different colors represent regions of the virion's outer protein shell, or capsid.

Table 22-1 **2019 CDC Antibiotic-Resistance Threats in the United States**

Microorganism	Threat Level	Annual Infections	Deaths
Carbapenem-resistant *Acinetobacter*	Urgent	8,500	700
Drug-resistant *Candida auris*	Urgent	323	
Clostridioides difficile	Urgent	223,900	12,800
Carbapenem-resistant *Enterobacterales*	Urgent	13,100	1,100
Drug-resistant *Neisseria gonorrhoeae*	Urgent	550,000	
Drug-resistant *Campylobacter*	Serious	448,400	70
Drug-resistant *Candida* Species	Serious	34,800	1,700
ESBL-producing *Enterobacterales*	Serious	197,400	9,100
Vancomycin-resistant *Enterococcus* (VRE)	Serious	54,500	5,400
Multidrug-resistant *Pseudomonas aeruginosa*	Serious	32,600	2,700
Drug-resistant nontyphoidal *Salmonella*	Serious	212,500	70
Drug-resistant *Salmonella* Serotype Typhi	Serious	4,100	Less than 5
Drug-resistant *Shigella*	Serious	27,000	Less than 5
Methicillin-resistant *Staphylococcus aureus* (MRSA)	Serious	323,700	10,600
Drug-resistant *Streptococcus pneumoniae*	Serious	9,000 (2014)	3,600 (2014)
Drug-resistant Tuberculosis	Serious	847	62
Erythromycin-resistant group A *Streptococcus*	Concerning	5,400	450
Clindamycin-resistant group B *Streptococcus*	Concerning	13,000	720

2 weeks after symptoms have abated and billions of viral particles are shed during that period. Routine and strict hand washing after using the restroom, washing food and preparing with careful attention to hygiene, and disinfection of all contaminated surfaces are the steps necessary in reducing transmission of these types of gastrointestinal viruses.

Two types of oral vaccines for prevention of rotavirus infections are available for children, starting at age 2 months. One type of vaccine is given in three doses at 2, 4, and 6 months of age, and the other is given in two doses at 2 and 4 months of age. There is no vaccine yet available for prevention of norovirus infections. Worldwide, norovirus infections have become the most common cause of acute gastroenteritis.

Researchers at Washington University in St. Louis have found potential promise in using antibiotic therapy to reduce the populations of enteropathogenic GI viruses. Although antibiotics have no effect on viruses, there is a symbiotic relationship between the bacteria that inhabit the intestines and the viruses that require viable bacterial hosts for replication and spread to other cells. The research theory revolves around the reduction of host bacteria causing elimination of the viral invaders; however, studies are ongoing.

Food-Borne Infections

Recurring food-borne infections continue to develop in multiple regions of the country and world from a variety of food sources, often gaining widespread media attention (see Figure 22-8). The most commonly seen infective agents are *Escherichia coli, Salmonella, Listeria, Cyclospora,* and *Vibrio.* The following list demonstrates the wide range of potential

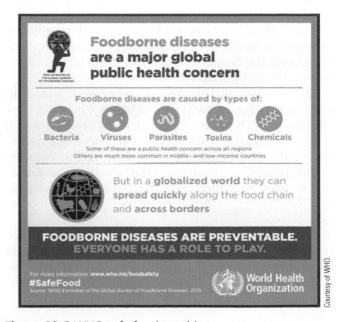

Figure 22-8 WHO safe food graphic

foodborne sources of infection. The list from the CDC is from 2021 and included:

- Seafood
- Italian-style meats
- Cake mix
- Pre-packaged salad
- Fully-cooked chicken
- Frozen cooked shrimp
- Raw frozen breaded stuffed chicken products
- Cashew brie
- Ground turkey
- Queso fresco

HIV/AIDS

Much has been written about the human immunodeficiency virus (HIV) and the subsequent disease it causes, acquired immunodeficiency syndrome (AIDS); however, HIV continues to be a serious global health issue and recurring disease. Chapter 8 also discusses HIV.

According to HIV.org, in the United States in 2019, there were an estimated 1.2 million cases of HIV, 34,800 of those being new and 15,815 deaths, however the cause of death may be from other causes. Globally in 2020, an estimated 37.6 million people were living with HIV and approximately 690,000 people died from AIDS-related illnesses, compared to 1.2 million in 2010.

According to the CDC, homosexual, bisexual, and other men who have sex with men (MSM) of all races and ethnicities remain the population most profoundly affected by HIV.

Many "urban myths" exist regarding HIV/AIDS and how it is transmitted. Unlike some other viruses, HIV does not remain viable outside the body for very long. It is only transmitted through intimate contact and not by activities such as shaking hands, closed-lip kissing, or through tears, sweat, or saliva. It is not transmissible by mosquitoes, ticks, water, or air. It cannot be contracted by sitting on a toilet seat used previously by someone with HIV.

Transmission of HIV through needle-stick injuries in healthcare settings is rare (1 percent chance); however, great care should still be taken when performing procedures with sharp objects such as scalpel blades, suture needles, hypodermic needles, and instruments with sharp points, including the following: Gelpi, Weitlaner, Senn, and skin hook retractors; K-wires, Steinman pins, drill bits, saw blades, perforators; bladed trocars, sharp-tipped scissors; and fine-toothed tissue forceps.

No-touch, neutral zone, or hands-free techniques reduce incidents of intraoperative sharps injuries and should be taught and practiced by all surgical technology students. These techniques are appropriate in all procedures to prevent potential transmission of other blood-borne pathogens as well.

Reappearing Diseases

Diseases previously considered under control have begun to reappear in the United States. This section discusses the preventable diseases that have been highlighted in the media and have created conversation and controversy.

Preventable Childhood Diseases

The phenomenon of herd immunity was discussed in Chapter 21 in reference to control of microbial disease when the vast majority of members of a population follow public health vaccination recommendations (see Figure 22-9). The reappearance of preventable diseases such as measles and whooping cough has gained media attention and has sparked vigorous debate about the rights and responsibilities of parents, citizens, and the medical community.

In response to the controversies caused by anti-vaccination groups and spread of misinformation; the CDC stepped up its public information campaigns. Some of the data they cite in support of childhood vaccinations include:

- Measles was declared eliminated from the United States in 2000 due to the success of the highly effective vaccination program. However, in many parts of the world, including some countries in Europe, Asia, Pacific island nations, and Africa, measles is still common. Worldwide, an estimated 20 million people contract measles and 142,000 people (mostly children) die from the disease each year.
- Measles is brought into the United States by unvaccinated travelers who get measles while they are in other countries. Anyone who is not vaccinated against measles is at risk.
- Measles is transmitted through the air when an infected person coughs or sneezes. It is so contagious that if one person has it, they can infect up to 10 others who are unvaccinated.
- A susceptible individual can get measles simply by breathing the air in a room where a person with measles has been, even up to 2 hours after that person has left the room.
- Infected individuals are contagious from 4 days before developing the measles rash through 4 days afterward.
- One in 5 individuals with measles must be hospitalized.
- One in 1,000 will develop serious meningitis or encephalitis.
- One or 2 per 1,000 will die from measles, even with medical treatment.

Pertussis, better known as whooping cough is caused by *Bordetella pertussis* bacteria, which cause serious inflammation of the respiratory tract in children, with infants typically

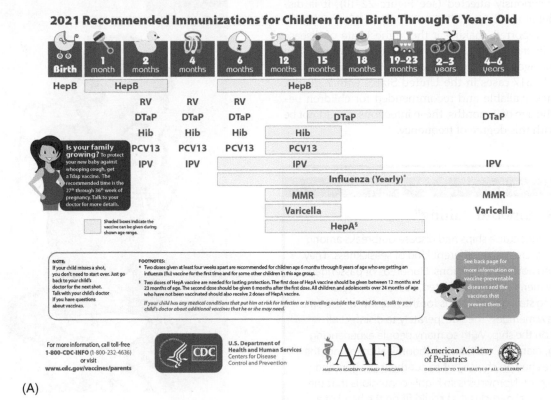

2021 Recommended Immunizations for Children from Birth Through 6 Years Old

Birth	1 month	2 months	4 months	6 months	12 months	15 months	18 months	19–23 months	2–3 years	4–6 years
HepB	HepB				HepB					
		RV	RV	RV						
		DTaP	DTaP	DTaP		DTaP				DTaP
		Hib	Hib	Hib	Hib					
		PCV13	PCV13	PCV13	PCV13					
		IPV	IPV		IPV					IPV
					Influenza (Yearly)*					
					MMR					MMR
					Varicella					Varicella
					HepA§					

Is your family growing? To protect your new baby against whooping cough, get a Tdap vaccine. The recommended time is the 27th through 36th week of pregnancy. Talk to your doctor for more details.

☐ Shaded boxes indicate the vaccine can be given during shown age range.

NOTE:
If your child misses a shot, you don't need to start over. Just go back to your child's doctor for the next shot. Talk with your child's doctor if you have questions about vaccines.

FOOTNOTES:
* Two doses given at least four weeks apart are recommended for children age 6 months through 8 years of age who are getting an influenza (flu) vaccine for the first time and for some other children in this age group.

§ Two doses of HepA vaccine are needed for lasting protection. The first dose of HepA vaccine should be given between 12 months and 23 months of age. The second dose should be given 6 months after the first dose. All children and adolescents over 24 months of age who have not been vaccinated should also receive 2 doses of HepA vaccine.

If your child has any medical conditions that put him at risk for infection or is traveling outside the United States, talk to your child's doctor about additional vaccines that he or she may need.

See back page for more information on vaccine-preventable diseases and the vaccines that prevent them.

For more information, call toll-free
1-800-CDC-INFO (1-800-232-4636)
or visit
www.cdc.gov/vaccines/parents

CDC   **U.S. Department of Health and Human Services** Centers for Disease Control and Prevention

AAFP AMERICAN ACADEMY OF FAMILY PHYSICIANS

American Academy of Pediatrics DEDICATED TO THE HEALTH OF ALL CHILDREN®

(A)

Vaccine-Preventable Diseases and the Vaccines that Prevent Them

Disease	Vaccine	Disease spread by	Disease symptoms	Disease complications
Chickenpox	Varicella vaccine protects against chickenpox.	Air, direct contact	Rash, tiredness, headache, fever	Infected blisters, bleeding disorders, encephalitis (brain swelling), pneumonia (infection in the lungs)
Diphtheria	DTaP* vaccine protects against diphtheria.	Air, direct contact	Sore throat, mild fever, weakness, swollen glands in neck	Swelling of the heart muscle, heart failure, coma, paralysis, death
Hib	Hib vaccine protects against *Haemophilus influenzae* type b.	Air, direct contact	May be no symptoms unless bacteria enter the blood	Meningitis (infection of the covering around the brain and spinal cord), intellectual disability, epiglottitis (life-threatening infection that can block the windpipe and lead to serious breathing problems), pneumonia (infection in the lungs), death
Hepatitis A	HepA vaccine protects against hepatitis A.	Direct contact, contaminated food or water	May be no symptoms, fever, stomach pain, loss of appetite, fatigue, vomiting, jaundice (yellowing of skin and eyes), dark urine	Liver failure, arthralgia (joint pain), kidney, pancreatic and blood disorders
Hepatitis B	HepB vaccine protects against hepatitis B.	Contact with blood or body fluids	May be no symptoms, fever, headache, weakness, vomiting, jaundice (yellowing of skin and eyes), joint pain	Chronic liver infection, liver failure, liver cancer
Influenza (Flu)	Flu vaccine protects against influenza.	Air, direct contact	Fever, muscle pain, sore throat, cough, extreme fatigue	Pneumonia (infection in the lungs)
Measles	MMR** vaccine protects against measles.	Air, direct contact	Rash, fever, cough, runny nose, pink eye	Encephalitis (brain swelling), pneumonia (infection in the lungs), death
Mumps	MMR**vaccine protects against mumps.	Air, direct contact	Swollen salivary glands (under the jaw), fever, headache, tiredness, muscle pain	Meningitis (infection of the covering around the brain and spinal cord), encephalitis (brain swelling), inflammation of testicles or ovaries, deafness
Pertussis	DTaP* vaccine protects against pertussis (whooping cough).	Air, direct contact	Severe cough, runny nose, apnea (a pause in breathing in infants)	Pneumonia (infection in the lungs), death
Polio	IPV vaccine protects against polio.	Air, direct contact, through the mouth	May be no symptoms, sore throat, fever, nausea, headache	Paralysis, death
Pneumococcal	PCV13 vaccine protects against pneumococcus.	Air, direct contact	May be no symptoms, pneumonia (infection in the lungs)	Bacteremia (blood infection), meningitis (infection of the covering around the brain and spinal cord), death
Rotavirus	RV vaccine protects against rotavirus.	Through the mouth	Diarrhea, fever, vomiting	Severe diarrhea, dehydration
Rubella	MMR** vaccine protects against rubella.	Air, direct contact	Sometimes rash, fever, swollen lymph nodes	Very serious in pregnant women——can lead to miscarriage, stillbirth, premature delivery, birth defects
Tetanus	DTaP* vaccine protects against tetanus.	Exposure through cuts in skin	Stiffness in neck and abdominal muscles, difficulty swallowing, muscle spasms, fever	Broken bones, breathing difficulty, death

* DTaP combines protection against diphtheria, tetanus, and pertussis.
** MMR combines protection against measles, mumps, and rubella.

Last updated February 2021 - CS322257-A

Courtesy of CDC.

(B)

Figure 22-9 (A) 2021 recommended immunizations for children from birth to six years old. **(B)** Vaccine-preventable diseases and the vaccines that prevent them.

being most seriously affected (see Figure 22-10). It is discussed in detail in Chapters 16 and 20. In 2012, there were 48,277 cases reported, making it the highest rate of disease since 1955. Twenty deaths, mainly in children younger than 3 months of age, were reported during that year. In 2019, there were 18,617 cases in the United States with 7 deaths. With vaccines available and recommended for children beginning at the age of 2 months, these infections should not be occurring with this degree of frequency.

MICRO NOTES

"Not So Smooth Sailing"

In 2019, eight cruise ships had disease outbreaks among passengers, creating a different kind of seasickness. They contracted norovirus infections. Hundreds of passengers and crew members were affected. Passengers were required to stay in their cabins for the majority of the time while crew members tried desperately to disinfect all surfaces on the ship. With so many people experiencing vomiting, diarrhea, and painful abdominal cramping, the cruise lines had no choice but to cut the trips short and return to port. Norovirus is so highly contagious that the number of viral particles that could fit on the head of a straight pin could infect 1,000 people, and it can live on inanimate objects for extended periods. So much for working on that suntan.

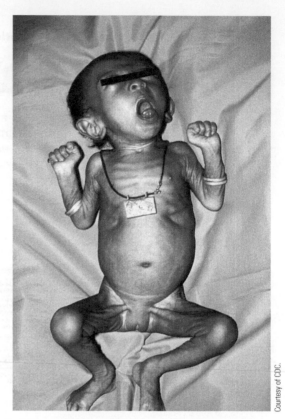

Figure 22-10 Female infant suffering from whooping cough caused by *Bordetella pertussis*

Courtesy of CDC.

 ## Under the Microscope

After returning from a wonderful medical mission trip to a medically-underserved area in Central America, several of the surgical team members complained of flu-like symptoms, despite having had their recommended travel immunizations prior to the trip. While there, the scope of illness in patients who have no access to healthcare became apparent as the team tried to treat severe conditions associated with vaccine-preventable infections as well as surgical conditions. Based in part on the range of illnesses endemic to the region, consider the following questions.

1. What types of diagnoses should be considered in the team members feeling ill?

2. Which types of diseases might the surgical team have seen in the patients due to lack of access to immunization or routine preventative healthcare?

3. Which modes of transmission might have contributed to the infections that team members are experiencing?

4. What factors should be considered when prescribing antibiotics, anti-fungals, or anti-viral medications for these possible infections?

5. What types of illnesses within the United States might be considered emerging, recurring, or reappearing diseases?

Abiogenesis: Also called the theory of spontaneous generation, this theory claimed that life could spontaneously arise from nonliving material.

Abscess: A localized collection of pus; a combination of body fluids and dead cells that result from an immune response to infection.

Abstinence: Voluntarily going without or refraining from doing something such as drinking alcohol or having sexual relations.

Acellular: Something which consists of or contains no cells or cell structure.

Acid-fast stain: A stain solution of carbolfuchsin which only fixes to bacteria that have a waxy chemical substance in their cell walls. Used to identify *Mycobacterium tuberculosis*. Also known as Ziehl-Neelsen method.

Adenocarcinoma: A type of malignant tumor originating in a glandular organ.

Adenosine triphosphate (ATP): A chemical compound of the nucleotide adenosine and three phosphoric acid groups which is present in all cells, however in larger number in muscle tissues. When the compound is split by enzymes, usable energy is produced.

Adherence: Attachment of a pathogen to the tissue of a host; a necessary step in the process of pathogenicity.

Aeration: The process of exchange of carbon dioxide for oxygen in the blood in the lungs.

Aerobic: Pertaining to an organism which lives and thrives in the presence of air and dies without it.

Aerosolized: Microscopic liquid or solid particles or microbes suspended or dispersed in a fine mist or gas.

Aerotolerant: Classification of microbes that do not require oxygen for growth and can survive in atmospheres containing small amounts of oxygen. Considered fermentative anaerobes, they grow best in the total absence of oxygen.

Agammaglobulinemia: The condition of an individual born without the ability to produce antibodies and whose blood therefore has no gammaglobulin.

Agar: A complex polysaccharide obtained from the red marine alga. Agar is added to a liquid medium to solidify the medium.

Alkaline: A substance with the properties of an alkali; base with a pH greater than 7.

Alveoli: Air cells of the lungs; singular: alveolus; sockets (hollows) of teeth; honeycomb-like depressions of gastric mucous membranes.

Amines: Organic compounds which are derivatives of ammonia, including cadaverine and putrescine, which are characterized by strong, foul odors.

Amoebas: Single-celled protozoa often found in soil and water which utilize pseudopods for movement. Also called amebas.

Anaerobic chamber: Laboratory equipment used when handling anaerobic bacteria; it is equipped with air locks to prevent oxygen from entering.

Anaerobic: Pertaining to an organism which lives and thrives in the absence of air and dies when exposed to it.

Anaphylaxis: Serious, potentially life-threatening, Type I immediate hypersensitivity (allergic) reaction to an antigen; may lead to systemic shock.

Aneurysm: Abnormal, localized dilatation of a blood vessel, commonly an artery; may be congenital or acquired and due to hypertension, trauma, or infection.

Angiogenesis: Creation or development of new blood vessels.

Annelides: Cells that produces conidia by growing longer, ending in a tapered tip.

Anomalies: Variations from normal, as in congenital anomaly, also known as birth defect.

Anoxygenic: Name of a microorganism which does not produce molecular oxygen during the process of photosynthesis.

Antibiotic: Substance produced naturally by bacteria or other organisms or synthetically produced in the laboratory, capable of killing or suppressing the growth of microorganisms and used clinically to fight infections.

Antibodies: Glycoproteins produced by B-lymphocytes that enter the circulatory system; the host's immune system is stimulated to produce antibodies when a specific bacteria or antigen enters the body. They bind with the bacteria or antigens.

Anticoagulant: Any agent which prevents or delays the coagulation (clotting) of blood.

Antigenic determinants: Also known as epitopes; specific parts of an antigen molecule to which antibodies and/or lymphocytes can bind.

Antisera: Solutions of antibodies that are commercially produced and used in the laboratory to identify particular microorganisms through qualitative slide agglutination; vaccine preparations given to impart acquired immunity to a specific disease.

Archaea: Category of microorganisms with ancient origins, which share characteristics of both prokaryotes and eukaryotes, however, are distinct from both groups. Many archaea inhabit extreme environments (e.g., thermophiles or acidophiles).

Arthralgia: Pain located in the joints.

Arthritis: An inflammatory disease of the joints, causing pain, edema, and restricted motion.

Arthroconidia: Square-like conidia formed by modified hyphal cells.

Arthropod vectors: Insect carriers, such as mosquitoes, that transmit microorganisms from an infected to a noninfected individual or animal.

Arthrospores: Segmented bacterial spores which have entered into a resting state.

Aseptate: The absence of septa; hyphae in certain kinds of molds that are not divided into sections or separate cells by walls called septa.

Aseptic techniques: Practices used by surgical technologists and other members of the surgical team to prevent transmission of pathogenic microorganisms; includes surgical scrub process or preoperative skin preparation of the patient among others.

Asymptomatic: Without symptoms; displaying no evidence of effects of a disease or infection.

Ataxia: Loss of or defective muscle coordination.

Atherosclerotic plaques: Deposits of lipids (fats) or other substances which adhere to and decrease the diameter of arterial blood vessels causing "hardening of the arteries."

Atrophic: Pertaining to atrophy which is a severe decrease in size of tissue such as muscle, or organs; wasting away.

Attenuated: Weakened in intensity, force, strength, or effect; types of vaccines which utilize live pathogens which are rendered non-pathogenic but produce an effective immune response.

Auscultation: Diagnostic method of listening to body sounds (commonly thoracic or abdominal) to detect abnormality.

Autoimmune disease: A disease in which the body produces antibodies to attack its own normal cells and tissues.

Autoinducers: Molecular chemical signals emitted from bacteria as a component of quorum-sensing communication within or between bacterial colonies which leads to alterations in gene expressions and regulation of physiologic processes in response

to environmental conditions. Also known as pheromones.

Auxotrophic: Pertaining to mutant microbe needing an alternate nutritional requirement from the parent cell.

Bactericidal: Destructive to bacteria; able to kill or destroy bacteria.

Bacteriocins: Any form of agent capable of killing bacteria.

Bacteriophages: Viruses which infect bacteria.

Bifurcated: Split, forked; having divisions or branches.

Bioburden: The presence of organic debris; amount or numbers of microorganisms present on any given object. Bioburden is removed during cleaning and decontamination and prior to sterilization procedures.

Biofilms: Microbial (typically bacterial) colonies that combine into dense colonies that adhere to surfaces and resist penetration or destruction by antibiotic therapy.

Bioleaching: Innovative method of extracting precious and base metals from ore by use of bacterial microorganisms rather than traditional heap leaching and smelting methods which produce large amounts of environmental pollutants.

Biological indicator: A type of process monitor for sterilization techniques which uses small populations of living microorganisms which are harmless to humans, however resistant to the form of sterilization used to verify the lethality of the process and demonstrate that all microorganisms were killed and sterility was achieved.

Bioprosthetic valves: Artificial replacement heart valves made with a combination of artificial and biological components from pigs (porcine), cattle (bovine), or horses (equine).

Bioremediation: A method of using microorganisms to clean up environmental contamination by pollutants such as oil, organic waste, and radiation.

Bioterrorism: The use of biological agents (bacteria or viruses) in terrorist attacks for the purposes of causing death or widespread disease in humans, animals, or plants.

Blastoconidium: A protuberance formed on the surface by a yeast parent cell during reproduction by budding; it eventually breaks away as a new daughter cell.

Blastomycosis: A rare fungal infection which causes inflammatory lesions of the skin, lungs, bones, central nervous system, or other internal organs caused by inhalation of *Blastomyces dermatitidis* conidia.

Blepharitis: Inflammation of the edges of eyelids which includes the hair follicles and glands; may be ulcerative caused by bacterial infection or non-ulcerative caused by allergens or environmental irritants.

Blood agar: A solid enriched medium that is a combination of nutrient agar and sheep erythrocytes (red blood cells).

Blood-borne pathogens (BBPs): Microorganisms capable of causing infection or disease which are spread through direct blood-to-blood contact via sharps injury, intravenous needle-sharing, unprotected sexual contact, contamination of mucous membranes, maternal-fetal circulation, or blood transfusion.

Boils: A large, raised, acutely inflamed skin lesions filled with pus; also known as furuncles.

Bronchospasm: Narrowing and obstruction of a bronchus or multiple bronchi caused by involuntary muscular contraction (spasm).

Bubonic plague: An acute, deadly, infectious disease also known as the Black Death in the Middle Ages; caused by *Yersinia pestis* carried and spread by infected rodents; and characterized by swollen lymph nodes that become hemorrhagic; the infection becomes systemic, resulting in a severe bacterial pneumonia with violent coughs.

Bullous: Characterized by eruption of blisters (bullae)/skin crusting without blisters; forms of the skin disease impetigo, with nonbullous impetigo being the more contagious form.

Candidemia: The presence of cells of the yeast *Candida* in the bloodstream.

Capnophiles: Microorganisms which thrive in or have a nutritional requirement for increased or high concentrations of carbon dioxide in the atmosphere.

Capsid: A protein covering that protects the RNA or DNA in a virus from destructive enzymes and promotes attachment to susceptible cells.

Capsomere: A protein molecule of a viral capsid.

Carbuncles: Circumscribed (focused) sites of staphylococcal subcutaneous tissue infection containing pus that eventually discharge to the surface of the skin.

Cardiac arrhythmia: Abnormal and irregular rhythm of cardiac contraction and relaxation caused by pathological or physiological disturbances of the electrical impulses of the sinoatrial (SA) node.

Cardiac tamponade: Serious to fatal pathological condition secondary to accumulation of fluid (blood, pus, clots) in the space between the myocardium and the pericardial sac (pericardium) causing compression and eventual cessation of function.

Cardiomyopathy: Primary disease of the myocardium (heart muscle).

Cardioverter-defibrillator: Implantable automated electronic device which corrects several types of cardiac arrhythmias /dysrhythmias and abnormal heart rates to prevent sudden cardiac arrest and death.

Catarrhal stage: The primary stage of pertussis (whooping cough) characterized by inflammation of the mucous membranes of the respiratory tract which causes excessive nasal discharge, low-grade fever, and coughing.

Cell theory: A scientific proposal first made by Robert Hooke following his observation of living units he termed "cells" which stated that all life was composed of these building blocks. Subsequent research by other scientists and biologists led to modification of the theory as scientists gained better understanding of how cells grow, multiply, and respond to environmental factors.

Cellulitis: Infection of solid tissue, especially the loose connective tissue just under the skin, commonly caused by *Haemophilus influenzae* type b.

Centrioles: Tiny cellular organelles. Two centrioles found within every cell lie perpendicular to the nucleus and at right angles to each other. They form spindle fibers to aid in cell division.

Cerebral Infarct: An area of the brain which becomes ischemic and necrotic due to disruption of blood supply; also known as ischemic stroke.

Cervical os: The funnel-shaped opening of the uterine cervix; which has internal or external components.

Cestodes: Tapeworms; intestinal parasites.

Chancre: A lesion that appears 10 to 60 days after the acquiring of syphilis; initially it is slightly red in appearance but eventually ulcerates, forming a slightly elevated oval lesion with a red rim.

Chemical indicator/integrators: Sterilization process monitors, which utilize strips, cards, or other devices impregnated with specific chemicals which change color when exposed to various sterilization methods to provide a visual indication that the items successfully went through the process; however, it does not prove that they are sterile.

Chemotaxis: Refers to the attraction of phagocytes to microbes, due to chemical stimuli secreted from injured tissue cells and other microbial products.

Chemotherapy: Treatment of disease with chemical substances or pharmaceutical agents which have a toxic or suppressive effect on the disease-causing microorganisms or neoplastic tissue.

Chlamydoconidia: Round, large conidia with a thick wall that are formed at the end, sides, or inside the hyphae.

Chlorophyll: A green photosynthetic pigment found in plants, algae, and cyanobacteria that accomplishes photosynthesis.

Chloroplasts: Small green bodies found in the cells of plant leaves and stems which possess stroma and pigments and are important in the photosynthesis process.

Chocolate agar: Both a selective and enriched medium, its name is given due to the brown color of the agar. It is a combination of nutrient agar and powdered hemoglobin.

Choroid plexus: An intracranial structure consisting of a group of specialized capillaries within the walls of the lateral ventricles of the brain which convert blood into cerebrospinal fluid (CSF).

Chromosomes: Linear strands of nucleoprotein hereditary structures within the nucleus of a cell composed of a double strand of DNA that determines inherited traits.

Ciliates: Type of single-celled microorganisms (protozoa), which have hair-like extensions (cilia) used for movement and capturing food particles.

Cirrhosis: Chronic condition of hardening of liver tissue due to disease or infection.

Cladistics: A classification system or taxonomy of organisms based on identification of common ancestors, phylogenic relationships, and evolutionary changes rather than on similar characteristics or morphology.

Coccidioidomycosis: Infection caused by inhalation of the fungus *Coccidioides immitis*, also known as Valley Fever.

Codon: A three-base (nucleotide) sequence in a strand of DNA or RNA which provides the genetic code for a specific amino acid.

Comatose: The condition of a patient in a coma or state of abnormal deep sleep stupor where patient cannot be aroused by external stimuli, usually due to head trauma, effects of drugs, or infections involving the brain (encephalitis) or meninges (meningitis).

Commensals: Types of organisms which develop a relationship in which one organism is benefited but the other is neither harmed nor benefits from the relationship.

Comorbidities: Disease states which coexist or occur simultaneously with a primary or other coincidental diseases.

Complement cascade: A biochemical sequence of reactions involving the C1 through C9 complement proteins acting as catalysts for each subsequent reaction culminating in the lysis of target cells.

Condenser: Located below the fixed stage of a compound light-microscope, it focuses the light onto the specimen to obtain a clear view.

Congestive heart failure: A chronic condition with signs and symptoms of shortness of breath, weakness, abdominal discomfort, and lower extremity edema from venous stasis.

Conidia: Asexual spores of fungi; singular: conidium.

Conidiophores: Types of asexual spores produced by fungi that are either unicellular or multicellular and not enclosed in sacs.

Conjugation: A coupling together or the process in which genetic information is transferred through cell-to-cell contact between bacteria.

Conjunctivitis: Inflammation of the conjunctiva of the eye caused by allergies, foreign bodies, or infection by various microorganisms.

Contractile vacuoles: Cavities in the cytoplasm of the cell that collect and expel the water that has entered the cell by osmosis, to keep the cell from lysing.

Convalescent stage: The stage of a disease or infection in which the individual is recovering and getting well.

Counterbalancing: The act of creating an equality of force or influence by eliminating an imbalance; making two sides comparable in weight, number, or power.

Covalent bonds: Types of strong chemical bonds in which atoms share pairs of electrons to create stability by having a fully filled outer electron shells.

Crepitus: The sound produced by gas in the intestines; pulmonary rales; popping sensation and sound produced by an arthritic, degenerated joint when flexed.

Creutzfeldt-Jakob Disease (CJD): A type of transmissible spongiform encephalopathy which affects humans and is caused by prions. CJD is a progressive, incurable, fatal central nervous system disease which is characterized by symptoms similar to dementia or Alzheimer's disease. Similar to "mad cow" disease in cattle.

Crohn's disease: Also called regional enteritis; inflammatory bowel disease which may include any part of the gastrointestinal system; chronic symptoms include abdominal pain, diarrhea, fever, and weight loss; causes may include autoimmune response, genetics, or environmental sources.

Culture media: A prepared substance which contains nutrients to grow microbes. Types of culture media include broths, gelatins, and agar and may be placed in Petri dishes or test tubes.

Culture: A population of microbes on a prepared culture medium conducive to their growth.

Cyst: A closed pouch or sac with a wall that contains fluid or other material; may be a congenital abnormality or a reaction to an infectious process.

Cystic fibrosis: A genetic (inherited) disorder caused by an autosomal recessive gene which primarily affects the respiratory and digestive systems, creating thickened mucous secretions which causing difficulty breathing or blockage of pancreatic ducts and may be life-threatening.

Cysticercosis: The condition of being infested or infected with one or more cysticercus larvae of *Taenia solium* which may infest any soft tissues of the body; most common parasitic central nervous system infection; resulting in episodes of basilar arachnoiditis, seizures, and hydrocephalus.

Cystogram: A diagnostic x-ray examination of the bladder using radiopaque contrast media.

Cytokines: Extracellular factors produced by various cells such as monocytes and lymphocytes; they include interleukins, some interferons, and tumor necrosis factor; important in controlling systemic and local inflammatory responses.

Cytopathic effects: Effects of viruses on the morphology of host cells in tissue cultures; used as one method of diagnosing a viral infection.

Cytotoxins: Exotoxins or antibodies that destroy host cells or affect their normal functioning.

Dacryocystitis: Inflammation of the mucous membranes of the lacrimal (tear) duct and sac which causes excessive tearing, redness, and pain in the area.

Debilitation: Gradual wasting away; a state of lacking physical strength; deterioration; weakening.

Debridement: Removal of dead or non-viable tissue, foreign material, or infected debris from a cavity, traumatic wound or surgical site infection.

Decontamination: The process of eliminating contamination; refers to the removal of living pathogens from any object, area, or person; also applies to removal of toxic or radioactive agents.

Degranulation: The digestive step of phagocytosis; refers to the decrease in number of granules in the granulocytes.

Dehydration: Removal of water; excessive loss of body fluids with reduction of electrolytes; process of becoming dry.

Dementia: Impairment of mental functioning (cognition) which may be acute or chronic (progressive over long periods) due to toxins, advanced age, infections of the central nervous system, or Alzheimer's disease.

Denatured: Loss, alteration, or inactivation of the natural qualities of a substance; enzymes denatured by heat or change in pH become inactive; denatured alcohol becomes unfit for human consumption while retaining its other functional properties; egg albumin is denatured by cooking and becomes solid and white.

Dental caries: Tooth decay, including cavities.

Dermatomes: Geographic areas of the skin of the body which are innervated by specific spinal or cranial nerves.

Desiccation: The process of removing water, completely drying up; method of preserving by dehydration.

Desiccator: A specialized laboratory container or chamber which removes water from chemicals, tissues, or other substances by use of dehydrating chemicals such as silica gel, sodium hydroxide, or calcium chloride and maintains a dry environment.

Determinants: Factors that determine the character, result, or outcome of something such as public health affected by factors such as poverty, access to care, cultural beliefs, etc.

Dialysis: The process of passing a solute through a membrane for filtration. Hemodialysis removes toxic materials from blood by diffusion through a semipermeable membrane.

Diatoms: Type of algae and phytoplankton found in aquatic environments; may be unicellular or found in colonies and have clear silica cell walls which provide incredible variability and intricacy in appearance.

Differential media: Types of media used to distinguish particular colonies of bacteria from other colonies that are growing on the same Petri dish.

Dimers: The combination of two identical molecules which form a single compound or molecule.

Dinoflagellates: Unicellular marine protozoa which produce red pigment toxic to fish and marine life; responsible for coastal "red tide" outbreaks.

Disinfection: The process of using chemical agents to kill most forms of pathogenic bacteria on the surfaces of inanimate objects.

Disseminated: Scattered over or distributed throughout a large area.

Diverticulitis: Inflammation of one or more diverticula (out-pouching sacs from the walls of the large intestine); may be chronic or acute and cause pain, constipation, and possible perforation.

Dormant: Condition of suspended activity, an inactive state with ability to be reactivated.

Double helix: The shape of DNA characterized by two spiral or coiled strands of deoxyribonucleic acid held together by hydrogen bonds between bases and creating a spiral staircase appearance.

Dysentery: Broad name for multiple viral, bacterial, or parasitic gastrointestinal infections characterized by inflammation of intestinal mucosal tissues.

Dysplasia: Abnormal development of tissue which may be congenital or acquired.

Dysuria: Difficult or painful urination which may indicate urinary tract infections.

Ecosystem: A complex or community of all living organisms and the interaction with their environment.

Ecthyma: An infection of the skin resulting in a crater-like ulcer often seen as a result of impetigo; occurs when the bacterial cells penetrate deep into the dermis.

Ectoparasites: Parasites such as a lice and ticks that reside outside the body and cause infestation.

Ectopic pregnancy: The implantation of a fertilized egg (ovum) outside of the uterus, often occurring in a fallopian tube (tubal pregnancy) which eventually ruptures and may cause pain and hemorrhage and require surgical excision.

Edematous: A condition or appearance of having edema (excessive amounts of fluid in tissues).

Electrophoresis: The use of electromotive force to cause movement of charged particles in a suspension through a medium such as paper or gel for analysis of protein mixtures and to separate mixed populations of DNA.

Electrosurgical smoke plume: Smoke produced by the interaction of high-frequency electrosurgical energy and tissues during surgical procedures; may contain aerosolized biological particles and toxic chemical fumes.

Emboli: Masses of undissolved solids (fat globules, infected tissues; plaques, foreign bodies), blood clots, or air/gas bubbles which travel through the bloodstream until they create an occlusion, leading to an infarct of the affected organ (lungs = pulmonary, cardiac arteries = coronary, etc.); singular: embolus.

Emetic: An agent or condition which produces vomiting.

Emphysema: Distention of tissues by gas or air; a chronic disease of the pulmonary system which causes shortness of breath with exertion.

Empyema: An accumulation of pus in a body cavity; usually in the pleural cavity, surrounding of a lung with purulent fluid as a result of a bacterial infection such as tuberculosis; may require surgical drainage.

Encephalitis: Inflammation of the brain parenchyma, often caused by a virus.

Endemic: Pertaining to an infectious disease that is constantly present in a region, community, or population, but involves relatively few numbers of people and low rates of mortality.

Endocarditis: Inflammatory infection of the inner (endocardial) lining of the heart valves or chambers.

Endocytosis: The ingestion (eating) of a foreign substance by a cell by a process of entrapment, surrounding, or invagination.

Endometriosis: A condition of endometrial tissue (mucous membrane which lines the inner surface of the uterus) occurring outside of the uterus in various locations within the pelvis and/or abdominal wall or viscera.

Endophthalmitis: Inflammation of the internal structures of the eye; may involve either or both chambers.

Endosome: During the process of endocytosis, the vacuole formed when material is absorbed in the cell.

Endospore: Thick-walled protective outer covering formed by bacteria as a means of surviving harsh environmental conditions; it represents the bacteria in "resting" stage until conditions for growth are favorable.

Endosymbiotic: Type of symbiosis in which one organism lives inside another. Endosymbiotic theory proposes that organelles of eukaryotic cells originated as free-living bacteria which took up residence inside other cells and created specialized functions.

Enriched media: Either a solid or broth mixture that contains nutrients which promote the growth of fastidious microbes.

Enteroaggregative: The ability of a microorganism to adhere to epithelial cells in a stacked brick-like pattern; pertains to EAEC: Enteroaggregative *Escherichia coli.*

Enterohemorrhagic: Type of microorganism which causes a severe bloody form of diarrhea called hemorrhagic colitis, pertains to EHEC: enterohemorrhagic *E. coli.*

Enteroinvasive: Strain of *E. coli* which penetrates and multiplies within the mucosal lining of the colon, causing severe diarrheal symptoms resembling shigellosis.

Enteropathogenic: Capable of causing disease in the intestinal tract; pertains to EPEC: enteropathogenic *E. coli* which infects infants, causing diarrhea and is characterized by the destruction of microvilli in the intestinal tract.

Enterotoxigenic: Containing or capable of producing substances toxic to intestinal tissues; pertains to ETEC: enterotoxigenic *E. coli* which causes "traveler's diarrhea," in which the bacteria adhere to the epithelial cells of the small bowel and produce exotoxins that produce the diarrheal symptoms.

Enteroviruses: Viruses which are members of the *Picornaviridae* family with two classes: polioviruses and non-polioviruses; primarily transmitted by the oral-fecal route but may also be transmitted through respiratory secretions and often invade other body tissues and organ systems.

Entomologists: Scientists who study insects; the branch of medical entomology and the spread of disease by insects to humans.

Entomopathogenic: Capable of causing disease in insects; including nematodes and fungi.

Enzyme: A complex protein with the ability to induce a chemical change without being changed itself; when secreted by a bacterium, it invades the host's cells and tissues to produce a reaction including breakdown of substances into simple compounds or causing disease.

Enzyme-linked immunosorbent assays (ELISAs) test: A laboratory test using antisera to identify a particular bacteria, antibodies, or hormones.

Epidemic: Pertaining to an infectious disease which occurs with a greater-than-normal incidence rate at the same time in a geographical area.

Epinephrine: A naturally occurring hormone secreted by the adrenal glands or synthesized pharmaceutical agent used for vasoconstriction, to treat cardiac arrhythmias, or relax bronchioles; also known as adrenaline.

Equilibrium: A state or condition of balance where competing forces are equal to one another.

Eradicated: Completely eliminated, as in the case of endemic or epidemic diseases.

ERCP: Endoscopic retrograde cholangiopancreatography; diagnostic procedure which uses endoscopy and fluoroscopy to examine and diagnose pathology of the biliary tract, including the gallbladder, pancreas, liver, and common bile duct and treat if indicated.

Erysipelas: A severe acute form of cellulitis usually caused by group A streptococci and accompanied by red patches on the skin, usually involving the face and head, high fever, and may progress to septicemia.

Erythema nodosum: Painful red nodules caused by inflammation of fat cells which develop primarily on the lower extremities; associated with a variety of medical conditions.

Erythematous: A condition or appearance of having erythema (capillary congestion resulting in redness of the skin).

Erythroblastosis fetalis: A hemolytic disease in fetuses or newborns caused by blood type or Rh factor incompatibility between mother and fetus in which the mother's immune system attacks the red blood cells (hemolysis) of the fetus resulting in anemia, jaundice, hepatomegaly, generalized edema (hydrops fetalis), or death.

Erythrocytic schizogony: A stage in the life cycle of parasitic *Plasmodium* species (cause of malaria) in which the parasite invades erythrocytes and undergoes asexual multiplication by means of multiple nuclear divisions which form progeny called merozoites that eventually cause the erythrocyte to rupture, spreading merozoites into the bloodstream.

Ethylene oxide: A chemical that is a frameshift mutagen and carcinogen; used for the sterilization of heat and moisture-sensitive surgical instruments.

Etiology: The cause or origin of something; typically used in medicine to describe the reason for a patient's illness or infection as part of the history and physical (H&P).

Eukaryotes: A classification of living cells that are more complex and contain a nucleus, including protozoa; fungi; green, brown, and red algae; and all plant and animal cells including human cells.

Eustachian tube: Also called the auditory tube; a mucous membrane-lined hollow tube which connects the middle ear to the pharynx. Blockage of the duct may lead to otitis media infections.

Exophthalmos: An abnormal bulging or protrusion of the eyeball.

Exoskeleton: Protective hard outer covering of some invertebrates such as arthropods and vertebrates such as turtles.

Exotoxins: Certain type of toxins (poisons) excreted primarily by living Gram-positive microbes into the surrounding tissues or media which enhance their pathogenicity.

Extrapulmonary: Existing or occurring outside of the lungs; as with extrapulmonary tuberculosis (TB infection occurring in tissues outside of the lungs).

Extremophiles: Types of microbes (including many types of archaea) which have adapted to and thrive in extreme conditions and environments (e.g., hydrothermal vents, salt marshes, arctic glaciers) which would kill most other types of organisms.

Exudate: Accumulation of fluid in a cavity; production of serum or pus.

Facultative: Possessing the ability to live in various conditions; types of bacteria which adapt to less ideal conditions such as anaerobes which live in moderate oxygen environments.

Fasciitis: Inflammation of the fascial layer of muscle, often caused by a bacterial infection. Severe progressive destruction and death of fascial tissue is called necrotizing fasciitis.

Fastidious bacteria: Bacteria which have complex and specific nutritional requirements for growth and survival.

Fermentation: An anaerobic process by which yeasts ferment sugar to alcohol; used for the production of food such as bread, beer, and wines.

Fibromyalgia: Condition or syndrome of widespread, diffuse pain, and sensitivity to pressure involving multiple muscles and joints.

Filaments: Fine threads or thread-like structures.

Filariasis: Chronic condition common in tropical countries caused by any of the filarial parasites that affect humans causing lymph node swelling and may result in elephantiasis or hydrocele formation.

Fistula: An abnormal tract that develops between two epithelium-lined surfaces and is open at both ends; may occur after bladder, bowel, anal, and vaginal procedures.

Flaccid myelitis: An acute neurologic illness characterized by symptoms of paralysis of arms or legs; first described and named by the CDC in 2014 following multiple incidents across the US in children with unknown etiology.

Flaccid paralysis: Caused by lesions of lower spinal cord motor neurons, a type of paralysis (loss of sensation or motor function) characterized by reduced muscle tone, tendon reflexes, muscle degeneration, and atrophy.

Flagella staining: A staining procedure that uses the stain carbolfuchsin and a mordant to thicken the diameters of the flagella so they can be seen through a light microscope.

Flagellates: Unicellular microorganisms which have a specialized organelle of cell motility; a long, thin structure attached to the outside of a cell; its whipping motion provides the cell a means of movement.

Fluoroscopy: The process of using ionizing radiation (x rays) to visualize internal body structures in movable, real-time images created by an image intensifier (C-arm) and monitor.

Folliculitis: An infection of hair follicles that causes the development of pustules.

Fomites: Any inanimate object containing potentially pathogenic microbes on its surface which can serve as a reservoir or point of transmission to an individual coming into contact with the inoculated surface.

Frameshift: A change in the reading frame of a DNA or mRNA sequence by the deletion or addition of one or more nucleotides, creating a genetic mutation.

Free radicals: Atoms or groups of atoms with unpaired electrons which, when they interact with a cell's DNA or cell membrane, can cause a chain of interactions resulting in cellular damage or death. Antioxidants can bind with free radicals to break or prevent chain reactions and cell damage.

Furunculosis: A condition of having large, raised skin lesions full of pus and surrounded by inflamed tissue; also known as boils.

Gallops: Abnormal increased numbers of heart sounds which mimic the sound of a galloping horse and may indicate the presence of heart disease.

Ganglion: A mass of tissues of the peripheral nervous system; a cystic tumor which develops on a tendon. Plural: ganglia.

Gas gangrene: A serious infection caused by *Clostridium perfringens* in which the bacterial cells enter through an opening in the skin caused by traumatic injury or surgical skin incision; the patient experiences intense pain, muscle necrosis, shock, renal failure, and possibly death; medical term is myonecrosis.

Gastroenteritis: Inflammation of the stomach and intestinal wall often associated with diarrhea.

Genome: The complete set of genetic material in an organism, including DNA, RNA, chromosomes, and/or genes.

Geosmins: Organic compounds responsible for the "earthy" flavor of some foods and distinct smell of fresh or wet soil.

Germ Theory of Disease: A scientific theory that pathogenic microbes are the cause of disease and illness.

Germ warfare: Military use of pathogenic microorganisms as a weapon against an enemy. Also known as biological warfare.

Glomerulonephritis: A type of nephritis (kidney inflammation) primarily involving the glomeruli (small structures of the kidney made up of capillaries).

Glutaraldehyde: A chemical in the aldehyde group used as a liquid disinfectant; may be used as a sterilant if moisture-stable, heat-sensitive items are fully immersed for 10 hours.

Glycocalyx: A layer of adhesive carbohydrates that covers the plasma membrane of a eukaryotic cell to strengthen the cell's surface and aid in cellular attachment.

Gram stain: A laboratory method developed by Hans Gram which involves the staining of bacteria with crystal violet, rinsing, staining with iodine solution, rinsing, counterstaining with carbolfuchsin, and rinsing again. Gram-positive bacteria retain the crystal violet stain and appear purple, while Gram-negative bacteria take on the counterstain and appear red. The differentiation demonstrates the type of cell membrane of the bacterium and which type of antibiotic would most likely be effective against it.

Gram-variable: Bacteria, in particular *Mycobacteriaceae*, that do not consistently stain purple or red.

Granulation tissue: A type of tissue that contains myofibroblasts and new capillaries to fill in a gaping wound that is left open to heal by second intention healing.

Granules: Small, grain-like structures; tiny masses in cells without obvious structure.

Granulocytopenia: Abnormally low number of granulocytes (polymorphonuclear leukocytes) in the blood.

Granuloma: A granular collection of lymphoid or epithelial cells creating a mass or tumor.

Greenhouse gases: Atmospheric gases such as carbon dioxide, methane, nitrous oxide, and ozone which occur naturally and man-made gases such as hydrofluorocarbons produced industrially which absorb and hold in atmospheric heat, adding to global warming or the greenhouse effect.

Guillain-Barré syndrome: Syndrome of unknown etiology, although often following a febrile illness, in which an individual's immune system attacks the body's own nervous system, resulting in pain, muscle weakness, or paralysis that can last for several weeks.

Gummas: Soft tissue or organ granulomatous tumors seen in the tertiary stage of syphilis.

Hallucinations: A false perception with no basis in reality; may be auditory, olfactory, or visual; may be caused by disease of sensory organs or by use of psychotropic drugs.

Halophilic: An affinity or strong attraction to salt or other halogen substances.

Heart murmur: An audible sound of blood flow in the heart heard on auscultation with a stethoscope which may indicate pathology in heart valve function.

Helminth: A parasitic or free-living worm-like organism including roundworms, flatworms, hookworms, and whipworms.

Hematuria: The presence of blood in the urine; may be visible or microscopic.

Hemodialysis: A medical procedure or process of mechanical filtration of an individual's blood by circulation through tubes made of semi-permeable membranes which remove metabolic waste and unwanted materials when kidneys are unable to perform the function.

Hemolysin: A condition or agent such as a bacterial exoenzyme that causes the lysis of erythrocytes.

Hemolytic anemia: Congenital or acquired condition of anemia (low red blood cell count) due to hemolysis (destruction or lysis of red blood cells).

Hemorrhagic fever: Any hemorrhagic disease (Dengue, Ebola, Lassa, or Marburg) caused by a filovirus; characterized by internal hemorrhaging and clotting; has a high mortality rate.

Hepatosplenomegaly: Abnormal enlargement of the liver and spleen often due to a disease such as typhoid fever, alcohol abuse, carcinoma, or other pathological conditions.

Histoplasmosis: A systemic fungal infection from inhalation of *Histoplasma capsulatum* which may affect multiple body systems, primarily the respiratory system, and symptoms may range from mild to fatal.

Homeostasis: The dynamic state of equilibrium of the body's internal environment maintained by feedback and regulation.

Host: An organism infected by a pathogen, often serving as the source of food supply to support the viability of the pathogen.

Humoral: Pertaining to body fluids or their chemical components.

Hybridization: The process of taking a single strand of DNA from one species to test its ability to bind (hybridize) with the DNA strand from another species; the stronger the degree of binding, the greater the similarity between the two species. Also combining two varieties or species of organisms to create a hybrid.

Hydrocele: Serous fluid accumulation in the tunica vaginalis testis creating a sac-like cavity and causing swelling of the scrotum.

Hydrocephalus: An abnormal accumulation of cerebrospinal fluid (CSF) within the ventricles of the brain; may be as a result of malabsorption, overproduction, or blocked foramina secondary to infection, injury, pathological or congenital disorders.

Hydrogen peroxide: A colorless liquid used as an antiseptic solution H_2O_2 which decomposes, releasing oxygen which causes effervescence (bubbling) and eventually reverting to H_2O (water).

Hydrolyze: To cause hydrolysis which is a chemical decomposition whereby a substance is split into smaller, simpler compounds by the elements of water; may be reversible.

Hyperbaric oxygen: Type of wound therapy which utilizes oxygen under greater pressure than normal atmospheric pressure. Patients who have non-healing wounds or bacterial infections are placed in a chamber that is airtight and contains the highly pressurized oxygen.

Hyperendemic: A high incidence of disease that is constantly present in a certain population, equal among all age groups.

Hypersensitivity: An abnormal sensitivity to any kind of stimulus. An immune response to exposure to an antigen that occurs after 24 hours and ranges from a mild to life-threatening reaction. Immediate hypersensitivity reaction is an abnormal immune response that occurs within a few seconds to 24 hours and ranges from a mild to a life-threatening reaction.

Hyperthyroidism: A medical condition caused by excessive secretion of thyroid hormones by the thyroid gland and characterized by increased basal metabolism and may result in exophthalmos and thyroid goiter (enlargement).

Hyphae: Long branching cytoplasmic filament of a fungus or mold, singular: hypha.

Hypotension: Abnormally low blood pressure; may be as a result of shock, hemorrhage, infection, anemia, etc., and may lead to death if untreated.

Hypothermia: The state of having a body temperature below normal; may be accidental or planned as in surgical procedures with high risk of major blood loss.

Hypovolemia: Diminished or lowered volume of blood plasma; may be due to hemorrhage, dehydration, or other factors.

Iatrogenic: Relating to an illness or adverse effect caused by medical treatment or a healthcare provider.

Icosahedral: Pertaining to an icosahedron; type of several morphological classifications of viruses with a capsid that is a regular polyhedron with 20 triangular faces and 12 corners and the capsomeres of each face form an equilateral triangle.

Idiopathic: Pertaining to unknown or unclear cause or origin of a disease, infection, or condition.

Idiosyncratic: Pertaining to an unusual or unexpected reaction to a drug, food, or other substance.

Immunity: The state of having a natural or acquired protection against an infectious disease.

Immunocompromised: The state or condition of having a lowered immune system, which makes an individual vulnerable to pathogenic and/or opportunistic infections.

Immunofluorescence: A technique for the identification of an antigen by exposing it to known antibodies. A fluorochrome is added that chemically combines with the antibodies; as the fluorescent antibodies bind to the antigens on the bacterial surface, the bacteria fluoresce.

Immunoglobulins: Any of a family of proteins which act as antibodies produced in response to specific antigens and can react with only that type of antigen.

Impetigo: A highly contagious streptococcal or staphylococcal skin infection characterized by isolated pustules that become crusted and rupture. May be bullous or non-bullous.

Indigenous flora: Microbes that normally reside in a region of the body such as the skin, gastrointestinal tract, or vagina; formerly called "normal flora."

Induction: The process of causing or producing and effect or result.

Infectivity dose: The amount or number of pathogenic organisms required to cause infection in susceptible individuals or hosts.

Inflammatory bowel disease: Chronic inflammation of the colon and rectum with unknown etiology; characterized by abdominal cramping, diarrhea, or constipation.

Infrastructure: The underlying foundation or framework of a system or organization.

Inoculation: The process of transmitting a pathogen to produce growth for analysis or transmitting an antigen, antitoxin, or antiserum to produce immunity to specific disease.

Inoculum: A small amount of a substance containing bacteria introduced into the body or tissues for purposes of vaccination, or culture medium for start of a new culture.

Interferons: Natural cellular proteins manufactured by specific cells of the human immune system in response to exposure to a virus; they inhibit the ability of that virus to replicate within the host's cells.

Interleukins: A group of polypeptides that cause the proliferation of T-cells.

Interstitial fluid: Fluid that surrounds living cells in tissues.

Intractable: Incurable, uncontrollable, or unresponsive to therapeutic treatment, as in some types of chronic pain syndromes.

Intubation: Procedure involving insertion of a tube into a hollow organ; in anesthesia administration: placement of a tube into the trachea through the mouth (endotracheal) or nose (nasotracheal) for airway maintenance and administration of anesthetic gases.

Invaginates: Pushes or enfolds inward to create a pouch; creates an indentation of the phagocytic membrane when ingesting foreign material.

Invasins: Types of proteins produced by bacteria which facilitate the pathogen's penetration into host cells by binding to special receptor sites.

Ionizing radiation: High energy radiation capable of freeing electrons from their orbits; commonly as x-rays;

overexposure to the radiation can cause mistakes in DNA replication and produce mutations.

Irreducible minimum: An amount which cannot be lowered further. Skin antisepsis is performed to remove transient microbes and lower the deep, resident skin microbial count to the lowest achievable number, as living skin cannot be sterilized and will always have microbes present.

Ischemia: Disruption of blood flow and oxygenation of areas of tissue due to obstruction of circulation.

Jaundice: A condition of excess bilirubin in the blood (hyperbilirubinemia) characterized by yellowing of the skin, mucous membranes, conjunctiva, and body fluids from deposition of bile pigment.

Keratin: A tough, fibrous protein produced by keratinocytes and found in two forms: hard (hair and nails) and soft (stratum corneum or top layer of the epidermis that sloughs off).

Keratitis: Inflammation of the cornea of the eye; may be due to infection, trauma, or immune response.

Kinins: Polypeptide substances released from tissue cells capable of causing vasodilation, hypotension, and influencing smooth muscle contraction.

Koch's Postulates: A sequence of steps established by the German physician Robert Koch for experimentally demonstrating in the laboratory that a specific microbe causes a specific disease.

Krill: Term for various species of tiny marine crustaceans found in all ocean environments which are important food sources for whales and other marine mammals.

Laryngospasm: Spasm (involuntary contraction) of the laryngeal muscles which may affect breathing or speaking.

Leavening: The process of incorporating air bubbles (fermentation) into dough to make it rise and have a lighter consistency by use of yeast or other leavening agents.

Leprosy: A disease caused by *Mycobacterium leprae* that infects the skin and peripheral nervous system, resulting in a severe and disfiguring skin rash with the loss of cutaneous sensation. Also known as Hansen's disease.

Lethargy: A condition of drowsiness, sluggishness, or stupor.

Leukocytes: White blood cells of two types: granulocytes and agranulocytes which are components of the immune system and help protect against infectious agents and foreign invaders.

Leukopenia: A condition characterized by an abnormal decrease of white blood cells in the blood, increasing risk for infection.

Lichens: Symbiotic relationship of algae and fungi which create a composite organisms commonly called lichens and scientifically called thalli (singular—thallus); in medicine, a form of papular skin disease.

Louse: Small ectoparasites which may infest humans in hair, in or on clothing, or in pubic hair; plural: lice.

Lumen: The space within a tubular structure such as a blood vessel, intestines, ureter, etc.; or device such as a catheter or drain.

Lymphadenopathy: Infected or diseased lymph nodes.

Lymphatic system: Body system that includes all structures (lymph capillaries, lacteals, lymph nodes, lymph vessels, and lymph ducts) that transport lymph fluid from the tissues to the bloodstream.

Lymphocytes: Cells present in blood and lymphatic tissues are derived from the stem cells which become blood cells and are important components of the immune response as B-cells and T-cells.

Lymphokines: A type of cytokine; a soluble protein released by sensitized lymphocytes; includes interleukins.

Lysis of adhesions: Surgical separation of tissue adhesions (stuck together) by sharp or blunt dissection.

Lysogeny: The interaction between a viral bacteriophage (prophage) and bacterium where the viral genetic material is introduced into the host bacterium and the viral DNA is replicated prior to release during the lytic phase.

MacConkey agar: A selective and differential medium that is a combination of bile salts, lactose, and crystal violet. The agar differentiates between lactose-fermenting and non-lactose-fermenting bacteria.

Macerated: Softened or separated into parts by soaking or steeping in liquid; decomposed by a solvent.

Macromolecule: A large molecule such as a polysaccharide, protein, nucleic acid, or polymer which contains greater than 100 atoms.

Malabsorption: Inadequate absorption of nutrients from the intestines; malabsorption syndrome is characterized by a number of symptoms to include anorexia, weight loss, abdominal pain, bone pain, and steatorrhea.

Mantoux test: The most accurate skin test for *Mycobacteria tuberculosis,* involving the intradermal injection of the antigen purified protein derivative (PPD) within the epidermal layer. Results are observed and recorded after 48 hours.

Mast cells: Cells found in connective tissues, around blood vessels, serous cavities, and in bone marrow which synthesize and store histamine; produce signs and symptoms of immediate hypersensitivity reactions such as anaphylaxis.

Mastectomy: Surgical removal of a breast by excision.

Mastoiditis: Inflammation of the mastoid air cells due to infection.

Meningitis: Inflammation of the meninges (protective dural covering) of the brain or spinal cord may be aseptic, caused by bacterial or viral infections, or as a result of trauma.

Metaplasia: Transformation of one type of tissue cell into another, regeneration of lost tissues by other types; or pathological replacement of tissue cells by another type of cells.

Metric system: A decimal system of measurement used in the scientific world and extensively used in European countries. It is based on units of 10.

Microaerophile: A classification of microbes that require oxygen for survival, however at a level lower than what is in ambient air—approximately 5%.

Microbiome: A group or community of microorganisms in a particular environment such as the human body or in specific body systems or areas (intestinal tract, respiratory tract, vagina, etc.). Sometimes called microbiota and previously called "normal flora."

Microtubules: Elongated hollow, tubular structures in cells which aid in maintaining cellular rigidity and transporting substances within the cell.

Microvilli: Microscopic hair-like projections on the surface of cell membranes.

Morbidity: The state or condition of being diseased; the incidence rate or statistical likelihood of disease in relationship to others in a group or population.

Mordant: A chemical added to a stain to increase the effectiveness of the stain.

Morphology: The study of the structure or form of organisms; the make-up (size, shape, and arrangements) of an organism used to categorize and classify it.

Mosaic: Spotted condition in plants such as tobacco, indicating disease; a design made of many pieces; tissues of different genetic kinds derived from the same cell.

Motility: The ability and power of a microbe or structure to move by itself.

Mutagen: An agent such as a chemical or ionizing radiation which causes a genetic mutation to occur.

Mutate: To change or cause to change in form, function, structure, or genetic make-up.

Myalgia: Muscle pains or tenderness.

Mycelium: The mass of hyphae that have branched and grown longer to form the vegetative body of fungi such as molds.

Myeloid progenitor stem cells: One of two types of stem cells derived from hematopoietic stem cells in bone marrow and includes the myeloid cells (monocytes and granulocytes) which play an important role in innate immunity.

Myocarditis: Inflammation of the muscle layer of the heart (myocardium); may be from viral, bacterial, or fungal infection, radiation, or heat stroke.

Myringotomy: The surgical incision in the tympanic membrane of the ear and placement of pressure equalizing polyethylene (PE) tubes to allow the drainage of infected fluid in patients who experience chronic otitis media.

Nephropathogenic: Capable of causing disease of the kidney; pertains to NPEC: nephropathogenic *E. coli*, a strain of *E. coli* responsible for causing urinary tract infection; this strain of bacteria has a capsule and pilus that add to its virulence factor.

Neti pots: Devices designed for administration of nasal irrigation.

Neuralgia: Sharp, severe pain associated with specific nerves of the body.

Neurotransmitter: Chemical substance such as dopamine, norepinephrine, or acetylcholine that crosses the synaptic gap from an excited axon terminal of a presynaptic neuron to a target cell in order to excite or inhibit its activity.

Neutralizes: Counteracts something such as a substance to make it harmless, as in adding a base to an acid to equalize and destroy the effects and particular properties of each agent.

Non-bullous: A form of impetigo which is more common and more contagious than bullous impetigo and may be caused by either *Streptococcus* or *Staphylococcus* species; characterized by a honey-colored crusted exudate from small, ruptured blisters.

Non-hemolytic: Pertaining to the lack of ability for or property of destruction of red blood cells.

Normal flora: Term previously used to describe the microbial population of a body system or other environment. Also called indigenous microflora, microbiome, or microbiota.

Obligate: Necessary or required; restricted to a specific set of conditions such as bacteria which are only able survive in strictly aerobic or anaerobic environments.

Ocular lens: The lens of a compound light microscope that is located in the eyepiece.

Oil immersion objective: A type of objective lens used with the compound light microscope. It is used to observe the characteristics of bacteria. The lens must be used with a drop of immersion oil between the specimen and objective lens.

Onychomycosis: Disease of fingernails or toenails due to a parasitic fungal infection.

Oocysts: A stage in sporozoan development in which, after fertilization, a zygote is produced that develops an enclosing cyst wall; oocysts of malarial parasites are often detected in the stomachs of infected *Anopheles* mosquitoes.

Opisthotonos: Chronic form of back spasm characterized by the bending back of the head and heels and body in an arched position; classic sign of a tetanus infection.

Opportunistic: Taking advantage of a given circumstance; common microbes may become opportunistic pathogens which cause infections in individuals whose immune systems are defective or compromised and unable to defend against invasion as those with normal immune systems would be able to do.

Optimum: The best or most favorable; as with environmental conditions for bacterial growth.

Organelles: Specialized structures within the cytoplasm of eukaryotes that carry out the functions of the cell controlled by the DNA formation; examples:

mitochondria, lysosomes, endoplasmic reticulum, Golgi apparatus, centrioles.

Osmosis: The movement of a solvent such as water from an area of lower solute concentration through a selectively permeable membrane, as in a microbial cell, to an area or solution with a higher concentration of dissolved solutes.

Osmotrophic: Description of a microorganism which obtains its nutritional requirements from surrounding solutions through osmotic absorption across membranes.

Osteomyelitis: Inflammation and chronic infection of the bone marrow and bone tissue often caused by *Staphylococcus aureus.*

Other potentially infectious materials (OPIMs): Acronym used by the Occupational Safety and Health Administration (OSHA) which describes potential exposure risks separate from blood-borne pathogens for healthcare workers. OPIMs include most body fluids, unfixed tissue specimens, and HIV or HBV-containing tissues, organs, or culture specimens.

Otitis externa: Inflammation of the outermost portion of the auditory canal.

Otitis media: Inflammation of the middle ear; often chronic due to infection.

Otorhinolaryngology: Medical specialty also called ENT (ear, nose, and throat) which involves the study and practice of otology (function and diseases of the ear), rhinology (function and diseases of the nasal structures), and laryngology (structures and diseases of the throat and surrounding structures).

Oxidative phosphorylation: The end result of a series of complex cellular energy transformations, which involve the electron transport system and mitochondria to produce ATP and collectively known as cellular respiration.

Pandemic: An infectious disease that occurs worldwide or in a majority of the population of a large geographic region.

Papillomas: Benign epithelial tumors of the skin or mucous membranes including warts, polyps, and condylomas.

Papule: Elevated area of skin with a reddened, solid, defined, circular lesion which may appear before pustular or vesicular lesions.

Paraphernalia: Any type of device, apparatus, or equipment designed for use in a specific activity. Drug paraphernalia refers to devices used in preparation and use of illicit drugs.

Parasitology: The branch of biological sciences or medicine that studies human pathogenic parasites, typically protozoa, helminths, and arthropods.

Parenchyma: The essential components of a bodily organ such as the brain, concerned with function.

Paroxysmal stage: The second stage of pertussis (whooping cough) characterized by numerous sudden bouts of rapid coughs which may lead to exhaustion and cyanosis.

Pasteurization: Named after Louis Pasteur, the process of using heat to kill bacteria without affecting the chemical composition or taste of a beverage such as milk.

Pathogenicity: The ability to or process of producing pathological changes or disease.

Pathological condition: Disease state or process; abnormal functioning.

Pellicle: A semi-rigid, thin film that surrounds flagellates and provides a more definitive shape, as compared to the less-defined shape of the amoeba.

Penicillin: The first antibiotic ever developed. Discovered and named by Alexander Fleming. Produced by the mold called *Penicillium notatum* and *P. chrysogenum.* Bactericidal and effective against many Gram-positive and certain Gram-negative bacteria.

Peracetic acid: A highly biocidal oxidizer used as a disinfectant and liquid chemical sterilant for heat-sensitive, moisture-stable surgical instrumentation.

Pericardiocentesis: An emergency procedure that involves needle aspiration (removal by suction) of fluid present in the pericardial sac in order to relieve compression of the heart.

Periodontitis: Untreated gingivitis that has become a chronic infection with inflammation.

Periodontium: The oral structures of the mouth which support the teeth; includes the periodontal ligament, gingivae, and alveolar bone of the mouth.

Peristalsis: The involuntary rhythmic movement of smooth muscles of tubular structures of the body, as in the manner by which food is pushed through the digestive tract or urine through the ureters.

Peristome: An anatomical region (channel or mouth) of flagellates and ciliates that assists in the ingestion of food.

Peritonitis: Inflammation of the serous membrane lining the walls of the abdominal and pelvic cavities (peritoneum).

Permeable: The property of the cell membrane to allow substances to enter and exit by crossing the plasma membrane; allowing passage of fluids or substances in solution.

Personal protective equipment (PPEs): Components of attire worn to protect against exposure to physical and biological hazards including masks, gloves, goggles/shields, respirators, gowns, lead aprons, and shoe covers.

Petechiae: Small hemorrhagic skin, mucous membrane, or serous tissue lesions which appear purple and may be due to blood clotting abnormality or as a result of certain types of fever such as typhus.

Petri dish: A round, shallow glass or plastic dish with a cover that contains solid culture media to grow microbes. Developed by Robert Koch's assistant Julius Petri.

Peyer's patches: Collection or aggregation of lymphatic nodules mainly in the ileum near the junction of the colon. In cases of typhoid fever, Peyer's patches may show hyperplasia (overgrowth) and become ulcerated.

Phage typing: A type of laboratory test used to determine to which bacteriophages a bacterium is susceptible to lysing, aids in determining the origin of a disease.

Phagolysosome: A digestive vacuole that contains enzymes to digest the material within it.

Phagosome: A membrane-bound vacuole of the phagocyte that contains material to be digested. Following digestion, the material is extruded by the phagosome to the exterior area.

Pharyngitis: Inflammation of the pharynx; may be chronic due to nasal/sinus pathology or smoking or acute as a result of streptococcal infection of the throat that causes fever, chronic pain, difficulty swallowing, and inflammation of the tonsils and pharynx; also known as strep throat.

Phenetics: Study and classification of organisms based on similar morphology and characteristics rather than comparative genetics; opposite approach from cladistics.

Pheromones: Signaling molecules emitted by bacteria as part of the communication mechanism seen in quorum sensing. See also "Autoinducers".

Phialide: In fungal organisms, a conidiogenous cell which does not change as new conidia are extruded and released to form chains.

Phlebovirus: Genus of the family *Bunyaviridae* transmitted by arthropod vectors and causes sandfly fever and Rift Valley fever.

Phlegm: Thick mucus secretions from the respiratory passages.

Photoreactivating: A type of bacterial enzyme that repairs the damage from ultraviolet light by breaking the abnormal thymine dimers and filling in the space with newly synthesized DNA that fits in the undamaged strand of DNA; this restores the original base-pair sequence.

Photosynthesizers: Any organisms, including green plants that synthesize chemical substances, especially carbohydrates, from atmospheric carbon dioxide and water. Light is used as an energy source and oxygen is liberated in the process.

Phototherapy: The use of natural or artificial light for therapeutic purposes; treatment for hemolytic anemia in newborns.

Phylogeny: The evolutionary pathway or history of organisms which are genetically related.

Pili: Filamentous, hair-like structures on the surface of some bacteria which enables attachment to other cells.

Plague: A widespread, deadly contagious disease; most often caused by *Yersinia pestis*.

Plaques: Clear spaces that appear on a Petri dish during phage typing which indicate where the bacteriophages have lysed the bacteria.

Plasma: The yellowish-straw-colored fluid portion of the circulatory system in which the blood cells circulate.

Plasmolysis: The result of cellular water loss due to osmosis, where the plasma membrane shrinks and pulls away from the cell wall.

Pleomorphic: Having many shapes; microorganisms with variety of appearance.

Pneumonia: An acute respiratory infection of the lung tissues and alveolar spaces, characterized by a collection of fluid within the lungs or pleural cavity; caused by a variety of pathogens, including bacteria, fungi, protozoa, and viruses.

Pollinators: Arthropod insects such as bees and butterflies which carry out plant fertilization (pollination) by the carrying of pollen from plant to plant.

Polymicrobial: Term used to describe a number of species of microbes.

Polymorphonuclear: Property of having a lobed nucleus which may appear to be multiple nuclei; pertains to white blood cells (leukocytes) with lobes of the nucleus connected by strands of chromatin.

Polyneuropathy: A condition involving disorder of multiple peripheral nerves, mainly non-inflammatory in nature.

Postpartum: The timeframe following childbirth.

Prions: Term short for "proteinaceous infectious particle"; non-living, abnormally folded beta-sheet, smaller than a virus and do not contain DNA or RNA. Responsible for transmissible spongiform encephalopathies including CJD in humans and mad cow disease in cattle.

Prodromal stage: The second of five stages of infection (incubation, prodromal, illness, decline, and convalescence) prior to characteristic symptoms appear and in which the pathogen is replicating rapidly, triggering the immune system response and causing vague, non-specific symptoms of fatigue and possibly low-grade fever.

Prokaryotes: A classification of living cells without a nuclear membrane or specialized organelles; includes bacteria and cyanobacteria.

Prostaglandins: Fatty acids produced at the site of injury and released by damaged cells to enhance the inflammatory process; also play a role in uterine contractions during labor.

Protoplasm: Organized, viscous, colloidal complex of organic and inorganic substances of a cell; includes the nucleus, cytoplasm, and mitochondria; fluid substance of the cell where metabolism and reproduction occur.

Pseudomembrane: A false membrane consisting of fibrin, bacteria, and leukocytes that forms in the throat of a patient suffering from diphtheria and causes respiratory difficulties.

Pseudomonad: An individual bacterium of the genus *Pseudomonas*.

Puerperal fever: A syndrome characterized by a systemic bacterial infection and septicemia suffered by a mother in the period immediately after childbirth.

Pure culture technique: A laboratory technique used to ensure the growth of only one type of microbe on a culture medium in a Petri dish or in a broth medium.

Purines: Chemical compounds required for synthesis of nucleotides (RNA and DNA); non-adenine-based purines (NABPs) promote cell proliferation and release of growth factors during wound healing.

Pustules: Skin lesions that are slightly raised and filled with lymph fluid or pus.

Pyelonephritis: Inflammation of the renal pelvis of the kidney often due to a bacterial infection.

Pyrimidines: Parent compounds of pyrimidine bases of nucleic acids; considered growth factors.

Pyrogen: Any substance or organism that induces fever.

Quarantine: A procedure utilized to protect the public by separating, isolating, and restricting the movement of individuals demonstrating symptoms of a contagious disease or those exposed to infectious disease in order to determine their status and potential transmissibility.

Radiofrequency: Oscillating (alternating) electromagnetic radio waves used to create heat for therapeutic purposes or, when applied to hydrogen peroxide gas in a chamber, to create a plasma state used for sterilization of heat-sensitive and moisture-sensitive surgical instruments.

Rales: Abnormal sounds produced by air passing through constricted bronchial passages during breathing and heard on auscultation of the chest with a stethoscope. Constriction of bronchi may be due to spasm, exudate, secretions, or thickening of bronchial walls.

Recombinant: The end result of a combining of genetic material from different sources; a type of DNA in which one or more segments or genes have been inserted naturally or artificially; an organism with a combination of alleles different from its parents.

Reducing media: A special laboratory medium used to culture anaerobic bacteria which contain agents that chemically combine with oxygen to eliminate it from the environment.

Refractive index: A measure of the relative velocity at which light passes through a material. The refractive index of microbes is altered through the use of various staining procedures.

Replication: Repetition; the reproduction or duplication of genetic material to create a new organism with the same genetic properties.

Replicon: A linear or circular section of RNA or DNA that replicates sequentially as a unit.

Resolution: The ability of the lens to produce image clarity by distinguishing two objects that must be at a particular distance apart; determines the amount of detail which can be seen.

Reticuloendothelial system (RES): Also known as the mononuclear system; the collection (system) of phagocytic cells that line the sinusoids of the spleen, lymph nodes, bone marrow, intestines, liver, and brain with diffuse immune system functions.

Retrovirus: Virus that contains the enzyme reverse transcriptase, which can synthesize DNA from an RNA template, the opposite of the usual process. HIV is a retrovirus.

Rheumatic fever: A rare serious and potentially life-threatening secondary inflammatory disease which may follow group A streptococcal infections and may affect the heart, brain, skin, and joints to varying degrees.

Rheumatism: A generalized term used to describe acute and chronic conditions of joint inflammation, soreness, muscle stiffness, and pain; includes arthritis, degenerative joint disease, and many other clinical conditions.

Rhinocerebral: Pertaining to the nasal sinuses and brain; type of mucormycosis fungal infection in immunocompromised individuals that spreads from the sinuses into the brain and has a high mortality rate.

Rhinovirus: Virus that causes the common cold.

Ribosomes: A structure of the cell formed within the cellular nucleus; it begins the production of proteins.

Ruminants: Any animals that have a stomach with four complete cavities. Undigested food is regurgitated from the first stomach (rumen) and masticated when the animal is at rest.

Sarcoidosis: A disease characterized by the production of multiple accumulations of inflammatory cells (nodules or granulomas); most common in the lungs, however, may involve any part of the body. Cause is unknown and signs may resolve or reappear without apparent cause.

Schwann cells: Supporting cells of the peripheral nervous system.

Selective media: Laboratory culture media which contain chemical inhibitors that prevent the growth of certain species of microbes while allowing the desired species to grow.

Septate: Having a dividing wall; as in hyphae that are divided into sections or separate cells by walls called septa.

Septicemia: Presence of bacterial pathogens in the bloodstream. A serious infection in which bacteria have spread throughout the body; also referred to as a systemic infection or sepsis.

Serovars/serotypes: Interchangeable terms for distinct differences or variations in serological reactions within species of bacteria, viruses, or other cells; the set of antigens common to and characteristic of a specific group of microorganisms.

Sharps injuries: Set of serious risk factors for healthcare workers which involves puncture of the skin and potential transmission of blood-borne pathogens by way of hypodermic or suture needles, scalpel or other blades, sharp-pointed instruments, wires, pins, or any other sharp objects used in patients' tissues.

Sheath: A close-fitting covering; typically an elongated structure of connective tissue which provides membrane coverage of tissues such as muscles and tendons.

Shingles: A disease caused by varicella-zoster virus, the same virus that causes chickenpox. The virus is latent (dormant) and then reactivated, possibly by stress, causing a new outbreak of the virus with painful vesicles similar to chickenpox except the infection follows cutaneous sensory nerve tracts.

Shock: A clinical condition of inadequate peripheral blood flow return to the heart creating lack of oxygenation to body organs and tissues which may be caused by traumatic hemorrhage, systemic infection (septic shock), drug interaction, myocardial infarction, poisoning, or severe dehydration.

Simple stain: Method of laboratory staining that involves the use of a single dye applied to the fixed smear.

Sinonasal: Pertaining to the facial sinuses and nasal passages.

Slants: Test tubes containing agar that has been allowed to solidify with the tube held at an angle.

Smelting: A method of extracting metals from ore by use of heat and chemical reduction and refining.

Solute: A substance that is dissolved in liquid.

Spastic paralysis: Constant excitatory synaptic activity which creates muscle rigidity accompanied by partial paralysis. May be caused by the tetanus toxin tetanospasmin that acts by blocking specific neurotransmitters.

Splenomegaly: Abnormal enlargement of the spleen usually caused by a disease or infection.

Sporangiospores: Specialized hyphae structures that support the sporangium of the asexual spore of a fungus. These asexual spores are produced only by the class of fungi called *Zygomycetes*.

Spores: A reproductive cell produced by plants and some protozoa; thick protective coating which allows certain spore-forming bacteria to survive harsh environmental conditions by remaining dormant until the conditions become favorable for growth.

Sporozoans: Any of four phyla of protozoans that are pathogenic parasites, nonmotile, and known to have alternating asexual and sexual life cycles; also called apicomplexa organisms.

Sporulates: Produces spores; the action of certain rod-shaped bacteria (bacilli) to form a protective endospore in response to unfavorable conditions for survival until conditions improve.

Stenosis: A narrowing or constriction of a tubular structure, passage, or orifice.

Sterilant: Any agent, physical (steam, heat, ionizing radiation) or chemical (liquid, gas, plasma vapor) capable of destroying all living microorganisms, including spores, to render an object sterile.

Sterilization: The process of using chemical or thermal methods to render free from or kill all microorganisms, pathogenic or non-pathogenic, including those capable of forming spore coats.

Steroids: Any of a large group of chemical substances related to sterols; anabolic steroids are similar to testosterone and used to build muscle tissue; corticosteroids are similar to hormones produced by the adrenal glands and used to reduce inflammation in disease and lesson the immune response in cases of tissue/organ transplantation

Sterols: Group of substances belonging to the lipoids; lipids that make up the cell membrane of fungi.

Subdural effusion: Abnormal accumulation of fluid between the brain and meninges; if fluid is infected, it is called subdural empyema.

Sub-pathogenic: Below the threshold of ability to cause disease or infection.

Subungual: Pertaining to the area beneath a fingernail or toenail.

Surface receptors: Molecular protein structures on the outside surfaces of cells which recognize and bind with certain chemical molecules to produce specific effects as a result of the interaction.

Surgical conscience: The honesty and moral integrity that the surgical technologist must possess in order to: always practice strict aseptic and sterile techniques; not hesitate to admit a mistake or break in technique; take corrective actions to prevent potential harm to the patient from acquiring a surgical wound infection or any other preventable injury.

Surgical site infection (SSI): An infection of an anatomical area following a surgical procedure; considered a type of healthcare-associated infection (HAI).

Susceptibility: The quality or condition of having inadequate resistance to infection or disease.

Symbiont: An organism that lives with an organism of a different species; both are symbionts.

Syncytial: Pertaining to a syncytium; description of a type of multinucleated cell produced by merging together and resulting in the cytoplasm of one cell being continuous with the cytoplasm of other cells. In Respiratory Syncytial Virus (RSV), a serious bronchial inflammation in babies, the virus passes from upper to lower respiratory structures by cell-to-cell transmission across intracytoplasmic bridges (syncytia).

Synergism: A relationship in which two organisms work together to achieve a result that cannot be achieved alone.

Synthesizing: The activity of producing or forming complex substances from simple compounds or elements.

Syphilomas: Gummas or syphilitic tumors.

Tachycardia: Abnormally fast heart rate (greater than 100 beats per minute in an adult).

Taxonomic hierarchy: A scientific system of subdivisions in which all living organisms are categorized in descending ranks (broadest to narrowest): kingdom, phylum, class, order, family, genus, species.

Taxonomy: The orderly scientific classification of organisms into appropriate categories (taxa), with application of suitable names.

Tenosynovitis: Infection of a tendon sheath, usually due to the direct inoculation of bacteria from a traumatic wound in the skin and spreads through the whole sheath, impairing nutrient flow and resulting in tendon necrosis; symptoms include pain, tenderness, and edema in the affected area.

Teratogen: An agent that causes birth defects.

Thrombocytopenia: Abnormal decrease in the number of blood platelets, often due to disease or bacterial infection.

Tracheostomy: Incision into and creation of an opening of the trachea to provide an alternative airway, often performed as an emergency surgical procedure due to tracheal obstruction or as replacement of long-standing endotracheal intubation.

Trachoma: Contagious infection of the eyelids caused by *Chlamydia trachomatis* which causes the inner eyelids to become rough and abrade the cornea; the leading cause worldwide of preventable blindness from bacterial infection.

Transfusions: Injections of blood or its constituent components into the bloodstream of an individual; may be direct or indirect and be from a donor or the individual's own previously collected blood.

Transmissible spongiform encephalopathy (TSE): A prion disease of the central nervous system that causes a degeneration of brain tissue, resulting in holes that produce a sponge-like appearance. In humans, it is called CJD. In cattle, it is called mad cow disease. In sheep and goats, it is called scrapie.

Trematodes: Flatworms commonly known as flukes, a class within the phylum Platyhelminthes.

Trivalent: On the molecular level, a combining with or replacement of three hydrogen atoms.

Typhoid fever: An infection caused by *Salmonella typhi;* symptoms include fever, headache, abdominal pain, constipation, and/or diarrhea; associated with poor sanitation, sewage disposal, and water treatment where human feces spread the bacteria. Some recovered patients become chronic carriers.

Ulcer: An open sore or lesion characterized by a depression in skin or organ tissue, such as the inner lining of the stomach, in which the tissue has been destroyed; most often due to trauma (pressure ulcer) or bacterial infection.

Ultraviolet light: A type of high-energy, short-wavelength radiation that is a component of normal sunlight beyond the visible light spectrum at the violet end; capable of therapeutic and mutagenic effects.

Urethral meatus: External opening of the urethra; distal-most structure of the urinary tract.

Vaccination: The procedure of producing immunity by administration of a vaccine through various means, such as intradermally or orally; also called immunization.

Vaginosis: A condition of an overgrowth of atypical bacteria causing increased vaginal discharge.

Vagotomy: Surgical procedure which entails ligation of one or more branches of the vagus nerve; often performed to reduce secretions of gastric acids in patients with or at risk of gastric ulcer.

Vasoconstrictors: Classification of drugs or other agents which constrict (narrow) blood vessels.

Vectors: In epidemiology: an insect arthropod, animal, or other organism that carries pathogens and infects other organisms; in virology: either a plasmid or a virus specifically used in genetic engineering to insert DNA into a cell; must be capable of replicating once in the cell.

Vegetative: Functioning involuntarily or passively as in comatose states; having the power to grow as in bacterial populations.

Ventilators: Mechanical devices used for artificial ventilation (breathing) of the lungs.

Ventriculitis: Inflammation of a ventricle.

Ventriculoatrial: A surgical approach used for insertion of a shunt to drain excess cerebrospinal fluid from the ventricles of the brain into the right atrium of the heart for reabsorption.

Ventriculoperitoneal: A surgical approach used for insertion of a shunt to drain excess cerebrospinal fluid from the ventricles of the brain into the peritoneal cavity for reabsorption.

Verotoxin: Also known as a Shiga-like toxin; one of the virulence factors of EHEC that destroys the endothelial cells that line the inner layer of blood vessels.

Vesicles: Small blister-like sacs containing fluid; small cellular organelles of protein molecules that break away from the smooth endoplasmic reticulum and travel to the Golgi complex.

Viability: The ability to survive, grow, develop, and potentially reproduce.

Viremia: The presence of viruses or viral particles in the bloodstream.

Virions: Mature viral particles; units of genetic materials which comprise the viral genome surrounded by a protein coat (capsid).

Viroid: Tiny infectious, naked molecules of RNA without protein coats (capsids) which are similar to viruses, however with much smaller genomes than viruses.

Virulence: The pathogenicity or degree to which a microbe can cause a disease.

Viruses: Non-living, infectious, obligate cellular parasites made up of DNA or RNA surrounded by a protein coat and may have an additional membrane called an envelope; require invasion of host cells for replication.

Zoonotic: Pertaining to diseases transmissible from animals to humans under natural conditions.

Zygospores: Thick-walled resting fungal or algal cells which are created by the fusion of two similar gametes in laboratory culture.

References

12th International Conference on Lyme Disease and Other Spirochetal and Tick-Borne Disorders. Day 1: April 9, 1999. (n.d.). Retrieved from http://www.actionlyme.org /BURGDORFER_CYST.htm.

2014 Ebola outbreak in West Africa-case counts. (2015). Retrieved from http://www.cdc.gov/vhf/ebola/outbreaks /2014-west-africa/case-counts.html

2014 Ebola outbreak in West Africa. Retrieved from http://www.cdc.gov/vhf/ebola/outbreaks/guinea/

5 babies test positive for TB in Texas exposure. (2014). Retrieved from http://medicalxpress.com/news/2014-09 -babies-positive-tb-texas-exposure.html

About coronavirus. (2014). Retrieved from http://www.cdc .gov/coronavirus/about/index.html. *Astrovirus.* (n.d.)

About HIV/AIDS. (2015). Retrieved from http://www.cdc.gov /hiv/basics/whatishiv.html

About pandemics. (n.d.). Retrieved from http://www.flu.gov /pandemic/about/index.html

About parasites. (2014). Retrieved from http://www.cdc.gov /parasites/about.html

About the USPHS Syphilis Study. (n.d.). Retrieved from http:// www.tuskegee.edu/about_us/centers_of_excellence /bioethics_center/about_the_usphs_syphilis_study.aspx

Accou-Demartin, M., Gaborieau, V., Song, Y., Roumagnac, P., Marchou, B., Achtman, M., & Weil, F. X. (2011). Salmonella enterica serotype typhi with nonclassical quinolone resistance phenotype. Retrieved from http://wwwnc.cdc.gov/eid/article/17/6/10-1242_article

Acharya, T. (6-24-2021). *Laboratory diagnosis of syphilis.* Retrieved from http://microbeonline.com/laboratory -diagnosis-of-syphilis/

Acharya, T. (6-25-2021). *Optochin test. Principle, procedure, expected results and quality control.* https://microbeonline .com/?s=optochin+test

Acharya, T. (6-21-2021). *Oxygen requirements for pathogenic bacteria.* Retrieved from http://microbeonline.com/oxygen -requirements-for-pathogenic-bacteria/

Acharya, T. (6-21-2021). *Enterobacteriaceae Family: Common Characteristics.* Retrieved from https://microbeonline.com/ enterobacteriaceae/Actinobacillus actinomycetemcomitans BRIAN HENDERSON,

MICHAEL WILSON, LINDSAY SHARP and JOHN M. WARD J. Med. Microbiol.—Vol. 51 (2002), 1013–1020 # 2002 Society for General Microbiology ISSN 0022-2615

Adam, S. A. (n.d.). *Mitochondrion.* Retrieved from http:// www.biologyreference.com/Ma-Mo/Mitochondrion.html

Aeromonas. (n.d). In *The Free Dictionary online.* Retrieved from http://medical-dictionary.thefreedictionary.com/Aeromonas.

Alcaligenaceae. (n.d.). Retrieved from http://www .medicalglossary.org/gramnegative_aerobic_rods_and _cocci_alcaligenaceae_definitions.html

Alexander, V., Dmitriev, A. V., & Chaussee, M. S. (2010). *The Streptococcus pyogenes proteome: maps, virulence factors and vaccine candidates.* Retrieved from http://www.ncbi .nlm.nih.gov/pmc/articles/PMC3092638/

Alexandraki, I. & Palacio, C. (2010). *Gram-negative versus Gram-positive bacteremia: what is more alarmin(g)?* Retrieved from http://www.ncbi.nlm.nih.gov/pubmed /20550728

Algae and algal blooms. (n.d.). Retrieved from http://www .algae.info/

Al-Nassir, W. (n.d.). *Brucellosis.* Retrieved from http:// emedicine.medscape.com/article/213430-overview

American Chemical Society. (2011). *The skinny on how shed skin reduces indoor air pollution.* Retrieved from http://www .sciencedaily.com/releases/2011/05/110509114034.htm

American Crystallographic Association. (2012). *Actinobacteria as the base of the evolutionary tree.* Retrieved from http:// www.sciencedaily.com/releases/2012/07/120726112729.htm

American Lung Association. (n.d.). *Understanding nontuberculous mycobacterium.* Retrieved from http://www .lung.org/lung-disease/nontuberculosis-mycobacterium /understanding-nontuberculous.html

American Society For Microbiology. (2004). *Doctor's Neckties: A Reservoir For Bacteria?* Retrieved from http://www .sciencedaily.com/releases/2004/05/040525062317.htm

American Society for Microbiology. (2021). ASM Membership. Retrieved from https://asm.org/ Membership/Home

Amoeba. (n.d.). In *Encyclopedia online.* Retrieved from http://www.encyclopedia.com/utility/printdocument .aspx?id=1G2:3438100043

Amoeba. (n.d.). In *Encyclopedia online*. Retrieved from http://www.encyclopedia.com/topic/amoeba.aspx

Ania, B. J. (n.d.). *Serratia*. Retrieved from http://emedicine.medscape.com/article/228495-overview#a0104

Anitori, R. P. (2012). *Extremophiles: Microbiology and biotechnology*.

Archaea, bacteria, viruses, and protists. Retrieved from http://www.uic.edu/classes/bios/bios104/mike/bacteria01.htm

Archer, D. L. & Young, F. E. (1988). *Contemporary issues: Diseases with a food vector*. Retrieved from http://www.ncbi.nlm.nih.gov/pmc/articles/PMC358061/

Arnold, C. (2014). *The man who rewrote the tree of life*. Retrieved from http://www.pbs.org/wgbh/nova/next/evolution/carl-woese/

Arthropod. (n.d.). In *Encyclopaedia Britannica online*. Retrieved from http://www.britannica.com/EBchecked/topic/36943/arthropod

ASM Journals. (May 2020) *Applied and Environmental Microbiology*. (Vol. 86, No. 11). A Nonlive Preparation of Chromobacterium sp. Panama (Csp_P) Is a Highly Effective Larval Mosquito Biopesticide. DOI: https://doi.org/10.1128/AEM.00240-20

Aspergillus flavus. (2005). Retrieved from http://www.aspergillusflavus.org/aflavus/index.html

Association of Surgical Technologists. (2018). *Surgical Technology for the Surgical Technologist* (5th ed.). United States: Cengage Learning.

Association of Surgical Technologists. (2021). *AST Guidelines for Best Practices in Bowel Technique*. Retrieved from https://www.ast.org/uploadedFiles/Main_Site/Content/About_Us/Standard_Bowel_Technique.pdf

Augus von Wassermann. (n.d.). In *Encyclopaedia Britannica online*. Retrieved from http://www.britannica.com/EBchecked/topic/636621/August-von-Wassermann

Autoimmune disease. (n.d.). Retrieved from http://www.ncbi.nlm.nih.gov/pubmedhealth/PMHT0022033/

Autoimmune diseases. (n.d.). Retrieved from http://immunologyinfo.weebly.com/autoimmune-diseases.html

Auyang, S. Y. (n.d.). *Reality and politics in the war on infectious diseases*. Retrieved from http://www.creatingtechnology.org/biomed/germs.htm

B10n3mber5: The database of useful biological numbers. (2009). Retrieved from http://bionumbers.hms.harvard.edu/bionumber.aspx?id5105093&ver53

B10n3mber5: The database of useful biological numbers. (2010). Retrieved from http://bionumbers.hms.harvard.edu/bionumber.aspx?&id5100649&ver54

Babcock, P. (n.d.). *12 reasons why adults need vaccines*. Retrieved from http://www.webmd.com/vaccines/features/why-adults-need-vaccines

Babcock, P. (n.d.). *12 reasons why adults need vaccines*. Retrieved from http://www.webmd.com/vaccines/features/why-adults-need-vaccines?page=3

Babu, E. & Oropello, J. (2011). "Staphylococcus Lugdunensis: The Coagulase-negative Staphylococcus You Don't Want to Ignore".

Bacillus bacteria. (n.d.). In *Encyclpaedia Britannica online*. Retrieved from http://www.britannica.com/EBchecked/topic/47965/bacillus

Bacillus. (n.d.). Retrieved from http://www.virology-online.com/Bacteria/Bacillus.htm

Bacteremia. (n.d.). In *The Free Dictionary online*. Retrieved from http://medical-dictionary.thefreedictionary.com/Blood+Stream+Infection

Bacteria live even in healthy placentas, says study. (2014). Retrieved from http://www.cbc.ca/news/health/bacteria-live-even-in-healthy-placentas-says-study-1.2650705

Bacteria. (n.d.). In *Encyclopaedia Britannica online*. Retrieved from http://www.britannica.com/EBchecked/topic/48203/bacteria#toc39333

Bacteria. (n.d.). Retrieved from http://www.microbexpert.com/bacteria.html

Bacteria. Retrieved from http://www.tutorvista.com/content/biology/biology-iii/kingdoms-living-world/bacteria.php#

Bacteria: The proteobacteria. (n.d.). Retrieved from http://mhhe.com/biosci/cellmicro/prescott/outlines/ch22.mhtml

Bacterial cell wall structure: Gram + and Gram -. (n.d.). Retrieved from http://www.scienceprofonline.com/microbiology/bacterial-cell-wall-structure-gram-positive-negative.html

Bacterial endocarditis. (n.d.). Retrieved from http://www.nmihi.com/e/endocarditis.htm

Bacterial endospores and vegetative cells.

Bacterial gastroenteritis. (n.d.). Retrieved from http://www.nlm.nih.gov/medlineplus/ency/article/000254.htm

Bacterial genomes. (n.d.). Retrieved from http://micro.cornell.edu/research/epulopiscium/bacterial-genomes

Bacterial strains: Enterobacteriaceae. (n.d.). Retrieved from http://www.globalrph.com/bacterial-strains-enterobacteriaceae.htm

Bailey, R. (n.d.). *Biology prefixes and suffixes: Staphylo-*. Retrieved from http://biology.about.com/od/prefixesandsuffixess/g/bls13.htm

Bailey, R. (n.d.). *Cellular respiration*. Retrieved from http://biology.about.com/od/cellularprocesses/a/cellrespiration.htm

Bailey, R. (n.d.). *Prokaryotes*. Retrieved from http://biology.about.com/od/cellanatomy/ss/prokaryotes.htm

Baorto, E. P. (n.d.). *Staphylococcus aureus infection treatment & management*. Retrieved from http://emedicine.medscape.com/article/971358-treatment

Bartlett, J. G. (2012). *Bacteroides fragilis*. Retrieved from http://www.hopkinsguides.com/hopkins/ub/view/Johns_Hopkins_ABX_Guide/540052/all/Bacteroides_fragilis

Bartlett, M. D., & John, G. (2014). "An Epidemic of Epidemics". Retrieved from http://www.medscape.com/viewarticle/821073

Bartlett, M. D., & John, G. (2014). "The 2014 Hit Parade: Infectious Disease Stories of the Year". Retrieved from http://www .medscape.com/viewarticle/835915

Basta M, Annamaraju P. *Bacterial Spores*. [Updated 2021 Feb 9]. In: StatPearls [Internet]. Treasure Island (FL): StatPearls Publishing; 2021 Jan.

Bates, T., Sheean, A. J., Kao, E., Bandino, J. P., Lynch, T. B., & Lybeck, D. (2021). Fulminant Pyoderma Gangrenosum After Outpatient Knee Arthroscopy. *Journal of the American Academy of Orthopaedic Surgeons*. Global research & reviews, 5(8), e21.00006. https://doi.org /10.5435/JAAOSGlobal-D-21-00006

BBB: Clostridium perfringens. (2014). Retrieved from http:// www.fda.gov/Food/FoodborneIllnessContaminants /CausesOfIllnessBadBugBook/ucm070483.htm

BBB: Clostridium perfringens. (2014). Retrieved from http:// www.fda.gov/Food/FoodborneIllnessContaminants/ CausesOfIllnessBadBugBook/ucm070000.htm

Beck, J. (2013). *Potential public health implications of periodontal disease and cardiovascular disease relationships*. Retrieved from http://www.cdc.gov/OralHealth/archive /conferences/periodontal_infections08.htm

Bedinghaus, T. (n.d.). *Pharyngoconjunctival fever*. Retrieved from http://vision.about.com/od /eyediseasesandconditions/g/Pharyn_Fever.htm

Beijerinck. M. W. (n.d.) In *Encyclopaedia Britannica online*. Retrieved from http://www.britannica.com/EBchecked /topic/58881/Martinus-W-Beijerinck

Bender, Eric. (2018). Getting cancer drugs into the brain. *Nature* 561, S46-S47. doi: https://doi.org/10.1038/d41586 -018-06707-4

Bennett, R. W. & Lancette, G. A. (2001). *BAM: Staphylococcus aureus*. Retrieved from http://www.fda.gov/Food/Food ScienceResearch/LaboratoryMethods/ucm071429.htm

Bergey's manual trust. (2018). *The Microbial Taxonomist*. Retrieved from http://www.bergeys.org/newsletter.html

Bigger brains: Complex brains for a complex world. (2015). Retrieved from http://humanorigins.si.edu/human -characteristics/brains

Biggest threats. (n.d). Retrieved from http://www.cdc.gov /drugresistance/biggest_threats.html

BIO230 microorganisms and bacteria.

Biology Dictionary. (2020). *Yersinia pestis*. Retrieved from https://biologydictionary.net/yersinia-pestis/

Bjornstad, O. N. & Harvill, E. T. (2005). *Evolution and emergence of Bortadella in humans*. Retrieved from http://www.cidd.psu.edu/research/synopses /evolution-and-emergence-of-bordetella-in-humans

Blaser, M. J. (2014). *Missing microbes: How killing bacteria creates modern plagues*. London, England: Oneworld Publications.

Blaser, M. J. (2014). *We kill germs at our peril. 'Missing microbes': How antibiotics can do harm*. Retrieved from http://www .nytimes.com/2014/04/29/health/missing-microbes-how -antibiotics-can-do-harm.html?_r=0

Blood differential. (n.d.). Retrieved from http://www.nlm.nih .gov/medlineplus/ency/article/003657.htm

Bloomberg.com. (2021). *Ethicon Plus Sutures Become First and Only Sutures With Antibacterial Protection Recommended for Use in NHS by NICE Medical*. Retrieved from https:// www.bloomberg.com/press-releases/2021-06-29 /ethicon-plus-sutures-become-first-and-only-sutures -with-antibacterial-protection-recommended-for-use-in -nhs-by-nice-medical

CDC. (2020). *Cutaneous anthrax*. Retrieved from https:// www.cdc.gov/anthrax/basics/types/index.html#cutaneous

Blutt, S. E., & Conner, M. E. (2013). *The gastrointestinal frontier: IgA and viruses*.

Boatman, E. S., & Kenny, G. E. (1971). *Morphology and ultrastructure of Mycoplasma pneumoniae spherules*.

Bocher, S., Tonning, B., Skov, R. L., & Prag, J. (2009). *Staphylococcus lugdunensis, a common cause of skin and soft tissue infections in the community*. Retrieved from http:// www.ncbi.nlm.nih.gov/pmc/articles/PMC2668335/

Bofinger, J. J., Fekete, T., & Samuel, R. (2007). *Bacterial peritonitis caused by Kingella kingae*. Retrieved from http://jcm.asm.org/content/45/9/3118.full

Botox. (n.d.). Retrieved from http://www.botox.com/

Bottone, E. J. (n.d.). *Bacillus cereus, a volatile human pathogen*. Retrieved from http://cmr.asm.org/content/23/2/382.full

Botulinum toxin. (n.d.). Retrieved from http://www.torticollis. org/botulinum-toxin-botox/

Botulism: Countering Common Clinical Misperceptions. *Medscape*. Apr 01, 2013.

Boundless. (2015). *The plasma membrane and the cytoplasm*. Retrieved from https://www.boundless.com/biology /textbooks/boundless-biology-textbook/cell-structure-4 /eukaryotic-cells-60/the-plasma-membrane-and -the-cytoplasm-314-11447/

Brandt, C. M. & Spellerberg, B. (n.d.). *Human infections due to Streptococcus dysgalactiae subspecies equisimilis*. Retrieved from http://cid.oxfordjournals.org/content /49/5/766.full

Brent, L. H. (n.d.). *Ankylosing spondylitis and undifferentiated spondyloarthropathy*.

Brook, I. (2014). *Bacteroides infection*. Retrieved from http:// emedicine.medscape.com/article/233339-overview

Broad Institute. (2021). *Questions and Answers About CRISPR*. Retrieved from https://www.broadinstitute.org/what-broad /areas-focus/project-spotlight/questions-and-answers -about-crispr

Brock, T. D. (1994). *Introduction to the Spirochetes*. Retrieved from http://www.ucmp.berkeley.edu/bacteria/spirochetes.html

Brooks, J. (2010). *On Cronobacter sakazakii. Brucella*. (n.d.). Retrieved from http://www.rightdiagnosis.com/medical /brucella.htm

Brouhard, R. (n.d.). *Causes of nausea and vomiting*. Retrieved from http://firstaid.about.com/od/abdominaldisorders /qt/06_nausea.htm

Brucellosis. (n.d.). Retrieved from http://www.cdph.ca.gov /HealthInfo/discond/Pages/Brucellosis.aspx

Brucellosis. (n.d.). Retrieved from http://www.nlm.nih.gov /medlineplus/ency/article/000597.htm

Brunner, J., Scheres, N., El Idrissi, N. B., Deng, D. M., Laine, M. L., van Winkelhoff, A. J., & Crielaard, W. (2010). *The capsule of Porphyromonas gingivalis reduces the immune response of human gingival fibroblasts*. Retrieved from http://www.biomedcentral.com/1471-2180/10/5

Brusch, J. L. (2014). *Infective carditis.* Retrieved from http://emedicine.medscape.com/article/216650-overview#a0104

Brusch, J. L. (2014). *Infective carditis.* Retrieved from http://emedicine.medscape.com/article/216650-overview #aw2aab6b2b3aa

Brusch, J. L. (2014). *Urinary tract infection in males.* Retrieved from http://emedicine.medscape.com/article/231574-overview #a0104

Brusch, J. L. (n.d.). *Infective endocarditis.* Retrieved from http://emedicine.medscape.com/article/216650-overview

Buchmayer, S., Sparen, P., & Cnattingisus, S. (2003). *Signs of infection* in Pap smears and risk of adverse pregnancy outcome.

Burrows, C. (n.d.). *Differences in bacillus and clostridium. Retrieved from* http://www.ehow.com/info_8270516 _differences -bacillus-clostridium.html

Bush, L. M. & Perez, M. T. (n.d.). *Acinetobacter infections.* Retrieved from http://www.merckmanuals.com /professional/infectious_diseases/neisseriaceae /acinetobacter_infections.html

Bush, L. M. & Perez, M. T. (n.d.). *Introduction to Neisseriaceae.* Retrieved from http://www.merckmanuals.com /professional/infectious_diseases/neisseriaceae /introduction_to_neisseriaceae.html

Caliciviridae. Retrieved from http://virology .microbiologyguide.com/834-Caliciviridae.html

Campylobacter jejuni. (n.d.). Retrieved from http://www .foodreference.com/html/fcampylobacter.html

Campylocater jejuni. (n.d). Retrieved from http://bioweb .uwlax.edu/bio203/s2013/rollins_tyle/classification.htm

Canny, G. O. & McCormick, B. A. (2008). *Bacteria in the intestine, helpful residents or enemies from within?* Retrieved from http://www.ncbi.nlm.nih.gov/pmc /articles/PMC2493210/

Carbon cycle. (n.d.). In *Encyclopedia online.* Retrieved from http://www.encyclopedia.com/topic/carbon_cycle.aspx

Cardiac tamponade. Retrieved from http://www.nlm.nih.gov /medlineplus/ency/article/000194.htm

Carey, J., Motyl, M., & Perlman, D. C. (2001). *Catheter-related bacteremia due to Streptomyces in a patient receiving holistic infusions.* Retrieved from http://wwwnc.cdc.gov/eid /article/7/6/01-0624_article

Catlin, K. (n.d.). *Yersinia pestis.* Retrieved from http://www .microbelibrary.org/library/bacteria/2787-yersinia-pestis

Causes of impetigo. (n.d.). Retrieved from http://www .rightdiagnosis.com/i/impetigo/causes.htm

Causes of *Moraxella catarrhalis* Pathogenicity: Review of Literature and Hospital Epidemiology Lucilene F. Tolentino, MD, FASCP, FCAP Lab Med. 2007;38(7):420–421. © 2007 American Society for Clinical Pathology.

Cavalca Cortelli, S., Oliveira Costa, F., Kawai, T., Romeiro Aquino, D., Nobre Franco, G. C., Ohara, K., Gonçalves Roman-Torres, C.V., & Cortelli, J. R. (2009). *Diminished treatment response of periodontally diseased patients infected with the JP2 clone of Aggregatibacter (Actinobacillus)*

actinomycetemcomitans. Retrieved from http://jcm.asm .org/content/47/7/2018.full

CDC Grand Rounds: The Growing Threat of Multidrug-Resistant Gonorrhea Weekly February 15, 2013 / 62(06);103–106. Reported by Edward W. Hook, III, MD, Univ of Alabama, Birmingham. William Shafer, PhD, Emory Univ, Atlanta, Georgia. Carolyn Deal, PhD, National Institute for Allergy and Infectious Disease, National Institutes of Health, Bethesda, Maryland. Robert D. Kirkcaldy, MD, Div of STD Prevention, National Center for HIV/AIDS, Viral Hepatitis, STD, and TB Prevention; John Iskander, MD, Office of the Associate Director for Science, CDC. Corresponding contributor: Robert D. Kirkcaldy, rkirkcaldy@cdc.gov, 404–639–8659.

CDC. (2002). *Enterobacter sakazakii infections associated with the use of powdered infant formula—Tennessee, 2001.* Retrieved from http://www.cdc.gov/mmwr/preview /mmwrhtml/mm5114a1.htm

CDC. (2010). *Klebsiella pneumoniae in health care settings.* Retrieved from http://www.cdc.gov/HAI/organisms /klebsiella /klebsiella.html#a1

CDC. (2010). *Staphylococcal food poisoning.* Retrieved from http://www.cdc.gov/nczved/divisions/dfbmd/diseases /staphylococcal/

CDC. (2010). *Syphillis: The facts.* Retrieved from http://www .cdc.gov/std/syphilis/the-facts/default.htm

CDC. (2011). *Gonococcal infections in adolescents and adults.* Retrieved from http://www.cdc.gov/std/treatment/2010 /gonococcal-infections.htm#gonopneopro

CDC. (2011). *Leptospirosis: Treatment.* Retrieved from http:// www.cdc.gov/leptospirosis/treatment/index.html

CDC. (2011). *Overview.* Retrieved from http://www.cdc.gov /bloodsafety/bbp/diseases_organisms.html

CDC. (2012). *Non-infectious meningitis.* Retrieved from http:// www.cdc.gov/meningitis/non-infectious.html

CDC. (2012). *Pulmonary Streptomyces infection in patient with sarcoidosis, France, 2012.* Retrieved from http://wwwnc .cdc.gov/eid/article/18/11/12-0797_article

CDC. (2012). *Resources for health professionals.* Retrieved from http://www.cdc.gov/parasites/babesiosis/health _professionals/index.html

CDC. (2012). *Symptoms.* Retrieved from http://www.cdc.gov /bartonella/symptoms/index.html

CDC. (2012). *Transmission.* Retrieved from http://www.cdc .gov/brucellosis/transmission/index.html

CDC. (2013). *Antibiotic-resistant gonorrhea.* Retrieved from http://www.cdc.gov/std/gonorrhea/arg/default.htm

CDC. (2013). *Arenaviridae.* Retrieved from http://www.cdc .gov/vhf/virus-families/arenaviridae.html

CDC. (2013). *Biology.* Retrieved from http://www.cdc.gov /parasites/leishmaniasis/biology.html

CDC. (2013). *CDC grand rounds: The growing threat of multidrug-resistant gonorrhea*

CDC. (2013). *Epidemiology and risk factors.* Retrieved from http://www.cdc.gov/parasites/chagas/epi.html

CDC. (2013). *Hansen's disease.* Retrieved from http://www .cdc.gov/leprosy/index.html

CDC. (2013). *Hantavirus pulmonary syndrome (HPS).* Retrieved from http://www.cdc.gov/hantavirus/hps/index.html

CDC. (2013). *Multidrug-resistant Bacteroides fragilis—Seattle, Washington, 2013.* Retrieved from http://www.cdc.gov /mmwr/preview/mmwrhtml/mm6234a2.htm

CDC. (2013). *Pertussis in other countries.* Retrieved from http://www.cdc.gov/pertussis/countries.html

CDC. (2013). *Pertussis: Summary of vaccine recommendations for health care professionals.* Retrieved from http://www .cdc.gov/vaccines/vpd-vac/pertussis/recs-summary.htm

CDC. (2013). *Symptoms, diagnosis, and treatment.* Retrieved from http://www.cdc.gov/anaplasmosis/symptoms/index.html

CDC. (2014). *Bacterial meningitis.* Retrieved from http:// www.cdc.gov/meningitis/bacterial.html

CDC. (2014). *C. neoformans infection.* Retrieved from http:// www.cdc.gov/fungal/diseases/cryptococcosis -neoformans/index.html

CDC (2014). *Gonorrhea.* Retrieved from http://www.cdc.gov /std/stats13/gonorrhea.htm

CDC. (2014). *Filoviridae.* Retrieved from http://www.cdc.gov /vhf/virus-families/filoviridae.html

CDC. (2014). *Fungal meningitis.* Retrieved from http://www .cdc.gov/meningitis/fungal.html

CDC. (2014). *Guillain-Barré syndrome.* Retrieved from http:// www.cdc.gov/flu/protect/vaccine/guillainbarre.htm

CDC. (2014). *Human Salmonella typhimurium infections linked to exposure to clinical and teaching microbiology laboratories.* Retrieved from http://www.cdc.gov/salmonella /typhimurium-labs-06-14/index.html

CDC. (2014). *Marburg hemorrhagic fever (MHF).* Retrieved from http://www.cdc.gov/vhf/marburg/

CDC. (2014). *Parasitic meningitis.* Retrieved from http://www .cdc.gov/meningitis/parasitic.html

CDC. (2014). *Transmission.* Retrieved from http://www.cdc .gov/chikungunya/transmission/index.html

CDC. (2014). *Types of healthcare-associated infections.* Retrieved from http://www.cdc.gov/HAI/infectionTypes.html

CDC. (2014). *Viral meningitis.* Retrieved from http://www .cdc.gov/meningitis/viral.html CDC. (2015). *Bacterial special pathogens branch (BSPB). Special bacteriology reference laboratory (SBRL).* Retrieved from http://www .cdc.gov/ncezid/dhcpp/bacterial_special/special_lab.html

CDC. (2015). *Buruli ulcer.* Retrieved from https://www.cdc .gov/buruli-ulcer/health-care-workers.html

CDC. (2015). *Chikungunya virus transmission.* Retrieved from http://www.cdc.gov/chikungunya/transmission/index.html

CDC. (2015). *Enterovirus D68.* Retrieved from http://www .cdc.gov/non-polio-enterovirus/outbreaks/EV-D68 -outbreaks.html

CDC. (2015). *For health care providers.* Retrieved from http://www.cdc.gov/mumps/hcp.html

CDC. (2015). *MERS in the U.S.* Retrieved from http://www .cdc.gov/coronavirus/MERS/US.html

CDC. (2015). *Summary of findings: Investigation of acute flaccid myelitis in U.S. children, 2014-15.* Retrieved from http:// www.cdc.gov/ncird/investigation/viral/sep2014 /investigation.html

CDC. (2016). *Nocardiosis Information for Healthcare Workers.* Retrieved from https://www.cdc.gov/nocardiosis/health -care-workers/index.html

CDC. (2016). *Tuberculosis (TB) Fact Sheet-Interferon-Gamma Release Assays (IGRAs)–Blood Tests for TB Infection.* Retrieved from https://www.cdc.gov/tb/publications /factsheets/testing/igra.htm

CDC. (2016). *Tuberculosis (TB) Fact sheet-Extensively Drug-Resistant Tuberculosis (XDR TB).* Retrieved from https:// www.cdc.gov/tb/publications/factsheets/drtb/xdrtb.htm

CDC. (2021). *Water, Sanitation & Environmentally-related Hygiene–Trachoma.* Retrieved from: https://www.cdc.gov /healthywater/hygiene/disease/trachoma.html

CDC. (2016). *Yersinia enterocolitica* (Yersiniosis). Retrieved from https://www.cdc.gov/yersinia/

CDC. (2017) Hanson's Disease (Leprosy). Retrieved from https://www.cdc.gov/leprosy/

CDC. (2017). *Hansen's Disease (Leprosy)–What is Hansen's Disease?* Retrieved from https://www.cdc.gov/leprosy /about/about.html

CDC. (2017). *Hanta Virus–Hemorrhagic Fever With Renal Syndrome (HFRS).* Retrieved from https://www.cdc.gov /hantavirus/hfrs/index.html

CDC. (2017). *Kingella denitrifians.* Retrieved from http:// www.cdc.gov/std/Gonorrhea/lab/Kden.htm

CDC. (2017). *Meningococcal Disease: Signs and symptoms.* Retrieved from http://www.cdc.gov/meningococcal /about/symptoms.html

CDC. (2017). *Pertussis.* Retrieved from http://www.cdc.gov /pertussis/about/causes-transmission.html

CDC. (2017). Smallpox-*Side Effects of Smallpox Vaccination.* Retrieved from https://www.cdc.gov/smallpox/vaccine -basics/vaccination-effects.html

CDC. (2018). Food Safety Staphylococcal food poisoning. Retrieved from https://www.cdc.gov/foodsafety/diseases /staphylococcal.html

CDC. (2018). *Immunization Schedules-Heplisav-B® (HepB-CpG) Vaccine.* Retrieved from https://www.cdc.gov /vaccines/schedules/vacc-updates/heplisav-b.html

CDC. (2018). *Parasites—Lymphatic filariasis.* Retrieved from http://www.cdc.gov/parasites/lymphaticfilariasis /disease.html

CDC. (2018). *Parasites—Schistosomiasis.* Retrieved from http://www.cdc.gov/parasites/schistosomiasis /disease.html

CDC. (2018). *Parasites-Toxoplasmosis (Toxoplasma infection).* CDC. (2018). *Tularemia.* Retrieved from http://www.cdc .gov/tularemia/

CDC. (2018). *Vaccines and Preventable Diseases-Shingles Vaccination.* Retrieved from https://www.cdc.gov/vaccines /vpd/shingles/public/shingrix/

CDC. (2019). *About the Division of Vector-Borne Diseases.* Retrieved from http://www.cdc.gov/ncezid/dvbd/about.html

CDC. (2019). *Acinetobacter in health care settings.* Retrieved from http://www.cdc.gov/HAI/organisms/acinetobacter.html

CDC. (2019). *Anaplasmosis.* Retrieved from http://www.cdc.gov/anaplasmosis/

CDC. (2019). *Antibiotic Resistance Threats in the United States 2019.* Retrieved from https://www.cdc.gov/drugresistance/pdf/threats-report/2019-ar-threats-report-508.pdf

CDC. (2019). *Ehrlichiosis.* Retrieved from http://www.cdc.gov/ehrlichiosis/

CDC. (2019). *Healthcare-associated Infections – Diseases and Organisms in Healthcare Settings.* Retrieved from https://www.cdc.gov/hai/organisms/organisms.html

CDC. (2019). Healthcare-associated Infections. *Carbapenem-resistant Enterobacterales (CRE).* Retrieved from https://www.cdc.gov/hai/organisms/cre/index.html

CDC. (2019). Healthcare-associated Infections. *Healthcare Facilities: Information about CRE.* Retrieved from https://www.cdc.gov/hai/organisms/cre/cre-facilities.html

CDC. (2019). *Japanese Encephalitis.* Retrieved from https://www.cdc.gov/japaneseencephalitis/index.html

CDC. (2019). *La Crosse encephalitis.* Retrieved from http://www.cdc.gov/LAC/

CDC. (2019). *Laboratory detection of coagulase-negative Staphylococcus species with decreased susceptibility to the glycopeptides vancomycin and teicoplanin.* Retrieved from https://www.cdc.gov/hai/settings/lab/labdetectioncoagulase_negative.html

CDC. (2019). *Lassa Fever.* Retrieved from https://www.cdc.gov/vhf/lassa/

CDC. (2019). *Leptospirosis.* Retrieved from http://www.cdc.gov/leptospirosis/

CDC. (2019). *Meningococcal Disease–Clinical Information.* Retrieved from https://www.cdc.gov/meningococcal/clinical-info.htmlCDC. (2019). *Meningococcal Disease - Meningococcal Disease in Other Countries.* Retrieved from https://www.cdc.gov/meningococcal/global.html

CDC. (2019). *Meningococcal Disease–Surveillance.* Retrieved from https://www.cdc.gov/meningococcal/surveillance/index.html

CDC. (2019). *Microsporidiosis.* Retrieved from http://www.cdc.gov/dpdx/microsporidiosis/

CDC. (2019). *Necrotizing fasciitis: A rare disease, especially for the healthy.* Retrieved from https://www.cdc.gov/groupastrep/diseases-public/necrotizing-fasciitis.html

CDC. (2019). *Parasites—American Trypanosomiasis (also known as Chagas disease).* Retrieved from https://www.cdc.gov/parasites/chagas/

CDC. (2019). *Parasites–Onchocerciasis (also known as River Blindness).* Retrieved from https://www.cdc.gov/parasites/onchocerciasis/

CDC. (2019). *Plague.* Retrieved from http://www.cdc.gov/plague/

CDC. (2019). *Rocky Mountain spotted fever.* Retrieved from http://www.cdc.gov/rmsf/

CDC. (2019). *Travelers' Health–Chapter 4-Helicobacter pylori.* Retrieved from https://wwwnc.cdc.gov/travel/yellowbook/2020/travel-related-infectious-diseases/helicobacter-pylori

CDC. (2019). *Types of fungal disease.* Retrieved from http://www.cdc.gov/fungal/diseases/

CDC. (2019). *Vaccines and Preventable Diseases–Meningococcal Vaccination.* Retrieved from https://www.cdc.gov/vaccines/vpd/mening/index.html

CDC. (2019). *Vibrio* Species Causing Vibriosis. Retrieved from https://www.cdc.gov/vibrio/index.html

CDC. (2019). *Yellow fever.* Retrieved from http://www.cdc.gov/yellowfever/

CDC. (2020). *Anthrax: What is Anthrax.* Retrieved from http://www.cdc.gov/anthrax/basics/index.html

CDC. (2020). Antibiotic / Antimicrobial Resistance (AR / AMR) *Lab Capacity: Antibiotic Resistance Laboratory Network (AR Lab Network).* Retrieved from https://www.cdc.gov/drugresistance/solutions-initiative/ar-lab-network.html?CDC_AA_refVal=https%3A%2F%2Fwww.cdc.gov%2Fdrugresistance%2Fsolutions-initiative%2Far-lab-networks.html

CDC. (2020). *Antibiotic Prescribing and Use-Antibiotic Stewardship Implementation Framework for Health Departments.* Retrieved from https://www.cdc.gov/antibiotic-use/training/state.html

CDC. (2020). *Antibiotic/antimicrobial resistance.* Retrieved from http://www.cdc.gov/drugresistance/index.html

CDC. (2020). *Arthritis: Rheumatoid arthritis.* Retrieved from https://www.cdc.gov/arthritis/basics/rheumatoid-arthritis.html

CDC. (2020). *Bartonella infection.* Retrieved from http://www.cdc.gov/bartonella/

CDC. (2020). *Candidiasis.* Retrieved from http://www.cdc.gov/fungal/diseases/candidiasis/

CDC. (2020). *Cholera-Vibrio cholerae infection-Sources of Infection & Risk Factors.* Retrieved from https://www.cdc.gov/cholera/infection-sources.html

CDC. (2020). *Cholera-Vibrio cholerae infection.* Retrieved from https://www.cdc.gov/cholera/

CDC. (2020). *Diphtheria Complications.* Retrieved from https://www.cdc.gov/diphtheria/about/complications.html

CDC. (2020). Disease or Condition of the Week. *Whooping cough (Pertussis)* Retrieved from https://www.cdc.gov/dotw/whoopingcough/

CDC. (2020). *Food Safety–Foodborne Germs and Illnesses.* Retrieved from https://www.cdc.gov/foodsafety/foodborne-germs.html

CDC. (2020). Fungal Diseases–*Blastomycosis.* Retrieved from https://www.cdc.gov/fungal/diseases/blastomycosis/index.html

CDC. (2020). *Fungal Diseases-C. neoformans infection.* Retrieved from https://www.cdc.gov/fungal/diseases/cryptococcosis-neoformans/index.html

CDC. (2020). *Fungal Diseases-Fungal nail infections.* Retrieved from http://www.cdc.gov/fungal/nail-infections.html

CDC. (2020). *Fungal Diseases-Histoplasmosis*. Retrieved from http://www.cdc.gov/fungal/diseases/histoplasmosis/

CDC. (2020). Fungal Diseases-*Symptoms of Valley Fever (Coccidioidomycosis)*. Retrieved from https://www.cdc.gov/fungal/diseases/coccidioidomycosis/symptoms.html

CDC. (2020). *Measles (Rubeola)-Top 4 Things Parents Need to Know About Measles*. Retrieved from https://www.cdc.gov/measles/about/parents-top4.html

CDC. (2020). *Meningococcal disease*. Retrieved from http://www.cdc.gov/meningococcal/index.html

CDC. (2020). *Mycetoma*. Retrieved from https://www.cdc.gov/fungal/diseases/mycetoma/index.html

CDC. (2020). *Neglected tropical diseases*. Retrieved from http://www.cdc.gov/globalhealth/ntd/

CDC. (2020). *Parasites—African Trypanosomiasis*. Retrieved from http://www.cdc.gov/parasites/sleepingsickness/

CDC. (2020). Parasites—Babesiosis. Retrieved from https://www.cdc.gov/parasites/babesiosis/gen_info/faqs.html

CDC. (2020). *Parasites-Cyclosporiasis (Cyclospora Infection)*. Retrieved from https://www.cdc.gov/parasites/cyclosporiasis/gen_info/faqs.html#what_cyclo

CDC. (2020). *Parasites—Cysticercosis*. Retrieved from http://www.cdc.gov/parasites/cysticercosis/

CDC. (2020). *Parasites–Echinococcosis*. Retrieved from https://www.cdc.gov/parasites/echinococcosis/index.html

CDC. (2020). *Parasites–Fasciola*. Retrieved from http://www.cdc.gov/parasites/fasciola/

CDC. (2020). *Parasites–Guinea worm*. Retrieved from https://www.cdc.gov/parasites/guineaworm/

CDC. (2020). *Parasites—Leishmaniasis*. Retrieved from https://www.cdc.gov/parasites/leishmaniasis/index.html

CDC. (2020). *Parasites-Naegleria fowleri-Primary Amebic Meningoencephalitis (PAM)-Amebic Encephalitis*. Retrieved from https://www.cdc.gov/parasites/naegleria/infection-sources.html

CDC. (2020). *Parasites—Soil-transmitted Helminths*. Retrieved from http://www.cdc.gov/parasites/sth/index.html

CDC. (2020). *Parasites*. Retrieved from http://www.cdc.gov/parasites/

CDC. (2020). Pneumococcal disease. Retrieved from https://www.cdc.gov/pneumococcal/global.html

CDC. (2020). *Pneumococcal Disease*. Retrieved from https://www.cdc.gov/pneumococcal/clinicians/clinical-features.html

CDC. (2020). Pneumococcal vaccination. Retrieved from http://www.cdc.gov/pneumococcal/vaccination.html

CDC. (2020). *Rabies*. Retrieved from https://www.cdc.gov/rabies/index.html

CDC. (2020). *Ringworm*. Retrieved from http://www.cdc.gov/fungal/diseases/ringworm/

CDC. (2020). *Scrub Typus*. Retrieved from https://www.cdc.gov/typhus/scrub/index.html

CDC. (2020). *Shigella–Shigellosis–Questions & Answers*. Retrieved from https://www.cdc.gov/shigella/general-information.html

CDC. (2020). *Shigella–Shigellosis*. Retrieved from https://www.cdc.gov/shigella/index.html

CDC. (2020). *Smallpox–History of Smallpox*. Retrieved from https://www.cdc.gov/smallpox/history/history.html

CDC. (2020). *Travelers' Health–Yersiniosis*. Retrieved from https://wwwnc.cdc.gov/travel/yellowbook/2020/travel-related-infectious-diseases/yersiniosis

CDC (2021). *Antibiotic / Antimicrobial Resistance (AR / AMR) – Biggest Threats Data*. Retrieved from https://www.cdc.gov/drugresistance/biggest-threats.html#pne

CDC. (2021) *Brucellosis*. Retrieved from https://www.cdc.gov/brucellosis/index.html

CDC. (2021) *Morbidity and Mortality Weekly Report (MMWR)-Tuberculosis—United States, 2020*. Retrieved from https://www.cdc.gov/mmwr/volumes/70/wr/mm7012a1.htm?s_cid=mm7012a1_w

CDC. (2021). *2019 Final Pertussis Surveillance Report*. Retrieved from https://www.cdc.gov/pertussis/downloads/pertuss-surv-report-2019-508.pdf

CDC. (2021). *Antibiotic / Antimicrobial Resistance (AR / AMR)–Biggest Threats and Data*. Retrieved from https://www.cdc.gov/drugresistance/biggest-threats.html

CDC. (2021). *Antifungal resistance*. Retrieved from http://www.cdc.gov/fungal/antifungal-resistance.html

CDC. (2021). *Botulism–Information for Health Professionals*. Retrieved from https://www.cdc.gov/botulism/health-professional.html

CDC. (2021). *Botulism–Kinds of Botulism*. Retrieved from https://www.cdc.gov/botulism/definition.html

CDC. (2021). Campylobacter (Campylobacteriosis) *Outbreak of Multidrug-resistant Campylobacter Infections Linked to Contact with Pet Store Puppies*. Retrieved from https://www.cdc.gov/campylobacter/outbreaks/puppies-12-19/index.html

CDC. (2021). *C. diff (Clostridioides difficile)-Information for Healthcare Professionals about C. diff*. Retrieved from https://www.cdc.gov/cdiff/clinicians/index.html

CDC. (2021). *C. diff (Clostridioides difficile)*. Retrieved from https://www.cdc.gov/cdiff/

CDC. (2021). *Campylobacter (Campylobacteriosis)*. Retrieved from https://www.cdc.gov/campylobacter/

CDC. (2021). *Chlamydia*. Retrieved from https://www.cdc.gov/std/chlamydia/default.htm

CDC. (2021). COVID-19-*Understanding mRNA COVID-19 Vaccines*. Retrieved from https://www.cdc.gov/coronavirus/2019-ncov/vaccines/different-vaccines/mrna.html

CDC. (2021). COVID-19–*Basics of COVID-19*. CDC. (2021). *Epidemiology and Prevention of Vaccine-Preventable Diseases–Pertussis*. Retrieved from https://www.cdc.gov/vaccines/pubs/pinkbook/pert.html#bordetella-pertussis

CDC. (2021). *Cronobacter*. Retrieved from https://www.cdc.gov/cronobacter/index.html

CDC. (2021). *Dengue Fever–About Dengue: What You Need to Know*. Retrieved from https://www.cdc.gov/dengue/about/index.html

CDC. (2021). *Dengue*. Retrieved from http://www.cdc.gov/dengue/

CDC. (2021). *E. coli (Escherichia coli)*. Retrieved from https://www.cdc.gov/ecoli/index.html

CDC. (2021). *E. coli (Escherichia coli)*. Retrieved from https://www.cdc.gov/ecoli/index.html

CDC. (2021). *Eastern equine encephalitis*. Retrieved from http://www.cdc.gov/EasternEquineEncephalitis/

CDC. (2021). *Epidemiology and Prevention of Vaccine-Preventable Diseases Tetanus*. Retrieved from https://www.cdc.gov/vaccines/pubs/pinkbook/tetanus.html

CDC. (2021). *Epidemiology and Prevention of Vaccine-Preventable Diseases–Diphtheria*. Retrieved from https://www.cdc.gov/vaccines/pubs/pinkbook/dip.html#Epidemiology

CDC. (2021). *Foodborne Outbreaks-List of Selected Multistate Foodborne Outbreak Investigations*. Retrieved from https://www.cdc.gov/foodsafety/outbreaks/multistate-outbreaks/outbreaks-list.html

CDC. (2021). *Foodborne Outbreaks–Multistate Outbreaks*. Retrieved from https://www.cdc.gov/foodsafety/outbreaks/multistate-outbreaks/index.html

CDC. (2021). *Fungal Diseases-About murcormycosis*. Retrieved from https://www.cdc.gov/fungal/diseases/mucormycosis/definition.html

CDC. (2021). *Fungal Diseases-Histoplasmosis: A Common Fungal Lung Infection*. Retrieved from https://www.cdc.gov/fungal/features/histoplasmosis.html

CDC. (2021). *Fungal Diseases-Valley Fever Awareness*. Retrieved from https://www.cdc.gov/fungal/features/valley-fever.html

CDC. (2021). *Fungal Diseases-Aspergillosis*. Retrieved from https://www.cdc.gov/fungal/diseases/aspergillosis/definition.html

CDC. (2021). *Genital herpes*. Retrieved from https://www.cdc.gov/std/herpes/default.htm

CDC. (2021). *Global HIV and TB–Combating the Global Tuberculosis Epidemic*. Retrieved from https://www.cdc.gov/globalhivtb/what-we-do/briefingbook/briefbook-combatglobaltb.html#combating-globaltb

CDC. (2021). *Global HIV and TB-Population-Based HIV Impact Assessments (PHIA)*. Retrieved from https://www.cdc.gov/globalhivtb/index.html

CDC. (2021). *Gonorrhea*. Retrieved from https://www.cdc.gov/std/gonorrhea/default.htm

CDC. (2021). *Gonorrhea: CDC Fact Sheet (Detailed Version)*. Retrieved from https://www.cdc.gov/std/gonorrhea/stdfact-gonorrhea-detailed.htm

CDC. (2021). *Haemophilus influenzae Disease (Including Hib)*. Retrieved from https://www.cdc.gov/hi-disease/clinicians.html

CDC. (2021). *Heartland virus*. Retrieved from https://www.cdc.gov/heartland-virus/index.html

CDC. (2021). *HIV*. Retrieved from https://www.cdc.gov/hiv/basics/statistics.html

CDC. (2021). *Human Papillomavirus (HPV)*. Retrieved from https://www.cdc.gov/std/HPV/STDFact-HPV.htm

CDC. (2021). *Salmonella*. Retrieved from https://www.cdc.gov/salmonella/index.html

CDC. (2021). *Immunization Schedules-Table 1. Recommended Child and Adolescent Immunization Schedule for ages 18 years or younger, United States, 2021*. Retrieved from https://www.cdc.gov/vaccines/schedules/hcp/imz/child-adolescent.html#note-mening

CDC. (2021). *Immunization Schedules*. Retrieved from https://www.cdc.gov/vaccines/schedules/hcp/imz/adult.html

CDC. (2021). *Influenza (Flu)*. Retrieved from https://www.cdc.gov/flu/prevent/vaccinesafety.htm

CDC. (2021). *Legionella (Legionnaires' Disease and Pontiac Fever) - Causes, How it Spreads, and People at Increased Risk*. Retrieved from https://www.cdc.gov/legionella/about/causes-transmission.html

CDC. (2021). *Listeria (Listeriosis)*. Retrieved from https://www.cdc.gov/listeria/faq.html

CDC. (2021). *Botulism Kinds of Botulism*. Retrieved from https://www.cdc.gov/botulism/definition.html

CDC. (2021). *Lyme disease*. Retrieved from http://www.cdc.gov/lyme/. CDC. (2019). *Other Spotted Fever Group Rickettsioses*. Retrieved from https://www.cdc.gov/otherspottedfever/

CDC. (2021). *Lyme disease*. Retrieved from http://www.cdc.gov/lyme/

CDC. (2021). *Malaria*. Retrieved from https://www.cdc.gov/malaria/about/faqs.html.

CDC. (2021). *Marburg–Marburg Virus Disease*. Retrieved from https://www.cdc.gov/vhf/marburg/.

CDC. (2021). *Measles (Rubeola) Measles Cases and Outbreaks*. Retrieved from https://www.cdc.gov/measles/cases-outbreaks.html

CDC. (2021). National Center for Health Statistics-*Whooping Cough or Pertussis*. Retrieved from https://www.cdc.gov/nchs/fastats/whooping-cough.htm

CDC. (2021). *Norovirus- Burden of Norovirus Illness in the U.S.* Retrieved from https://www.cdc.gov/norovirus/trends-outbreaks/burden-US.html

CDC. (2021). *Parasites–American Trypanosomiasis (also known as Chagas disease)*. Detailed FAQs. Retrieved from https://www.cdc.gov/parasites/chagas/gen_info/detailed.html#intro

CDC. (2021). *Plague. Maps and Statistics*. Retrieved from https://www.cdc.gov/plague/maps/

CDC. (2021). *Plague*. Retrieved from https://www.cdc.gov/plague/

CDC. (2021). *Pneumococcal Disease Fast Facts You Need to Know about Pneumococcal Disease*. Retrieved from https://www.cdc.gov/pneumococcal/about/facts.html

CDC. (2021). *Powassan virus*. Retrieved from http://www.cdc.gov/powassan/

CDC. (2021). *Salmonella*. Retrieved from https://www.cdc.gov/salmonella/

CDC. (2021). *Sexually Transmitted Disease Surveillance 2019-National Overview*. Retrieved from https://www.cdc.gov/std/statistics/2019/overview.htm#Gonorrhea

CDC. (2021). *Sexually Transmitted Diseases (STDs)-Sexually Transmitted Infections Prevalence, Incidence, and Cost*

Estimates in the United States. Retrieved from https://www
.cdc.gov/std/statistics/prevalence-2020-at-a-glance.htm

CDC. (2021). *Sexually Transmitted Infections Treatment
Guidelines, 2021-Gonococcal Infections Among Neonates.*
Retrieved from https://www.cdc.gov/std/treatment
-guidelines/gonorrhea-neonates.htm

CDC. (2021). *Sexually Transmitted Infections Treatment
Guidelines, 2021–Syphilis.* Retrieved from https://www
.cdc.gov/std/treatment-guidelines/syphilis.htm

CDC. (2021). *Sexually Transmitted Infections Treatment
Guidelines, 2021 Diseases characterized by genital, anal, or
perianal ulcers.* Retrieved from https://www.cdc.gov/std
/treatment-guidelines/genital-ulcers.htm

CDC. (2021). *Sexually-Transmitted Diseases (STDs) -
Gonococcal Isolate Surveillance Project (GISP).* Retrieved
from https://www.cdc.gov/std/gisp/default.htm

CDC. (2021*). St. Louis encephalitis.* Retrieved from http://
www.cdc.gov/sle/

CDC. (2021). *Syphilis.* Retrieved from https://www.cdc.gov
/std/syphilis/default.htm

CDC. (2021). *Trichomoniasis.* Retrieved from http://www.cdc
.gov/std/trichomonas/stdfact-trichomoniasis.htm

CDC. (2021). *Trichomoniasis.* Retrieved from https://www
.cdc.gov/std/trichomonas/default.htm

CDC. (2021*). West Nile virus.* Retrieved from http://www.cdc
.gov/westnile/

CDC. (2021). *Zika Virus–Zika in the US.* Retrieved from
https://www.cdc.gov/zika/geo/index.html

CDC. (n.d.). *Osteomyelitis/septic arthritis caused by Kingella
kingae among day care attendees—Minnesota, 2003.*
Retrieved from http://www.cdc.gov/mmwr/preview
/mmwrhtml/mm5311a4.htm

CDC. (n.d.). *The Targeted Neglected Tropical Diseases (NTDs).*
Retrieved from https://www.cdc.gov/globalhealth/ntd
/resources/targeted_ntds.pdf

Cell motility determination. Retrieved from http://www
.microscopesblog.com/2010/05/cell-motility
-determination.html

Centers for Disease Control and Prevention. (2021). *CDC
Timeline.* Retrieved from https://www.cdc.gov/museum
/timeline/index.html

Centers for Disease Control and Prevention. *Campylobacter*
(Campylobacteriosis). 12-23-2019. Retrieved from
https://www.cdc.gov/campylobacter/faq.html

Centers for Disease Control and Prevention. *HIV in the
United States and Dependent Areas.* (Last reviewed 8-9-
2021). Retrieved from https://www.cdc.gov/hiv/statistics
/overview/ataglance.html

Centers for Disease Control and Prevention. *HIV Surveillance
Report, 2019; vol.32. (May 2021).* Retrieved from https://
www.cdc.gov/hiv/library/reports/hiv-surveillance/vol-32
/index.html

Centers for Disease Control and Prevention. *Immunization
Schedule. Heplisav-B® (HepB-CpG) Vaccine.*
(April 24, 2018). Retrieved from https://www
.cdc.gov/vaccines/schedules/

Centers for Disease Control and Prevention. *Norovirus.*
(March 5, 2021). Retrieved from https://www.cdc.gov
/norovirus/trends-outbreaks/burden-US.html

Centers for Disease Control and Prevention. *Three Rotavirus
Outbreaks in the Postvaccine Era—California, 2017.
Morbidity and Mortality Weekly Report.* (April 27, 2018).
Retrieved from https://www.cdc.gov/mmwr/volumes/67
/wr/mm6716a3.htm

Centers for Disease Control and Prevention. (2021). *Variant
Creutzfeldt-Jakob Disease (vCJD).* Retrieved from https://
www.cdc.gov/prions/vcjd/about.html

Cerebral blood flow. (n.d.). Retrieved from http://www
.vascularneurosurgery.com/cbf.html

Chamberlain, N. R. (2009). *From sepsis to septic shock.*
Retrieved from http://www.atsu.edu/faculty/chamberlain
/website/lectures/lecture/sepsis2007.htm

*Chapter 6 metabolism: Fueling cell growth. Retrieved
from* http://www.life.umd.edu/classroom/bsci424
/BSCI223WebSiteFiles /LectureSummaries
/SummaryLectures7thru9.htm

*Chapter 8: Identification and characterization of Streptococcus
pneumoniae* (2012). Retrieved from http://www.cdc.gov
/meningitis/lab-manual/chpt08-id-characterization
-streppneumo.html

Charlson, E. S. (n.d.). *The human respiratory tract microbiome
in health and disease.* Retrieved from http://repository
.upenn.edu/dissertations/AAI3542787/

Chater, K. F. (2006). *Streptomyces inside-out: a new perspective
on the bacteria that provide us with antibiotics.* Retrieved
from http://www.ncbi.nlm.nih.gov/pmc/articles
/PMC1609407/

Chemolithotroph. (n.d.). In *The Free Dictionary online.*
Retrieved from http://medical-dictionary.
thefreedictionary.com/chemolithotroph

Cheprasov, A. (n.d.). *What are viruses?—Definition, structure
& function.* Retrieved from http://education-portal.com
/academy/lesson/what-are-viruses-definition-structure
-function.html#lesson

Cheshire, S. (2014). *Vibrio vulnificus: A summertime bacteria.*
Retrieved from http://www.cnn.com/2014/08/07/health
/vibrio-vulnificus-bacteria/index.html

Cheung, W.Y. (2007). *Fusobacterium.* Retrieved from http://
www.ncbi.nlm.nih.gov/pmc/articles/PMC2234623/

Choudhary, A. (2015). *Biological indicator for moist heat
(steam) sterilization processes.* Retrieved from http://www
.pharmaguideline.com/2011/06/biological-indicator-for
-dry-heat.html

*Chromobacterium violaceum and its important metabolites—
review.* (n.d.). Retrieved from http://www.bioportfolio
.com/resources/pmarticle/136147/Chromobacterium
-Violaceum-And-Its-Important-Metabolites-Review.html

Chronic fatigue syndrome. (n.d.). Retrieved from http://www
.mayoclinic.org/diseases-conditions/chronic-fatigue
-syndrome /basics/causes/CON-20022009

Clark, D. P., Pazdernik, N. J., & McGehee, M. R. (2019).
Chapter 24 - Viruses, Viroids, and Prions. *Molecular*

Biology (3rd ed. pp. 749-792). ISBN 9780128132883, https://doi.org/10.1016/B978-0-12-813288-3.00024-0

Classification by morphology, biochemistry, and other features. (n.d.). In *Encyclopaedia Britannica online.* *Retrieved from* http://www.britannica.com/EBchecked /topic/48203/bacteria/39371/Classification-by -morphology-biochemistry-and -other-features

Classification of algae. (n.d.). In *Encyclopaedia Britannica online.* Retrieved from http://www.britannica.com /EBchecked/topic/14828/algae/31725/Classification -of-algae

Classification. (2007). Retrieved from http://bioweb.uwlax. edu/bio203/s2008/kitzmann_step/Classification.htm

*Claverie, J. M., Abergel, C., & Ogata, H. (2009). Mimiv*irus. Retrieved from http://www.ncbi.nlm.nih.gov /pubmed/19216436

Cleveland Clinic. (2017). *Sty (Stye)*. Retrieved from https:// my.clevelandclinic.org/health/diseases/17658-sty-stye

Clostridium difficile, Pediatr Pharm. 2000;6(6) © 2000 Children's Medical Center, University of Virginia.

CNN Wire Staff. (2011). *Retracted autism study an elaborate fraud, British journal finds.* Retrieved from http://www .cnn.com/2011/HEALTH/01/05/autism.vaccines/index .html

Coban, A., Matur, Z., Hanagasi, H. A., & Parman, Y. (2010). *Iatrogenic botulism after botulinum toxin type A injections.* Retrieved from http://www.ncbi.nlm.nih.gov/pubmed /20150804

Cohen-Poradosu, R., Jaffe, J., Lavi, D. Grisariu-Greenzaid, S., Nir-Paz, R., Valinsky, L., Dan-Goor, M., Block, C., Beall, B., & Moses, A. E. (2004). *Group G streptococcal bacteremia in Jerusalem.* Retrieved from http://wwwnc.cdc.gov/eid /article/10/8/03-0840_article

Coleman, R. (2010). *Bacterial & fungal infections and heart disease.* Retrieved from http://www.livestrong.com /article/258408-bacterial-fungal-infections-and-heart -disease/

Combs, Sydney. National Geographic. *She discovered coronaviruses decades ago—but got little recognition. April17, 2020.* https://www.nationalgeographic.com/history/article /june-almeida-discovered-coronaviruses-decades-ago -little-recognition#close

Common colds: Protect yourself and others. (2015). Retrieved from http://www.cdc.gov/Features/Rhinoviruses/

Complement system. Retrieved from http://courses .washington.edu/conj/inflammation/complement.htm

Complement. (n.d.). In *Encyclopaedia Britannica online.* Retrieved from http://www.britannica.com/EBchecked /topic/129861/complement

Complement. (n.d.). Retrieved from http://www.nlm.nih.gov /medlineplus/ency/article/003456.htm

Condyloma. (n.d.). Retrieved from http://www.colonrectal .org/services.cfm/sid:6682/Condyloma/index.html

Conrad Stoppler, M. (n.d.). *Staph infection facts.* Retrieved from http://www.medicinenet.com/staph_infection /article.htm

Constantinescu, M. (2014). *Moraxella catarrhalis infection treatment & management.*

Constantinescu, M. (2014). *Moraxella catarrhalis infection.* Edmondson DG, Hu B, Norris SJ. Long-Term In Vitro Culture of the Syphilis Spirochete *Treponema pallidum* subsp. *pallidum.* mBio. 2018 Jun 26;9(3):e01153-18. doi: 10.1128/mBio.01153-18. PMID: 29946052; PMCID: PMC6020297.

Crohn's disease: Topic overview. (n.d.). Retrieved from http://www.webmd.com/ibd-crohns-disease/crohns -disease/tc/crohns-disease-topic-overview

Cucinotta D, & Vanelli M. WHO Declares COVID-19 a Pandemic. Acta Biomed. 2020 Mar 19;91(1):157-160. doi: 10.23750/abm.v91i1.9397. PMID: 32191675; PMCID: PMC7569573

Culvera, R. (2021). Protozoa: Explained. Microscope Clarity. Retrieved from https://microscopeclarity.com/protozoa -explained/

Cunha, B. A. (n.d.). *Acinetobacter.* Retrieved from http:// emedicine.medscape.com/article/236891-overview

Cunha, J. P. (n.d.). *Rhogam side effects center.* Retrieved from http://www.rxlist.com/rhogam-side-effects-drug -center.htm

Cytoplasm of prokaryotic cells. (2014). Retrieved from http:// www.scienceprofonline.com/cell-biology/cytoplasm -prokaryotic-biological-cells.html

Dash, P. (n.d.). *Blood brain barrier and cerebral metabolism.* Retrieved from http://neuroscience.uth.tmc.edu/s4 /chapter11.html

Davis, C. P. (1996). *Normal flora.* Retrieved from http://www .ncbi.nlm.nih.gov/books/NBK7617/

Davis, C. P. (n.d.). *Listeriosis (Listeria monocytogenes infection).* Retrieved from http://www.medicinenet.com/listeria /article.htm

Davis, C. P. (n.d.). *Salmonella.* Retrieved from http://www .emedicinehealth.com/salmonella/article_em.htm

Davis, C. P. (n.d.). *Scarlet fever.* Retrieved from http://www .medicinenet.com/scarlet_fever_scarlatina/article.htm

Davis, C. P. (n.d.). *Scarlet fever.* Retrieved from http://www .medicinenet.com/scarlet_fever_scarlatina/article.htm

Declining Guillain-Barré Syndrome after Campylobacteriosis Control, New Zealand, 1988–2010 Michael G. Baker, Amanda Kvalsvig, Jane Zhang, Rob Lake, Ann Sears, and Nick Wilson Emerging Infectious Diseases • www.cdc .gov/eid • Vol. 18, No. 2, February 2012.

Definition of enterococcus. (n.d.). Retrieved from http://www .medicinenet.com/script/main/art.asp?articlekey=20162

Definition of vector. (2012). Retrieved from http://www .medicinenet.com/script/main/art.asp?articlekey=5968

Denistry Today. (2011). *Porphyromonas gingivalis linked to atherosclerosis.* Retrieved from http://www.dentistrytoday .com/clinical-update/4435-porphyromonas-gingivalis -linked-to-atherosclerosis

Difference between innate and adaptive immunity. (2012). Retrieved from http://www.differencebetween.com/ difference-between-innate-and-vs-adaptive-immunity/

Difference between rheumatic fever and scarlet fever. (2011). Retrieved from http://www.differencebetween.net /science/health/difference-between-rheumatic-fever -and-scarlet-fever/

Dmitri Iosifovich Ivanovsky. (n.d.). In *Encyclopedia online.* Retrieved from http://www.encyclopedia.com/topic /Dmitri _Iosifovich_Ivanovsky.aspx

DNA sequencing. (2015). Retrieved from http://www.genome .gov/10001177

Doem, C. D., Burnham, & C.-A. D. (2010). *It's not easy being green: The viridans group streptococci, with a focus on pediatric clinical manifestations.* Retrieved from http://www.ncbi.nlm.nih.gov/pmc/articles /PMC3020876/

Drug discovery potential of natural microbial genomes. (2014). Retrieved from http://health.ucsd.edu/news/releases /Pages/2014-01-22-natural-microbial-genomes.aspx

Dugdale, D. C. III. (2012). *Nocardia infection.* Retrieved from http://www.nlm.nih.gov/medlineplus/ency /article/000679.htm

Dzeing-Ella, A., Szwebel, T. A., Loubinoux, J., Coignard, S., Bouvet, A., Le Jeunne, C., & Aslangul, E. (2009). *Infective endocarditis due to Citrobacter koseri in an immunocompetent adult.* Retrieved from http://www.ncbi.nlm.nih.gov/pmc /articles/PMC2786675/

Ebola data and statistics. (n.d.). Retrieved from http://apps .who.int/gho/data/view.ebola-sitrep.ebola-summary -latest?lang=en

ECHO virus. (n.d.). Retrieved from http://www.nytimes.com /health/guides/disease/echo-virus/overview.html

Ectoparasites. (2014). Retrieved from http://ratguide.com /health/integumentary_skin/ectoparasites.php

Edward Jenner. (n.d.). In *Encyclopaedia Britannica online.* Retrieved from http://www.britannica.com/EBchecked /topic/302579/Edward-Jenner

Elasticity and Hooke's Law. (1-7-2021). GK Scientist. https:// gkscientist.com/elasticity-and-hookes-law/

Emerging and reemerging infectious diseases. (n.d.). Retrieved from http://www.medscape.com/resource/infections

Emerging infectious diseases/pathogens. (2010). Retrieved from http://www.niaid.nih.gov/topics/emerging/Pages /introduction.aspx

Endocarditis. (n.d.). Retrieved from http://www.medicinenet .com/endocarditis/article.html

Endocarditis. (n.d.). Retrieved from http://www.nlm.nih.gov /medlineplus/ency/article/001098.htm

Endocarditis: Topic overview. (n.d.). Retrieved from http:// www.webmd.com/heart-disease/tc/endocarditis -topic-overview

Endosymbiotic theory. (n.d.). Retrieved from http://www.bio -medicine.org/biology-definition/Endosymbiotic_theory/

Energy and nutrient requirements for prokaryotes. Retrieved from https://www.boundless.com/biology/textbooks /boundless -biology-textbook/prokaryotes-bacteria-and -archaea-22/prokaryotic-metabolism-142/needs-of -prokaryotes-564-11777/

Enterobacteriaceae summary. (2000). Retrieved from http://www.life.umd.edu/classroom/bsci424 /PathogenDescriptions/Enterobacteriaceae.htm

Enterobacteriaceae. (n.d.). In *Encyclopedia online.* Retrieved from http://www.encyclopedia.com/topic /Enterobacteriaceae.aspx

Enzyme lab. Retrieved from http://biologycorner.com /worksheets/enzyme_lab.html

EPA. (n.d.). *Aeromonas detection: What does it mean?* Retrieved from http://water.epa.gov/lawsregs/rulesregs/sdwa/ucmr /data_aeromonas.cfm

Epclusa. Common Epclusa Side Efects. (n.d.). Retrieved from https://www.epclusa.com/common-side-effects?utm _source=bing&utm_medium=cpc&utm_campaign =USA_MA_SEM_NB_EX_Epclusa-DTP-Consideration -RLSA&utm_content=Medication+-+Exact&utm_term= hepatitis+c+medication&gclid=bda2d81da5741a3235ddb 90f7b220f4e&gclsrc=3p.ds&msclkid=bda2d81da5741a32 35ddb90f7b220f4e

Epidemiology. (n.d.). Retrieved from http://www.who.int /topics/epidemiology/en/

Errington, J. (2013). *L-form bacteria, cell walls and the origins of life.*

Erythema nodosum. (n.d.). Retrieved from http://www.nlm .nih.gov/medlineplus/ency/article/000881.htm

Eske, Jamie. Medical News Today. *The Five stages of infection explained.* (March 3, 2021). Retrieved from https://www .medicalnewstoday.com/articles/5-stages-of-infection

Eukaryote. (n.d.). In *Science Daily* online. Retrieved from http://www.sciencedaily.com/articles/e/eukaryote.htm

Eukaryotic cell vs. prokaryotic cell. (n.d.). Retrieved from http://www.diffen.com/difference/Eukaryotic_Cell_vs _Prokaryotic_Cell

Eukaryotic cells. (n.d.) Retrieved from http://www.nature .com/scitable/topicpage/eukaryotic-cells-14023963

Fact sheets. (n.d.). Retrieved from http://www.nfid.org /factsheets/

Facts about botulism. (2001). Retrieved from http://emergency .cdc.gov/agent/botulism/factsheet.asp

FAMeS. (n.d.). Retrieved from http://fames.jgi-psf.org/

Fankhauser, D. B. (n.d.). *Bacterial morphology.* Retrieved from http://biology.clc.uc.edu/fankhauser/Labs/Microbiology /Bacterial_Morphology/Bacterial_Morphology.htm

Fastidious gram-negative bacilli. (n.d.). Retrieved from http:// www.buddycom.com/bacteria/gnr/gnrfastid.html

Fastidious. (n.d.). In *Merriam-Webster online.* Retrieved from http://www.merriam-webster.com/medical/fastidious

Fatal familial insomnia. (2014). Retrieved from http:// rarediseases.info.nih.gov/gard/6429/fatal-familial -insomnia/resources/1

FDA. (2014). *Raw oyster myths.* Retrieved from http://www .fda.gov/Food/ResourcesForYou/HealthEducators /ucm085385.htm

FDA. (n.d.) *Bad Bug Book: Foodborne pathogenic microorganisms and natural toxins handbook: Aeromonas hydrophila.* Retrieved from http://www.fda.gov/Food

/FoodborneIllnessContaminants/ CausesOfIllnessBadBugBook/ucm070523.htm

Fernández Guerrero, M. L., Goyenechea, A., Verdejo, C., Roblas, R. F., & de Górgolas, M. (2007). *Enterococcal endocarditis on native and prosthetic valves: a review of clinical and prognostic factors with emphasis on hospital-acquired infections as a major determinant of outcome.* Retrieved from http://www.ncbi.nlm.nih.gov/ pubmed/18004181

Fine, D. H., Markowitz, K., Furgang, D., & Velliyagounder K. (2010). *Aggregatibacter actinomycetemcomitans as an early colonizer of oral tissues: Epithelium as a reservoir?* Retrieved from http://jcm.asm.org/content/48/12/4464.full

Flores, R., Gas, M.-E., Molina-Serrano, D., Nohales, M.-A., Carbonell, A., Gago, S., De la Pena, M., & Daros, J.-A. (2009). *Viroid replication: Rolling-circles, enzymes, and ribozymes.* Retrieved from http://www.ncbi.nlm.nih.gov /pmc/articles/PMC3185496/

Food spoilage organism: psychrotrophs. (2013). Retrieved from http://www.foodscience-avenue.com/2013/10/food -spoilage-organism-psychrotrophs.html

Foster, C. S. (2014). *Stevens-Johnson syndrome.* Retrieved from http://emedicine.medscape.com/article/1197450 -overview #aw2aab6b2b4

Fox, A. (2014). *Bacteriology—chapter twelve. Streptococci: Groups A, B, D, and others. Enterococcus faecalis.* Retrieved from http://www.microbiologybook.org/fox /streptococci.htm

Fraser, S. L. (2015). *Enterococcal infections.* Retrieved from http://emedicine.medscape.com/article/216993-overview

Fraser, S. L. (n.d.). *Enterobacter infections.* Retrieved from http://emedicine.medscape.com/article/216845 -overview#aw2aab6b2b3

Frassetto, L. A. (2015). *Corynebacterium infections.* Retrieved from http://emedicine.medscape.com/article/215100 -overview

Frey, J. & Kuhnert, P. (2002). *RTX toxins in Pasteurellaceae.* Retrieved from http://www.ncbi.nlm.nih.gov/pubmed /12398206

Frith, J. *Journal of Military and Veterans' Health.* (Volume 20 No. 4, 2012). "Syphilis–Its early history and Treatment until Penicillin and the Debate on its Origins". Retrieved from https://jmvh.org/article/syphilis-its-early-history -and-treatment-until-penicillin-and-the-debate-on -its-origins/

Fuerst, J. A. (2010). *Beyond prokaryotes and eukaryotes: Planctomycetes and cell organization.* Retrieved from http://www.nature.com/scitable/topicpage/beyond -prokaryotes-and-eukaryotes-planctomycetes-and -cell-14158971

Fujinami S, Fujisawa M. Industrial applications of alkaliphiles and their enzymes–past, present and future. Environ Technol. 2010 Jul-Aug;31(8-9):845-56. doi: 10.1080/09593331003762807. PMID: 20662376.

Fungal diseases. (2012). Retrieved from http://www.cdc.gov /fungal/diseases/other/exserohilum-rostratum.html

Fungi. (n.d.). Retrieved from http://www.microbeworld.org /types-of-microbes/fungi

Galeziok, M., Roberts, I., & Passalacqua, J. (2009). *Bordetella bronchiseptica pneumonia in a man with acquired immunodeficiency syndrome: a case report.* Retrieved from http://www.jmedicalcasereports.com/content/3/1/76

Gan, S. H. (2014). *How do periodontal infections affect the onset and progression of Alzheimer's disease.* Retrieved from http://www.academia.edu/6958904/How_Do_Periodontal _Infections_Affect_the_Onset_and_Progression_of _Alzheimer_s_Disease

Gander, Kashmira. (8-21-2018). *How Does an Iron Lung Work? Polio Survivor, 82, Among Last to Use Breathing Equipment.* Newsweek. Retrieved from https://www .newsweek.com/how-does-iron-lung-work-polio -survivor-last-us-1083104

Garcia, Patricia, et al. "Coagulase-negative staphylococci: clinical, microbiological and molecular features to predict true bacteraemia", *Journal of Medical Microbiology* (2004), 53, 67–72.

Garden, J. M., O'Banion, M. K., Bakus, A. D., & Olson, C. (2002). *Viral disease transmitted by laser-generated plume (aerosol).* Retrieved from http://www.ncbi.nlm.nih.gov /pubmed/12374535.

Gas gangrene. Retrieved from http://www.nlm.nih.gov /medlineplus/ency/article/000620.htm

Genetics. (n.d.). In *Encyclopedia online.* Retrieved from http:// www.encyclopedia.com/topic/genetics.aspx#2

Genital herpes—CDC fact sheet. (2014). Retrieved from http:// www.cdc.gov/std/herpes/STDFact-herpes.htm

Genus Bacillus. (n.d.). Retrieved from http://www.bacterio .net/bacillus.html

Gerlach, G. & Reidl, J. (2006). *NAD+ utilization in Pasteurellaceae: Simplification of a complex pathway.* Retrieved from http://www.ncbi.nlm.nih.gov/pmc /articles/PMC1595515/

Gerstmann-Straussler-Scheinker disease. Retrieved from http:// rarediseases.info.nih.gov/gard/7690/gerstmann -straussler-scheinker-disease/case/21304/case-questions

Ghasemi, M., Norouzi, R., Salari, M., & Asadi, B. (2012). *Iatrogenic botulism after the therapeutic use of botulinum toxin-A: a case report and review of the literature.* Retrieved from http://www.ncbi.nlm.nih.gov/pubmed/22986799

Ghosh, W., Alam, M., Roy, C., Pyne, P., George, A., Chakraborty, R., Majumder, S., Agarwal, A., Chakraborty, S., Majumdar, S., & Das Gupta, S. K. (2013). *Genome implosion elicits host-confinement in Alcaligenaceae: Evidence from the comparative genomics of tetrathiobacter kashmirensis, a pathogen in the making.* Retrieved from http://www.ncbi.nlm.nih.gov/pmc/articles/PMC3669393/

Giardiasis. (2014). Retrieved from http://www.webmd.com /hw-popup/giardiasis-giardia

Girolama Fracastoro. (n.d.). In *Encyclopaedia Britannica online.* Retrieved from http://www.britannica.com /EBchecked/topic/215496/Girolamo-Fracastoro

Global disease detection (GDD) operations center. (2015). Retrieved from http://www.cdc.gov/globalhealth/healthprotection/ghsb/gddopscenter/default.htm

Godoy, Maria. (August 25, 2020). *Africa Declares Wild Polio Is Wiped Out — Yet It Persists In Vaccine-Derived Cases.* National Public Radio Goats and Soda. Retrieved from https://www.npr.org/sections/goatsandsoda/2020/08/25/905884740/africa-declares-wild-polio-is-wiped-out-yet-it-persists-in-vaccine-derived-cases

Gonzalez, G. (n.d.). *Proteus infections workup.* Retrieved from http://emedicine.medscape.com/article/226434-workup.

Good teeth, good memory. (2013). Retrieved from http://www.wellbeing.com.au/newsdetail/Good-teeth,-good-memory_000989

Gram stain. (n.d). Retrieved from http://labtestsonline.org/understanding/analytes/gram-stain/tab/test

Gram stain. Retrieved from http://labtestsonline.org/understanding/analytes/gram-stain/tab/test

Gram-negative aerobic activity. (n.d.). Retrieved from http://www.labome.org/topics/organisms/bacteria/gram/gram-negative-aerobic-bacteria-2401.html

Gram-negative aerobic cocci. (n.d.). Retrieved from http://education.med.nyu.edu/modules/nyu/microbiology/infect-disease/Gram_Neg_Aerobic_Cocci3.html

Gram-negative bacteria. (n.d.). Retrieved from http://www.fpnotebook.com/ID/Bacteria/GrmNgtvBctr.htm

Gram-negative bacterial cell wall. (n.d.). Retrieved from http://www.scienceprofonline.org/microbiology/gram-negative-bacteria-cell-wall.html

Grave's disease. (n.d.). Retrieved from http://www.nlm.nih.gov/medlineplus/ency/article/000358.htm

Griffin, R. M. (n.d.). *Staying healthy with HIV. Retrieved from* http://www.webmd.com/hiv-aids/staying-healthy-10/hiv-aids-treatment?page=1

Group C streptococcal infections. (n.d.). Retrieved from http://www.rightdiagnosis.com/medical/group_c_streptococcal_infections.htm

Gueudry, J., Leclercq, M., Saadoun, D., & Bodaghi, B. (2021). Old and New Challenges in Uveitis Associated with Behçet's Disease. *Journal of clinical medicine,* 10(11), 2318. https://doi.org/10.3390/jcm10112318

Gupta, R. S. (2002). *What are archaebacteria: life's third domain or monoderm prokaryotes related to Gram-positive bacteria? A new proposal for the classification of prokaryotic organisms.* Retrieved from http://onlinelibrary.wiley.com/doi/10.1046/j.1365-2958.1998.00978.x/abstract

Gutiérrez-Venegas, G., Kawasaki-Cárdenas, P., Portillo Garcés, C., Román-Alvárez, P., Barajas-Torres, C., & Contreras-Marmolejo, L. A. (2007). *Actinobacillus actinomycetemcomitans adheres to human gingival fibroblasts and modifies cytoskeletal organization.* Retrieved from http://www.sciencedirect.com/science/article/pii/S1065699507000960

Haddrill, M. (2014). *Conjunctivitis: Bacterial, viral, allergic and other types.* Retrieved from http://www.allaboutvision.com/conditions/conjunctivitis-types.htm

Haiti's cholera outbreak tied to Nepalese U.N. peacekeepers. (2013). Retrieved from http://www.npr.org/templates/story/story.php?storyId=211434286

Hale, C. (2013). *Microbiology: Gram-positive: Streptococcus species.* Retrieved from http://www.pathologyoutlines.com/topic/microbiologystreptococci.html

Hand hygiene project. (n.d.). Retrieved from http://www.centerfortransforminghealth care.org/projects/detail.aspx?Project=3

Handa, S. (2014). *Cholera.* Retrieved from http://emedicine.medscape.com/article/962643-overview

Handa, S. (2014). *Propionibacterium infections.* Retrieved from http://emedicine.medscape.com/article/226337-overview

Hanging drop method—procedure and interpretation. Retrieved from http://www.laboratorystack.com/hanging-drop-method-procedure-interpretation/

Hao, W. L. & Lee, Y. K. (2004). *Microflora of the gastrointestinal tract: a review.* Retrieved from http://www.ncbi.nlm.nih.gov/pubmed/15156063

Haydon, D. T., Cleaveland, S., Taylor, L. H., & Laurenson, M. K. (2002). *Identifying reservoirs of infection: a conceptual and practical challenge.* Retrieved from http://wwwnc.cdc.gov/eid/article/8/12/01-0317_article

Healthcare Infection Control Practices Advisory Committee (HICPAC). *2007 Guideline for isolation precautions: Preventing transmission of infectious agents in health care settings.* (n.d.). Retrieved from http://www.cdc.gov/hicpac/2007IP/2007isolationPrecautions.html

Healthcare-associated infections (HAIs). (n.d.). Retrieved from http://www.cdph.ca.gov/programs/hai/Pages/Health careAssociatedInfections.aspx

Healthcare-associated infections. (n.d.). Retrieved from http://www.healthypeople.gov/2020/topics-objectives/topic/health care-associated-infections

Healthcare-associated infections. (n.d.). Retrieved from http://www.medicare.gov/hospitalcompare/Data/Health care-Associated-Infections.html?AspxAutoDetectCookieSupport=1

Healthcare-associated infections. (n.d.). Retrieved from http://doh.dc.gov/page/health care-associated-infections

Healthcare-associated infections. (n.d.). Retrieved from http://www.healthypeople.gov/2020/topics-objectives/topic/health care-associated-infections

Health Resources and Services Administration (HRSA). (2021). *National Hansen's Disease (Leprosy) Program Caring and Curing Since 1894.* Retrieved from https://www.hrsa.gov/hansens-disease/index.html

Healy, B., Cooney, S., O'Brien, S., Iversen, C., Whyte, P., Nally, J., Callanan, J. J., & Fanning, S. (2010). *Cronobacter (Enterobacter sakazakii): an opportunistic foodborne pathogen.* Foodborne pathogens and disease, 7(4), 339–350. https://doi.org/10.1089/fpd.2009.0379

Helmenstine, A. M. (n.d.). *What is the chemical composition of air? Retrieved from* http://chemistry.about.com/od/chemistryfaqs/f/aircomposition.htm

Hemolytic disease of the newborn. (n.d.). Retrieved from http://umm.edu/health/medical/ency/articles/hemolytic-disease-of-the-newborn

Henry, R. (2019). Etymologia: Poliomyelitis. *Emerging Infectious Diseases,* 25(8), 1611. https://doi.org/10.3201/eid2508.et2508.

HPV and men — fact sheet. (2015). Retrieved from http://www.cdc.gov/std/hpv/stdfact-hpv-and-men.htm

Hentges, D. J. (n.d.). *Chapter 17: Anaerobes:* General characteristics. Retrieved from http://*www.ncbi.nlm.nih.gov/books/NBK7638/*

Hepatitis D. (2015). Retrieved from http://www.cdc.gov/hepatitis/HDV/index.htm

Herchline, T. E. (n.d.). *Staphylococcal infections.* Retrieved from http://emedicine.medscape.com/article/228816-overview

Herpes simplex virus 1 & 2. (n.d.). Retrieved from http://www.clinicaladvisor.com/herpes-simplex-virus-1–2/slideshow/1258/#0

Hess, L. C. (2012). *Cell wall deficient bacteria and common diseases.* Retrieved from http://www.wellbodyfield.com/blog/cell-wall-deficient-bacteria-and-common-diseases

Hess, L. C. (n.d.). *Cell wall deficient bacteria and common diseases.* Retrieved from http://www.wellbodyfield.com/blog/cell-wall-deficient-bacteria-and-common-diseases

HICPAC *Guideline for Isolation Precautions: Preventing Transmission of Infectious Agents in Healthcare Settings (2007) [Updated July 2019].* CDC. Retrieved from https://www.cdc.gov/infectioncontrol/pdf/guidelines/isolation-guidelines-H.pdf

Hidalgo, J. A. (2014). *Candidiasis treatment and management.* Retrieved from http://emedicine.medscape.com/article/213853-treatment

Hiremath, P. S., & Bannigidad, P. (2011). *Identification and classification of cocci bacterial cells in digital microscopic images.* Retrieved from http://www.ncbi.nlm.nih.gov/pubmed/21778559

Histiocyte. (n.d.). Retrieved from http://www.nlm.nih.gov/medlineplus/ency/article/002374.htm

HIV.gov. (2021). *Global Statistics.* Retrieved from https://www.hiv.gov/hiv-basics/overview/data-and-trends/global-statistics

HIV.gov. (2021). *U.S. Statistics.* Retrieved from https://www.hiv.gov/hiv-basics/overview/data-and-trends/statistics

HLA gene family. (2015). Retrieved from http://ghr.nlm.nih.gov/geneFamily/hla

Ho, H. (2013). *Gas gangrene.* Home page. (n.d.). Retrieved from http://infantbotulism.org/

Ho, H. (2014). *Vibrio infections.* Retrieved from http://emedicine.medscape.com/article/232038-overview

Hoen, B. (2015). *Clinical manifestations, diagnosis, and treatment of infections due to group D streptococci (Streptococcus bovis/Streptococcus equinus complex).* Retrieved from http://www.uptodate.com/contents/clinical-manifestations-diagnosis-and-treatment-of-infections-due-to-group-d-streptococci-streptococcus-bovis-streptococcus-equinus-complex

Holshue ML, DeBolt C, Lindquist S, Lofy KH, Wiesman J, Bruce H, Spitters C, Ericson K, Wilkerson S, Tural A, Diaz G, Cohn A, Fox L, Patel A, Gerber SI, Kim L, Tong S, Lu X, Lindstrom S, Pallansch MA, Weldon WC, Biggs HM, Uyeki TM, Pillai SK; Washington State 2019-nCoV Case Investigation Team. First Case of 2019 Novel Coronavirus in the United States. *N Engl J Med.* 2020 Mar 5;382(10):929-936. doi: 10.1056/NEJMoa2001191. Epub 2020 Jan 31. PMID: 32004427; PMCID: PMC7092802

Homepage. Retrieved from http://www.sciences360.com/index.php/what-are-the-four-phases-of-bacterial-growth-18035/

Horn, C. C. (2008). *Why is the neurobiology of nausea and vomiting so important?* Retrieved from http://www.ncbi.nlm.nih.gov/pmc/articles/PMC2274963/

How do prokaryotes perform cellular respiration without membrane bound organelles? Retrieved from http://biology.stackexchange.com/questions/5430/how-do-prokaryotes-perform-cellular-respiration-without-membrane-bound-organelle

Human skin alive with bacteria. (n.d.). Retrieved from http://www.webmd.com/skin-problems-and-treatments/news/20090528/human-skin-alive-with-bacteria?page=2

Humoral theory. (n.d.). *The Free Dictionary online.* Retrieved from http://medical-dictionary.thefreedictionary.com/humoral+theory

Humors. (2002). Retrieved from http://www.pbs.org/wnet/redgold/basics/humors.html

Ignaz Philipp Semmelweis. (n.d.). In *Encyclopaedia Britannica online.* Retrieved from http://www.britannica.com/EBchecked/topic/534198/Ignaz-Philipp-Semmelweis

Immunodeficiency disorders. (n.d.). Retrieved from http://www.nlm.nih.gov/medlineplus/ency/article/000818.htm

Immunoglobulin. (n.d.). Retrieved from http://www.ebioscience.com/knowledge-center/antigen/immunoglobulin.htm

Impetigo (Infantigo): Causes, Symptoms and Treatments. (n.d.). Retrieved from http://www.medicalnewstoday.com/articles/162945.php

Impetigo. (n.d.). Retrieved from http://www.nlm.nih.gov/medlineplus/ency/article/000860.htm

Impetigo: Topic overview. (n.d.). Retrieved from http://www.webmd.com/skin-problems-and-treatments/tc/impetigo-overview?page=2

Infant botulism. (n.d.). Retrieved from http://www.nlm.nih.gov/medlineplus/ency/article/001384.htm

Infections of the teeth, gingivae, and jaws. (2013). Retrieved from http://www.atsu.edu/faculty/chamberlain/website/lectures/lecture/gi2.htm

"Infectious diseases lessons" Posted by Nabil Khoury MD.

InformedHealth.org [Internet]. Cologne, Germany: Institute for Quality and Efficiency in HealthCare (IQWiG); 2006. The innate and adaptive immune systems. [Updated 2020 Jul 30]. Available from https://www.ncbi.nlm.nih.gov/books/NBK279396/.-

International Committee of Systematics of Prokaryotes. *Homepage*. Retrieved from http://www.icsp.org/

International Journal of Systematic and Evolutionary Microbiology. (2009). International Code of Nomenclature of Prokaryotes. Appendix 9: Orthography, 59, 2107–2113.

Introduction to the cyanobacteria: Architects of the earth's atmosphere. Retrieved from http://www.ucmp.berkeley.edu/bacteria/cyanointro.html

Ito, S., Kobayashi, T., Ara, K., Ozaki, K., Kawai, S., & Hatada, Y. (1998). *Alkaline detergent enzymes from alkaliphiles: enzymatic properties, genetics, and structures*. Retrieved from http://link.springer.com/article/10.1007/s007920050059

Ivermectin. (n.d.). Retrieved from http://livertox.nlm.nih.gov/Ivermectin.htm

Janda, J. M., & Abbott, S. L. (2021). The Changing Face of the Family *Enterobacteriaceae* (Order: "Enterobacterales"): New Members, Taxonomic Issues, Geographic Expansion, and New Diseases and Disease Syndromes. *Clinical microbiology reviews*, 34(2), e00174-20. https://doi.org/10.1128/CMR.00174-20

Javid, M. H. (2014). *Campylobacter infections clinical presentation*. Retrieved from http://emedicine.medscape.com/article/213720-clinical

Javid, M. H. (2014). *Campylobacter infections*. Retrieved from http://emedicine.medscape.com/article/213720-overview

Javid, M. H. (2014). *Meningococcemia*. Retrieved from http://emedicine.medscape.com/article/221473-overview

Johns Hopkins University Coronavirus Research Center (May 16, 2021). Retrieved from https://coronavirus.jhu.edu/map.html

Johnson, E. K. (2015). *Urinary tract infections in pregnancy*. Retrieved from http://emedicine.medscape.com/article/452604-overview#aw2aab6b2b3aa

Jurtshuk, P. (1996). *Bacterial metabolism*. Retrieved from http://www.ncbi.nlm.nih.gov/pubmed/21413278

Kaakoush, N. O., Holmes, J., Octavia, S., Man, S. M., Zhang, L., Castaño-Rodríguez, N., Day, A.S., Leach, S. T., Lemberg, D. A., Dutt, S., Stormon, M., O'Loughlin, E. V., Magoffin, A., & Mitchell, H. (2010). *Detection of Helicobacteraceae in intestinal biopsies of children with Crohn's disease*. Retrieved from http://www.ncbi.nlm.nih.gov/pubmed/21073612

Kahn, A. (2012). *Gram stain or urethral discharge*. Retrieved from http://www.healthline.com/health/gram-stain-of-urethral-discharge#Symptoms2

Kahn, Z. Z. (2013). *Yersinia enterocolitica*. Retrieved from http://emedicine.medscape.com/article/232343-overview

Kaiser, G. E. (2014). *The prokaryotic cell: Bacteria*. Retrieved from http://faculty.ccbcmd.edu/courses/bio141/lecguide/unit1/shape/shape.html

Kashani, Mitra. *International Microorganism Day*. 10 Unsung Heroines of Microbiology. August 24, 2020. Retrieved from https://www.internationalmicroorganismday.org/blog/10-women-microbiologists-you-dont-know-about-but-should

Katz, D. S. (2010). *Coagulase test protocol*. Retrieved from http://www.microbelibrary.org/index.php/library/laboratory-test/3220-coagulase-test-protocol

Keep Listeria out of your kitchen. (2015). Retrieved from http://www.fda.gov/ForConsumers/ConsumerUpdates/ucm274114.htm

Keita, A.K., Koundouno, F.R., Faye, M. et al. Resurgence of Ebola virus in 2021 in Guinea suggests a new paradigm for outbreaks. *Nature* 597, 539–543 (2021) https://doi.org/10.1038/s41586-021-03901-9

Kelly, C. P. (2015). *Clostridium difficile in adults: Treatment*. Retrieved from http://www.uptodate.com/contents/clostridium-difficile-in-adults-treatment

Khan, Z. Z. (2014). *Group A streptococcal infections*. Retrieved from http://emedicine.medscape.com/article/228936-overview

King Abdullah University of Science & Technology (KAUST). *New Biosensor Technology Makes Coronavirus Testing Quick and Easy*. May 28, 2021.

Klappenbach, L. (n.d.). *How animals are classified: A history of high-order taxonomy*. Retrieved from http://animals.about.com/od/scientificdisciplines/a/classifyinganim_4.htm

Klochko, A. (2014). *Salmonellosis*. Retrieved from http://emedicine.medscape.com/article/228174-overview

Koenig, A. (n.d.). *Acidithiobacillus thiooxidans*. Retrieved from http://web.mst.edu/~microbio/BIO221_2010/A_thiooxidans.html

Koo, I. (n.d.). *Strep throat diagnosis: How diagnostic tests for strep throat work*. Retrieved from http://infectiousdiseases.about.com/od/respiratoryinfections/a/Strep_diagnosis.htm

Koonin, E.V. (2010). *The two empires and three domains of life in the postgenomic age*. Retrieved from https://www.academia.edu/22649841/The_Two_Empires_and_Three_Domains_of_Life_in_the_Postgenomic_Age

Koonin, E.V. (2010). *The two empires and three domains of life in the postgenomic age*. Retrieved from http://www.nature.com/scitable/topicpage/the-two-empires-and-three-domains-of-14432998

Kozarov, E.V., Dorn, B. R., Shelburne, C. E., Dunn Jr, W. A., & Progulske-Fox, A. (2005). *Human atherosclerotic plaque contains viable invasive Actinobacillus actinomycetemcomitans and Porphyromonas gingivalis*. Retrieved from http://atvb.ahajournals.org/content/25/3/e17.full

Kuman, M. R. (2012). *Chromobacterium violaceum: A rare bacterium isolated from a wound over the scalp*. Retrieved from http://www.ncbi.nlm.nih.gov/pmc/articles/PMC3657989/

Kurdgelashvili, G. (2015). *Nocardiosis*. Retrieved from http://emedicine.medscape.com/article/224123-overview#a0199

Lactobacillus. (2015). Retrieved from http://www.nlm.nih.gov/medlineplus/druginfo/natural/790.html

Lactobacillus. (n.d.). Retrieved from http://www.webmd.com/vitamins-supplements/ingredientmono-790-LACTOBACILLUS.aspx?activeIngredientId=790&activeIngredientName=LACTOBACILLUS

Lamivudine. (2012). http://www.nlm.nih.gov/medlineplus /druginfo/meds/a696011.html

Lancefield grouping of streptococci. Retrieved from http://www .medical-labs.net/lancefield-grouping-of-streptococci -1306/

Lentino, J. R. (2013). *Overview of anaerobic bacteria.* Retrieved from http://www.merckmanuals.com /professional/infectious _diseases/anaerobic_bacteria /overview_of_anaerobic_bacteria.html

Leprosy elimination. Retrieved from http://www.who.int/lep /microbiology/en/

Leprosy in the United States. (n.d.). Retrieved from http:// diseases.emedtv.com/leprosy/leprosy-in-the-united -states.html

Leprosy overview. (n.d.). Retrieved from http://www.webmd .com/skin-problems-and-treatments/guide/leprosy -symptoms-treatments-history

Leptospiraceae. (n.d.). Retrieved from http://medicine .academic.ru/135733/Leptospiraceae

Levy, D. (2013). *Necrotizing soft tissue infection.* Retrieved from http://www.nlm.nih.gov/medlineplus/ency /article/001443.htm

Lewis, L. S. (n.d.). *Impetigo treatment and management.* Retrieved from http://emedicine.medscape.com/article /965254-treatment

Lewis, R. E. (2011). *Current concepts in antifungal pharmacology.* Retrieved from http://www.ncbi.nlm.nih.gov/pmc/articles/ PMC3146381/

Leyssen, P., De Clerq, E., & Neyts, J. (2000). *Perspectives for the treatment of infections with Flaviviridae.* Retrieved from http://www.ncbi.nlm.nih.gov/pmc/articles/PMC88934/

L-form bacteria. Retrieved from http://mpkb.org/home /pathogenesis/microbiota/lforms

L-form. (n.d.). In *Merriam Webster Dictionary online.* Retrieved from http://www.merriam-webster.com/dictionary/l-form

Li, Z., & Nair, S. K. (2012). *Quorum sensing: How bacteria can coordinate activity and synchronize their response to external signals.* Retrieved from http://www.ncbi.nlm.nih.gov /pmc/articles/PMC3526984/

Listeria: Definition. (2013). Retrieved from http://www.cdc .gov/listeria/definition.html

Listeriosis: Topic overview. (n.d.). Retrieved from http://www .webmd.com/a-to-z-guides/listeriosis-topic-overview

Liu, H., Zhu, J., Hu, Q., & Rao, X. (2016). *Morganella morganii,* a non-negligent opportunistic pathogen. *International journal of infectious diseases: IJID: official publication of the International Society for Infectious Diseases,* 50, 10–17. https://doi.org/10.1016/j.ijid.2016.07.006

Liu, Y., Song, Y., Hu, X., Yan, L., & Zhu, X. (2019). Awareness of surgical smoke hazards and enhancement of surgical smoke prevention among the gynecologists. *Journal of Cancer,* 10(12), 2788–2799. https://doi.org/10.7150 /jca.31464

Lopez-Goni, I. & O'Callaghan, D. (n.d.). *Brucella: Molecular microbiology and genomics.* Retrieved from http://www .horizonpress.com/brucella

Louis Pasteur. (n.d.). In *Encyclopaedia Britannica online.* Retrieved from http://www.britannica.com/EBchecked /topic/445964/Louis-Pasteur

Louis Pasteur. Retrieved from http://science.howstuffworks.com /dictionary/famous-scientists/chemists/louis-pasteur-info.htm

Loynachan, T. (2008). *Soil actinomycetes.* Retrieved from http://www.microbelibrary.org/library/fungi /3180-soil-actinomycetes

Luhmann, N., Holley, G. & Achtman, M. BlastFrost: fast querying of 100,000s of bacterial genomes in Bifrost graphs. *Genome* Biol 22, 30 (2021). https://doi.org/10.1186/ s13059-020-02237-3

Magori, K. & Drake, J. M. (2013). *The population dynamics of vector-borne diseases.* Retrieved from http://www.nature .com/scitable/knowledge/library/the-population -dynamics-of-vector-borne-diseases-102042523

Mancini, R., Nigro, M., Ippolito. G. "Lazzaro Spallanzani and His Refutation of the Theory of Spontaneous Generation." *Le Infezioni in Medicina* 15 no. 3 (2007): 199–206. Retrieved from https://bio.libretexts.org/ Courses/Portland_Community_College/Cascade _Microbiology/03%3A_The_Cell/3.1%3A_Spontaneous _Generation

Mandal, A. (n.d.). *Vaccine immunity.* Retrieved from http:// www.news-medical.net/health/Vaccine-Immunity.aspx

Markowitz, V. M., Korzeniewski, F., Palaniappan, K., Szeto, E., Werner, G., Padki, A., Zhao, X., Dubchak, I., Hugenholtz, P., Anderson, I., Lykidis, A., Mavromatis, K., Ivanova, N., & Kyrpides, N. C. (2005). *The integrated microbial genomes (IMG) system.* Retrieved from http:// www.ncbi.nlm.nih.gov/pmc/articles/PMC1347387/

Mase, Sundari. (2014). *New Drug Available to Treat Multidrug-Resistant Tuberculosis. Medscape.* Retrieved from https://www.medscape.com/viewarticle/822098?src =par_cdc_stm_mscpedt&faf=1

Mathew, A. (n.d.). *Hypogammaglobulinemia.* Retrieved from http://www.hxbenefit.com/hypogammaglobulinemia .html

Mayo Clinic Staff. (2014). *Complications.* Retrieved from http://www.mayoclinic.org/diseases-conditions /tuberculosis/basics/complications/con-20021761

Mayo Clinic. Hepatitis C. Diagnosis–Screening for hepatitis C. March 20, 2020. Retrieved from https://www.mayoclinic .org/diseases-conditions/hepatitis-c/diagnosis-treatment /drc-20354284

McNamara LA, Potts C, Blain AE, et al. Detection of Ciprofloxacin-Resistant, β-Lactamase–Producing Neisseria meningitidis Serogroup Y Isolates—United States, 2019–2020. *MMWR Morb Mortal Wkly Rep* 2020;69:735–739. DOI: http://dx.doi.org/10.15585/mmwr .mm6924a2

McQuiston, J. (2015). *Rickettsial (spotted and typhus fevers) and related infections (anaplasmosis and ehrlichiosis).* Retrieved from http://wwwnc.cdc.gov/travel /yellowbook/2014/chapter-3-infectious-diseases-related

-to-travel/rickettsial-spotted-and-typhus-fevers -and-related-infections-anaplasmosis-and-ehrlichiosis

MDLinx. (2020). *5 viruses more dangerous than the new coronavirus.* Retrieved from https://www.mdlinx.com /article/5-viruses-more-dangerous-than-the-new -coronavirus/7wQzXjJudXjqIZVb8eU6LI

Medline Plus. (2021). Necrotizing Enterocolitis. Retrieved from Ronald, A. R. & Alfa, M. J. (1996). *Chapter 97 microbiology of the genitourinary system.* Retrieved from http://www .ncbi.nlm.nih.gov/books/NBK8136/

Medscape (2019). *What is the worldwide incidence of pertussis (whooping cough)?* Retrieved from https://www.medscape .com/answers/967268-63385/what-is-the-worldwide -incidence-of-pertussis-whooping-cough

Melia, M. (n.d.). *Streptococcus species.* Retrieved from http:// www.hopkinsguides.com/hopkins/ub/view/Johns _Hopkins_ABX_Guide/540525/all/Streptococcus_species

Melina, R. (2011). *Why does hydrogen peroxide fizz on cuts?* Retrieved from http://www.livescience.com/33061-why -does-hydrogen-peroxide-fizz-on-cuts.html

Meningitis in children. (n.d.). Retrieved from http://www .emedicinehealth.com/meningitis_in_children/page2 _em.htm

Meningitis symptoms. (n.d.). Retrieved from http://www .meningitis.org/symptoms.

Meningitis: meningococcal. (n.d.). Retrieved from http://www .nlm.nih.gov/medlineplus/ency/article/000608.htm

Merriam-Webster Dictionary. *Replicon.* (n.d.) Retrieved from https://www.merriam-webster.com/dictionary/replicon

Mersch, J. (n.d.). *Impetigo.* Retrieved from http://www .medicinenet.com/impetigo/article.htm

Metabolism. (n.d.). In *Encyclopaedia Britannica online.* Retrieved from http://www.britannica.com/EBchecked/topic/377325 /metabolism

Miao, V. & Davies, J. (2010). *Actinobacteria: the good, the bad, and the ugly.* Retrieved from http://www.ncbi.nlm.nih. gov/pubmed/20390355

Microbial genetics. (n.d.). In *Encyclopedia online.* Retrieved from http://www.encyclopedia.com/topic/Microbial _genetics.aspx

Microbial genetics. (n.d.). Retrieved from http://www .encyclopedia.com/doc/1G2-3409800382.html

Microbial spore formation. Retrieved from http://archives .microbeworld.org/know/spore.aspx

Microbiologists. (2014). Retrieved from http://www.bls.gov /ooh/life-physical-and-social-science/microbiologists htm

Microbiology. (n.d.). In *Encyclopaedia Britannica online.* Retrieved from http://www.britannica.com/EBchecked /topic/380246/microbiology

Micrococcus luteus. (n.d.). Warbleton Council. Retrieved from https://warbletoncouncil.org/micrococcus-luteus-1578

Micrococcus. (2010). Retrieved from http://microbewiki .kenyon.edu/index.php/Micrococcus

Miller, J. R. (n.d.). *Morganella infections.* Retrieved from http://emedicine.medscape.com/article/222443-overview

Miller, K. (2013). *How mushrooms can save the world.* Retrieved from http://discovermagazine.com/2013 /julyaug/13-mushrooms-clean-up-oil-spills-nuclear -meltdowns-and-human-health

Miller, Y. M. & Grima, K. M. (2013). *Eligibility criteria: Alphabetical.* Retrieved from http://www.redcrossblood .org/donating -blood/eligibility-requirements/eligibility -criteria-alphabetical-listing#arc5

Mobed, A, & Sepehri Shafigh, E. Biosensors promising bio-device for pandemic screening"COVID-19". *Microchem J.* 2021 May;164:106094. doi: 10.1016/j.microc.2021.106094. Epub 2021 Feb 19. PMID: 33623173; PMCID: PMC7892310. *Rapid strep test for strep throat.* (2012). Retrieved from http://www.webmd.com/oral-health /rapid-strep-test-for-strep-throat

Modifications to radical prostatectomy: Feasibility study. (2014). Retrieved from http://clinicaltrials.gov/ct2/show /NCT00928850

Modric, J. (n.d.). *What is Staphylococcus aureus?* Retrieved from http://www.healthhype.com/staphylococcus-aureus.html

Monitoring psychrotrophic lactic acid bacteria contamination in a ready-to-eat vegetable salad production environment. (2015). Retrieved from http://www.bioportfolio.com /resources/pmarticle/1027527/Monitoring-psychrotrophic -lactic-acid-bacteria-contamination-in-a-ready-to-eat -vegetable.html

Moraxella catarrhalis. (n.d.). Retrieved from http://www .bionity.com/en/encyclopedia/Moraxella_catarrhalis.html

Moraxella spp. (n.d.). Retrieved from http://www.msdsonline .com/resources/msds-resources/free-safety-data-sheet -index/moraxella-spp.aspx/

Morris, J. G. & Hornerman, A. (2014). *Aeromonas infections.* Retrieved from http://www.uptodate.com/contents /aeromonas-infections

Morse, S. A. (n.d.). *Neisseria, moraxella, kingella and eikenella.* Retrieved from http://www.ncbi.nlm.nih.gov/books /NBK7650/

Moyer, C. L., & Morita, R. Y. (2007). *Psychrophiles and psychrotrophs.* Retrieved from http://www.els.net /WileyCDA/ElsArticle/refId-a0000402.html

Muccari, R., Chow, D., & Murphy, J. (January 1, 2021). Coronavirus timeline: Tracking the critical moments of Covid-19. *NBC* News. https://www.nbcnews.com/health /health-news/coronavirus-timeline-tracking-critical -moments-covid-19-n1154341

Murcormycosis. (n.d.). Retrieved from http://www .medicinenet.com/mucormycosis/article.htm

MUTATION: Basic feature and "Joshua and Esther Lederberg's experiment." Retrieved from https://acbr12.wordpress .com/2012/08/04/mutation-basic-feature-and -joshua-and-esther-lederbergs-experiment-2/

Mutualism. (n.d.). Retrieved from http://www.cas.miamioh .edu/mbi-ws/BiodiversitySymbiosis/mutualism.htm

Mycologoy—Fungi. (2011). Retrieved from http://www .microbexpert.com/blog/category/mycology-fungi

Mycoplasma infection (walking pneumonia, atypical pneumonia). (2011). Retrieved from http://www.health.ny.gov/diseases /communicable/mycoplasma/fact_sheet.htm

Mycoplasma pneumoniae. Retrieved from http:// mycoplasmapneumoniae.org/

Myocarditis. (n.d.). Retrieved from http://www.webmd.com /heart-disease/myocarditis

Nadell, C. D., Xavier, J. B., Levin, S. A., & Foster, K. R. (2008). *The evolution of quorum sensing in bacterial biofilms.* Retrieved from http://www.plosbiology.org/article /info%3Adoi%2F10.1371%2Fjournal.pbio.0060014

Natural killer cell. (n.d.). Retrieved from http://www .sciencedaily.com/articles/n/natural_killer_cell.htm

Nau, R., Sorgel, F., & Eiffert, H. (2010). *Penetration of drugs through the blood-cerebrospinal fluid/blood-brain barrier for treatment of central nervous system infections.* Retrieved from http://www.ncbi.nlm.nih.gov/pmc/articles /PMC2952976/

Necrotizing fasciitis (flesh-eating bacteria). (n.d.). Retrieved from http://www.webmd.com/skin-problems-and -treatments/necrotizing-fasciitis-flesh-eating-bacteria

Necrotizing Fasciitis: A Rare Disease, Especially for the Healthy. (2015). Retrieved from http://www.cdc.gov/features /NecrotizingFasciitis/

Nicolson, Garth L, *Chronic Bacterial and Viral Infections in Neurodegenerative and Neurobehavioral Diseases*, Lab Med. 2008;39(5):291-299.

Nicolson, Garth L. PhD, *Chronic Bacterial and Viral Infections in Neurodegenerative and Neurobehavioral Diseases* Lab Med. 2008;39(5):291–299. © 2008 American Society for Clinical Pathology.

NIH, *Emerging and Re-emerging Infectious Diseases* (2012). Retrieved from science.education.nih.gov /supplements/nih1 /diseases/guide/pdfs/NIH

NIH. (2012). *Bacteria on skin boost immune cell function.* Retrieved from http://www.nih.gov/researchmatters /august2012/08132012skin.htm

NIH. (2014). *Features of an immune response.* Retrieved from http://www.niaid.nih.gov/topics/immunesystem/Pages /features.aspx

NIH. (2014). *Immune cells.* Retrieved from http:// www.niaid.nih.gov/topics/immunesystem/Pages /immuneCells.aspx

NIH. (2014). *Klebsiella.* Retrieved from http://rarediseases. info.nih.gov/gard/10085/klebsiella/resources/1

NIH. (2015). *Handout on health: scleroderma.* Retrieved from http://www.niams.nih.gov/Health_Info/Scleroderma /default.asp

NIH. (2015). *Myasthenia gravis fact sheet.* Retrieved from http://www.ninds.nih.gov/disorders/myasthenia_gravis /detail_myasthenia_gravis.htm

Nixon, R. (2010). *5 dangerous vaccination myths.* Retrieved from http://www.livescience.com/35163-dangerous -vaccination -myths.html

Noonan, L. (2015). *Bacillus cereus and other non-anthracis Bacillus species.* Retrieved from http://www.uptodate.com /contents/bacillus-cereus-and-other-non-anthracis -bacillus-species

Nørskov-Lauritsen, N., Claesson, R., Birkeholm Jensen, A., Åberg, C. H., & Haubek, D. (2019). *Aggregatibacter Actinomycetemcomitans:* Clinical Significance of a Pathobiont Subjected to Ample Changes in Classification and Nomenclature. Pathogens (Basel, Switzerland), 8(4), 243. https://doi.org/10.3390/pathogens8040243

Okulicz, J. F. (2014). *Actinomycosis clinical presentation.* Retrieved from http://emedicine.medscape.com/article /211587-clinical #a0218

Okulicz, J. F. (2014). *Actinomycosis.* Retrieved from http:// emedicine.medscape.com/article/211587-overview#a0104

Organelles of a eukaryotic cell. (n.d.). Retrieved from http:// thecellorganelles.weebly.com/centrioles-microtubules -vacuole-peroxisomes.html

Osteomyelitis. (n.d.). Retrieved from http://www.webmd .com/pain-management/ osteomyeltis-treatment-diagnosis-symptoms

Overdorf, J. (2011). *India: bouncing back from the plague.* Retrieved from http://www.globalpost.com/dispatch /news/regions/asia-pacific/india/110928/india-surat -gujarat-plague-health-economy

Oza, N. (2011). *List of Gram-negative bacteria and their functions.* Retrieved from http://www.brighthub.com /science/medical/articles/114554.aspx

Palm, E., Khalaf, H., & Bengtsson, T. (2013). *Porphyromonas gingivalis downregulates the immune response of fibroblasts.* Retrieved from http://www.ncbi.nlm.nih.gov/pmc /articles/PMC3717116/

Parasitic diseases. (n.d.). Retrieved from http://www .humanillnesses.com/original/Pan-Pre/Parasitic -Diseases.html

Parija, S. C. (n.d.). *Parainfluenza virus.* Retrieved from http:// emedicine.medscape.com/article/224708-overview

Parise, M. E., Hotez, P. J., & Slutsker, L. (2014). *Neglected parasitic infections in the United States: Needs and opportunities.* Retrieved from http://www.ajtmh.org /content/90/5/783.full

Pasteurellaceae. (2013). Retrieved from http://www.slideserve .com/Lucy/lecture-26

Pasteurellaceae. (n.d.). Retrieved from http://www.fpnotebook .com/ID/Bacteria/Pstrlc.htm

Pasteurellaceae. (n.d.). Retrieved from https://pediaview.com /openpedia/Pasteurellaceae

Patel, P., Weiner-Lastinger, L., Dudeck, M., Fike, L., Kuhar, D., Edwards, J., . . . Benin, A. (2021). Impact of COVID-19 pandemic on central-line–associated bloodstream infections during the early months of 2020, *National Healthcare Safety Network. Infection Control & Hospital Epidemiology*, 1-4. doi:10.1017/ice.2021.108.

Patel, R. (n.d.). *Staphylococcus lugdunensisem biofilm formation.* Retrieved from http://www.mayo.edu/research/labs /infectious-diseases/staphylococcus-lugdunensisem -biofilm-formation

Patterson, D. J. & Sogin, M. L. (2000). *Eukaryotes. Eukaryota, organisms with nucleated cells.* Retrieved from http://tolweb.org/Eukaryotes/3/2000.09.08

Paul Ehrlich-biographical. Retrieved from http://www.nobelprize.org/nobel_prizes/medicine/laureates/1908/ehrlich-bio.html

Penicillium. (2006). Retrieved from http://www.biology-online.org/dictionary/Penicillium

Periodontal Disease and Rheumatoid Arthritis The Evidence Accumulates for Complex Pathobiologic Interactions Clifton O. Bingham III; Malini Moni Curr Opin Rheumatol. 2013;25(3):345–353. © 2013 Lippincott Williams & Wilkins.

pH. (n.d.). In *The Free Dictionary online.* Retrieved from http://medical-dictionary.thefreedictionary.com/pH

Phages. (n.d.). Retrieved from http://phages.org/temperate-phages/

Philip, K., Teoh, W.Y., Muniandy, S., & Yaakob, H. (2009). *Pathogenic bacteria predominate in the oral cavity of Malaysian subjects.* Retrieved from http://scialert.net/fulltext/?doi=jbs.2009.438.444

Phillips, T. (n.d.). *Thermophilic.* Retrieved from http://biotech.about.com/od/glossary/g/thermophilic.htm

Phototherapy for Jaundice in Newborns—Topic Overview. (n.d.). Retrieved from http://www.webmd.com/parenting/baby/tc/phototherapy-for-jaundice-in-newborns-topic-overview

PLOS. (2014). *A gut bacterium that attacks dengue and malaria pathogens and their mosquito vectors.* Retrieved from http://www.sciencedaily.com/releases/2014/10/141023142208.htm

Pneumovax23. (n.d.). Retrieved from http://www.pneumovax23.com/what-is-pneumococcal-disease/?utm_source=bing&utm_medium=cpc&utm_term=about%20pneumococcal%20bacteria&utm_campaign=Unbranded+2014&utm_content=RBFzaaOt|pcrid|5902573503

Pokhrel, G. (n.d.). *Gram-positive bacteria.* Retrieved from http://www.scribd.com/doc/95259006/Gram-Positive-Bacteria#scribd

Pollan, M. (2013). *Some of my best friends are germs.* Retrieved from http://www.nytimes.com/2013/05/19/magazine/say-hello-to-the-100-trillion-bacteria-that-make-up-your-microbiome.html?pagewanted%3Dall&_r=0

Popat, R., Crusz, S. A., Messina, M., Williams, P., West, S. A., & Diggle, S. P. (2012). *Quorum-sensing and cheating in bacterial biofilms.* Retrieved from http://cid.oxfordjournals.org/content/47/8/1070.long

Porphyromonas gingivalis accelerates inflammatory atherosclerosis in a mouse model. (2011). Retrieved from http://www.sciencedaily.com/releases/2011/01/110104101344.htm

Porphyromonas gingivalis. (n.d.). Retrieved from http://www.rightdiagnosis.com/medical/porphyromonas_gingivalis.htm

Post-streptococcal glomerulonephritis. (n.d.). Retrieved from http://www.nlm.nih.gov/medlineplus/ency/article/000503.htm

Pottumarthy, S., Schapiro, J. M., Prentice, J. L., Houze, Y. B., Swanzy, S. R., Fang, F. C., & Cookson B. T. (2004). *Clinical isolates of Staphylococcus intermedius masquerading as methicillin-resistant Staphylococcus aureus.* Retrieved from http://www.ncbi.nlm.nih.gov/pmc/articles/PMC535261/

Pregnancy: Preeclampsia and eclampsia. (n.d.). Retrieved from http://www.medicinenet.com/pregnancy_preeclampsia_and_eclampsia/article.htm

Preventing norovirus outbreaks. (2014). Retrieved from http://www.cdc.gov/vitalsigns/norovirus/index.html

Protein synthesis. In *Encyclopedia online.* Retrieved from http://www.encyclopedia.com/topic/Protein_Synthesis.aspx

Proteobacteria. (2012). Retrieved from http://biology-forums.com/definitions/index.php/Proteobacteria

Protista. (n.d.). Retrieved from http://www.microbeworld.org/types-of-microbes/protista

Protozoa. (n.d.). In *Encyclopedia online.* Retrieved from http://www.encyclopedia.com/topic/Protozoa.aspx

Protozoa. (n.d.). Retrieved from http://www.biologyreference.com/Po-Re/Protozoa.html

Protozoa. (n.d.). Retrieved from http://www.microbeworld.org/types-of-microbes/protista/protozoa

Protozoa. (n.d.). Retrieved from http://www.scienceclarified.com/Ph-Py/Protozoa.html

Protozoa: Ciliates. (n.d.). Retrieved from http://www.micrographia.com/specbiol/protis/cili/cili0100.htm

Pujari, S. (n.d.). *Plasma membrane—Structure and function of plasma membrane.* Retrieved from http://www.yourarticlelibrary.com/science/plasma-membrane-structure-and-functions-of-plasma-membrane/22977/

Pum, D., Toca-Herrera, J. L., & Sleytr, U. B. (2013). *S-layer protein self-assembly.* Retrieved from http://www.ncbi.nlm.nih.gov/pmc/articles/PMC3587997/

Quereshi, S. (2014). *Klebsiella infections.* Retrieved from http://emedicine.medscape.com/article/219907-overview

Questions and Answers on the Executive Order Adding Potentially Pandemic Influenza Viruses to the List of Quarantinable Diseases. (2014). Retrieved from http://www.cdc.gov/quarantine/qa-executive-order-pandemic-list-quarantinable-diseases.html

Quorum-sensing and cheating in bacterial biofilms. Proc Biol Sci. 2012 Dec 7; 279(1748): 4765–4771. Published online 2012 Oct 3. doi: 10.1098/rspb.2012.1976.

Racaniello, V. (2008). *Discovery of viruses.* Retrieved from http://www.virology.ws/2008/12/23/discovery-of-viruses/

Rahaman, S. (n.d.). *Top 10 most dangerous viruses for your health.* Retrieved from http://alltoptens.com/top-10-most-dangerous-viruses-for-your-health/

Ramirez, J. L., Short, S. M., Bahia, A. C., Sariva, R. G., Dong, Y., Kang, S., Tripathi, A., Miambo, G., & Dimoupolos, G. (2014). *Chromobacterium Csp_P reduces malaria and Dengue infection in vector mosquitoes and has entomopathogenic and in vitro anti-pathogen activities.*

Retrieved from http://journals.plos.org/plospathogens /article?id=10.1371/journal.ppat.1004398

Reactive arthritis. (n.d.). Retrieved from http://www.nlm .nih.gov/medlineplus/ency/article/000440.htm

Reboli, A. C. (n.d.). *Erysipelothrix infection.* Retrieved from http://www.uptodate.com/contents/erysipelothrix-infection

Reiner, K. (2010). *Catalase test protocol.* Retrieved from http://www.microbelibrary.org/library/ laboratory-test/3226-catalase-test-protocol

Reiner, K. (n.d.). *Catalase test protocol.* Retrieved from http://www.microbelibrary.org/library/ laboratory-test/3226-catalase-test-protocol

Renier, S., Micheau, P., Talon, R., Hebraud, M., & Desvaux, M. (2012). *Subcellular localization of extracytoplasmic proteins in monoderm bacteria: Rational secretomics-based strategy for genomic and proteomic analyses.* Retrieved from http://www.ncbi.nlm.nih.gov/pmc/articles/PMC3415414/

Renom, F., Garau, M., Rubí, M., Ramis, F., Galmés, A., & Soriano, J. B. (2007). *Nosocomial outbreak of Corynebacterium striatum infection in patients with chronic obstructive pulmonary disease.* Retrieved from http://jcm.asm.org/content/45/6/2064.full

Researchers identify workings of L-form bacteria. (2009). Retrieved from http://www.sciencedaily.com/releases /2009/10/091013105811.htm

Reuters. (2015). *Disneyland measles outbreak linked to low vaccine rate.* Retrieved from http://www.nydailynews.com /life-style/health/disneyland-measles-outbreak-linked -vaccine-rate-article-1.2151859

Rh incompatibility. (n.d.). Retrieved from http://www.nlm .nih.gov/medlineplus/ency/article/001600.htm

Ribavirin for respiratory syncytial virus (RSV) infection. (n.d.). Retrieved from http://www.webmd.com/a-to-z-guides /ribavirin -for-respiratory-syncytial-virus-rsv-infection

Ribosomes—Protein construction teams. Retrieved from http:// www.biology4kids.com/files/cell_ribos.html

Riedmann, E. M., & Mylonakis, E. (2012). *Virulence: Three years and counting.* Retrieved from http://www.ncbi.nlm .nih.gov/pmc/articles/PMC3545930/

Rise and fall. Models shed new light on what fuels an exploding star. (n.d.). Retrieved from http://microbialgenomics .energy.gov/

Robert Hooke. (n.d.). In *Encyclopaedia Britannica online.* Retrieved from http://www.britannica.com/EBchecked /topic/271280/Robert-Hooke

Robert Koch - biographical. Retrieved from http://www .nobelprize.org/nobel_prizes/medicine/laureates/1905 /koch-bio.html

Robert Koch. Retrieved from http://ocp.hul.harvard.edu /contagion/koch.html

Rodrigues, C., Siciliano, R. F., Zeigler, R., & Strabelli, T. M. (2012). *Bacteroides fragilis endocarditis: a case report and review of literature.* Retrieved from http://www.ncbi.nlm .nih.gov/pubmed/22358367

Rogers, G. B., Hoffman, L. R., Whiteley, M., Daniels, T. W. V., Carroll, M. P., & Bruce, K. D. (2010). *Revealing the dynamics of polymicrobial infections: implications for antibiotic therapy.* Retrieved from http://www.ncbi.nlm .nih.gov/pmc/articles/PMC3034215/

Role of Actinobacillus (aggregatibactor) actinomycetemcomitans in periodontal diseases. (n.d.). Retrieved from http:// periobasics.com/role-of-actinobacillus-aggregatibactor -actinomycetemcomitans-in-periodontal-diseases.html

Role of staphylococcus enterotoxins in human diseases health essay. (n.d.). Retrieved from http://www.ukessays.com /essays/health/role-of-staphylococcal-enterotoxins-in -human-diseases-health-essay.php

Rosenberg, J. (n.d.). *1918 Spanish flu pandemic.* Retrieved from http://history1900s.about.com/od/1910s/p/ spanishflu.htm

Rosenberg, J. (n.d.). *Typhoid Mary.* Retrieved from http:// history1900s.about.com/od/1900s/a/typhoidmary_2.htm

Rotavirus basic research. (n.d.). Retrieved from http://www .niaid.nih.gov/topics/rotavirus/Pages/research.aspx

Rotavirus in the U.S. (2014). Retrieved from http://www.cdc .gov/rotavirus/surveillance.html

Rotavirus. (n.d.). Retrieved from http://www.niaid.nih.gov /topics/rotavirus/Pages/default.aspx

Roth, F. B. & Pillemer, L. (1953). *The separation of alpha toxin (Lecithinase) from filtrates of Clostridium Welchii.* Retrieved from http://www.jimmunol.org/content/70/6/533.abstract

Routes of transmission. (n.d.). Retrieved from http://www .microbiologyonline.org.uk/about-microbiology /microbes-and-the-human-body/routes-of-transmission

Roxby, A. C., Greninger, A. L., Hatfield, K.M., et al. Detection of SARS-CoV-2 Among Residents and Staff Members of an Independent and Assisted Living Community for Older Adults — Seattle, Washington, 2020. *MMWR Morb Mortal Wkly Rep* 2020;69:416–418. DOI: http://dx.doi .org/10.15585/mmwr.mm6914e2external icon

Ruder, K., & Winstead, E. R. (n.d.). *A quick guide to sequenced genomes.* Retrieved from http://www .genomenewsnetwork.org/resources/sequenced _genomes/genome_guide_p1.shtml

Ruoff, K. L. (2002). *Miscellaneous catalase-negative, Gram-positive cocci: Emerging opportunists.* Retrieved from http://www.ncbi.nlm.nih.gov/pmc/articles/PMC140404/

Saccharomyces cerevisiae final risk assessment. (1997). Retrieved from http://www.epa.gov/biotech_rule/pubs /fra/fra002.htm

Saint-Joanis, B., Garnier, T., & Cole, S. T. (1989). *Gene cloning shows the alpha-toxin of Clostridium perfringens to contain both sphingomyelinase and lecithinase activities.* Retrieved from http://link.springer.com/article /10.1007%2FBF00259619

Sakurai, J., Nagahama, M., & Oda, M. (2004). *Clostridium perfringens alpha-toxin: characterization and mode of action.* Retrieved from http://www.ncbi.nlm.nih.gov /pubmed/15632295

Salmonella enterocolitis. (n.d.). Retrieved from http://www .nlm.nih.gov/medlineplus/ency/article/000294.htm

Salmonella information. (n.d.). Retrieved from http://salmonella.org/info.html.

Salmonellosis: Topic overview. (n.d.). Retrieved from http://www.webmd.com/food-recipes/food-poisoning/salmonellosis-topic-overview

Sanchez, R. (2014). *Viruses: Tiny teachers of biology.* Retrieved from http://uanews.org/story/viruses-tiny-teachers-of-biology?utm_source=uanow&utm_medium=email&utm_campaign=biweekly-uanow

Sanders, M. E., Norcross, E. W., Robertson, Z. M., Moore, Q. C., III, Fratkin, J., & Marquar, M. E. (2011). *The Streptococcus pneumoniae capsule is required for full virulence in pneumococcal endophthalmitis.* Retrieved from http://www.ncbi.nlm.nih.gov/pmc/articles/PMC3053111/

Santacroce, L. (2014). *Helicobater pylori infection.* Retrieved from http://emedicine.medscape.com/article/176938-overview

Sarcomastigophora. (n.d.). Retrieved from http://www.itis.gov/servlet/SingleRpt/SingleRpt?search_topic=TSN&search_value=43781

Scapini, J. P., Flynn, L. P., Sciacaluga, S., Morales, L., & Cadario, M. E.. (2008). *Confirmed Mycoplasma pneumoniae Endocarditis.* Retrieved from http://www.ncbi.nlm.nih.gov/pmc/articles/PMC2609863/

Schoepe, H., Pache, C., Neubauer, A., Potschka, H., Schlapp, T., Wieler, L. H., & Baljer, G. (2001). *Naturally occurring Clostridium perfringens nontoxic alpha-toxin variant as a potential vaccine candidate against alpha-toxin-associated diseases.* Retrieved from http://iai.asm.org/content/69/11/7194.full

Schrager, H. M., Rheinwald, J. G., & Wessels, M. R. (1996). *Hyaluronic acid capsule and the role of streptococcal entry into keratinocytes in invasive skin infection.* Retrieved from http://www.ncbi.nlm.nih.gov/pmc/articles/PMC507637/

Seenivasan, M. H. (2012). *Treponema pertenue, Treponema carateum, Treponema endemicum (Yaws, Pinta, Bejel).* Retrieved from http://antimicrobe.org/b247.asp

Sepsis (blood infection) and septic shock. (2014). Retrieved from http://www.webmd.com/a-to-z-guides/sepsis-septicemia-blood-infection

Sepsis. (n.d.). Retrieved from http://www.nlm.nih.gov/medlineplus/ency/article/000666.htm

Septicemia and systemic inflammatory response syndrome. (n.d.). Retrieved from http://faculty.ccbcmd.edu/courses/bio141/labmanua/lab12/diseases/blood/septicemia.html

Sewell, D. (n.d.). *Enterococcus and group D streptococcus.* Retrieved from http://www.thefreelibrary.com/Enterococcus+and+group+D+streptococcus.-a0109740701

Sheppard, Y. D., Middleton, D., Whitfield, Y., Tyndel, F., Haider, S., Spiegelman, J., Swartz, R. H., Nelder, M. P., Baker, S. L., Landry, L., MacEachern, R., Deamond, S., Ross, L., Peters, G., Baird, M., Rose, D., Sanders, G., & Austin, J.W. (2012). *Intestinal Toxemia Botulism in 3 Adults, Ontario, Canada, 2006–2008.* Retrieved from http://www.ncbi.nlm.nih.gov/pmc/articles/PMC3310098/

Shiel Jr, W. C. (2002). *Blood, how much do we have?* Retrieved from http://www.medicinenet.com/script/main/art.asp?articlekey=21474

Shiel Jr, W. C. (n.d.). *Vasculitis.* Retrieved from http://www.medicinenet.com/vasculitis/article.htm

Shoeb, H. (2010). *Examination for motility by hanging drop technique.* Retrieved from http://www.microbelibrary.org/library/laboratory-test/3139-examination-for-motility-by-hanging-drop-technique

Siegel, R. (1998). *Paramyxoviridae.* Retrieved from http://virus.stanford.edu/paramyxo/paramyxo.html

Signs of an eye infection. (n.d.). Retrieved from http://www.webmd.com/eye-health/signs-of-an-eye-infection

Sinave, C. P. (2014). *Streptococcus group D infections.* Retrieved from http://emedicine.medscape.com/article/229209-overview.

Small Intestinal Bacterial Overgrowth Prevalence, Clinical Features, Current and Developing Diagnostic Tests, and Treatment E. Grace; C. Shaw; K. Whelan; H. J. N. Andreyev Aliment Pharmacol Ther. 2013;38(7):674–688. © 2013 Blackwell Publishing.

Smallpox. (n.d.). Retrieved from http://www.emedicinehealth.com/smallpox/page4_em.htm

Smith, A. C. & Hussey, M. A. (n.d.). *Gram stain: Gram-variable rods and cocci.* Retrieved from http://www.microbelibrary.org/library/gram-stain/2858-gram-stain-gram-variable-rods-and-cocci

Spelman, D. (2014). *Treatment of nocardiosis.* Retrieved from http://www.uptodate.com/contents/treatment-of-nocardiosis

Spirochete. (n.d.). In *Encyclopaedia Britannica online.* Retrieved from http://www.britannica.com/EBchecked/topic/560509/spirochete

Spirochetes and spirilla. Retrieved from http://www.cliffsnotes.com/sciences/biology/microbiology/the-bacteria/spirochetes-and-spirilla

Spirochetes. (n.d.). In *Encyclopedia online.* Retrieved from http://www.encyclopedia.com/topic/Spirochetes.aspx

Spirochetes. (n.d.). Retrieved from http://virology-online.com/Bacteria/Spirochaetes.htm

Staph aureus food poisoning. (n.d.). Retrieved from http://www.mch.com/gastrointestinal/staph-aureus-food-poisoning.aspx

Staphylococcal skin infections. (n.d.). Retrieved from http://www.dermnetnz.org/bacterial/staphylococci.html

Staphylococcus aureus adheres to human intestinal mucus but can be displaced by certain lactic acid bacteria Satu Vesterlund, 1 Matti Karp, 2 Seppo Salminen 1 and Arthur C. Ouwehand Microbiology (2006), 152, 1819–1826 DOI 10.1099/mic.0.28522–0 Printed in Great Britain.

Staphylococcus. (n.d.). Retrieved from http://pusware.com/testpus/bug_Staphylococcus.html

Staphylococcus. (n.d.). Retrieved from http://www.emedicinehealth.com/staphylococcus/article_em.htm

Staphylococcus. Retrieved from http://www.medical-labs.net/?s=staphylococcus&x=4&y=8

Statistics about toxic shock syndrome. (n.d.). Retrieved from http://www.rightdiagnosis.com/t/toxic_shock_syndrome/stats.htm

Statistics overview. (2015). Retrieved from http://www.cdc.gov/hiv/statistics/basics/index.html

Steenhuysen, J. (2014). *CDC says more lab workers may have been exposed to anthrax.* Retrieved from http://www.reuters.com/article/2014/06/20/us-usa-anthrax-scare-idUSKBN0EV2FJ20140620.

Stevens, D. L. (n.d.). *Streptococcus pyogenes.* Retrieved from http://antimicrobe.org/b239.asp

Stout, J. (2015). *Tuberculosis pericarditis.* Retrieved from http://www.uptodate.com/contents/tuberculous-pericarditis

Stratton, C. W. (2015). *Infections due to the Streptococcus anginosus (Streptococcus milleri) group.* Retrieved from http://www.uptodate.com/contents/infections-due-to-the-streptococcus-anginosus-streptococcus-milleri-group

Strep throat: Cause. (n.d.). Retrieved from http://www.webmd.com/oral-health/tc/strep-throat-cause

Streptococcal skin infections. (2014). Retrieved from http://www.dermnetnz.org/bacterial/streptococcal-disease.html

Streptococcus mutans. (n.d.). Retrieved from http://www.mimg.ucla.edu/faculty/shi/smutans.htm

Streptococcus pneumoniae. (2014). Retrieved from http://www.niaid.nih.gov/topics/pneumococal/Pages/Pneumococcal Disease.aspx

Streptococcus. (2014). Retrieved from http://www.encyclopedia.com/topic/streptococcus.aspx

Structure. Retrieved from http://bioweb.uwlax.edu/bio203/s2007/wojtowic_trav/Structure.htm

Summary of biochemical tests. Retrieved from http://www.uwyo.edu/molb2210_lab/info/biochemical_tests.htm

Sureshbabu, J. (2014). *Shigella infection.* Retrieved from http://emedicine.medscape.com/article/968773-overview

Sutton, S. (n.d.). *The Gram stain.* Retrieved from http://www.microbiol.org/resources/monographswhite-papers/the-gram-stain/

Sutyak, K. (n.d.). *Yersinia pestis.* Retrieved from http://web.uconn.edu/mcbstaff/graf/Student%20presentations/Y.%20pestis/Yersinia%20pestis.html

Symbiosis. (n.d.). Retrieved from http://www.bio-medicine.org/Biology-Definition/Symbiosis/

Systemic lupus erythematosus. (n.d.). Retrieved from http://www.nlm.nih.gov/medlineplus/ency/article/000435.htm

Szczepanski, K. (n.d.). *Black death in Asia: bubonic plague.* Retrieved from http://asianhistory.about.com/od/asianenvironmentalhistory/p/Black-Death-In-Asia-Bubonic-Plague.htm

Tabes Dorsalis. (n.d.). In *Encyclopedia online.* Retrieved from http://www.encyclopedia.com/topic/Tabes_Dorsalis.aspx

Takami, H., Nakasone, K., Takaki, Y., Maeno, G., Sasaki, R., Masui, N., Fuji, F., Hirama, C., Nakamura, Y., Ogasawara, N., Kuhara, S., & Horikoshi, K. (2000). *Complete genome sequence of the alkaliphilic bacterium Bacillus halodurans and genomic sequence comparison with Bacillus subtilis.* Retrieved from http://www.ncbi.nlm.nih.gov/pmc/articles/PMC113120/

Taldir, G., Parize, P., Arvis, P., & Faisy, C. (2013). *Acute right-sided heart failure caused by Neisseria meningitidis.* Retrieved from http://www.ncbi.nlm.nih.gov/pmc/articles/PMC3536187/

Tan, J. S. & File, T. M. (n.d.). *Streptococcus species (group G and group C streptococci, viridans group, nutritionally variant streptococci).* Retrieved from http://www.antimicrobe.org/b241.asp

Temaru, E., Shimura, S., & Karasawa, T. (2005). *Clostridium tetani is a phospholipase (Lecithinase)-producing bacterium.* Retrieved from http://jcm.asm.org/content/43/4/2024.full

The determinants of health. (n.d.). Retrieved from http://www.who.int/hia/evidence/doh/en/

The energetics of chemolithotrophy. (2015). Retrieved from https://www.boundless.com/microbiology/textbooks/boundless-microbiology-textbook/microbial-metabolism-5/chemolithotrophy-50/the-energetics-of-chemolithotrophy-319-8021/

The evolution of the cell. (n.d.). Retrieved from http://learn.genetics.utah.edu/content/cells/organelles/

The History of Vaccines. The College of Physicians of Philadelphia. (January 2018). Retrieved from https://www.historyofvaccines.org/content/articles/history-anti-vaccination-movements

The Human Genome Project completion: Frequently asked questions. (2010). Retrieved from http://www.genome.gov/11006943

The infection prevention and HAI portal. (n.d.). Retrieved from http://www.jointcommission.org/hai.aspx

The influenza epidemic of 1918. Retrieved from http://www.archives.gov/exhibits/influenza-epidemic/

The Salmonella/E. coli mutagenicity test or Ames test. (n.d.). Retrieved from http://ntp.niehs.nih.gov/testing/types/genetic/invitro/sa/index.html

Therapy. (n.d.). Retrieved from http://www.ohsu.edu/xd/research/centers-institutes/neurology/blood-brain-barrier/patients-and-caregivers/therapy.cfm

Timeline of microbiology. Retrieved from http://timelines.ws/subjects/Microbiology.HTML

Titer testing. (n.d.). Retrieved from https://requestatest.com/titer-testing

Todar, K. (n.d.). *Bacillus cereus Food Poisoning.* Retrieved from http://textbookofbacteriology.net/B.cereus.html

Todar, K. (n.d.). *Bacterial endotoxin.* Retrieved from http://textbookofbacteriology.net/endotoxin.html

Todar, K. (n.d.). *Bacterial structure in relationship to pathogenicity.* Retrieved from http://textbookofbacteriology.net/BSRP_2.html

Todar, K. (n.d.). *Bordetella pertussis and whooping cough.* Retrieved from http://textbookofbacteriology.net/pertussis.html

Todar, K. (n.d.). *Diphtheria.* Retrieved from http://textbookofbacteriology.net/diphtheria.html

Todar, K. (n.d.). *Diphtheria.* Retrieved from http://textbookofbacteriology.net/diphtheria_2.html

Todar, K. (n.d.). *Diversity of metabolism in prokaryotes.* Retrieved from http://textbookofbacteriology.net/metabolism_5.html

Todar, K. (n.d.). *Immune defense against bacterial pathogens: Adaptive or acquired immunity.* Retrieved from http://textbookofbacteriology.net/adaptive.html

Todar, K. (n.d.). *Immune defense against bacterial pathogens: Innate immunity.* Retrieved from http://textbookofbacteriology.net/innate_3.html

Todar, K. (n.d.). *Immune defense against bacterial pathogens: Innate immunity.* Retrieved from http://textbookofbacteriology.net/innate.html

Todar, K. (n.d.). *Important groups of procaryotes.* Retrieved from http://textbookofbacteriology.net/procaryotes_6.html

Todar, K. (n.d.). *Introduction to the Spirochetes.* Retrieved from http://www.textbookofbacteriology.net/Lyme.html

Todar, K. (n.d.). *Listeria monocytogenes.* Retrieved from http://textbookofbacteriology.net/Listeria.html

Todar, K. (n.d.). *Mechanisms of bacterial pathogenicity.* Retrieved from http://textbookofbacteriology.net/pathogenesis_4.html

Todar, K. (n.d.). *Pathogenic neisseriae: Gonorrhea, neonatal ophthalmia and meningococcal meningitis.* Retrieved from http://textbookofbacteriology.net/neisseria_5.html

Todar, K. (n.d.). *Salmonella and salmonellosis.* Retrieved from http://textbookofbacteriology.net/salmonella.html

Todar, K. (n.d.). *Staphylococcus aureus and Staphylococcal Disease.* Retrieved from http://www.textbookofbacteriology.net/staph.html

Todar, K. (n.d.). *Staphylococcus.* Retrieved from http://textbookofbacteriology.net/staph_2.html

Todar, K. (n.d.). *Streptococcus pneumoniae.* Retrieved from http://www.textbookofbacteriology.net/S.pneumoniae.html

Todar, K. (n.d.). *Streptococcus pyogenes and streptococcal disease.* Retrieved from http://www.textbookofbacteriology.net/streptococcus.html

Todar, K. (n.d.). *The genus Bacillus.* Retrieved from http://www.textbookofbacteriology.net/Bacillus.html

Todar, K. (n.d.). *The Genus Bacillus.* Retrieved from http://www.textbookofbacteriology.net/Bacillus.html

Todar, K. (n.d.). *The normal bacterial flora of humans.* Retrieved from http://textbookofbacteriology.net/normalflora.html

Toner, C. B. (2014). *Pseudomonas folliculitis.* Retrieved from http://emedicine.medscape.com/article/1053170-overview#a0199

Toxic shock syndrome. (n.d.). Retrieved from http://www.mayoclinic.org/diseases-conditions/toxic-shock-syndrome/basics/definition/CON-20021326

Toxic shock syndrome. (n.d.). Retrieved from http://www.medicinenet.com/toxic_shock_syndrome_tss/page4.htm#what_is_the_prognosis_of_toxic_shock_syndrome

Toxic shock syndrome. (n.d.). Retrieved from http://www.nlm.nih.gov/medlineplus/ency/article/000653.htm

Tran, M.P., Caldwell-McMillan, M., Khalife, W., & Young, V. B. (2008). *Streptococcus intermedius* causing infective endocarditis and abscesses: a report of three cases and review of the literature. Retrieved from http://www.biomedcentral.com/1471-2334/8/154

Transmission of blood borne pathogens. (n.d.). Retrieved from http://www2.lbl.gov/ehs/biosafety/BBP_Training/html/bbp_transmission.shtml

Treatment of hepatitis C in the near future. (n.d.). Retrieved from http://www.hepatitiscnewdrugresearch.com/2014-treatment-of-hepatitis-c-in-the-near-future.html

Trowbrige Fillipone, P. (n.d.). *Why buy oysters in months with the letter "r"?* Retrieved from http://homecooking.about.com/od/cookingfaqs/f/faqoysterseason.htm

Tsakok, T., Tsakok, M., Damji, C., & Watson, R. (2011). *Washout after lobectomy: Is water more effective than normal saline in preventing local recurrence?* Retrieved from http://www.ncbi.nlm.nih.gov/pmc/articles/PMC3279979/

Tsutsumi, T., Hiraoka, E., Kanazawa, K., Akita, H., & Eron, L. J. (2010). *Diagnosis of E. coli tricuspid valve endocarditis: A case report.* Retrieved from http://www.ncbi.nlm.nih.gov/pmc/articles/PMC3071200/

Tuazon, C. U. (n.d.). *Bacillus species.* Retrieved from http://www.antimicrobe.org/new/b82.asp

Tuberculin skin test. (n.d.). Retrieved from http://www.webmd.com/a-to-z-guides/tuberculin-skin-tests

Tuberculosis. (n.d.). Retrieved from http://www.cedars-sinai.edu/Patients/Health-Conditions/Tuberculosis-TB.aspx

Tuuminen, T., Suomala, P., & Vuorinen, S. (2013). *Sarcina ventriculi in blood: the first documented report since 1872.* Retrieved from http://www.biomedcentral.com/1471-2334/13/169

Type 1 diabetes: Overview. (2013). Retrieved from http://www.ncbi.nlm.nih.gov/pubmedhealth/PMH0072523/

Types of fungal diseases. (n.d.). Retrieved from http://www.cdc.gov/fungal/diseases/index.html

Types of fungal nail infection—topic overview. (n.d.). Retrieved from http://www.webmd.com/a-to-z-guides/types-of-fungal-nail-infection-topic-overview

Types of growth media used to culture bacteria. (n.d.). Retrieved from http://www.scienceprofonline.org/microbiology/types-culture-media-for-growing-bacteria.html

Types of influenza viruses. (2014). Retrieved from http://www.cdc.gov/flu/about/viruses/types.htm

Types of vaccines. (2012). Retrieved from http://www.niaid.nih.gov/topics/vaccines/understanding/Pages/typesVaccines.aspx

Typhoid fever. (n.d.). Retrieved from http://www.cdc.gov/nczved/divisions/dfbmd/diseases/typhoid_fever/

U.S. FDA. (2021). *Recommendations for Investigational COVID-19 Convalescent Plasma.* Retrieved from https://www.fda.gov/vaccines-blood-biologics/investigational-new-drug-applications-inds-cber-regulated-products/recommendations-investigational-covid-19-convalescent-plasma

U.S. Food and Drug Administration. *FDA-Approved Dermal Fillers.* (11-9-2020). Retrieved from https://www.fda.gov/medical-devices/aesthetic-cosmetic-devices/fda-approved-dermal-fillers

U.S. Preventative Services Task Force. *Hepatitis C Virus Infection in Adolescents and Adults: Screening.* March 2, 2020. Retrieved from https://www.uspreventiveservicestaskforce.org/uspstf/document/RecommendationStatementFinal/hepatitis-c-screening.

Uchino, M., Mizuguchi, T., Ohge, H., Haji, S., Shimizu, J., Mohri, Y., Yamashita, C., Kitagawa, Y., Suzuki, K., Kobayashi, M., Kobayashi, M., Sakamoto, F., Yoshida, M., Mayumi, T., Hirata, K., & SSI Prevention Guideline Committee of the Japan Society for Surgical Infection (2018). *The Efficacy of Antimicrobial-Coated Sutures for Preventing Incisional Surgical Site Infections in Digestive Surgery: a Systematic Review and Meta-analysis.* Journal of gastrointestinal surgery: official journal of the Society for Surgery of the Alimentary Tract, 22(10), 1832–1841. https://doi.org/10.1007/s11605-018-3832-8

UNAIDS. *Global HIV and AIDS Statistics–Fact sheet.* (2021). Retrieved from https://www.unaids.org/en/resources/fact-sheet

Understanding foodborne diseases. (2014). Retrieved from http://www.niaid.nih.gov/topics/foodborne/Pages/Default.aspx

Understanding toxic shock syndrome: The basics. (n.d.). Retrieved from http://www.webmd.com/women/understanding-toxic-shock-syndrome-basics

Updates on CDC's polio eradication efforts. Retrieved from http://www.cdc.gov/polio/updates/

Urbina, P., Flores-Díaz, M., Alape-Girón. A., Alonso, A., & Goni, F. M. (2009). *Phospholipase C and sphingomyelinase activities of the Clostridium perfringens alpha-toxin.* Retrieved from http://www.ncbi.nlm.nih.gov/pubmed/19428363

Ureaplasam. In *The Free Dictionary online.* Retrieved from http://medical-dictionary.thefreedictionary.com/Ureaplasma

Vancomycin-resistant enterococcus (VRE) infection. (2011). Retrieved from http://www.cdc.gov/HAI/organisms/vre/vre-infection.html

Variant Creutzfeldt-Jakob disease. Retrieved from http://www.cdc.gov/prions/vcjd/index.html

Vasculitis. (n.d.). Retrieved from http://www.nlm.nih.gov/medlineplus/vasculitis.html

Vashi, S. (n.d.). *FDA approves first at-home HIV test.* Retrieved from http://www.webmd.com/hiv-aids/news/20120703/fda-approves-first-at-home-hiv-test

Ventura, M., Canchaya, C., Tauch, A., Chandra, G., Fitzgerald, G. F., Chater, K. F., & van Sinderen, D. (2007). *Genomics of Actinobacteria: tracing the evolutionary history of an ancient phylum.* Retrieved from http://www.ncbi.nlm.nih.gov/pubmed/17804669

Verheij, J., Jaspars, E. H., van der Valk, P., & Rozendaal, L. (2009). *Russell bodies in a skin biopsy: A case report.* Retrieved from http://www.ncbi.nlm.nih.gov/pmc/articles/PMC2783049/

VeryWellHealth. (2021). *The Anatomy of the Eustachian Tube.* Retrieved from https://www.verywellhealth.com/what-is-the-eustachian-tube-1192115

Viral diseases. (n.d.). Retrieved from http://www.news-medical.net/health/Viral-Diseases.aspx

Viral hepatitis—hepatitis E information. (2015). Retrieved from http://www.cdc.gov/hepatitis/HEV/index.htm

Viral size. (n.d.). Retrieved from https://www.boundless.com/microbiology/textbooks/boundless-microbiology-textbook/viruses-9/virus-overview-117/viral-size-611-5404/

Virulence factors—Biotech, pharma, and life science channel. (n.d.). Retrieved from http://www.bioportfolio.com/channels/virulence-factors

Virulence factors of pathogenic bacteria. Retrieved from http://www.mgc.ac.cn/cgi-bin/VFs/status.cgi

Virulent bacteriophages and T4. (2015). Retrieved from https://www.boundless.com/microbiology/textbooks/boundless-microbiology-textbook/viruses-9/viral-diversity-123/virulent-bacteriophages-and-t4-636-7343/

Virus Taxonomy. The ICTV Report on Virus Classification and Taxon Nomenclature. (2021). Retrieved from https://talk.ictvonline.org/ictv-reports/ictv_online_report/

Viruses. (n.d.). Retrieved from http://www.microbeworld.org/types-of-microbes/viruses

Vyan, J. M. (2014). *Meningitis: pneumococcal.* Retrieved from http://www.nlm.nih.gov/medlineplus/ency/article/000607.htm

Waites, K. B. (n.d.). *Mycoplasma infections.* Retrieved from http://emedicine.medscape.com/article/223609-overview#a0104

Wapner, J. (2014). *We now have the cure for hepatitis C, but can we afford it?* Retrieved from http://www.scientificamerican.com/article/we-now-have-the-cure-for-hepatitis-c-but-can-we-afford-it/.

Ward, B. *What is a Compound Microscope?* Microscope Clarity. (2021). Retrieved from https://microscopeclarity.com/microscope-magnification-explained/

Warnecke, F., Sommaruga, R., Sekar, R., Hofer, J. S., & Pernthaler, J. (2005). *Abundances, identity, and growth state of actinobacteria in mountain lakes of different UV transparency.* Retrieved from http://www.ncbi.nlm.nih.gov/pmc/articles/PMC1214628/

Watanabe, T., Furukawa, S., Hirata, J., Koyama, T., Ogihara, H., & Yamasaki, M. (2003). *Inactivation of Geobacillus stearothermophilus spores by high-pressure carbon dioxide treatment.* Retrieved from http://www.ncbi.nlm.nih.gov/pmc/articles/PMC309949/

Watson, R. (n.d.). *Summary of biochemical tests.* Retrieved from http://www.uwyo.edu/molb2210_lab/info/biochemical_tests.htm

WBC count. (n.d.). Retrieved from http://www.nlm.nih.gov/medlineplus/ency/article/003643.htm

Weagant, S. D. (2001). *BAM: Yersinia enterocolitica.* Retrieved from http://www.fda.gov/Food/FoodScienceResearch/LaboratoryMethods/ucm072633.htm

WebMD. (2021). *What is otomycosis?* Retrieved from https://www.webmd.com/a-to-z-guides/what-is-otomycosis

Weil syndrome. (2015). Retrieved from http://www.webmd.com/children/weil-syndrome

Weinstein, R. A., Gaynes, R., & Edwards, J. R. (2005). *Overview of nosocomial infections caused by Gram-negative bacilli.* Retrieved from http://cid.oxfordjournals.org/content/41/6/848.long

Weiss, D. (n.d.). *Meningococcal meningitis.* Retrieved from http://www.austincc.edu/microbio/2704r/nm.htm

Wessels, M. R. (n.d.). *Group C and group G streptococcal infection.* Retrieved from http://www.uptodate.com/contents/group-c-and-group-g-streptococcal-infection

Wessner, D. R. (2010). *Discovery of the giant mimivirus.* Retrieved from http://www.nature.com/scitable /topicpage/discovery-of-the-giant-mimivirus-14402410

What is a genome? (n.d.). Retrieved from http://ghr.nlm.nih .gov/handbook/hgp/genome

What is a pandemic? What is an epidemic? (2014). Retrieved from http://www.medicalnewstoday.com /articles/148945.php

What is phenotyping? (n.d.) Retrieved from http://www .hopkinsmedicine.org/mcp/PHENOCORE /What_is_phenotyping

What is Staphylococcus aureus? (n.d.). Retrieved from http://www.ehagroup.com/resources/pathogens /staphylococcus-aureus/

White, S. (2014). *Are you a man or a microbe?* Retrieved from http://www.brevis.com/blog/tag/microbial-genes/

WHO. (2011). *Campylobacter.* Retrieved from http://who.int /mediacentre/factsheets/fs255/en/

WHO. (2014). *Vector-borne diseases.* Retrieved from http://www.who.int/mediacentre/factsheets/fs387/en/

WHO. (2015). *Meningococcal meningitis.* Retrieved from http://www.who.int/mediacentre/factsheets/fs141/en/

WHO. (2018). *Zika virus.* Retrieved from https://www.who .int/news-room/fact-sheets/detail/zika-virus

WHO. (2020). *Chikungunya.* Retrieved from https://www .who.int/news-room/fact-sheets/detail/chikungunya

WHO. (2021). Cholera. Retrieved from https://www.who.int /news-room/fact-sheets/detail/cholera

WHO. (2021). Schistosomiasis. Retrieved from https://www .who.int/news-room/fact-sheets/detail/schistosomiasis

WHO. (2021). *WHO Coronavirus (COVID-19) Dashboard.* Retrieved from https://covid19.who.int/

Why viruses are referred to as obligate parasites. (n.d.). Retrieved from http://www.sciences360.com/index .php/why-viruses-are-referred-to-as-obligate -parasites-6665/

Wickman, F. (n.d.). *Fact-checking Spock: Was the 'enemy of my enemy' guy really killed by his 'friend'?* Retrieved from http://www.slate.com/blogs/browbeat/2013/05/16/star _trek_into_darkness_fact_checked_was_the_enemy_of _my_enemy_guy_really.html

Wiley Online Library. (April 2015). *Bergey's Manual of Systematics of Archaea and Bacteria (BMSAB).* Online ISBN: 9781118960608| DOI: 10.1002/9781118960608. Retrieved from https://www.onlinelibrary.wiley.com/doi /book/10.1002/9781118960608

Willingham, E., & Helft, L. (2014). *What is herd immunity.* Retrieved from http://www.pbs.org/wgbh/nova/body /herd-immunity.html

Wong, M.Y., Lau, S.K. P., Tang, S. C. W., Curreem, S. O. T., Woo, P. C.Y., & Yuen, K.Y. (2012). *First report of peritoneal dialysis-related peritonitis caused by Citrobacter amalonaticus.* Retrieved from http://www.ncbi.nlm.nih .gov/pmc/articles/PMC3525409/

Woods, C. J. (n.d.). *Streptococcus group B infections.* Retrieved from http://emedicine.medscape.com/article/229091 -overview

World Health Organization. (October 24, 2019). *Two out of three wild poliovirus strains eradicated.* Retrieved from https://www.who.int/news-room/feature-stories/detail /two-out-of-three-wild-poliovirus-strains-eradicated

World Organization for Animal Health. (2021). *Yersinia pseudotuberculosis Aetiology Epidemiology Diagnosis Prevention and Control-Potential Impacts of Disease Agent Beyond Clinical Illness References.* Retrieved from https://www.oie.int/app/uploads/2021/05/yersinia -enterocolitica-infection-with.pdf

Xu, S. X., & McCormick, J. K. (2012). *Staphylococcal superantigens in colonization and disease.* Retrieved from http://www.ncbi.nlm.nih.gov/pmc/articles/PMC3417409/

Yaeger, R. G. (1996). *Chapter 77. Protozoa: Structure, classification, growth, and development.* Retrieved from http://www.ncbi.nlm.nih.gov/books/NBK8325/

Yagupsky, P., Porsch, E., & St. Geme, J. W. III. (n.d.). *Kingella kingae: An emerging pathogen in young children.* Retrieved from http://pediatrics.aappublications.org/content/127/3 /557.full

Yardley, W. (2012). *Carl Woese dies at 84; Discovered life's "Third Domain."* Retrieved from http://www.nytimes. com/2013/01/01/science/carl-woese-dies-discovered-lifes -third-domain.html?_r=0

Yip, K. H. K. & Smales, R. J. (2012). *Implications of oral biofilms in medically at risk persons.* Retrieved from http:// www.ncbi.nlm.nih.gov/pmc/articles/PMC3596074/

Young Karris, M., Litwin, C. M., Dong, H. S., & Vinetz, J. (2011). *Bartonella henselae infection of prosthetic aortic valve associated with colitis.* Retrieved from http://www .ncbi.nlm.nih.gov/pmc/articles/PMC3216094/

Your microbes and you. (2012). Retrieved from http:// newsinhealth.nih.gov/issue/nov2012/feature1

Zhong, ZP., Tian, F., Roux, S. et al. Glacier ice archives nearly 15,000-year-old microbes and phages. *Microbiome* 9, 160 (2021). https://doi.org/10.1186/s40168-021-01106-w

Zimmer, C. (2013). *Comfortable in the cold: Life below freezing in an Antarctic lake.* Retrieved from http://www.pbs.org/wgbh /nova/next/nature/seeking-psychrophiles-in-antarctica/

Zimmer, C. (2014). *A tiny emissary from the ancient past.* Retrieved from http://www.nytimes.com/2014/09/25/ science/a-tiny-emissary-from-the-ancient-past.html

Zimmer, C. (2014). *In 1918 flu pandemic, timing was a killer.* Retrieved from http://www.nytimes.com/2014/04/30/science /in-1918-flu-pandemic-timing-was-a-killer.html?_r=0

Zimmer, C. (2014). *Viruses as a cure.* Retrieved from http:// www.nytimes.com/2014/11/19/science/viruses-as-a-cure. html?_r=0

Index

Boldface type indicates illustration/photo.

A

Abscess, 119, 124, 148, 150, 188, 189, 247, 255, 256, 265
Abstinence, 302
Acellular organism, 22
Acetylcholine, 180, 182
Achromobacter xylosoxidans, 218
Acid-fast stain, 34, 191
Acidophile, 67
Acinetobacter, 225
Acinetobacter baumannii, 225
Acne, 250, **251**
Acquired immunodeficiency syndrome (AIDS)
    circumcision and, 13
    description of, 101–102
    first diagnosis of, 12
    fungal infections and, 147–148
    rapid testing for, 37
    yeast infections of, 147, 148, 151–152
Actinobacillus, 225, 227
Actinobacteria, 188
Actinomyces, 188–189
Actinomyces bovis, 188–189
Actinomyces israelii, 188, **189**
Actinomycosis, 188–189
Active adaptive immunity, 293–294
Active carrier, 110
Active process, 57
Active tuberculosis, 192
Acute fulminating meningococcal septicemia, 205
Acute necrotizing ulcerative gingivitis (ANUG), 261
Adaptive immunity, 293–295
Adenine, 76, 77
Adenocarcinoma, 262
Adenosine diphosphate (ADP), 59
Adenosine triphosphate (ATP), 57, 59, 69
Adenovirus, **87**, 95
Adenylate cyclase, 218
Adherence, 112, 118, 123
Adhesin, 112, 120, 226
Adhesion, 109, 120
Adipose tissue, 246
Adult intestinal toxemia botulism, 180, 181

Aeration, 306
Aerobic organism, 44, 157
Aeromonadaceae, 228
Aeromonas, 228
Aeromonas caviae, 228
Aeromonas hydrophila, 228
Aeromonas sobria, 228
Aerosolized bacteria, 130, 192
Aerotolerant anaerobe, 48, 69
African fruit bat, 312
Agammaglobulinemia, 295, 301
Agar, 36, 40, 46, 73
Aggregatibacter actinomycetemcomitans, 227
Agranulocyte, 117
AIDS. *See* Acquired immunodeficiency syndrome
Airborne precautions, 16
Alcaligenaceae, 218
Alcohol, 260, 285–286
Algae, 58, 61
Alkaline conditions, 67, 222
Alkaliphile, 67
Allergic reaction, 278, 298–299
Alpha interferon, 120
Alpha proteobacteria, 216
Alpha streptococcus, 163
Alpha toxin, 179
Alveoli, **280,** 285
Amblyomma americanum, 130
Amebiasis, 124
Ames, B., 83
Ames test, 83, **84**
Amikacin, 194
Amine, 270
Amino acid, 69
Amino acid sequencing, 39
Amoeba, 61
    cell wall of, 58
    definition of, 61
    description of, 123
    life cycle of, 123–124, **124**
Amoxicillin, 213
Amphitrichous, **52**
Anaerobic chamber, 37
Anaerobic organism, 7, 44

Ventriculoperitoneal shunt, 234
Verotoxin, 263
Vesicle, 59, **248,** 253
V factor, 226
Viability, 47, 66–70
Vibrio, 45–46, **46,** 227, 266
Vibrio cholerae, 114, 227, 266
Vibrionaceae, 227
Vibrio parahaemolyticus, 227
Vibrio vulnificus, 46, 227, 251
Vincent's angina/infection, 261
Violacein, 217
Viral conjunctivitis, 277
Viral meningitis, 92, 97
Viremia, 312
Viridans group streptococci, 168
Virion, 311–313, 316
Viroid, 102
Virology, 86
Virulence, 72, 109, 112, 113, 118
Virulent phage, 78
Virus. *See also specific viruses;* specific viruses
   antibiotics for, 86, 91
   characteristics of, 87–89
   common types of, 88, 93–102, 283–284
   cytopathic effects of, 115–116
   description of, 22
   diseases caused by, 86, 87
   domains of, 21–22
   emergence of, 311–314
   examples of, **24**
   infection by, 89
   origin of, 88
   pathogenicity of, 115–116
   replication of, 88–89, **90**
   size of, 29, **87**
   taxonomy of, 24–25, **25**
   transmission of, 94
   treatment of, 92
   vaccines for, 92
Volunteerism, 122
Von Behring, E., 10
Von Wassermann, A., 10
Vulvovaginal candidiasis, 269

W

Wakefield, A., 301
Warren, J. R., 12

Wart, 253, 271
Washer-sterilizer, 305, **305**
Washington, G., 209
Wasserman test, 211
Waterhouse-Friderichsen syndrome, 205, 240
Watson, J., 12
Wax, 191–192
Waxing skin, 250
Weil, A., 214
Weil's disease, 214
Wells, H. G., 307
Western blot, 213
West Nile virus
   description of, 130
   first documentation of, 11
   outbreaks of, 13
Wheal, **248**
Whipworm, 140
Whirlpool, 250
White blood cell, 59, 117, 149, 160, 232–243.
    See also Leukocyte
Whitehead, 250
Whittaker, R., 21
Whooping cough, 218, 282, 283, 294, 318, 320
Woese, C., 21
Wound botulism, 180
Wound healing, 69–70

X

X factor, 226

Y

Yaws, 208, 211
Yeast, 62, 63, 144–146, 151–153
Yeast infection, 147, 152–153, 269
Yellow fever, 130
Yersinia, 224, 265
Yersinia enterocolitica, 235, 265
Yersinia pestis, 112, 115, 130, 224–225
Yersinia pseudotuberculosis, 224, 266

Z

Zoonosis, 110
Zoonotic infection, 217
Zygomycete, 146
Zygospore, 146, 147